Personal Health Choices

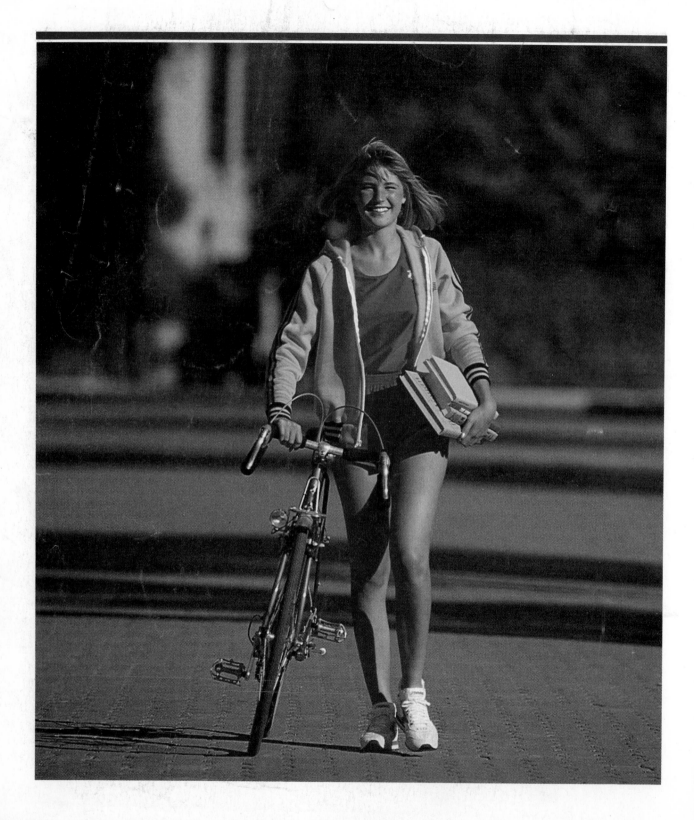

Personal Health Choices

Sandra F. Smith
Cabrillo College

Christopher M. Smith

JONES AND BARTLETT PUBLISHERS
Boston

Editorial, Sales, and Customer Service Offices
JONES AND BARTLETT PUBLISHERS
20 PARK PLAZA
BOSTON, MA 02116

Printed in the United States of America
10 9 8 7 6 5 4 3 2 1

Library of Congress Cataloging-in-Publication Data

Smith, Sandra Fucci.
   Personal health choices / Sandra Smith, Christopher Smith.
     p. cm.
   Includes bibliographical references.
   ISBN 0-86720-130-4
   1. College students—Health and hygiene.   I. Smith, Christopher,
1935– , II. Title.
RA777.3.S65 1990   89-26866
613'.0434—dc20   CIP

Graphic Design: Janet Bollow
Production Coordinator: Christopher M. Smith
Composition: Alphatype
Cover Design: Rafael Millán
Front and Back Cover Photographs: Rafael Millán, Kathryn J. Kraus, Clayton E. Jones

Photo/Illustration Credits and Acknowledgments Follow the Index.

In writing this text the authors and publisher have made every attempt to follow current health care practices and to ensure that suggested health and wellness programs are up-to-date and conform with current recommendations and practices at time of publication. However, it is the responsibility of the reader to validate health practices and treatment with a physician or health service.

Contributors

CHAPTER CONTRIBUTORS

W. Henry Baughman, HSD
Western Kentucky University

Christine Freeman, BA

Ralph Manchester, MD
University of Rochester

Susan North, RN, PhD

James Rothenberger, MPH
University of Minnesota

Beverlie Conant Sloane, PhD
Dartmouth College

Christopher Smith, MBA

Sandra Smith, RN, MS
Cabrillo College

SECTION CONTRIBUTORS

Lida Chase, RN, PhD
University of Hawaii

Marilyn Manning, PhD

Beverly Meyer, RN, MS
University of Oregon
Health Sciences Center

Emmett Miller, MD

Barney Nielson, DDS

Trish Ratto, BS, RD
University of California at Berkeley

Tarah Smith, Student
University of California at Berkeley

Diane Sussman, BA, RT

Barbara Thomas, PhD
National University

Claire Walsh, PhD
University of Florida

STUDENT ADVISORS

Perrin Brew, Dartmouth College

Scott Hellar, University of Southern California

Carol Kenny, UCLA

Don Marek, UCLA

Katherine Nino, University of San Francisco

Doug Robinson, UC Berkeley

Tarah Smith, UC Berkeley

Lise Starner, Duke University

Catherine Wachter, Northwood Institute (MI)

Mary Wachter, Purdue University

Contents in Brief

Contents

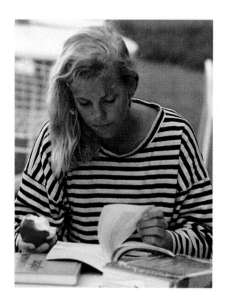

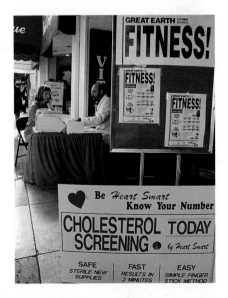

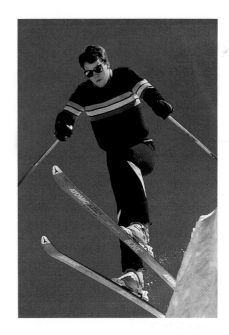

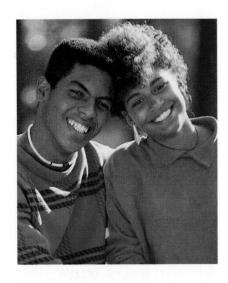

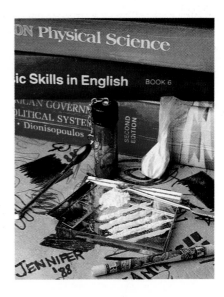

CHAPTER 13

The AIDS Crisis   329

CHAPTER 14

Pregnancy, Childbirth and Parenting   353

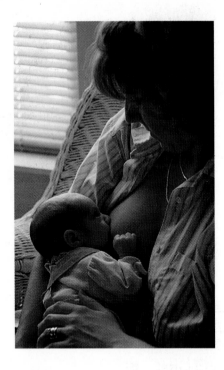

CHAPTER 15

Alcohol and Other Drugs   385

CHAPTER 16

Health Hazards of Tobacco   427

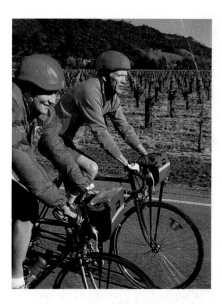

Preface

Managing your health is a challenge—a continual process that requires you to adapt as your own needs change. You face health decisions each day: diet, stress, relationships, exposure to disease, risk of injury, and many others. To meet these challenges, you need accurate and timely information, the discipline to say no at the appropriate times, and the ability to weigh risks against benefits. **Personal Health Choices** is a valuable resource to assist you in making informed choices when managing your health and wellness in the 1990s.

Topics of Current Interest and Unique Focus

Subjects selected for coverage in **Personal Health Choices** include health topics of current concern to college students. We have used "National Health Objectives for the Year 2000," published by the U.S. Department of Health and Human Services, as one of our important guidelines. Other sources for timely information presented in this text include medical journals and newsletters, health-oriented textbooks, health and wellness periodicals, agencies of the federal government, and national health education and promotion foundations.

Chapter 13 answers the questions most often asked by college students about AIDS and includes the latest statistics on this deadly disease. Chapter 21 discusses current environmental health issues, including air and water pollution, acid rain, and global warming. The Surgeon General's latest research on the health hazards of tobacco is covered in Chapter 16. Finally, Chapters 7 and 8, nutrition and weight management, incorporate the findings published in the 1989 report, "Diet and Health," by the National Research Council.

Throughout this text you will find many unique topics that, although vital to your health and well-being, are often overlooked. Chapter 10 discusses personal image and the importance of looking and feeling good in order to lead a healthy, happy life. Chapter 6 addresses the topic of time management and provides helpful suggestions for setting goals and efficiently budgeting your valuable time. Chapter 5 discusses eating and sleep disorders and includes advice on how to recognize and cope with these health threats. Other problems on college campuses, such as depression, suicide, acquaintance rape, and alcohol abuse, are discussed in a sensitive manner with the objective of helping you avoid them.

Special Features

Each chapter of **Personal Health Choices** includes special features to help you make informed choices and apply the information. One feature, "Seeking Professional Help," provides guidelines for recognizing when to ask for qualified assistance. Another feature, "Beyond the Text," poses thought-provoking questions that ask you to relate important health issues to your own life.

Learning Aids

To help the reader better understand the materials, each chapter of the text contains numerous learning aids, including the following:

- Chapter overviews, which summarize the material to be presented in a concise and readily understandable format
- Chapter outlines, which list all major topics and subtopics to be covered in the chapter
- Interesting boxed material, such as quotes and statistics, set aside from the main text of the book

- Listing of key terms in every chapter
- End-of-chapter glossary of the key terms
- Short list of suggested supplemental readings that extend the focus and provide additional up-to-date information

Student Advisors

A diverse group of 10 college students from across the country reviewed all the material in the text. The input of the student advisors has been instrumental in developing an easy-to-read, lively student-oriented text. Many of the interesting short-subject topics in the text are a direct result of suggestions from the student advisors, including: "Sweaty Palms and Other Signals of Stress," "Drugs and Academics," "Test Anxiety," "Confronting the Grizzly Bears in Your Life," "Dining Hall Eating," "External Time Wasters," and "Acquaintance Rape."

Supplements to Accompany This Text

1. **Instructor's Resource Manual** An indispensable resource to assist every instructor teaching a personal health course.
2. **Instructor's Test Bank** Approximately 2,000 questions in true/false, matching, multiple-choice, and short answer format (hard copy).
3. **Instructor's Computerized Text Bank** Available in IBM format which allows the instructor to create, edit, add, or delete questions, and also to print an answer key to the test.
4. **Jones and Bartlett Telephone Test Preparation Service** Allows an instructor without access to a computer to create a customized test. Available to all adopters by calling toll-free (1-800-832-0034). The customized test and answer key is then sent by regular mail within 48 hours.
5. **Jones and Bartlett Health Video Library** Free videos are available to all adopters of the book. The number of videos available depends on the number of books purchased from Jones and Bartlett:

Copies Per Semester	Number of Free Videos
50	1
100	2
200	3
400	4
800	5
1000	6

Adopters can choose from a wide selection of videos including: *The Addicted Brain*; *Kicking Cocaine*; *Alcohol Addiction*; *Kick the Habit*; *Sexual Roulette: AIDS and the Heterosexual*; *Our Aching Backs*; *Teen Suicide*; *Stress Management*; *Anorexia and Bulimia*; *Emergency*; *Navratilova on Nutrition, Sports and Fitness*; and *The Nutritional Advocate*. Please contact the Jones and Bartlett College Marketing Department (1-800-832-0034) for a current listing, as the availability of videos may vary.

6. **Instructor's Transparencies** Fifty colored acetates taken from illustrations in the text, as well as additional charts and figures. One set is free to adopters of 50 copies or more.
7. **Classroom Handout Masters and Health Assessment Masters** An ideal source for assessing the reader's health before and after completing the course.
8. **Health Assessment Software** User-friendly software that allows students to assess and continually monitor their own health. Available in IBM format to adopters of 50 copies or more.
9. **Nutritional Analysis Software** User-friendly software that allows students to assess and monitor their nutritional habits. Available in IBM format to adopters of 50 copies or more.
10. **Classroom Audiotapes on Stress Reduction and Relaxation** An excellent source of information from a leading expert in this field. Available to adopters of 50 copies or more.

Sandra F. Smith   Christopher M. Smith
Cabrillo College

February 1990

Choosing Wellness

The way we view health is changing. Even the terms we use to describe health have changed; new terms like *holistic health* and *high-level wellness* are being heard more frequently in both medical and nonmedical circles. In the past, good health meant the absence of disease. The new definition, holistic health, goes beyond physical health to encompass the health of the whole person, including mental, emotional, and spiritual health. In fact, the definition of health has broadened so much in the past decade that many people now include the health of the planet as well as the people living on it. A recent poll found that people cited "living in an environment with clean air and water" as their third top health concern.

A holistic redefinition of health emphasizes high-level wellness, or going beyond the absence of disease toward one's maximum health potential. This chapter focuses on the mind/body/spirit/environment connection and discusses how you can use this connection to reach your possible highest level of health and wellness.

Contents

Key Terms

Disease

Health

Holism

Holistic

Holistic paradigm

Immune system

Peak experience

Psychoneuroimmunology

Self-actualization

Shaman

Spiritual values

Wellness

A New Definition of Health

The 1990s are witnessing a significant growth in a new dimension of health—a holistic approach. As shown in a recent Gallup survey completed for *American Health Magazine*, many people in our society now include a very broad range of issues in their concept of personal health. Certainly their top health concern is still oriented toward the individual body—"staying free of disease." However, their third-highest priority—"living in an environment with clean air and water"—expresses a much more global health perspective. Many of their top concerns show that they regard not only physical status but also mental and emotional status as important parts of personal health. Today's significant health goals include having a positive outlook on life and sharing love with friends and family.

This contemporary focus on health has shaped the issues covered in this book. These values probably also influence how you will interpret and use what you read here. Toward that end, this book has two major objectives: first, to give you the information you need to protect yourself from major health risks, such as physical trauma, alcohol and drug abuse, sexual disease, smoking, and so forth; second, to present tools to help you strengthen your own inner natural tendencies to develop your fullest potential. You can go far beyond just the absence of illness to true wellness—a life full of thoughts and actions oriented toward a positive, satisfying sense of self and relationships with others. Wellness can be thought of as a state of being; holistic health is the means of achieving it.

The World Health Organization (WHO) formulated a definition of health in 1970 that has had a great impact on the medical model of health care. WHO described health as "a state of complete physical, mental and social well-being, not merely the absence of disease or infirmity." What made this definition innovative is that it took into account the mind as well as the body. In fact, this new interpretation of health almost enters the spiritual dimension. Though critics have pointed out that by this definition no one would be truly healthy, it is the beginning of a view of health as an open system in a holistic framework.

The Concept of Holistic Health

The history of how people view health and disease varies as much as tribes and cultures have throughout the ages. Holistic health began with the shamans, healers in ancient cultures who viewed healing as a process of bringing the body back into balance. The ancient Greeks believed in the holistic concept of health, for they recognized that disharmony in the mind can create illness. The word holistic actually comes from the Greek, holos, which means whole.

From early primitive peoples to the nineteenth century, many societies believed in a split between mind and body. In Western civilization, the mind-body division began in the early 1600s with René Descartes, who viewed nature as two separate parts of reality—mind and matter.

The great error in the treatment of the human body is that physicians are ignorant of the whole. For the part can never be well unless the whole is well.

Plato

2

In recent decades, a new and far more encompassing paradigm has developed in Western thought. In 1926, South African Jan Smuts coined the word *holism*. He used this term to refer to the tendency in nature to synthesize and organize toward greater wholes. He wrote that the meaning of the whole organism is greater than the sum of the parts. His theory suggests that we think of the human organism not as separate parts, but rather as the sum of all its parts—physical, psychological, social, and spiritual; in this way, the whole person becomes the focus of healing. Holistic medicine postulates a constant interchange between mind and body, psyche and soul.

In the modern era, Carl Jung was one of the first therapists to discuss the prevention of illness in terms of utilizing one's inner resources. He discussed the inner self and themes of self-renewal in relation to growth, spirituality, and health. As our body of research knowledge grows, more and more physicians are utilizing spiritual growth techniques as a health tool. For example, Dr. Carl O. Simonton and Stephanie Simonton have been using meditation and imagery as adjunct therapy for patients with cancer. Dr. Joan Borysenko at the Harvard Mind-Body Clinic is using meditation as a medical tool; Dr. Norman Shealy, founder of the American Holistic Medical Association and founder of the Shealy Institute for Comprehensive Pain and Health Care, has used alternative methods of health care for many years. The current literature, much of it authored by prominent physicians, exemplifies today's trend toward the holistic model. Well-known proponents include Bernard Siegel, MD, professor at Yale University and author of *Love, Medicine & Miracles*; C. Norman Shealy, MD, PhD, co-author with Caroline M. Myss of the *The Creation of Health*; Richard Gerber, MD, author of *Vibrational Medicine, New Choices for Healing Ourselves*; John W. Farquhar, MD, author of *The American Way of Life Need Not Be Hazardous to Your Health*; and Mike Samuels, MD, and Nancy Samuels, authors of *The Well Adult*.

Treatment, Prevention, and Promotion

The holistic paradigm suggests that the body, psyche, and environment are one. This idea can assist us to view our personal health from a new dimension. In the holistic view, health care includes three types of actions—treatment, disease and injury prevention, and health promotion—with emphasis on the second two types.

Treatment   Treatment covers care after illness or injury has occurred. Western doctors use techniques such as diagnosis, medications, surgery, and other care procedures to guide the body away from illness or injury and back toward normal function.

These advances have brought many benefits, but they do not always aid us as toward recovery. Although millions of people successfully undergo surgery every year, a small number develop infection or other complications from surgery that are more serious than the original problem for which they entered the hospital.

New Focus Predicted

In 1976, John Knowles, former president of the Rockefeller Foundation, suggested a new focus for health care. Over 99 percent of us are born healthy, but many suffer premature death and disability only as a result of personal misbehavior and environmental conditions. Mr. Knowles predicted that the next major advance in the health of the American people would result from the assumption of individual responsibility for one's own health, requiring a change in lifestyle for the majority of Americans.

Source: *Time*, August 1976

Many physicians prescribe medication because they feel the patient wants it rather than because this is the only effective treatment. Miraculous medications save millions of lives each year; however, they lead to unwanted drug side effects in thousands of others. Nearly 5 percent of hospital admissions are due to drug reactions. In the hospital, 20 percent of patients receive either the wrong dose or wrong medications, or experience an adverse drug reaction. Such occurrences run counter to a constructive wellness model.

As the patient, you should discuss alternative treatments with your physician. These may include treatments that require involvement on your part, such as changes in eating patterns and other lifestyle behaviors, or other physical treatments, such as acupuncture, vitamin therapy, and so forth. If you take the initiative and assume responsibility for your own health, your physician can guide you to various health care options.

Truly holistic treatment involves an integrated assessment of all aspects of your health. For example, if you practice generally healthy behaviors but still feel depressed much of the time, WHO's holistic definition of health would find you not healthy. You may wish to look for ways to bring yourself further along on the wellness continuum. The holistic perspective encourages you to consider other possible causes of the depression; for example, a deficiency in certain vitamins or amino acids, a long-term anxiety with which you have not yet dealt consciously, or even a chemical imbalance or ingestion of an environmental toxin.

Health prevention and promotion can help you avoid much of the

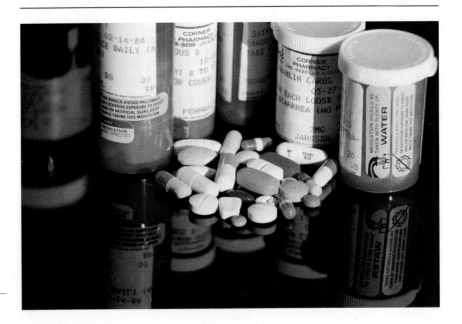

pain, death, and financial burden that the treatment-based approach entails. These two types of action are the cornerstones for much of the holistic approach to health.

Disease and Injury Prevention   During the past twenty years, a tremendous shift has occurred away from treating disease and toward preventing it. The latest research now shows that a few changes in lifestyle habits can prevent 80 percent of deaths in midlife. Middle-aged men can greatly reduce their risk of death from heart disease, the biggest killer in their age range, by practicing good nutritional habits, proper exercise, stress management, avoiding smoking, and treating hypertension. Many of these same lifestyle habits also affect your chance of contracting many forms of cancer, the second major cause of death in this age range. Avoiding alcohol abuse can decrease rates of alcohol addiction, liver disease, organ deterioration, and accidents. The more we reduce or eliminate the risk behaviors for the major killers in our society, the more we will prevent or reduce the incidence of these diseases.

Health Promotion   The U.S. Department of Health and Human Services has made a commitment to the philosophy and practice of individual health promotion. The process of health promotion combines educational, organizational, and economic tools to inform the public about a particular health issue (such as the dangers of smoking). Health promotion bases such actions on the premise that correct information may motivate individuals to moderate or avoid risky behaviors.

This philosophy of health promotion was initiated by the Carter Administration in 1980 when the U.S. Department of Health and Human Services published major national health goals for the year 1990. Then, in late 1989, the federal government issued revised and updated health promotion and disease prevention objectives for the year 2000. These objectives have been defined in terms of health promotion, health protection, and preventive services. Each of the current 21 priority areas is presented with measurable objectives for the year 2000, supported by recommended strategies to be implemented during the decade of the 1990s.

High priority health promotion areas include nutrition, physical fitness, tobacco, alcohol and other drugs, and sexual behavior, all of which are important concerns of the college population. Priorities for health protection focus on environmental health, occupational safety, and prevention of unintentional injuries. Disease prevention objectives have been established for critical conditions, including HIV infection, high blood cholesterol, cancer, and mental and behavioral disorders.

This text discusses these and other health risks and healthy lifestyle behaviors throughout the chapters. You probably encounter health promotion information almost wherever you go. Certainly it appears in education courses and texts, but also in magazines, television programs and advertisements, political debates, and casual conversations. Though much of this information has significant value, you should evaluate the

---

Prevention Can Save Money

Robert Blank, author of **Rationing Medicine**, stated that if the United States does nothing to change our health care system by the year 2000, we will be spending $1.9 trillion on health costs per year. Our health care system emphasizes curative medicine. However, 80 percent of illness in our nation is linked to individual behavior (smoking, diet, alcohol, obesity, and other high-risk activities). If we would allocate our resources to prevention, we would save billions of dollars.

Source: *Holos' Practice Report*, June 1989

Health Objectives for the Year 2000

National health priorities are defined in terms of measurable health objectives. Examples include the following:

- **Risk reduction:** reduce occasions of heavy drinking of alcoholic beverages among college students to no more than 28 percent by the year 2000. (Baseline: 43 percent in 1987)
- **Public awareness:** increase to 75 percent the proportion of people age 18 and older who know that saturated fat raises blood cholesterol. (Baseline: 56 percent in 1988)
- **Protection:** eliminate exposure to tobacco product advertising and promotion among youths age 18 and younger. (Baseline: 100 percent of youth are presently exposed)

10 Leading Causes of Death: United States, 1987

Rank	Cause of Death	Number	Percent of Total Deaths
1*	Heart diseases	759,400	35.7
	(Coronary heart disease)	(511,700)	(24.1)
	(Other heart disease)	(247,700)	(11.6)
2*	Cancers	476,700	22.4
3*	Strokes	148,700	7.0
4**	Unintentional injuries	92,500	4.4
	(Motor vehicle)	(46,800)	(2.2)
	(All others)	(45,700)	(2.2)
5	Chronic obstructive lung disease	78,000	3.7
6	Pneumonia and influenza	68,600	3.2
7*	Diabetes mellitus	37,800	1.8
8**	Suicide	29,600	1.4
9**	Chronic liver disease and cirrhosis	26,000	1.2
10*	Atherosclerosis	23,100	1.1
	All causes	2,125,100	100.0

*Causes of death in which diet plays a part.

**Causes of death in which excessive alcohol consumption plays a part.

Source: Estimates from the National Center for Health Statistics, *Monthly Vital Statistics Report*, vol. 37, no. 1, April 25, 1988.

source and content of each warning, reassurance, or promotional message.

You could spend your entire life learning and worrying about health risks, but you have other things to do with your time as well. Concentrate on the behaviors that place you and others at greatest risk. Consider each potential risk in the context of all the risks you believe you face. Why consider moving out of earthquake country if you don't consistently wear your seatbelt in the car? Why worry about the level of residual pesticides in your apple juice if you get so drunk on Saturday night that you pass out?

> The art of medicine consists of amusing the patient while nature cures the disease.
>
> Voltaire, 1694–1778

Goals of Holistic Health

If you follow holistic health principles, you may make progress toward several goals: high-level wellness, self-responsibility, and viewing health challenges as opportunities for growth.

High-Level Wellness

High-level wellness, a term coined by Dr. John Travis, means more than the absence of disease. It implies a state of being healthy in body, mind, and spirit. In this state you are happy with the direction of your life and you have mutually productive relationships. True wellness means living in a state in which you are maximizing your potential. You feel good physically, your emotions are almost always stable, you like yourself, and your relationships with others are positive and rewarding. You handle the stressors in your life successfully; when you encounter major stress, you have constructive ways of coping. You feel intellectually productive. You enjoy living, creating, and achieving.

Abraham Maslow spent decades trying to discover how human beings develop their potential. As a result of his search, he formulated the concept of "self-actualization," the highest level of growth. Self-actualization implies that an individual has fulfilled his or her higher human potential for creativity, love, charity, and happiness. For most people, this fulfillment becomes possible only after more basic needs for food, affection, shelter, and self-respect are met.

When Maslow described people he perceived as self-actualized, he used terms such as creative, successful, independent, accepting of themselves and others, living life to the fullest, democratic in their attitudes, and experiencing reciprocal interpersonal relationships. Some of the people Maslow described in this way were Abraham Lincoln, Henry David Thoreau, Albert Einstein, and Eleanor Roosevelt. Maslow observed that the healthiest individuals are those who are self-actualized. Researchers who have continued Maslow's work have further observed that the more self-actualized you become, the more you make "growth" choices rather than destructive choices. As you become more self-actualized, your life becomes happier, healthier, and more vital.

Self-Responsibility

Adopting a holistic view of health includes taking personal responsibility for the state of your physical, emotional, and spiritual health. You do not blame other people or circumstances for your health status; rather, you acknowledge that you alone take responsibility for your life.

Many believe that viruses, bacteria, and other parasites are the causes of illness. This view places health in the hands of fate. But you've certainly noticed that not everyone in your residence hall or apartment building catches a cold when one goes around, and some people (always the same ones, it seems) develop more severe cases than others. Clearly, an external organism has only a limited influence in determining illness; the individual plays a very important role.

If your immune system is strong and your body is in a state of true wellness, you can resist these invasions. The lower your resistance, the higher your potential for illness. When your actions, thought patterns, or beliefs create a negative health status, you provide a welcome host for disease.

The Healthiest Nation

The healthiest nation in the world? Not the United States or Sweden. The correct answer is Japan. Japan now has the world's longest life expectancy (81 years for women and 75 years for men compared with 78 for American women and 71 for American men). The Japanese also boast the lowest infant mortality rate, almost half of the United States' death rates. You might assume that Japan spends the most money on medical care—not so. The Japanese spend less than half of what we spend per person annually. The Japanese see a physician three times as often as the average American. Since prevention is less expensive than medical treatment, the medical treatment applied earlier to illness is less expensive than treatment begun late, this may account for the state of Japanese health.

Source: *Johns Hopkins Medical Letter*, March 1989

The more responsibility we take for our choices, the more they work for us rather than against us.

The key to health is prevention, taking actions that do not allow bacteria, fungi, or viruses an opportunity to find a home in your body.

Even if you have a genetic predisposition or medical history that increases your susceptibility to certain health problems, you can take charge of your health to minimize this vulnerability. Pay attention to what you need to maximize your wellness.

Health Challenges as Opportunities for Growth

Holistic health encompasses the view that illness can be a positive opportunity for growth. Though this idea seems bizarre at first, if you do consider this point of view when you are ill or injured, you may find yourself able to give up a self-pitying attitude and substitute openness and exploration.

Sometimes you may clearly not be responsible for creating a health challenge that arises. A drunk driver may run a red light and hit a car in which you are a passenger, sending you to the hospital. Remaining angry or depressed about your injuries, pain, and loss does not help with your recovery. By following a holistic philosophy and working through these negative attitudes, you can focus your mental energy on physical healing. You also learn more about the process of letting go of negative feelings, so you can suffer less from such emotions in the future. You may also gain insights about what is really important to you in life.

Wellness in Body, Mind, and Spirit

As was stated earlier, high-level wellness results from health in body, mind, and spirit in relation to your overall environment. Each of these aspects has particular health implications that, when considered as a whole, can lead you to holistic wellness.

Wellness for the Body

For many years the traditional medical model focused on the body; when physical symptoms appeared, physicians treated the affected body part. If a disease occurred in the body, they suspected infection or trauma as the cause. This medical model has been responsible for invaluable advances in medical knowledge, techniques and treatments. However, it has not brought us all the answers, as evidenced by our nation's consistently high rates of cancer, infant mortality, and other health weaknesses.

A holistic approach allows us to treat the diseased body part as part of the whole rather than a separate entity. For example, the body may manifest an unhealthy condition arising from an emotional upheaval, such as depression, anxiety, or poor self-esteem, rather than from a bacteria invasion. A growing body of information from both traditional Western medicine and holistic practitioners is helping us expand and integrate our understanding of the relationships between certain types of behaviors and our total health.

What you eat may not only give you energy and contribute to growth, but also affect virtually every aspect of your health, such as mental fitness, sleep patterns, stamina, and susceptibility to illness. Keeping physically fit not only improves your appearance and strength, it also aids in preventing heart disease, hypertension, and obesity. A 1989 study published in *The Journal of the American Medical Association* points out that existing as a "couch potato" ranks second only to smoking as a risk factor for heart disease and cancer. Physical exercise improves self-image, emotional well-being, and, for some, a sense of spiritual focus. We have learned a great deal, but still have more to uncover about the physical manifestations of illnesses as caused by weight problems, alcohol and drug abuse, and stress. It is clear that taking care of our bodies helps us take care of our mind and spirit as well.

Mind and Wellness

In the holistic view, your mental status may act as an indicator of your overall health. Strong positive or negative mental attitudes can influence not only your emotional, but also your physical health.

To achieve high-level wellness, you must pay attention to your intellectual performance and your emotional well-being. Intellectual performance may have particular importance to your well-being during college years. If you are having trouble academically, you may have trouble sleeping, drink more, or feel more physical symptoms of stress, such as an upset stomach. To maintain your health, you need to solve the underlying problem, seeking help if necessary. As long as work or academic issues remain unresolved, they drain energy that you need to keep yourself strong and balanced. Often stress management techniques, time management techniques, or academic counselling can help.

Many college students occasionally face challenges such as depression, loneliness, anxiety, and fear. Of course, such problems may surface at any period in your life, as may grief, troubled or unresolved relationships, or thoughts of suicide. Though most of us can handle our emotional load most of the time, if it starts to get the better of you, evaluate the situation as soon as possible. As described in later chapters in this book, counselling (as well as other techniques) can often mean the difference between an emotional challenge that strengthens and one that causes long-term pain and damage. Taking care of the health of your emotions is part of striving toward high-level wellness.

Mind and wellness have another connection as well: What you believe about yourself has the power to become reality. A decade ago, only so-called "fringe physicians" and "holistic quacks" believed in the dramatic effect of the mind on the immune system. Then the prestigious *New England Journal of Medicine* published an article by Pulitzer Prize winner Norman Cousins entitled "Anatomy of an Illness." Cousins chronicled his experience with a debilitating, incurable disease and its remission. He had

One of my problems is that I internalize everything. I can't express anger; I grow a tumor instead.

Woody Allen

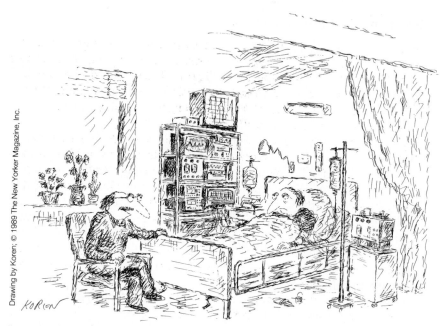

"Milt, I'm beginning to think that your illness is a disharmony of life energy."

wondered whether, if stress and negative emotions produce chemical changes in the body that lead to a disease, perhaps positive emotions could produce balancing chemical changes to reverse the illness. Indeed, when he filled his life with laughter (by watching reruns of Candid Camera and other amusing films), he experienced less pain. To this laughter, Cousins added high doses of Vitamin C. Before long, his disease went into complete remission. A miracle? No, just programming the mind to believe it can influence the body, creating the physiological circumstances that enhance the immune system.

Cousins' article sparked tremendous interest and controversy about the power of the mind over the body. Like any breakthrough theory, this approach still needs more study, documentation, and experiential learning. For the past ten years, thousands of researchers have been examining the immune system and human ability to exert voluntary control over it. The new area of scientific research that explores this connection is called psychoneuroimmunology. More and more people, on their own and in clinical settings, have overcome illness and improved their health through such techniques as imagery-visualization, biofeedback, hypnosis, meditation, and positive thinking. The possible implications for your own health status make this knowledge extremely valuable. If you can control your own immune system through stress reducers, laughter, love, forgiveness, and other mental and emotional actions, why not give it a try?

Spirit and Wellness

Spirit is that part of yourself that is connected to some larger existence, some larger set of values. For some individuals, this perspective comes from the tenets of an established religion. Others find it in a personal philosophy or a set of ethics. You may consider yourself religious, atheist, agnostic, humanist, Eastern, Western, or iconoclastic, and still be in touch with your spirit and its effect on your health.

Our spirit is the essence of our being. When we experience a sense of unity with the cosmos or oneness, we are able to have what Maslow calls a "peak experience." A peak experience, according to Maslow, occurs when your mind is totally still—centered on a single object or thought to the exclusion of all thoughts or perceptions. This may occur when you are watching a sunset, running, focusing on a piece of music, sitting on a mountain top, praying, or working in the garden. Maslow correlated these times with creativity, personality integration, and personal satisfaction. Maslow believed that the more peak experiences you have, the more complete your life becomes.

Beliefs serve as a foundation for your thought patterns and subsequently your emotional and physical reactions. If your personal philosophy strengthens and centers you, then the thoughts derived from this philosophy will lead you toward self-actualizing emotional and physical conditions. The more you maintain a positive spirit, the more you can connect with your most capable, self-nurturing energy. This energy gives you strength to overcome health challenges in other areas of your life, as well as the motivation to avoid negative, self-destructive behaviors.

Become aware of your spiritual values. Then consider how well they are working for you, how they affect your overall health. If you have a weak or negative personal philosophy, your thoughts may produce negative emotional and physical reactions. For example, if you believe people are not trustworthy, that they want to manipulate and use you, then you may have unfulfilling relationships. This, in turn, may result in feelings of isolation, even depression, which may result in physical problems, such as loss of appetite, or, in serious cases, suicide. On the other hand, if you believe in the inherent goodness of others and trust them, you may experience profound interpersonal relationships that enhance your emotional well-being.

If your spiritual orientation is threatening your physical or mental health in some fashion, such as leading to thoughts of alienation or fear, then you may wish to consider whether you are choosing the most constructive path. You may want to try some alternatives, perhaps some simple contemplative techniques that can help you relieve stress and increase your awareness of your spirit. Useful methods include meditation, biofeedback, and visualization, as well as several others discussed later in this book. Some people attend churches, synagogues, or temples. Others find a spiritual teacher, follow a spiritual path, join prayer groups, practice spiritual disciplines on their own, or practice no specific discipline. They simply shape their own personal values and live according to them.

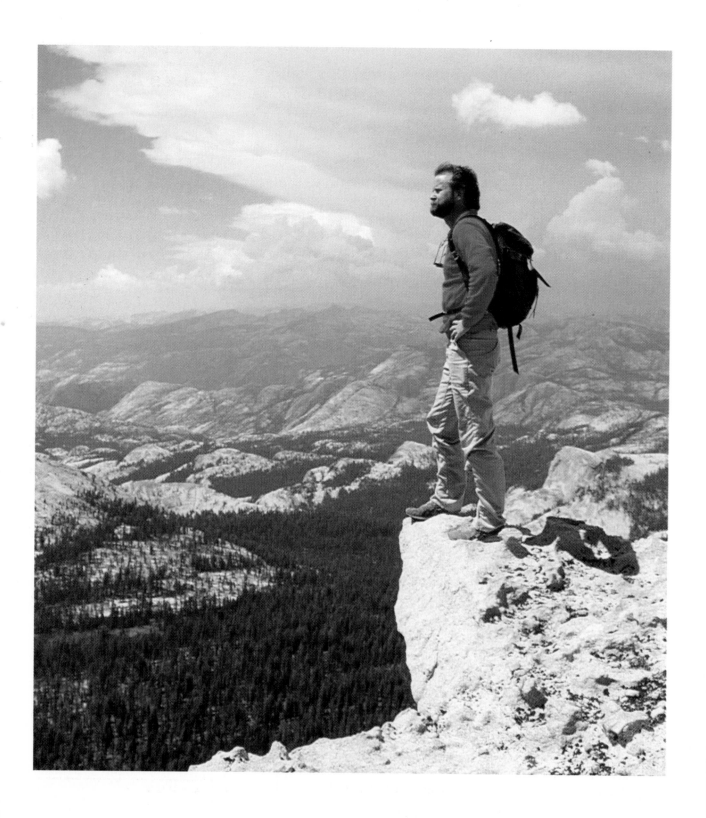

Building a positive relationship with your spirit has numerous positive results. Many people who work at such connections report that they cope better with stress, are more peaceful and happy, and have a better sense of self. By becoming able to detach yourself from the busy world, you can develop a sense of humor and a more loving and nonjudgmental attitude toward others. All these benefits fit into the framework of wholeness.

Health is Choice, Not Chance

Fundamental to college life is choice. During your college career you will have many opportunities for making choices: your academic major, extracurricular activities, social life, relationships, and so forth. Many of your daily decisions affect your health and their importance should not be underestimated.

Health Choices During College

The college environment presents many special choices that affect your health. In general, colleges insist only that you fulfill academic requirements; sometimes you are not even required to attend classes, as long as you obtain passing grades. For many students, the unstructured nature of college life presents as many perils as opportunities. The freedom of college life contrasts with parental management at home and with the stricter disciplines of full-time employment. How many days would you need to miss work due to hangovers from overconsumption of alcohol before your employer would fire you? On the other hand, how many days could you skip classes for the same excuse before the college would expel you? Colleges usually allow more latitude on such issues than do employers. In recent years, the AIDS crisis has influenced sexual attitudes of college students and added a new dimension to decision-making regarding sexual activities.

As individuals, we grow by accepting and meeting challenges. Benjamin Franklin stated, "Those things that hurt, instruct." You face health challenges every day from friends and family, chance events, the media, and your environment. When faced with challenges, you have choices. You can choose to avoid, delay, procrastinate, or ignore issues. Or you can choose to meet the challenges, take on the problems, and direct your life toward positive goals. Do you choose to be:

- Holistically conscious of your body?
- Physically fit?
- Nutritionally aware?
- Emotionally balanced?
- Part of a loving relationship?
- Responsibly aware of the environment?
- Sexually responsible?
- Moderate in your use of alcohol, nicotine and caffeine?
- Drug free?

How to Make Effective Decisions

1. Decide whether you will make the decision alone or with someone else.
2. Gather all the information you can.
3. Define the problem.
4. Brainstorm—generate as many alternatives as possible.
5. Pick the best alternatives and consider the consequences of each.
6. Actually make a choice.
7. Plan your implementation.
8. Evaluate your choice; do some follow-up research, and alter your plan, if necessary.

Remember, usually there is not just one "right" choice. Most decisions made with knowledge and implemented with conviction will probably turn out well, so don't dilute your resolve with worry about whether or not you made the right choice. If you made it, it was right! And don't forget to reinforce the decision-making successes in your life. Reward yourself for a choice well made.

The direction of our lives is determined by our choices.

Choosing Wellness

CHAPTER 1

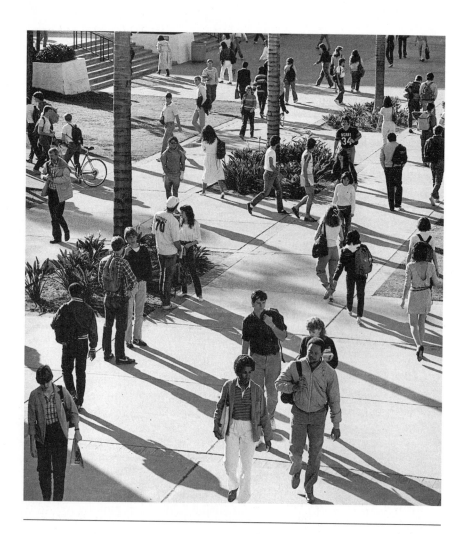

When you assume responsibility for managing your life, you take on the process of choosing lifestyle behaviors that influence your overall health and well-being. Your health is too valuable to be left to chance or uninformed choice. When faced with challenges, learn to make informed choices.

The Process of Choice

In his book, *Profound Simplicity*, psychiatrist Will Schutz, PhD, discusses the process of choice. He suggests that all of us make choices on the basis of options, but that sometimes we are not aware of our options nor fully aware of how we make our choices. He compares our unaware choices to unconscious desires. For example, you assume you will fail a midterm exam because you have not done the reading, so you attend a party the night before the test. You choose partying over studying without knowing or acknowledging why you didn't do the reading in the first place. To make conscious rather than unconscious choices, become more aware of your options and their consequences. As the philosophy of health promotion suggests, you must be aware of the need to change your behavior before any change can take place.

- *Define how important wellness is for your life.* To do so, consider the goals you have in your life, both short-term and long-term. Recognize how high-level wellness can help you achieve your goals. This chapter has provided some guidance in this area; the rest of the book frequently touches on wellness in relation to your overall lifestyle.
- *Learn how your actions affect your health.* Read about these issues, talk with your healthcare providers and develop a network of health resources. This book provides guidelines in virtually every chapter for health-related behaviors. Health has too many facets to rely solely on experience and hearsay.
- *Evaluate your health status.* To do so, you might complete a health risk appraisal form, a questionnaire designed to quantify your potential for major disease. Your personal physician or campus health educator may have various assessment tools. This step helps identify which behaviors pose the greatest risk and changes that may offer the greatest benefit.
- *Prioritize your health goals.* After identifying behaviors that increase your health risk, prioritize them in the order you would like to change them. It is unrealistic to change all at once, but with planning and patience you can meet your health goals. Decide on one behavior you really want to change. First comes clarity; then comes commitment. Before embarking on a plan for change, be sure you really are ready to do it; then, tell yourself you truly can do it. If you believe that you can reach a goal, you will. In fact, belief in yourself can overcome many obstacles you may encounter on your path toward behavior changes.
- *Plan how you will accomplish your goals.* Setting both long-term and intermediate goals is often more manageable than being grandiose with your planning. For example, if one of your goals is to lose 20 pounds, perhaps a more realistic intermediate goal is to lose 5 pounds. A possible strategy might be to cut down on high-calorie foods while substituting nonfood rewards for yourself. Strategies for goal achievement should be realistic, practical, and manageable.

Each of the relevant chapters in this book offers concrete suggestions about techniques that can aid you to achieve true wellness. Believing in or adhering to a holistic health philosophy is just the beginning. As an individual, you are responsible to incorporate health principles into your daily life by modifying unhealthy behaviors or by developing positive lifestyle habits that will enhance your level of health and wellness. Remaining passive will allow chance to erode your choices and your health.

Seeking Professional Help

Many of us are reluctant to seek professional help because we do not want to admit that we have a problem or be categorized as "sick." As outlined in this introductory chapter, many of today's health challenges are complicated, potentially dangerous, and frequently threaten both our physical and emotional well-being.

A health care professional may be able to assist you to recognize your real problem (sometimes symptoms are confused with underlying causes), explore alternatives, and guide you toward informed choices. Perhaps you wish to avoid a problem but you lack accurate and reliable information about what to do. Again, a health care specialist or educator may be able to help. Colleges recognize that students need professional help, and most institutions provide an array of health education, care, and counseling facilities.

Each chapter in this text includes a special section, Seeking Professional Help, to assist you. If you need help beyond what the specific chapter offers, then consider the suggestions for obtaining professional assistance.

Beyond the Text

1. Respond to the following statement: The mind and the body are separate entities and never the twain shall meet.

2. Is it possible to experience gain from an illness or injury?

3. Your roommate runs five miles every day and looks healthy, yet she is socially isolated and harried. Is she healthy?

4. Respond to the following statement: Human beings are separate from their environment.

5. Respond to the following statement: Good health is just good luck. It's a roll of the dice. You don't really have control over illness.

6. How can spiritual values and your attitude toward them affect your health?

7. Few medical doctors describe themselves as "holistic" physicians. Do you believe that holistic health should be a required subject at medical school?

8. The American way of life is hazardous to your health. Respond to this statement.

Supplemental Readings

Healing From Within by Dennis T. Jaffee, PhD. New York: Fireside, 1980. A holistically oriented book that shows you how to develop a program of self-healing in concert with your physician. Techniques, such as meditation, stress-management, imagery, and biofeedback, assist you to gain control over your own health.

Health for the Whole Person by Arthur C. Hastings, PhD, editor, et al. Boulder, CO: Westview Press, 1980. A complete guide to holistic medicine, this comprehensive sourcebook will answer your questions on alternative health practices and present you with possibilities for enhancing your health.

Holistic Medicine by Kenneth Pelletier. New York: Delacorte Press, 1974. An early classic book that introduces the concept of holistic medicine and takes you from coping with stress to optimum health. Offers current research, stress-control techniques, nutrition practices, and exercise as the vital components of holistic health care.

Minding the Body, Mending the Mind by Joan Borysenko, PhD. Reading, MA: Addison-Wesley, 1987. The book is a tool that will allow you to take control of your physical and emotional well-being for health enhancement. Exercises for both the mind and the body will teach you how to use the power of your mind to promote health in your body—a classic in mind-body medicine.

The Creation of Health by C. Norman Shealy, MD, PhD and Caroline M. Myss, MA. Walpole, NH: Stillpoint Publishing, 1988. Presenting a holistic framework, one of the first books to truly encompass the spiritual dimension and how it relates to disease. A noted physician and an intuitive combine their talents to present a framework for how we can consciously create a healthy life though a case study approach.

The Healer Within: The New Medicine of Mind and Body by Steven Locke, MD, EP, and Douglas Colligan. New York: E. P. Dutton, 1986. Discusses the evidence that the mind and body are intimately connected.

The Healing Heart. Antidotes to Panic and Helplessness by Norman Cousins. New York: W.W. Norton and Co., 1983. The author shares his experiences of recovering from a massive heart attack as well as his strategies for summoning the regenerative processes needed to overcome illness and reduce panic.

Key Terms Defined

disease pathological process in the body having a characteristic set of signs and symptoms

health state of physical, psychological, sociological, and spiritual well-being

holism term coined by Jan Smuts to refer to the tendency in nature to synthesize and organize toward greater wholes

holistic way of looking at individuals and organisms as a whole; the notion that physical, mental, social and spiritual aspects of a person's life must be viewed as an integrated whole

holistic paradigm model or system of thought (paradigm) that encompasses a way of considering an individual as whole—mind, body, and spirit

immune system the group of organs and tissues that protect the body from disease

peak experience unique human experience that occurs when the mind is still and the person connects to a universal power

psychoneuroimmunology new specialty area of medicine that focuses on the connection between the brain, mind, and the immune system

self-actualization term coined by Abraham Maslow who assigned five levels to human needs; the most basic is physiological, the most advanced, self-actualization; fully achieving one's potential

shaman healers from ancient cultures; also nontraditional healers today such as Indian medicine men

spiritual values relating to the essential philosophy or beliefs each of us has about God, the universe, human nature, and the significance of life and relationships

wellness state of physical, psychological and sociological well-being of a whole person; synonym for *health*

Coping with Stress

For most students, college is a time of stress. College offers exciting new opportunities, but with them come new pressures to succeed academically, socially and, for many, financially as well. New freedoms, chances to experiment, and the absence of daily parental supervision demand that you deal with many difficult and stressful situations. Some students cope with college stress with ease, while others are driven to anxiety, depression and suicide. Burnout—the hopeless, helpless feeling that results in emotional and physical exhaustion is a common problem. As many as 25 percent of today's college students may suffer from enough stress to make them consider dropping out.

Stress can affect your behavior and, ultimately, your health. Your ability to cope with stress and maintain control of your life is fundamental to college success. You can learn to handle stress effectively and minimize its damaging effects by channeling pressure into a productive force and using stressors as motivators for positive action. Such techniques, known as stress management, can be a valuable asset for you throughout college and can contribute to your future career and personal success.

Contents

Key Terms

Adaptation
Anxiety
Autogenic training
Biofeedback
Endorphin
Eustress
Fear
Homeostasis

Meditation
Relaxation response
Stress
Stressor
Type A personality
Type B personality
Yoga

The process of coping with stress starts with a self-assessment. You have a sense of your personal relationship to stress when you answer the following questions either negatively or positively.

Am I in control of my life?

Do I have reasonable, attainable goals?

Am I willing to keep trying when my goals are blocked, or do I give up?

Do I have adequate coping methods to handle stress?

How effective is my ability to manage time?

Can I help my friends manage their stress?

These assessments are all relative, but their answers give clues to how much you may need an effective stress management program. If your lifestyle borders on chaos and you frequently exhibit and suffer from stress, you are a prime candidate for a stress management program.

Because stress is an individual experience, you need a personal plan for stress management. What bothers you may not faze your friend. Some students handle academic stress with ease but become totally unnerved when facing certain social situations. Others who are comfortable meeting new people at parties are stressed when taking an important exam. This chapter describes the four steps to coping successfully with stress:

1. Understand what stress is and learn how to recognize the signs of stress in your life.
2. Identify the most frequent and significant sources of stress for you: academic, social, lifestyle, environmental.
3. Determine which stressors are within your control and which are not.
4. Develop techniques that help you reduce the physiological and psychological effects of stress.

Understanding Stress: From Classroom to Boardroom

Current research continues to confirm a direct relationship between the amount of stress encountered in everyday life and sickness, premature aging, and poor performance in work, academics and athletics. Everywhere from college classrooms to corporate boardrooms, people discuss and complain about stress. Many of us confuse stress with nervous tension or anxiety; although those feelings may be a part of stress, they are not the whole picture. Whether you have stress-related symptoms now as a student or in the future as a professional, you court the possibility of suffering from stress or a stress-related disorder; so it's important to understand what stress is and what happens to your body when you experience it.

Confronting the Grizzly Bears in Your Life

Dr. Hans Selye, Canadian endocrinologist and world-famous researcher and author, defined stress as "the nonspecific response of the body to any

The Three Stages of Stress: Academic Deadline

Stage 1: Alarm	Your economics term paper deadline is two days away, but you haven't started your research or writing. You mobilize your resources and get started because you need a good grade in this course. With liberal support from coffee (caffeine) and snacks (sugar/starch), you stay up late on the first night to work.	The body mobilizes its defenses to meet the stressor. Hormonal levels increase; the autonomic nervous system operates.
Stage 2: Resistance	On the second day, you skip a couple of meals to continue working on the material. On the third day you finish inputting copy on your PC at 3:30 AM. The printer takes another half hour.	The body successfully adapts to carrying the burden of the stressor. Biochemical responses to stress wear off.
Stage 3: Exhaustion	You have trouble dragging yourself out of bed to deliver your paper at 9 AM, hurrying to grab a donut and coffee on the way. During classes, you can't seem to focus consistently. Cutting the rest of your morning classes, you stumble back to your room and fall into bed. You wake up with a sore throat, headache and congested nose.	The body becomes too fatigued to maintain resistance. Continued stress weakens the adaptation response. After your response wears down, it wears out. When your resistance cannot maintain an adequate defense, the usual results are physical illness or emotional distress such as depression.

demand made on it." The demand can be physical (confronting a grizzly bear), or it can be psychological (your parents are pressuring you to declare a pre-med major, but you prefer art history). *Nonspecific* means your body reacts regardless of whether your stressor is potentially harmful or helpful to your well-being. As illustrated on the accompanying chart, Selye described reaction to stress as having three stages: alarm, resistance and exhaustion.

Exhaustion leading to physical or mental breakdown is not inevitable. An alternative ending to the economics term paper saga described in the chart could have been as follows: You hand in the paper on time (barely), and feeling relieved and pleased, fall into bed and sleep for several hours. Waking up reasonably rested, you are motivated to think about your next assignments. Your body naturally moves back to a state of equilibrium, or balance. This phenomenon is known as **homeostasis**.

Researcher and author Dr. Walter B. Cannon described the human reaction to stress as "fight or flight." Modern man continues to display survival instincts and reactions that originated in primitive times. The following scenario illustrates Cannon's "fight or flight" theory:

You are walking alone at night to your car which is parked at the far end of a poorly lit campus parking lot. You are several yards away when you notice movement in your car. Is someone stealing your stereo unit, hot wiring your car, or waiting to attack you? Perhaps all three! Your heartbeat quickens, muscles tense, pupils

Coping with Stress

CHAPTER 2

dilate; your breathing becomes shallow and fast to provide more oxygen to your large muscles. Suddenly, adrenaline released into your bloodstream provides you with a sense of energy and alertness. In extreme situations, your bladder may relax to the point where you wet your pants. You have just experienced Cannon's flight or fight response, regardless of whether you approach your car to confront the stranger or beat a hasty retreat. Then, a split-second later, you recognize a friend getting out of your car. "I need a ride home; my battery is dead. By the way, don't you ever lock your car?" The stressor is gone, but when your body returns to its normal state, you will probably feel exhausted._

Not all stressful situations are as dramatic as the parking lot episode. Many are hardly noticeable at the time. Others occur so often that you don't give them a second thought—but they can wear you down. Stress is cumulative; that is, you may cope with a major stressor (a broken relationship), then you have a second stressor (a crucial final exam), but when a third one appears (you lose your lecture notes), you suddenly cease to cope. One plus two can add up to more than three when stress is the problem.

In *Successfully Managing Stress*, Lynn Brallier observed, "If you think about the incredibly wide range of stressors—the forces of change that tamper with homeostasis—you may find it remarkable that you are still alive and alert enough to read these words." This might appear to be an overstatement. However, when one realizes that stress has the potential to ultimately kill its subject, it is amazing that our minds and bodies can adapt to multiple stressors at the same time. We must adapt or die, stated Selye. In reality, as we fail to adapt effectively, we begin to suffer and become ill or exhibit a behavioral dysfunction.

Sweaty Palms and Other Signals of Stress

When dealing with stress, you can look at the problem from two angles. First, consider what physiological or behavioral symptoms you frequently exhibit. Then, work backwards to link them to their sources. Do you experience one or more of the signals of stress that are listed in the accompanying chart? It may surprise you to learn that stress is probably at the root of many of your problems. A disadvantage of this approach is that by the time you react to the stressor and rebound from its impact, the situation or event may have passed. Perhaps a disagreement with a friend or professor flared into an argument. Hours later, you are still fuming! You have a headache and can't concentrate on your studies. You experience the signals but can't resolve the problem. In frustration, you release anger or impatience toward the next "innocent" person who enters your space. Perhaps you overconsume alcohol or binge on food. Now, you have another problem, and so forth. A minor stressful situation often grows into a major crisis.

A second and perhaps more constructive approach to dealing with stress is to consider how stressors common to college life actually affect

If we encounter too much stress in our lifetime, we lose our ability to adapt to new stress altogether.

Dr. Hans Selye

Coping with Stress

Signals of Stress

Physiological

Fatigue, lethargy

Muscle tension—neck, back, legs, and so forth

Frequent headaches—tension, migraine

Shaking, trembling, spasms

Cold extremities, poor circulation

Digestion disturbances—acid, nausea, ulcers, gas cramps

Eating disorders—compulsive eating, loss of appetite

Elimination disorders—diarrhea, constipation

Sleep problems—insomnia, nightmares, excessive sleep, early awakenings

Pain—backache, teeth grinding

Excessive sweating

Heart problems—palpitations, racing, variable heartbeat, chest pain

Breathing complications—hyperventilation

High blood pressure

Skin eruptions—rash, hives, itching, eczema, acne

Sexual difficulties—impotence, low libido (desire), non-orgasmic, vaginitis

Amenorrhea (absence of menstrual period)

Psychological

Feelings	*Behavioral Indicators*
Anxiety	Restlessness
Panic disorder	Loss of memory, poor concentration
Depression	Nervous mannerisms—tics, grimaces, finger tapping, hair twisting
Pessimism	
Melancholy	Speech difficulties—stuttering, stammering
Impatience	Hyperactivity
Anger	Disorganization
Irritability	Passivity
Boredom	Aggressiveness
Confusion	Indecisiveness
Helplessness	Tardiness
Apathy	Inflexibility
Alienation	Nonproductivity
Isolation	Poor problem-solving
Numbness	Alcohol and drug abuse
Self-consciousness	Phobic responses
Purposeless	Overeating

you. Events that stress you may not affect your friends or roommate. For example, living in a messy room may upset you but not concern your sloppy roommate in the least. Perhaps you are reluctant to confront your roommate regarding the situation because interpersonal conflicts are difficult for you to handle. Now you have two sources of stress, environmental and behavioral.

Common Sources of Student Stress

Researchers at Marquette University (Wisconsin), Radford University (Virginia), and Arizona State University categorized the sources of stress most frequently listed by students: academic and social situations, environment and lifestyle. Noted researcher Richard Lazarus concluded that of the multitude of anxieties with which students have to cope, they feel most overwhelmed and anxious about wasting time, meeting high standards, and being lonely. Here are common college stressors.

Academic and Social Situations	Separation from home and parents
	Rejection by fraternity or sorority
	Failure to earn the grade expected on an important examination
	Serious conflict with roommate
	Victim of theft (bike, stereo)
	Sexual assault/acquaintance rape
Environment	High noise level
	Overcrowded living or classroom space
	High level of air pollution
	Inadequate lighting for study area
Lifestyle	Eating or sleeping disorder
	Increased use of alcohol or other drugs
	Substantial weight gain
	Increased dependence on caffeine

The examples listed above are negative stressors. Your body reacts to positive as well as negative stressors. Positive stressors could include receiving a surprisingly high grade, becoming very attracted to a new friend, being accepted by the Greek society of your choice, and so forth. Naturally, the positive ones are usually easier to deal with, and your body returns to a natural state of equilibrium more rapidly. It might be helpful for you to list 10 to 12 negative stressors that you've experienced in the past few months. See if they tend to fall into one of the categories men-

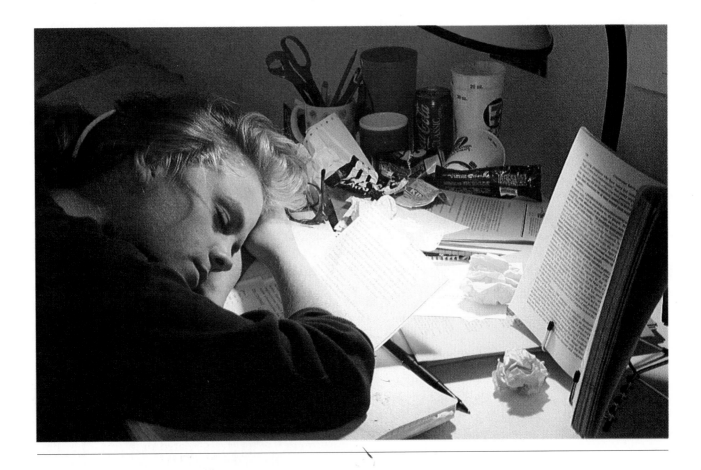

tioned above. Then ask yourself, "How much control do I have over these stressors?"

Stressors: Within or Beyond Your Control?

A crucial step in coping with stress is learning which stressors you can influence or control and which ones you cannot. Academic deadlines, such as midterms, are normally **beyond** your control. Getting assignments done on time is **within** your control. Requesting extension of a term paper deadline is an attempt to influence the situation.

You may be able to resolve some of your more critical stress situations by thinking in terms of problem, cause and remedy; for example:

- *Problem*: Excessive fatigue due to sleep deprivation.
- *Cause*: Your study time does not begin until late evening due to procrastination.
- *Remedy*: Establish a routine Sunday through Thursday to go to the library for two hours every afternoon and work undistracted on your assignments.

Coping with Stress

Effective coping includes isolating the part of a situation you can influence. This process is not an "either/or" proposition. Many environmental stressors cannot be changed, but you may be able to avoid some and rectify others. How much control can you exert? Sometimes, a small amount of control provides substantial stress relief.

Stress and Your Personality

Your roommate's taste in rock music leaves you feeling kicked out of your own room. Your friends drink too much alcohol and become obnoxious. It's easy to blame other people for your stress, but sometimes your personality is responsible. For instance, if you happen to be a perfectionist who works for so many hours on one term paper that you fail to complete other assignments, who is responsible? If you can't get organized or motivated, you'll face the crunch of covering an entire term's readings in only a few nights. Before concluding that your stress is caused by others, try to consider how your own personality traits may contribute to stressful conditions or hinder your ability to cope. When you take responsibility, you are in control and have the ability to change situations.

One popular method of labeling personality is based on Type A versus Type B. Individuals who set high goals for themselves and have high self-expectations are Type A. They are impatient, competitive, aggressive, ambitious, and hard-working. People who are calm, relaxed, balanced, and generally laid back are Type B. Not surprisingly, Type A's are more likely to suffer from stress. Type A's often look for an achievement payoff, but the added stress keeps them from reaching their goals. Type B personalities are at much lower risk for stress-related problems. They have more modest, realistic and, therefore, attainable goals. However, the overly enthusiastic Type B may relax to the point of missing academic deadlines.

Few of us are pure A or B; we have aspects of both. These labels cannot be interpreted literally, and you are not trapped in the stress patterns of your personality profile. If you are more Type B, you probably already have skills and attitudes that help you cope with stress successfully. If Type A seems more like you, and you value your high-achievement orientation, you can reduce stress-inducing aspects without compromising your academic goals. Change your work goal from "Can I work longer?" to "Can I work more efficiently?" If you find yourself studying nearly every waking hour, join an extracurricular activity or organization whose focus interests you.

Coping with Collegiate Stress

Stress is an integral part of college life. Once you assess the stress in your life, you can decide how to modify your reactions to it. The following section outlines steps for coping with specific stressors. It is important to understand that stressors can originate from several different sources at the same time. Frequently, it is difficult to identify precisely the type or intensity of a stressor. You sense that part of your life is out of control and you want to take positive steps to regain a more comfortable equilibrium.

Social Stress: Invigorating to Devastating

Social stress in college can be invigorating, devastating or somewhere in between. Upon entering college, you may be living away from home for the first time. Separated from friends and family, you face myriad potentially stressful situations, including:

Sense of belonging: Do you identify with your new school?

Personal relationships: Is it easy for you to make new friends?

Isolation: Do you feel separated from the majority of students due to differences in race, economic status, religion, sexual preference, or some other reason?

Social pressure: Are you being pushed to join new groups or engage in social behaviors that make you uncomfortable?

Competition: Do you feel like a small fish in a big pond, or like a big fish in a small pond with lots of other big fish?

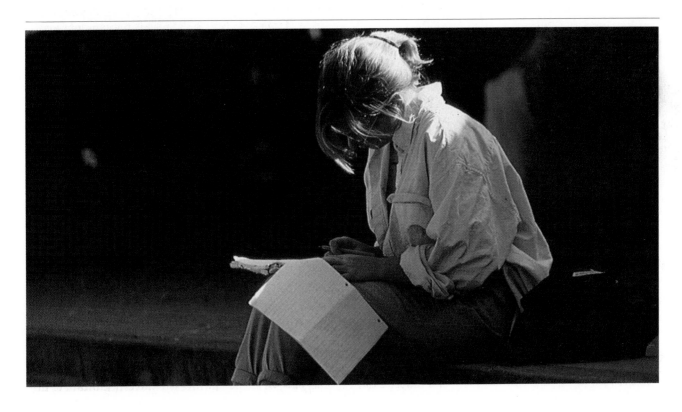

Student Stress Scale

The Student Stress Scale represents an adaptation of Holmes and Rahe's *Life Events Scale*. It has been modified to apply to college-age adults and should be considered a rough indicator of stress levels and health consequences.

In the Student Stress Scale, each event, such as beginning or ending school, has been assigned a score that represents the amount of readjustment a person has to make in life as a result of that event. In some studies, people with serious illnesses have been found to have high scores on such scales. People with scores of 300 or higher have a high health risk. Subjects scoring between 150 and 300 points have about a 50-50 chance of serious health change within two years. Subjects scoring below 150 have a 1 in 3 chance of serious health change.

To determine your stress score, add up the number of points corresponding to the events you have experienced in the past six months or are likely to experience in the next six months.

	Past		Future
Death of a family member	☐	100	☐
Death of a close friend	☐	73	☐
Diagnosed as HIV positive	☐	65	☐
Parents become divorced	☐	63	☐
Serious personal injury	☐	63	☐
Marriage	☐	58	☐
Pregnancy	☐	50	☐
Fired from job	☐	47	☐
Contracted a STD	☐	45	☐
Failed important academic course	☐	45	☐
Wallet with credit cards lost or stolen	☐	44	☐
Problems with alcohol or other drugs	☐	40	☐
Serious argument with close friend	☐	39	☐
Change in financial status	☐	39	☐
Major disagreement with parents	☐	39	☐
Illness of a family member	☐	38	☐
New romantic attachment	☐	37	☐
Substantial increase in academic load	☐	36	☐
First quarter/semester at college	☐	35	☐
Personal achievement in sports or academics	☐	31	☐
Living quarters burglarized	☐	30	☐
Low grades threaten academic progress	☐	29	☐
Change of residence	☐	29	☐
Serious disagreement with instructor	☐	29	☐
Sleeping problems	☐	28	☐
Citation for moving violation	☐	26	☐
Significant weight gain	☐	26	☐
Bicycle lost or stolen	☐	25	☐
Change in social activities	☐	24	☐
Awarded multiple parking tickets	☐	23	☐

Total _____

Though most students are quite well prepared for the academic pressures of college, you may sometimes feel rather overwhelmed by the new social experiences, choices and pressures you encounter. A helpful method of assessing social stressors on your life is to measure the impact of life event changes. One popular tool is the Holmes and Rahe Social Readjustment Rating Scale, first published in 1967. This scale, adapted for students, identifies events that cause stress. By listing and compiling a total, you can derive a general measure of the social stress experienced during the past year. Holmes and other researchers concluded that higher stress scores indicate a higher probability that you will experience illness during the following year. Though no tool or scale is 100 percent accurate in its predictions, these exercises point out when you should seriously regard the potential impact of social stressors. As you develop more capacity to cope with stressors, you minimize their damaging potential.

Sometimes a friend may suffer from social stress. If your roommate has recently experienced the loss of a close relative, the manifestations of this personal loss may not show. You know that this event, when coupled with a low course grade or rejection by a campus organization, may result in your roommate suffering significant stress. As an understanding friend, you can provide sensitive support and help your roommate cope more effectively.

Academic Stress

Academic achievement and preparation for a career after college are two of the most central purposes of your college experience. The capacity to cope with academic stress may prove critical to achieving your academic goals. Sources of academic stress include fulfilling the expectations of your professors and parents, meeting your own goals, dealing with your school's academic system, peer pressure, and all the decisions that you must make for yourself. Academic stress is pressure: you have substantial work assigned but limited time; passing grades are prerequisite to earning a degree; and competition for top grades may be intense. Recognizing the constancy of such stress is the first step in coping.

Your Major and Career   "Have you declared your major yet?" "What graduate schools have you applied to?" "How did the job interview go?" Even when friends and family are just curious, you may feel pressured to have some definite response. It's not considered cool to say, "I have no idea what I want to do in life." If you suspect you have made poor decisions about your major and college courses, you may feel trapped and unable to change direction without adding a semester or year of additional classes, with associated expenses.

A highly competitive environment for graduate school admission may influence you to specialize early in your college career. If you arrive at college committed to a major or profession your parents have chosen for you, you may feel obligated to pursue this path, especially if your family is paying your college expenses. Refusing their wishes while they hold financial leverage over you can be very stressful. And, if you are quite sure that your long-term goals are now different, the situation may be even more difficult to handle.

If declaring your major seems like a familiar stressor, try to determine whether it stems from peer pressure, parental influence, or lack of career definition. You can respond to your friends and relatives through rational discussion. Lack of career direction during freshman and sophomore

Stress vs. Anxiety

A stressor is a "demand" to which your body responds in a variety of ways—Selye's "nonspecific response." Anxiety is a general feeling of apprehension or impending doom. You sense that something is wrong, but there is no specific source or cause. Anxiety, like stress, is manifested by a variety of physical symptoms such as sweaty palms, "butterflies" in the stomach, dizziness, pounding heart, and diarrhea.

years has advantages. You have the opportunity to explore many options. Intensely interesting courses become good clues concerning your possible future direction. Professors whom you find particularly stimulating are good resources for career and graduate school advice.

Academic Skills   To achieve academic success, you need to master important skills—in listening, concentrating and notetaking, in reading and writing, and in test-taking. You can improve in any of these areas and, through that improvement, increase your academic success. If you lack confidence in your ability to grasp a certain course, find a tutor. This might threaten your self-image temporarily, but you can tolerate it. Attend special sessions when offered; spend time with peers who have mastered the material. If you have weak writing skills, or never mastered the rules of grammar, find someone to help you edit your papers before submitting them. Most colleges have learning skills centers where you can get help in many of these areas. Your academic advisor should be able to direct you to these resources on campus. As you develop academic skills, your confidence increases, and anxiety regarding academic success decreases. You are now better equipped to channel your energy into positive, rewarding experiences and away from stress-provoking negative thinking.

Test Anxiety   Anxiety can exert a powerful effect on your academic success. As a positive motivator, test anxiety mobilizes you to review for exams early. You concentrate more intensely on your assigned material, and you are "sharper" and more focused when you take the test. On the negative side, test anxiety can lead to postponed study sessions, poor concentration, and perhaps that sinking feeling when your mind goes blank at the beginning of the test. This type of stress reaction can have a damaging effect on your academic performance.

Many students feel nervous, tense and apprehensive just before taking tests. Some experience nausea, trembling, dizziness and even heart palpitations. Why should the sight of a test booklet cause sweaty palms and other reactions, and why don't all students react the same way?

The answer stems from each person's unique set of anxiety reactions. **As in other forms of anxiety, the crucial aspect is not the actual threat but how you perceive the threat.** If you usually become anxious concerning important events, the prospect of taking an exam will probably evoke an anxiety response. Or, if past experience with taking tests was negative, you may need to develop a new "mind set."

Research shows that test anxiety has two components: emotion and worry. Your emotional response to test taking results in unpleasant physiological reactions (pounding heart, sweaty palms, and so forth). These reactions usually do not impair your performance but rather increase your ability to concentrate on the immediate task. This is analogous to an athlete who is "up" for a competitive event. When you worry, you spend energy on the negative consequences of failure rather than preparing *not* to fail. Once you see yourself as failing, you may lose con-

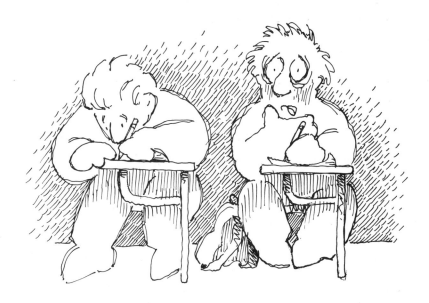

fidence in your ability to succeed on future tests. Test worry often stems from how you perceive others will react to your poor performance.

If your reaction to preparing for or taking tests involves the worry component of anxiety, the following steps will help you to reduce it:

1. Learn to recognize and separate your emotional reactions from your worry.
2. Reconsider your concerns about how others view your performance. Perhaps your perception of their view is not accurate; their opinions might be based on their own needs rather than yours. Let go of anxiety caused by what you cannot control, such as the reactions of other people.
3. Increase your self-confidence about test-taking by requesting help from your counseling center on campus or by using a special rehearsal technique for tests. Close your eyes and visualize yourself walking into the test feeling confident and calm. Next, picture yourself taking the test, doing well, and feeling rewarded. Students report remarkable results from positive image rehearsal. Their test performances are enhanced because they have less negative thinking to cloud their recall ability. Analyzing your own reactions and undertaking a program of positive visualization can be very effective in neutralizing this stressor.
4. And, of course, prepare adequately. If you don't know the material, test anxiety is rather realistic.

Coping with Stress

Time Management   College has many time-related stresses. Academic deadlines cause constant pressure, made worse by professors who warn you that late papers will receive lower or failing grades. Students who work at outside jobs or volunteer for community service must juggle many commitments. This requires organization and dedication. At times, you may have to choose between part of your social life and academic goals. In fact, the ability to effectively manage your time is so important to college success that this book has an entire chapter focused on the subject. Managing your time effectively begins with setting realistic goals for yourself. Planning how to achieve these goals forces you to prioritize your efforts and allocate your resources, including time. This process relieves you of dealing with the stress of drifting through college without definite purpose or commitment.

Stress and Your Lifestyle

Along with the academic pressures of college life, college students also experience a special set of living circumstances that involve stress producers such as poor eating habits, fatigue and heavy use of caffeine, alcohol and other drugs. Daily activities strongly influence your stress level. For example, eating properly helps you stay well, but unhealthy eating can contribute to your becoming sick. This creates additional anxiety when you miss deadlines, classes and job commitments. One of the most effective ways to reduce your stress level is to pay attention to your lifestyle. The following will help you determine which aspects of your lifestyle may be contributing to your stress level and how to minimize such negative effects. Additional information on these topics is contained in separate chapters throughout this book.

Eating, Nutrition and Stress   The quality and quantity of the food you eat influences your body's susceptibility to stress. When you eat well, your body has the nutrients, vitamins and minerals you need to spring back from the rigors of stressful events.

In fact, the body needs more careful attention to nutrition when you are under stress. Stressful periods deplete certain nutrients from the body, particularly Vitamin C, several of the B vitamins, and also potassium, zinc, copper, and magnesium. Stress interferes with your body's ability to absorb calcium from food. This potential calcium problem is particularly significant for women who participate in active physical fitness activities such as aerobics and running.

Of course, it's when you are under stress that your eating patterns go the most haywire. Some eat more when under stress. As one student stated, "During finals week, my motto is 'If you can't sleep, eat pizza.' " Others don't eat enough or even forget to eat. And most students react to pressure by substituting fast foods for regular meals and junk foods for nutritious snacks.

> **No matter how ambitiously we work on controlling external stressors, we undermine our efforts by overeating, underexercising, and consuming alcohol, caffeine and other drugs.**

To keep stress at bay, follow the basics for good nutrition—eat regular meals, consume healthy foods, and minimize unhealthy snacking. Remember, a "Big Mac attack" can occur at any hour, and certain foods high in sugar, fats, salt, and caffeine are in themselves stressors. This includes many chocolate snacks, soft drinks, potato chips, corn nuts, and other packaged snacks. When under academic stress, the last thing you need is to eat or drink stress.

Fatigue One of college's most persistent stressors is fatigue. Late nights and early morning classes can result in sleep deprivation. Research indicates that you can recover quite easily from a few nights of little or no sleep. However, when stress causes you to suffer from insomnia or some other sleep disorder, you have a problem that calls for attention.

Caffeine Substances that contain the chemical stimulant caffeine— coffee, tea, chocolate, soft drinks, and over-the-counter pep and diet pills—increase the adrenaline level in your bloodstream. If you pour on the caffeine when you're already under stress, you get a double dose of adrenaline. Your heart, hormonal systems, and nerves become twice as stressed. The results can include (1) increased reliance on sweets to fuel your system, (2) caffeine withdrawal symptoms, (3) digestive complications, and (4) sleep problems. **Behavioral symptoms of heavy caffeine drinkers are often indistinguishable from people having an anxiety attack.** By gradually shifting to caffeine-free drinks, you can enjoy the ritual of drinking coffee, sodas and so forth without experiencing the stress associated with excess caffeine.

Entire college lives have been powered by caffeine.

Alcohol and Other Drugs A common method of stress relief is through the use of alcohol and other drugs. Our culture teaches us that alcohol and drugs make us more comfortable, elevate our mood, and make it easier to have fun. In fact, however, alcohol and other drugs can increase stress levels and decrease your capacity for handling stress. Alcohol is a depressant. After a certain quantity, it makes you sluggish, more prone to negative feelings, and less self-assured. Inappropriate use of alcohol or other drugs interferes with your ability to perform important functions. These may include judging risks, behaving in a socially acceptable manner, fulfilling expectations of your friends, and even engaging in daily activities such as studying efficiently, attending classes, and eating properly. Failure increases stress, partially due to alcohol or drugs as a stressor and partially due to personal guilt.

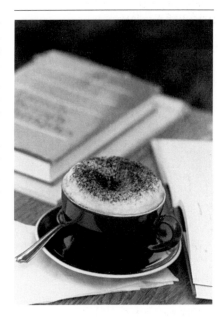

Stress and Illness Stress lowers your resistance, so you are more susceptible to infection, injury and other physical breakdowns. On the other hand, being seriously or chronically ill can cause so much mental stress that your body can't fight back effectively against the original physical problem. Some people seem to catch a cold, suffer from allergies, or experience a headache just when they most need to study extra hard for exams. If you are caught in such an illness/stress syndrome, here are some techniques that will help.

- Make the commitment to take control of your health and well-being. This includes eating well, getting sufficient sleep, and staying physically fit.
- Get high-quality medical attention for persistent symptoms or ongoing medical problems. Your college health service is staffed to provide you with diagnosis, treatment and, as appropriate, referrals.
- Harness the power of your mind to focus on wellness not illness. Visualization techniques work particularly well on certain chronic conditions associated with stress: tension headaches, digestion problems, sleep disorders, allergies, and so forth.
- If excessive use of alcohol, caffeine or other substances is interfering with your ability to accomplish your goals, talk with a counselor at your health service or get in touch with a support group that has helped others with the same condition. Talking with others who understand about practical and emotional issues can relieve substantial amounts of stress. Remember, your college health service is prepared to help you, as are various on-campus counseling programs.

Environmental Stress

Every student who starts college on a new campus encounters a new environment. You are a stranger and must "learn your way around." If you move from home to a campus residence or to off-campus housing, you face even more complex environmental changes. Crowded living conditions, lack of privacy, noise pollution, and concern for personal safety and security of belongings can cause frustration and stress. You may experience a new climate as well. A major change in your physical environment stresses your body; it may also stress your mind. Some you can avoid; others you can reduce. Begin with general preventive measures, such as:

- Even before you start school, find out what environmental changes you will encounter. Talk to others who have attended that campus and seek their advice.
- Create a comfortable, efficient personal space for yourself. With minimal investment you can do this whether you live in a residence hall, apartment or house and whether you live alone or with roommates.

Here are some helpful hints on how to reduce specific environmental stresses you may find at your college:

Air and Water Pollution   Certain areas of the country, such as Denver, Los Angeles, and New York, experience potentially dangerous air pollution levels on certain days and generally obnoxious levels on many others. If you move from a rural area to an urban campus, you will probably notice a higher level of vehicle exhaust fumes. Your residence hall or

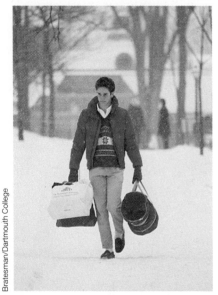

Bratesman/Dartmouth College

apartment building may have an inadequate air circulation system. You cannot change these conditions, but a small electrostatic air purifier might keep the air in your room cleaner and fresher.

If your water is particularly high in chlorine or fluoride or is otherwise unpalatable, use a portable water filter or bottled water. Residence hall students sometimes share the cost of bottled water delivered weekly to their floor. The more "good" water you drink every day—at least six to eight glasses—the more toxins will be flushed from your system and the less internal stress you will experience.

Noise   The subject of frequent complaints is stress-producing noise. It originates from many sources, including street traffic, loud voices, a snoring roommate, and amplified music. Noise has a cumulative negative effect on your body. Headaches and muscle tension are usual reactions, but insomnia, irritability and loss of concentration are also common.

If noise pollution bothers you, try foam earplugs or play relaxing music with headphones that cover your ears. Find a quiet place to study. If your roommate persists in disrupting your study and sleep, discuss your frustration openly and try to reach a mutually acceptable arrangement.

Safety and Stress   College is not always an idyllic, secure place. From petty theft to murder, crime threatens student safety and security on virtually every campus. In 1988, *USA Today* reported that one third of 764 colleges and universities surveyed admitted to an increase in all types of violence, including rape, robbery and assault. More than half of violent acts on campus are linked to alcohol. College women indicate an alarmingly high incidence of manipulation or force on the part of male students to persuade them to commit sexual acts. Because so many rapes go unreported, an accurate measure of the problem is not possible.

Theft of bicycles, stereo equipment, cash, and jewelry runs rampant on campuses throughout the United States. The majority of campus crime, including homicides, is perpetrated by fellow students, not outsiders. Although schools are taking steps to bolster security, you must assume responsibility for your own safety. Protecting yourself and your possessions requires awareness and vigilance. Experiencing a theft is a very stressful event, especially when your room or apartment has been violated. Lock your living quarters (including windows) when you're out. Don't leave valuables in plain sight. Use a sturdy lock to attach your bike to a secure structure so that no one can carry away a wheel, your lock, or your entire bike. If you have an automobile or motorcycle, determine where you can park safely, and always leave your car locked.

At night, when returning from the library or elsewhere to your room, use escort services. Many colleges now provide shuttle buses or personal escort services for safe transportation throughout the campus and to off-campus residences during evening hours. Whether you live on campus or off, get to know your neighbors and keep a watchful eye on each other

Negative Ions Can Lower Your Stress Level

Negatively charged particles affecting your stress level sounds like 21st century science. You breathe in (and out) at least 10,000 liters of air daily. Whether this air is positively or negatively charged makes a difference. In the last few years, scientists have learned that negatively charged air enhances your mood, makes your skin healthier, and protects you against premature aging. The natural source of negative ions in the air is water. The pounding ocean surf, a swiftly moving river, and the mist beneath waterfalls create a negative charge in surrounding air. A morning shower does the same thing. When you feel stressed, depressed, or generally out of sorts, spend ten minutes in the shower and let the negatively ionized air improve your mood. Or, buy a negative ionizer for your room. The improvement in your daily moods will be the telling difference.

At the Pennsylvania dormitory where a female student was raped and murdered, students had propped a door open to allow for a late-night pizza delivery. A male student was convicted of murder and sentenced to death.

and for suspicious people in or near your living quarters. Keep the telephone number of campus or city police near your phone. You don't have to be neurotic about these precautions, but preventive measures may help you avoid undue stress.

Stress and Your Personal Space College living space is usually crowded, especially when you share living quarters with one or more roommates. Lack of privacy is confining. You need space exclusively yours for study, sleeping, relaxation, and storage. Talk to your roommates about respecting each other's privacy and possessions.

Environment and mood are closely related. Arranging and decorating your space to your own taste is a method of self-expression and a means of achieving efficiency and comfort. Your space planning should feature adequate lighting and ventilation, practical and comfortable furniture, and pleasing colors. Research has shown that colors have a definite effect on your personality, health and mood.

Light also profoundly influences your mood. Most of us feel more energetic in bright, sunny weather. When constantly surrounded by artificial light, we tend to feel tired and depressed. Try to avoid fluorescent lighting, a most unnatural form of light. For your study space, buy full-spectrum lights, which simulate daylight. If you study in a library during daylight hours, try to find a location that has outside light. In your own living quarters, place your desk near a window. And, get out into the sun—your body needs full-spectrum light and Vitamin D from the sun for at least 20 minutes per day.

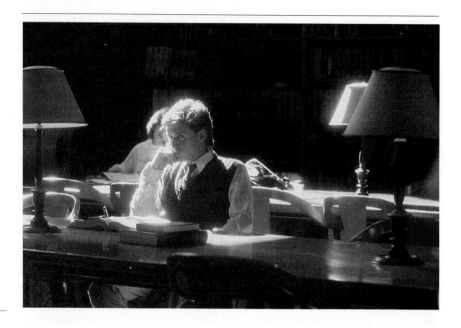

Coping with Stress

Good air ventilation is essential to good health. Central heating, cigarette smoke, and overcrowding charge the air with positive ions, which have a "downer" effect on your mood. Higher suicide rates have been associated with an environment highly charged with positive ions. In addition, these ions increase your susceptibility to asthma, hay fever and headaches. An ionizer will help keep your room air fresh, clear and charged with healthy negative ions. And, negative ions are considered to be stress reducing.

Roommates often disagree about open versus closed windows. The individual who craves fresh air suffers considerable frustration and stress when confined to a hot, stuffy environment. Excessively dry air triggers sinus, throat and respiratory disorders. Though electronic humidifiers are effective, a more practical approach is to open the windows for a short time each day or keep some well-watered plants in your room.

Furniture at college is easily taken for granted, especially if you live in a furnished space or "inherit" furnishings. A hand-me-down bed may seem to be a great bargain, but an uncomfortable mattress can cause sleeping problems or back pain. A desk too high or low, a chair that fails to provide good back support, a lamp that provides inadequate light—all contribute to discomfort and stress. With minimal investment, you can obtain comfortable, stress-reducing furniture. Organization of your furniture and possessions is important when customizing your space. Clutter and lack of organization create mental stress, especially when you waste time and get frustrated searching for misplaced items.

Personal Strategies for Stress Reduction

Even if you reduce your stress level by eliminating unnecessary stressors, you will still frequently feel stressed. Midterms approach, grad schools have application deadlines, friends move away, romances wane. You can learn to minimize the damaging effect of stress on your mind and body. Effective stress reduction strategies range from everyday activities to more disciplined techniques. Descriptions of several possibilities follow.

Invite Stress Management into Your Daily Life

Every day you engage in activities having effective stress-reduction potential, such as walking, taking a shower, or listening to music. Note which activities you associate with relaxation and feeling good. You are the best person to discover what is stress-relieving for you. Stretching, deep breathing and exercising are quick, easy and more effective than sugar or caffeine.

Ten Quick Tips for Stress Reduction

1. Spend quiet time—be alone with you.
2. Concentrate on one problem or project at a time. Don't get scattered.
3. Enjoy your food and the eating environment.
4. Take life one day at a time. When you survive, feel good about it.
5. Stay with your emotions. Don't avoid, repress or negate them. They are an important part of you.
6. Take time off from stress. Relax, lay back, "veg out," exercise, laugh, eat something healthy.
7. Avoid uptight, stressed friends. Anxiety is catching, so stay away.
8. Spend time with healthy, put-together friends. They will enhance, not decrease, your good feelings.
9. Praise yourself daily. Soon you will believe it and so will those around you.
10. Provide support to help others cope with their stress.

A brisk 10–15 minute walk is an energizer and stress reliever. Your body responds to this physical exercise. As your heartbeat increases, more oxygen circulates to your brain and all your body systems pick up the tempo. Your craving for snack foods decreases and your mental outlook takes on a positive note.

Physical Fitness   The many potential benefits of physical fitness include its ability to provide relief from stress. This is accomplished in several ways:

1. As stress-related tension builds, your muscles build up stores of lactic acid, sometimes to the point where you experience neck tension and headaches. Aerobic exercise, such as running or cycling, gets your cardiovascular system functioning and relieves this tension.
2. Vigorous aerobic exercise increases the release of endorphins, brain chemicals that contribute to a sense of well-being. Their euphoric effect lasts for some time after you have exercised. For this reason, afternoon workouts will help you approach evening study with confidence, energy and determination.
3. Long hours of work at a table or computer terminal put strain on your back. Proper exercises, including stretching, can strengthen your lower back muscles, improve your posture, and help you resist this physical stress.
4. Competitive sports, such as volleyball, softball and tennis, help alleviate academic and other stressors. Attending intercollegiate sports events provides diversion from studies and stimulates enthusiasm.
5. Physical fitness can result in physical or psychological stress if you go overboard. Constantly pushing yourself to go faster or harder cancels out the stress-relieving benefits of exercise. For example, excessive running to lose weight or divert your mind from resolving difficult situations can result in injury and even more stress.

Vitamins and Minerals   As already discussed, stress comes from many sources, but one of the most common is a deficiency in adequate nutrition. This deficiency may either be the cause or the result of stress. In either event, the solution is to provide the body with essential vitamins and minerals.

Nutrition experts, such as Dr. Hans Fisher of Rutgers University and Dr. Neil Solomon of Johns Hopkins University School of Medicine, believe that additional vitamins and minerals will help combat stress. They suggest a program that includes doubling the U.S. Recommended Daily Allowances (RDA) for fourteen vitamins and minerals. This does not mean that you should change your diet. The following nutrients are in addition to a healthy, well-balanced diet:

Daily RDA Dose Doubled (mg)

Vitamin C	120	Biotin	0.6
Vitamin B_1	3	Panothenic acid	20
Vitamin B_2	3.4	Iron	36
Niacin	40	Zinc	30
Vitamin B_6	4.4	Magnesium	800
Vitamin B_{12}	0.01	Manganese	10
Folic acid	0.8	Calcium	2000

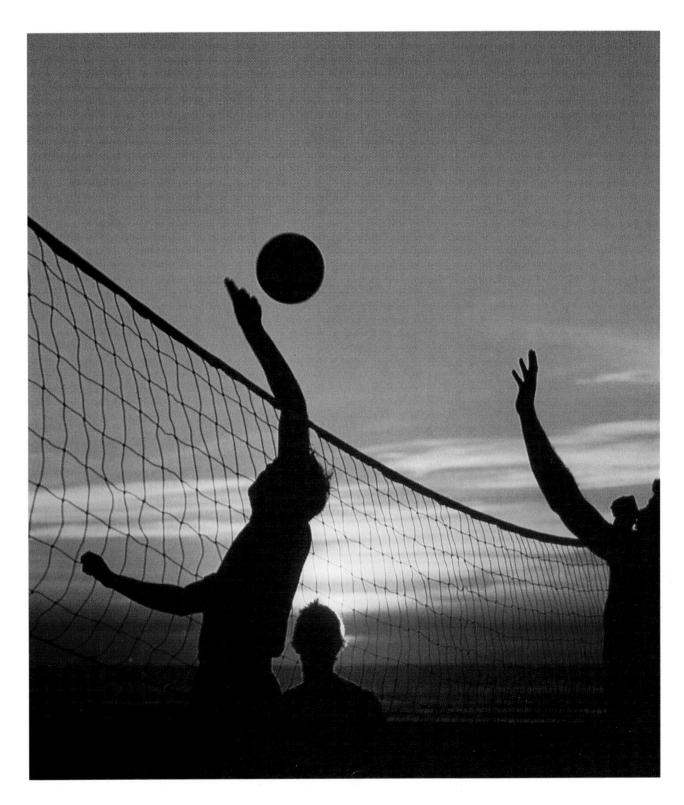

How can you tell whether you're feeling temporarily stressed and overwhelmed or if you're experiencing symptoms severe enough to call for professional attention? Most stress periods resulting from life's hassles last just a few weeks; these you can manage through concerted effort. If your physical or emotional discomfort lasts longer than that, seems to be intensifying, or occurs with increasing frequency, you may benefit from exploring other options. The Signals of Stress listed earlier in this chapter provide helpful indicators of physical symptoms that may be caused by stress.

Begin by getting a physical exam. A clinician can help discover or rule out physical causes for your condition and can help assess the extent of physical damage you may have incurred through stress. Remember, prolonged stress can result in a vast variety of debilitating physical problems. If the exam doesn't reveal conclusive answers, you may want to consult a counselor, psychologist or psychiatrist who has experience in treating stress-related disorders. Most campuses provide student psychological services which are free, informal and helpful. Your student health center may also provide peer counselors.

Most of these vitamins and minerals are contained in a multi-vitamin supplement. Follow this plan for a week. If you feel better, continue with the RDA doses, and when you are under stress again, increase the doses to the higher levels listed above.

Positive Attitude   The villain is not stress per se; stress actually adds spice to your life; the right type and amount of stress revitalizes and motivates you to achieve your best. Your goal should be to function with the right level of stress for your personality.

Confidence in facing a situation plays a large part in determining how much stress that situation produces in you. One skier stepping off the top of a chairlift may feel exhilaration at the challenge of heading down the steep slope. The next skier may have equal skiing skills but experience acute fear to the point of immobility when facing this same situation.

You can turn attitude into a stress-reduction tool. But you must take charge. Here are some hints for creating a positive attitude that reduces stress:

1. Become aware of your most important goals and develop a plan to reach them. Individuals who have a greater sense of control over their lives remain healthier than those who feel controlled by external forces. With goals and plans, you will have an easier time making decisions rather than being influenced by others.
2. Make a commitment to what matters to you. People who feel committed to their daily activities usually can handle stress effectively. The busy student who works hard academically and participates in extracurricular activities usually has little time to worry about stress, much less to get sick.
3. Remain open to the unexpected; serendipity often enhances your life. Perceive new situations as opportunities rather than threats.
4. Accept that happiness comes from within yourself. Don't depend on other people to provide for your happiness. When you are positive, people will respond to you in the same way.

Humor   How often do you experience a situation in which the tension mounts unbearably until someone cracks a joke and frees everyone from their nervousness? Laughter and a good sense of humor are so wonderfully elusive that they seem to be frightened away when sober scientists analyze them. E. B. White said, "Humor can be dissected, as a frog can, but the thing dies in the process and the innards are discouraging to any but the pure scientific mind."

A good sense of humor fosters well-being. Although wit slides out from under the microscope, some scientific facts emerge; laughter increases endorphin levels (those marvelous brain chemicals that make fans of physical fitness feel on top of the world), relaxes the body, and reduces the stress response. "Laughter gives a person a different perspective on life," maintains Vera Robinson, educator and humor researcher at California State University at Fullerton. "When you laugh, you let go of anxiety, fear, embarrassment, hostility, and anger." If you are not a stand-up comic, you can derive these benefits as an armchair humor booster with videotapes, movies, the Saturday Night Live cast, and perhaps friends who have the wonderful talent of turning your frustrating experiences into humorous anecdotes. Laughter is one of the best stress reducers available. Notice how much better you feel after a good laugh.

Social Support Is Crucial

Stressful situations confront students daily and multiply as the term progresses. One reason why some students handle stressors more effectively than others is that they have a social support network. Facing stressful situations alone is difficult. Roommates, friends, discussion group members, RA's, professors, TA's, coaches, deans, and counselors can help you by discussing options and just listening. Students who lapse into depression usually are found to have few close friends and weak social support.

Stressed Out on Monotony

Monotony is stressful. Although most students are victims of the stresses resulting from overstimulation, understimulation is equally insidious. Do you feel unhappy, purposeless or stagnant during semester breaks or other periods of decreased activity? If so, increasing your stress will help replace your lost vitality. The human mind and body were designed to be used, so vigorous physical activity is one effective remedy for stagnation. Ironically, sometimes the best prescription for the stress of boredom and inactivity is stress.

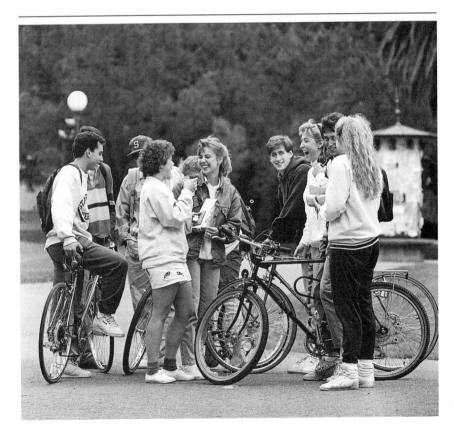

Coping with Stress

Stress and a Satisfying Life

Understanding stress teaches you critical principles for creating a healthy and satisfying life. Consider the following principles, and reflect on how you can use stress in your life to positive advantage.

- **Stress does not come from the outside; you generate it totally within yourself.** In Hans Selye's definition, stress is the nonspecific reaction to any demand. An upcoming exam may be a stressor; your reaction may or may not be stress. A specific response to the exam (assuming you want to get a good grade in the course) is to study extra hard. But non-specific reactions, which do not serve specifically to resolve the imbalance of having an upcoming exam and wanting to do well, may also include a certain amount of fear, even panic. You might eat more, smoke cigarettes, pace the floor, or have difficulty sleeping. You yourself, not the exam, have generated these reactions—they are the symptoms of stress.

- **You cannot see stress directly; you can only experience its symptoms.** No one can see love, but we all know its symptoms: the fluttering heart, butterflies in the stomach, inability to concentrate on other things, tendency to think about a loved one all the time. You must discover your personal characteristic symptoms of stress. You might overeat or get headaches or skin rashes. You might become short-tempered. Learn to recognize your symptoms as not actual problems but bodily warning lights signalling an imbalance. Merely seeking immediate relief from the symptoms through drugs, sex, or other distractions is like painting over the warning light to keep it from bothering you. You must look deeper within your system to discover and correct the imbalance.

- **Your attitude plays a significant role in illness and wellness.** While working at the University of Chicago with professionals who experienced constant pressure, researcher Susanne Kobasa demonstrated that the primary difference between those who became ill and those who stayed well was attitude. Those who stayed well tended to be committed to their jobs, viewed problems as challenges not obstacles, and felt a sense of control—they believed their actions and presence actually made a difference. Your attitude, beliefs, and conceptualization of what is happening to you determine your internal reaction to those events and, therefore, determine your stress level.

The challenge is to shift your attitudes so that you look for the positive side of events—not a phoney positive attitude that turns one into a "Pollyanna" who fails to recognize painful situations or major problems, but a "can do" attitude.

- **Stress is essential to everything you enjoy.** We all love the feeling of victory, and this feeling of achievement is proportional to the challenge. Think about what makes you feel happiest, most excited and enthusiastic. Having your team win a football game in the final two minutes is more exciting and memorable than when the team wins by a large margin over a poor team. When you have learned a subject well, how much better it feels to handle successfully a challenging set of final exam problems rather than a bunch of boring multiple-choice questions that test only a small part of what you've learned in the course.

Coping with stress requires exploring the inner you, utilizing and reinforcing your creativity, skill, and strength. Stressful events and periods in our lives can help us grow to be better able to make the most of our lives. Learning to truly celebrate your successes will increase your joy, personal satisfaction, and enthusiasm.

- **A healthy life is a balance of stress and relaxation.** In nature, stress and tension alternate with relaxation. Your heart contracts and relaxes to keep your blood flowing. Your breath enters and leaves. Your busy, complex world provides plenty of stress; most of us must work diligently to find relaxation techniques and time to balance this stress. Few aspects of our culture really encourage us to acknowledge the importance of relaxation. Can you imagine one of your professors, as the assignment is being collected, asking if you made sure to do your 20-minute meditation last night?

- **You must take responsibility for your own life, including its stress.** Only you can really make your life better. No one else can feel or deal with your symptoms of stress. Take responsibility for dealing effectively with stressors. Focus on wellness, not illness. Practice self-awareness, self-education, and self-responsibility. Create a stress management program, motivate yourself to follow it, and update it regularly until it becomes an automatic part of your life.

Emmett E. Miller, MD

Emmett E. Miller, MD, is a leading practitioner of psychophysiological medicine, which relates mental processes to physical health and optimal performance. Dr. Miller has developed a unique series of self-improvement audio tapes and experiential videotapes relating to stress management, self-improvement, and health and wellness. He is a frequent guest speaker at health conferences and workshops. Dr. Miller maintains a private practice in hypnotherapy, preventive medicine, and psychotherapy in Menlo Park, California.

Techniques for Relaxation and Visualization

Stress experts have carefully studied the effects of deep relaxation on the mind and body. They found that individuals who regularly practice relaxation exercises experience less stress than people who don't. The **relaxation response** is actually the physiological opposite of the **stress response**. People adept at invoking the relaxation response use their minds to control their autonomic nervous system—oxygen consumption, respiratory rate, heart rate, blood pressure, and muscle tension. Their alpha brain waves, the waves associated with feelings of well-being, increase. Effective body relaxation techniques have existed for centuries. Several have gained significant popularity in recent years. The following short descriptions will familiarize you with the leading techniques. The end of the chapter lists relevant additional resources.

Deep breathing is emphasized by virtually all relaxation exercises as a core concept. When you are tense, your breathing becomes rapid, irregular and shallow. Healthy deep breathing increases the amount of oxygen in your blood, cleanses your system of carbon dioxide and other waste chemicals, relaxes your muscles, and encourages your heart rate to return to normal. When you learn how to take deep, slow, full breaths and exhale completely, you will have mastered a key relaxation technique. B. K. S. Iyengar, a world-class yoga teacher, suggests a breathing technique for stress reduction. Try it for yourself:

- Inhale as you normally do.
- Exhale as you normally do.
- Pause as long as comfortable.
- Repeat the first three steps.

Simple? Yes. Effective? Yes. This technique allows your lungs to empty more completely, continuing the normal exhalation process. Why is this simple exercise effective? Because the completed exhalation enables the mind to quiet—a rest from the jumble of one thought upon another. Iyengar says that if you learn this "secret," you can control stress. And, it also provides the foundation for meditation.

In **autogenic training**, you visualize warmth and heaviness, two physical sensations associated with the relaxed state. The warmth represents increased blood flow throughout the body, and heaviness is perceived as relaxation of the skeletal muscles. During **progressive relaxation**, you tense and release specific muscles or groups of muscles throughout your body. This technique is especially effective when your body feels stiff and sore from protracted study sessions. A detailed relaxation exercise is included later in this chapter.

Meditation, originating thousands of years ago, is based on Eastern cultures and religions. The effects of meditation are similar to those associated with deep relaxation. Meditation is the process of bringing the mind to stillness. It sounds easy, but if you have tried meditation, you know from experience how difficult and frustrating this process can be. There are many methods, from the traditional transcendental meditation

---

Thoughts That Help You Cope with Stress

Preparation

There's nothing to worry about.
I've succeeded with this before.
I know I can do these tasks.
It's easier once I get started.

Confronting the Stressful Situation

Stay organized.
Take it step by step.
Any tension I feel is a signal to use my coping exercises.
I can get help if I need it.
If I get tense, I'll take a breather and relax.

Coping with Pressure

Relax now!
Just breathe deeply.
There's an end to it.
I've survived this before.

Reinforcing Success

I did it!
Next time I won't have to worry as much.
I am able to relax away anxiety.

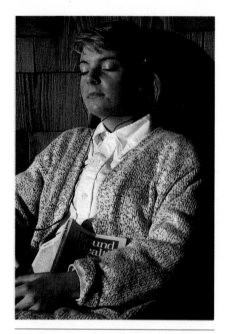

(TM) and Zen meditation to the repetition of a word such as "one," advocated by Dr. Herbert Benson of Harvard University. TM is a structured form of meditation popularized in the United States in the 1960s by Maharishi Mahesh Yogi. In TM, you select a mantra (a word or sound) that you repeat mentally while seated quietly in a tranquil place.

Perhaps the easiest meditation technique is to sit in a comfortable position with your spine straight (the lotus position is perfect if your legs can stand it), close your eyes, and relax. Concentrate on relaxing your muscles and organs throughout your body, then focus on your breathing. Inhale fully, then exhale, watching the breath come out "in your mind's eye." If a thought comes in, let it slip away. Continue inhaling and exhaling, watching your breath. The objective of meditation is to quiet the mind. No thoughts rush in to break your concentration.

Visualization is a proven technique for healing, stress management, and positive goal attainment. When you create a mental picture, your body can respond as if it were a real experience. Visualization can help you perform better on tests, speak more effectively in class, discuss difficult situations with others, and act more confident in any circumstance filled with uncertainties.

Yoga is an ancient Indian discipline that begins with postures, or asanas, that stretch and strengthen muscles. It progresses to meditative relaxation or breathing techniques. Yoga is not sport or exercise as such; nor does it have to be a religion. The system was devised completely for health and well-being. The best way to begin yoga is to find an experienced teacher who can correct your postures and guide you through the breathing and relaxation exercises.

T'ai Chi Ch'uan, a soft Chinese technique for relaxation, is actually a system to both stimulate and balance your subtle life energies. Thirty minutes a day devoted to this gentle, flowing movement is relaxing, centering and invigorating—a great way to relax and an interesting alternative to energetic Western exercise.

Biofeedback is the use of an instrument to monitor physiological processes of the body and to "feed back" measurements to the individual being monitored. A scale, thermometer and pulse monitor are common feedback devices, as are more technically sophisticated machines having electronic sensors and digital readouts. Recent research has confirmed that many people can influence or control their autonomic processes (heart rate, temperature, digestive functions, and so forth). As you become more adept at controlling your body's responses, the need to use monitoring devices decreases—and the mental tools become your own.

Color is much more than a background; it influences your mind and emotions. Although schools have not yet decorated classrooms or examination centers in colors known to relax students, you can use color to its best effect in your own environment. In *Color Meditation*, S. G. J. Ourseley identifies green, indigo and midnight blue as having a calming, restful effect. Baker-Miller pink is now being used in jails and mental hospitals to relax inmates and patients. If college is driving you slightly crazy, and you paint your room pink, make sure it is Baker-Miller.

Music, like color, influences your mind and emotions. One of the most

Rainbow Visualization

A body relaxation and visualization experience is an effective stress reducer. When you are anxious or stressed, your muscles and organs become tense. When the tension is drained out, your body is relaxed. Physiologically, as you become relaxed, you become less anxious. Try it and see. The following process is an example of a stress-reducing experience.

Find a quiet place where you can be comfortable.

Sit in a chair with a straight back, lie down on the floor, or sit in the lotus position with your legs crossed.

Become comfortable in your chair, turn on your tape, and close your eyes.

Breathe in deeply through your nostrils, allowing the air to fill your lungs.

Exhale slowly through your mouth, letting all of the air flow out.

Pause at the end of the breath—neither breathing in nor out.

Good. This pause lets your mind come to quietness.

Repeat breathing in and out. Watch the breath as it goes in and comes out during each cycle. Find yourself becoming more and more relaxed.

Feeling relaxed and at peace, mentally look into your body and see if there are any areas of tenseness, tightness. Let this tension go. Again, look through your body in your mind's eye. Relax any muscle that appears tight or tense.

Now, feeling totally relaxed and serene, imagine a rainbow in the distance. In your mind's eye, visualize this rainbow as it gracefully curves over a mountain. See all of the colors—brilliant, vivid colors blending into one another.

Join this rainbow now; experience the different color vibrations as they move through your body. If you are attracted by a particular color, remain in its aura for a few moments. Each color has its own vibration

and if one especially appeals to you, it may mean that your body and spirit require this specific energy at this time.

Good. Now, softly move through the colors: red, orange, yellow, green, blue, purple, violet, and finally white on the outer edge.

As you leave the rainbow, experience the sun as it warms your body—lending its warmth and brilliance to your body. Remain here for a few moments, letting the sun bathe your body with its healing rays. As you leave this visualization, remember the feeling of well-being, health and peace.

Whenever you are ready, leave the sun but bring these peaceful and relaxed feelings with you. Return to the room, then open your eyes, feeling energized but serene.

---

effective and convenient stress reduction tools is audio tapes. These range from movie soundtracks and classical selections to "new age" artists and specially recorded tapes with subliminal messages. Music with a tempo of about 60 beats per minute tends to synchronize with your natural physiologic rhythms, especially your heart beat, and promotes a relaxed body state. Another popular practice among relaxation zealots is listening to sounds of nature such as gently falling rain or ocean surf. Just as rock music helps to set a party mood, certain selections have proven effective to enhance the relaxation/visualization process. The following list is only a small sample of the many available possibilities.

Movie Soundtracks	Classical Works	Instrumental Artists
Love Story	Pachelbel's "Cannon in D"	Steven Halpern
Out of Africa	Vivaldi's "Four Seasons"	Kitaro
Doctor Zhivago	Tchaikovsky's "Swan Lake"	George Winston

Beyond the Text

1. How does physical or mental stress affect you at college? How can you cope more effectively?

2. Is it possible to avoid most stressors in your daily life? Should you concentrate on responding to them as they arise?

3. Can you recognize Type A and Type B personality traits in yourself and your friends? Is it possible to change from one to the other and why would you want to?

4. The life events scale (presented earlier in this chapter) has been criticized by those who say that stress-induced illness is more a result of ongoing daily hassles than significant isolated events. Do you agree?

5. Techniques of body relaxation and imagery are widely used by athletes prior to important performances. How can you use these techniques in your own life, such as during final examinations?

6. Respond to this statement: If you have no stress in your life, you're not living.

Supplemental Readings

Beyond The Relaxation Response by H. Benson and W. Proctor. New York: Times Books, 1984. An update on the classic introduction to the health benefits of relaxation and how to achieve it.

How to Stubbornly Refuse to Make Yourself Miserable About Anything—Yes, Anything! by Albert Ellis, PhD. New York: Lyle Stuart, 1988. Clear, no-nonsense advise from a nationally respected psychologist and author.

Mind as Healer, Mind as Slayer by Kenneth Pelletier. New York: Delta, 1977. A summary of the author's views on the role of stress in causing illness and ways to prevent it.

Resilience: Discovering a New Strength at Times of Stress by Frederic Flach, MD. New York: Fawcett Columbine, 1988. Common sense approach to developing resilience, which the author feels is the key to reintegrating one's life in times of great stress.

Software for the Mind by Emmet E. Miller, MD. Belmont, CA: Celestial Arts, 1987. Practical exercises for using visualization to release tension, lower anxiety levels, and create new attitudes and experiences in life.

Tai Chi by Chia Siew Pang and Goh Ewe Hock. Reno, NV: CRCS Publications, 1985. As a review or learning guide, this book covers 44 Chinese tai chi positions.

The Relaxed Body Book by Daniel Goleman and Tara Bennet Goleman. New York: Doubleday and Co., 1986. The editors of American Health magazine have assembled a series of gentle, easy-to-learn relaxation exercises using a variety of techniques.

Key Terms Defined

adaptation changes in response to a new situation

anxiety feeling of uneasiness, apprehension, or dread

autogenic training a method of deep muscle relaxation that enables one to reduce the stress response, regain homeostasis, and prepare to handle additional stress

biofeedback training technique that utilizes monitoring instruments to assist subjects to control stress-related disorders through self-regulation of internal functions

endorphin group of brain substances that bind to opiate receptors in various areas of the brain and thereby raise the pain threshold

eustress positive stress; usually causing one to feel excited or happy

fear unpleasant emotional state consisting of physical and psychological responses to a threat or danger

homeostasis the body's natural state of internal balance

meditation process of bringing the mind to stillness; used as a stress-reduction technique

relaxation response physiological opposite of the stress response, characterized by metabolic reduction and increased sense of calm

stress nonspecific response to the body to demands placed upon it

stressor any agent or situation that produces the stress response

Type A personality characterized by impatient, aggressive, and fast-paced lifestyle; associated with heart disease

Type B personality characterized by patient, unhurried, relaxed attitude

yoga ancient system of postures and breathing techniques known for producing a calming effect

Mental Fitness

As a human being, you are an integral unit of body, mind, and spirit; what affects one part of this triad affects the whole. To maximize your physical, spiritual, and intellectual energy and achievement, mental health is a prerequisite. Mental fitness refers to the state of having a healthy mind, with the ability to adapt to and cope with the circumstances of life.

Mental fitness manifests on a continuum. If you are mentally healthy, you will be able to cope with stress, adjust to changing circumstances, form healthy relationships, and enjoy life. Toward the other end of the continuum, you may experience minor coping problems, have limited but manageable symptoms, or perhaps have major mental or emotional problems such as panic attacks, generalized anxiety, or compulsive behavior. This chapter begins with the concept of self-esteem, essential for mental health, and guidelines for maintaining mental fitness. It continues with a discussion on how to manage minor as well as major anxiety problems, and how to renew your spirit when you feel over-whelmed.

Contents

Key Terms

Agoraphobia

Anxiety

Compulsion

Hypnotic

Obsession

Obsessive-compulsive disorder

Panic attack

Phobia

Premenstrual syndrome (PMS)

Psychotherapy

Self-esteem

Tranquilizers

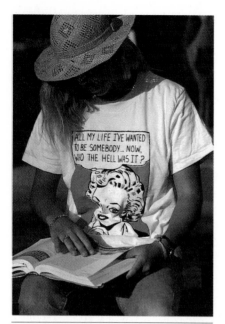

Self-Esteem

Self-esteem is how you feel about yourself. Underneath the acts you perform for others and behind the image you project to the world is the real you. How you feel about this you is a critical component of how you handle life—its stressors, failures, successes, and ultimately the joy, happiness and meaning of life. If you see yourself as worthy, lovable, likeable, trustworthy, dependable and so forth, you have what psychologists call a positive self-esteem. If, on the other hand, you feel you are a failure because you cannot meet expectations, you don't see yourself as very likeable, much less lovable, or you are not too dependable, you have poor self-esteem.

The way you view yourself has a profound effect on the way you carry out your daily life. People with a positive sense of self-worth typically display poise, confidence and self-assurance. This section will discuss several components of self-esteem: accepting yourself, setting realistic goals, and developing personal power. An important part of the foundation of your self-esteem is the beliefs and values you have acquired.

Accepting Yourself

Learning to accept yourself is one of those things that you know you're supposed to do, but you don't always know how. (If you're like many people, you start feeling bad about yourself for not feeling good about yourself—how can you win?!) Accepting yourself does not mean feeling OK "as soon as" you get over your shyness, lose weight, get your grades up, or change whatever else you don't like about yourself. Accepting yourself doesn't even mean liking all the ways that you are manifesting yourself in the world right now, or giving up the desire to change some things.

Accepting yourself means being OK with yourself right this instant, imperfect as you may recognize yourself to be. It means (among other things) being patient with yourself while you try to figure out what "being

Nobody can make you feel inferior without your consent.

Eleanor Roosevelt

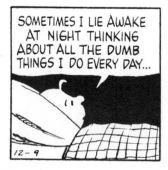

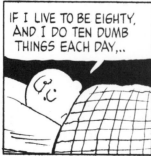

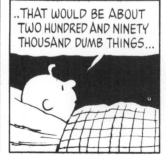

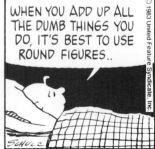

OK with yourself" really means, and tolerant of feeling that there are some things you just can't imagine feeling OK about.

Accepting Your Strengths and Weaknesses   It's important to realize that all characteristics have a double edge.

- Those who don't like spending time alone worry that they need too much from other people, while those who want a lot of time alone worry that they don't give enough to others.
- Those who make changes easily worry that they can't make commitments, while those who commit easily worry that they settle for too little.
- Those who find it difficult to feel really special with a person who seems to love everyone, and hard to feel really safe with a person who is very discriminating.
- Those who worry about being "too sensitive," because it's more difficult for them than for others to maintain emotional equilibrium. Being sensitive can be understood as being like an FM rather than an AM band on the radio—the signals are more complex, take longer to adjust and require more monitoring, but when tuned properly, you hear something of real quality and precision.

As you become more aware of your particular characteristics and understand that your strengths and weaknesses are integrally related to one another, it gets easier to accept who you are and make the most of it. You expect to have weaknesses—the flip sides of your strengths. And you can look for strengths hidden behind what you usually regard as your weaknesses. Now, as you work at developing the things you like about yourself and changing the things you don't like, you can stand on a foundation of basic self-acceptance. And the more you accept yourself, the less other people will feel invited to judge you, but will instead expand their own concept of what is considered acceptable.

Understanding that all characteristics have advantages and disadvantages can help you to accept them in yourself. Value the advantages and be tolerant of the disadvantages that go with your characteristics.

To truly accept yourself, you may need to experience who you are underneath your pleasant or unpleasant, "good" or "bad," behavior in any given moment, and to appreciate your intrinsic value. Rather than struggling endlessly and compulsively for enough "achievement" to make you feel OK, you can begin to search for the kinds of experiences and relationships that support your feelings of intrinsic worth—your self-esteem.

- Don't let the criticisms of others affect you as a person. Instead, evaluate those specific actions the criticisms addressed. When this evaluation exposes an area that needs improvement, accept feedback as constructive.
- Don't stay around "friends" or situations that consistently make you feel inadequate. This may be a sign that such "friends" are not right for you.

Dr. Sidney Simon Talks About Self-Esteem

Self-esteem, according to Dr. Simon, includes both the image of yourself and your opinion of that image. If you have a consistent high self-esteem, you feel a sense of empowerment. For example, if you see yourself as bright and smart and have a positive opinion of your intellectual ability, then, in this area, you will have high self-esteem. In turn, this view of yourself gives you a sense of power allowing you to make choices that challenge your potential. As in any circular pattern, the more you exercise choices and reaffirm your view of yourself, the higher your self-esteem.

Dr. Simon reports that we all have to take risks, and every risk that we take and master increases our self-esteem. You can take an intellectual risk—join a class on a subject you know nothing about; take an emotional risk—form a new relationship and tell another person you love him or her without the assurance you are loved in return; you might also take a physical risk—join a group for rock climbing or river rafting—in which you have to stretch to the limits of your physical skill and endurance. Take a risk and increase your self-esteem. Researchers are increasingly becoming aware of the importance of self-esteem—in finding harmony and vitality in your life, and especially in coping with life's adversities. Perhaps the critical question is if we have it (high self-esteem), where did it come from? And if we don't have it, how can we develop it?

47

Shyness

You stand outside the circle and
wonder why you feel left out,
Unaware that you need your OWN
permission to join the others—not
theirs.

Rusty Berkus from *Appearances*

You are not alone in feeling
shy—but it probably feels that
way. Shyness is considered a
social disease. Millions suffer
from it and there is no miracle
cure. This traumatic, painful and
even debilitating condition forces
people into isolation and loneliness. According to Philip Zimbardo, foremost researcher on the
subject of shyness and originator
of the revolutionary Shyness
Clinic in Palo Alto, California,
"shyness is an insidious personal
problem that is reaching epidemic
proportions." Further, he believes
that trends in our society will only
make the problem worse.
Zimbardo studied 5000 American
college students in an attempt to
determine what shyness is and
what can be done about it.

Shyness, as a concept and as an
experience, is difficult to define. It
seems to be a form of social
anxiety where the individual may
experience a range of feelings
from mild anxiety in the presence
of others to actual fear to a pronounced anxiety disorder. For a
person experiencing shyness, it is
often anxiety-producing to have
to interact with others and, at the
same time, the loneliness of
limited relationships is profoundly
painful.

Shyness seems to be an
all-encompassing phenomena in
that the person experiences
definite feelings, exhibits certain

behaviors and, physiologically,
manifests certain symptoms. If
you are one of the 84 million
adults in the U.S. who experience
shyness, you will be more than
familiar with the behaviors and
feelings that accompany this
condition.

Behaviors

Reluctance to talk

Difficulty in making eye contact

Avoidance of others

Failure to take the initiative to
act

Speaks in low, almost inaudible
voice

Inability to make speeches

Difficulty in volunteering

Feelings

Self-consciousness

Feelings of embarrassment

Feelings of insecurity

Attempts to keep a low profile

Feelings of inferiority

Physical Symptoms

Blushing

Butterflies in the stomach

Sweaty hands

Increased pulse

Pounding heart

Dry mouth

Trembling

Shyness relates to one's
exaggerated sense of self—it
implies that a self-conscious
person is conscious about self;

this, in fact, seems to be true. Shy
individuals are absorbed in the
self and constantly focused on
how they affect others and how
others feel about them. They
worry about themselves and
become so absorbed in their own
discomfort and inadequacies that
they cannot focus on or feel
toward others. This cycle serves to
futher isolate shy people from the
mainstream of warm, giving
relationships.

Imagine yourself as a shy
person, (if you have never
experienced extreme shyness),
having to approach a new group
of people. What would it feel like?
Would you do anything rather
than place yourself here? Are you
feeling extreme embarrassment
and self-consciousness? Are you
blushing, feeling butterflies in
your stomach; is your heart
pounding? Just imagining this
experience is bad enough—think
if you really had to live it. Now,
you may begin to have an idea of
what true shyness is all about and
to have compassion for anyone
who suffers from this condition.

Since shyness is now being
recognized as a major social
problem in our society, social
scientists are devoting considerable resources toward identifying
ways to help shy people. New
shyness clinics incorporate
methods of treatment that range
from building social and cognitive
skills to assertiveness training,
techniques to reduce anxiety and
systematic desensitization.

Loneliness

"It is no new thing to be lonely. It comes to all of us sooner or later . . . if we face it, if we remember that there are a million others like us, if we try to reach out to comfort them and not ourselves, we find in the end we are lonely no longer. We are in a new family, the family of man . . ."

Morris L. West,
The Devil's Advocate

Loneliness is caused not by being alone, but by being without close relationships. It is an unpleasant, at times acutely painful, feeling of isolation.

Aloneness, on the other hand, is a state of being that can be growth-producing and desirable. "Being alone" is not the same experience as feeling separated from others; it is not the empty feeling of being lonely. We all need "time out" from others. It is important to include alone time in your busy college schedule.

Loneliness can result from rejection, misunderstanding, separation, illness, or tragedy. Certain personal characteristics increase the level of loneliness a person may experience. These include poor social skills, negative attitudes, low self-esteem, insecurity, and mistrust.

To deal effectively with loneliness, you must first admit to yourself that you are lonely. Then you can try to understand what would help alleviate it. Though loneliness itself may cause stress and anxiety, the anxiety of loneliness increases if you attempt to eliminate it by constantly keeping busy or seeking activity with others. Being out of touch with yourself and your needs only prolongs the pain of loneliness.

If your loneliness stems primarily from a lack of social skills, a number of resources on campus can help you develop those skills. These include social clubs, support groups, self-help campus groups and workshops. You will find recommendations in this chapter on how to deal with insecurity and low self-esteem also apply to alleviating loneliness through increasing positive social interactions. Take the initial step to reach out to someone; this helps you avoid feeling hopeless and powerless. Look for the similarities between you and those around you rather than dwelling on the differences. Loneliness may provide the catalyst to lead you to new and fulfilling relationships and a more complete life.

- Allow yourself time to be alone. Communicate with yourself; enjoy activities you can do alone. This will help you become more comfortable.
- Try meditation or a religious path that is meaningful to you.
- Spend time alone in nature, finding your place in the scheme of things.
- Pay attention to people in your life who seem to value you more than you value yourself—what do they see? Look at yourself this way.
- Watch other people to get ideas on how to change the parts of you with which you are not satisfied. If one approach isn't working, try another. More of the same approach usually just creates more of the same effects.
- Formulate achievements so that they become something you pursue only to the degree that enhances your experience of living.
- Approach projects and goals with the philosophy that you can accomplish what you set out to do—the power of positive thinking takes you more than halfway to achievement.
- Finally, a professional counselor might be helpful for evaluating your alternatives, experiencing yourself in a positive way, and raising your self-esteem so that you really like the person you are.

Mental Fitness

Mental Fine-Tuning

Your body, your mind and your spirit all face significant challenge during college. To meet these challenges with focused, positive energy, you need to be mentally fit. If your body is mildly out of condition, you can take steps on your own to regain physical fitness. On the other hand, if your body is in poor physical condition, you should begin by consulting a physician for guidance about how to improve your physical health without risking greater injury. Similarly, the degree of mental discomfort you may be experiencing determines whether self-help alone can solve your problem or whether you should seek professional guidance.

How's Your Mental State?

You don't think everyone's out to get you, you aren't hearing voices, and you don't believe you're the reincarnation of John Lennon. But are you really healthy? To determine where you are on a mental fitness continuum, answer the questions in the accompanying chart, Are You Going Sane? If you answer yes to most questions, congratulations; you are among the select group that is considered mentally fit. If your answers are not as positive as you would like, you can take action to build a more comfortable mindset. If you answer no more often than yes, this chapter may provide helpful suggestions. You may also want to find a professional counselor with whom you can talk. Often, just talking about the obstacles in your life will help to resolve them.

Because mental fitness is a continuum, understanding a friend's seemingly disturbed behavior (or even your own) may be difficult. The accompanying chart, How To Tell Who Is OK and Who Is Not, gives you some general guidelines about which behaviors may be "normal" or OK, and which may be cause for concern. The behaviors that are labeled "maybe not OK" do not in themselves imply that a person is disturbed or "crazy"; if you suspect or even wonder if certain behavior signals a significant problem, it may be better to get a professional opinion.

Stressors and Mental Discomfort

Stress is frequently a catalyst for both minor and major mental discomfort. The more stressors present in your life, the more your mental fitness is affected. To understand the source of emotional or mental distress in your life, take a look at your lifestyle; notice which parts are working poorly and creating stress for you. The following stress factors can impair your mental state.

Emotional stress—an unhappy relationship with a lover or a roommate; no close friends, especially one who serves as a confidant; poor interactions with family and siblings.

Mental stress—heavy academic demands; work pressure; not enough time for yourself to be alone and quiet; feeling scattered due to many demands on your time.

Are You Going Sane?

Positive answers to the following questions mean you're in pretty good shape mentally. If your answers are more negative than positive, a professional counselor can help you learn how to feel better.

1. Do you have a positive image of yourself and other people? Do you have more happy thoughts than negative ones?
2. Do you wake up each morning feeling good? Are you excited and full of positive anticipation when you think of the day ahead?
3. Do you meet each new task, homework assignment or problem as an opportunity or lesson rather than an obstacle almost impossible to surmount?
4. Do you laugh a lot and maintain your sense of humor even when life gets heavy?
5. Do you rarely feel irritated or express anger toward those around you?
6. Do you take responsibility for who you are and what happens to you rather than placing blame on others or fate?
7. Do you feel grateful for your life circumstances, friends and family, rather than playing the "poor me" role?
8. Are you able to think clearly, complete your homework efficiently, and communicate in a clear, open way?
9. Do you have the energy to complete the day? If you miss a night's sleep, can you continue to function?
10. Do you have goals or a vision of the future that you have every intention of achieving?

How to Tell Who Is OK and Who Is Not

This chart is a quick way to assess behavior, either your own or a friend's. If you recognize yourself or a friend as maybe being not OK, you may choose to talk over your observations with someone.

Probably OK	Maybe Not OK
Tends to be secretive and demands privacy.	Secretive about experiencing severe emotional distress.
Ventilates feelings and concerns to friends.	Has no real friends with whom to communicate these feelings.
Experiences varying degrees of loneliness; may feel loved but not understood.	Suffers profound loneliness; feels total lack of loving; has no meaningful relationships. DANGER OF SUICIDE.
Feels need for friends; very conscious of peer pressure. Usually has at least one person who is loving and supportive (a best friend).	May be friendless; does not socialize well. May act indifferent about making friends. Usually alone or considered a "loner."
Experiences varying degrees of conflict, overt or covert, with family; continues to feel he or she is loved.	Views family as not caring or loving. Family has severe, long-term conflicts that cannot be resolved.
College achievement varies but work does get done. Not immobilized.	Poor school achievement and work seldom gets completed and turned in.
Impulse control varies; usually exercises good judgment and decision-making ability.	Poor impulse control (usually from lack of positive role model). Behavior may include drug or alcohol abuse, even violent or criminal acts.
Self-esteem varies; struggles to find own identity but basically feels OK about self.	Poor self-esteem; extreme difficulty in working out own identity. Cannot use conflicts with family to work out internal struggles.
Develops personal goals; makes plans for the future.	Unable to develop personal goals; feels future will not change things.
May have vague physical ailments that come and go; no long-term symptoms that persist.	May present physical symptoms of chronic stress: frequent headaches, panic attacks, ulcers, constipation.
Usually has few, infrequent, major losses while growing up.	Has suffered many losses (parents, friends, lovers).
Varying levels of depression that are really bouts of sadness or gloom.	Long-standing depression that may show up as withdrawal from others, isolation, hopeless attitudes, or even reckless or acting-out behaviors. DANGER OF SUICIDE.

Mental Illness in the United States

In 1988, more than 40 million people, 9.5 million of them children, suffered from a form of mental illness, including anxiety, depression, schizophrenia, and the effects of drug use.

Mental Fitness

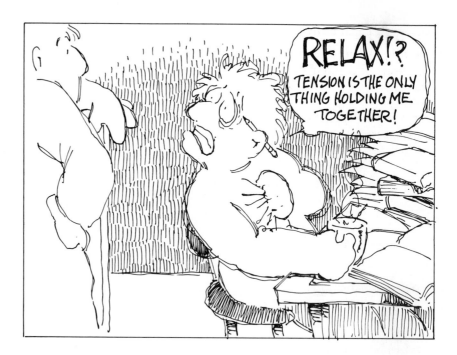

- *Social stress*—no close group of friends; pressure from your social group to act in certain ways that make you uncomfortable; too many social demands and distractions.
- *Environmental stress*—no space of your own, lots of noise and confusion; contaminants, such as smoke in the air.
- *Physical stress*—overdoing or underdoing physical exercise; allotting exceptional time or energy to sports or other activities.
- *Health stress*—inappropriate types or amounts of alcohol or other drugs; too much caffeine, sugar, junk food, highly processed or fast food; not enough water (six to eight glasses a day); and finally, and very important, lack of a nutritionally well-balanced diet, especially without vitamin or mineral supplements to fill in the nutritional gaps.

How You Respond to Mental Distress

When the stresses, choices and changes at college get to be a bit too much, each student has his or her own individual way of responding. You may feel more anxious or confused, sleep less well, eat erratically, or feel alienated from your surroundings. Your mental distress may have physical symptoms. If you frequently experience fatigue, lethargy, headaches, digestive complaints, PMS, or unexplained pain in various parts of your body, don't ignore these patterns. Too often, people ignore or rationalize nonspecific, vague symptoms that are the body's way of telling you that something is not right.

Boosting Mental Fitness

According to Chinese medicine (contemporary Western medicine has a lot to learn from ancient traditions), free energy flow is an essential key to health. Your body has a tremendous capacity for self-regulation. When conditions are right, your body functions perfectly. However, when stress is high and constant, the body moves out of homeostasis, using up its energy reserve. You can take steps to boost your energy and regain and maintain mental fitness.

Practice Good Nutrition   When stress mounts, your body requires more of certain nutrients. A supportive diet includes eating a well-balanced array of foods and eliminating substances that create stress, such as alcohol, caffeine, sugar, and tobacco. Read **Nutrition** for a complete picture of healthy nutrition, including the relationship between stress and nutrition.

Get Plenty of Vigorous Exercise   A sluggish system and toxic build-up drain energy and cause you to feel fatigued and sluggish. Exercise stimu-

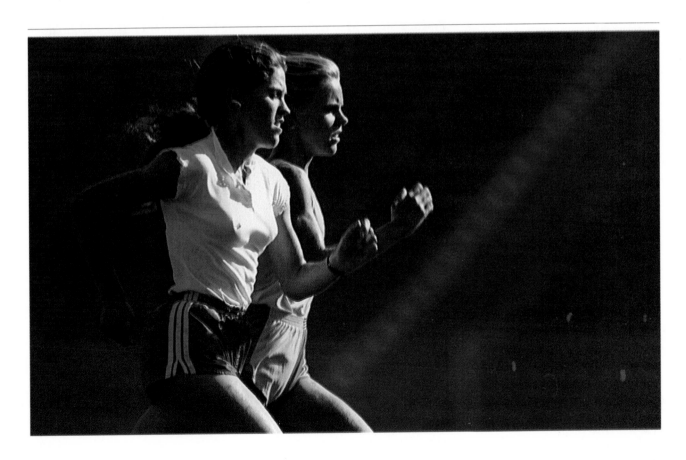

lates lymph and blood flow so nutrients are carried to your cells and toxins are flushed out. It also increases your metabolic rate, which converts calories to energy more efficiently; and with adequate exercise, you will look and feel better. If you are physically tired, you will sleep more soundly and restfully. **Physical Fitness** more fully explains the importance of exercise in your lifestyle.

Get Sound and Adequate Sleep   Frequent poor quality sleep, insomnia or restlessness depletes energy reserves to a dangerous level. If sleep is a problem for you, follow the suggestions in the section on **Sleep Disorders**. Alcohol or sleeping medications are not a solution; they only become another problem.

Determine the Cause of Your Distress   If your mental distress is moderate, not intense, you can often relieve your discomfort and constructively refocus your energy by working directly to reduce the issues that are causing the problem. Talking with someone else is often a good way to get to the root of a problem. Whether you talk with a professional counselor, friend or religious advisor, you'll probably feel better after talking with someone.

Practice Stress Management and Time Management   These techniques are described in earlier chapters.

Time for Professional Involvement

If you try these approaches but still do not feel OK, or if you also experience frequent physical symptoms, such as infections, long-term and painful headaches, recurring insomnia, and faintness, or if you are depressed, feel isolated or have bizarre thoughts, it is time to visit your health practitioner. Though stress may be causing these conditions (you aren't really losing your mind), they are serious. Don't take chances with your health.

   Prevention is the best treatment, but once serious mental problems occur, the best approach is professional help. Your doctor or your health practitioner will refer you to the best resource for help. You have to initiate change. No one will be aware that you need help right now unless you tell them.

Anxiety: The Nameless Fear

The word "anxiety" conjures up many painful pictures for most of us. Maybe you asked someone you liked to go to a movie and he or she turned you down. Maybe you drive miles out of your way to avoid having to cross a certain bridge. To be alive is to be vulnerable to anxiety. This section explains how anxiety can be both constructive and destructive, what its symptoms are, and how to help yourself or someone else deal with anxiety. It includes a discussion of anxiety-related conditions experienced by many college students: generalized anxiety disorder, panic disorder, phobias, and obsessive-compulsive disorder.

Anxiety may be broadly defined as diffuse apprehension that is vague in nature and associated with feelings of uncertainty and helplessness.

Understanding Anxiety

Many of the symptoms of stress are also recognized as symptoms of anxiety. What is the difference between stress and anxiety? Stress is a complex reaction to some potential threat. If you interpret that threat as dangerous or threatening, anxiety develops. Anxiety is measured by the degree of threat, the person's perception of that threat, and the person's reaction to the perceived threat.

Anxiety can be either realistic or unhealthy. For example, you are startled as someone begins to follow you when you are walking from the library to the dorm at night. Your heart pounds, you want to run, you feel afraid. This is normal anxiety. However, if you are standing in line at registration and have those reactions—fear, pounding heart, sweaty palms—and you feel like you are going to faint unless you "get away," this is unhealthy anxiety. You can channel realistic anxiety constructively. To be without anxiety would mean going through life in a stupor and without a necessary warning system for avoiding danger.

Anxiety is different from fear. Fear has a specific source or object that can be identified and described. The degree of fear is proportionate to the degree of real danger. When a person walks down a dark street at night, he may experience fear. This person's apprehension is realistic when one considers the high urban crime rate. A person who experiences anxiety may be afraid of socializing, trying anything new, or taking any risks. The rationale behind the anxiety is vague, diffuse and subjective; it may even be denied. Anxiety and fear do have similarities: physical reactions may feel alike and both may interfere with a person's life and ability to function. Either reaction triggers the release of adrenaline as you prepare to meet the real or imaginary threat.

As the chapter on **Stress** explains, your physiological reactions are preparing you for "fight or flight." Your body reacts the same way to a frightening dream or a close call on the freeway. Some of the most common symptoms of anxiety are feeling tense, jumpy and unable to relax. Your hands may be sweaty, your heart racing, and you find you can't concentrate and fear losing control.

Take a moment now and consider if you have felt any of these symptoms. Ask yourself the following questions.

Mental Fitness

CHAPTER 3

Do I see myself as a nervous person?

Do most things worry or upset me?

Do I worry about failure even though I have never really failed?

Do I daydream frequently?

Do I have frequent physical complaints: headaches, fatigue, vague pains?

Do I react to every event as though it were a life-or-death situation?

Do I keep my fears and feelings to myself?

Do I lack close friends?

Do I get physical exercise infrequently?

Do I have difficulty concentrating?

Do I eat too much or too little when I'm upset?

Do I seldom see myself as a worthwhile person?

Do I see myself as a person who has few rights and can't say "no" to others?

Do I have a secret that I do not want anyone to know?

If you answered yes to more than half the questions, you probably have frequent, chronic feelings of anxiety that affect your school performance and overall satisfaction with life. Everyone experiences periods of anxiety from time to time, but the duration and the intensity of your anxiety is what determines whether it controls you life.

John, a straight-A freshman student, is approaching first semester finals. He is the first person in his family to go to college and everyone is "proud" of his success. Recently, John has experienced irritability, lightheadedness, difficulty concentrating, and bouts of diarrhea. The morning before his first final, John suddenly becomes blind. He nonchalantly calls his roommate, who has an anxiety attack of his own, but who takes John to the student health service. John is immediately hospitalized. After extensive medical testing, the physician concludes that John's blindness is not due to anything physical; rather it is an extreme anxiety reaction to the threat of college examinations and possibility of failure.

John is unconcerned about the blindness and responds, "Well, the one good thing is that I won't have to take the finals this week." John's mind strangely and wondrously has directed all his anxiety into the blindness; therefore, he did not seem observably anxious about his academic problem.

Most students do not have to go this far to avoid the anxiety of examinations. John's case is rare, but all students experience the feelings and physical symptoms of anxiety at one time or another. A recent Wisconsin study found that 65 percent of all panic disorders began between the ages of 15 to 29. Share this with your professor next time you get a particularly challenging term paper assignment or face three midterms on the same day.

Mental Fitness

Causes of Anxiety

Anxiety may stem from many possible sources—genetic, physical, psychological, or drug-induced.

Innate Reactions   Situations arise that human beings seem to innately fear, probably for survival purposes. The most common include fear of snakes, being looked at, heights, or enclosed spaces.

Heredity   Genetic transmission has been documented to play an important role as a cause of anxiety, especially panic attacks. A genetic link may explain why twice as many women as men suffer panic attacks and agoraphobia.

Physical Illness   Disease or illness may lead to severe anxiety symptoms. The illnesses that most commonly have these effects are premenstrual syndrome (PMS), diabetes, thyroid disease, anemias, hypoglycemia, and asthma. If you experience extreme levels of anxiety, it is essential that you have a physical examination and laboratory workup to rule out a physical cause.

Drugs   Many drugs, both illegal and legal, may contribute to anxiety symptoms. Even a small amount of a substance to which you are sensitive can trigger a panic attack. Stimulants (such as amphetamines, cocaine, and caffeine) are the most likely to have such effects.

Traumatic Events   Early life traumas, such as parental abandonment or rejection, may lead to later phobias or panic attacks. Childhood loss sets up a pattern of insecurity and lack of trust that may manifest as a panic attack when a subsequent loss occurs.

Interpersonal Conflicts   People who try to sacrifice their own best interests for the sake of avoiding interpersonal conflict may develop anxiety. Highly anxious people often have low self-esteem, are very critical of themselves, and have unconscious negative beliefs to engender anxiety.

Threats to the Self System   When expectations are not met, and needs for status, prestige and being special are not fulfilled, an anxiety attack may occur.

Anxiety Disorders

Jill, a 22-year-old graduate student, came to the student health center after hearing a lecture on panic disorders. She recognized herself in the symptoms the professor was describing. Jill complained of recurrent episodes of lightheadedness, heart palpitations, upset stomach, and occasionally feeling unreal. Although these feelings

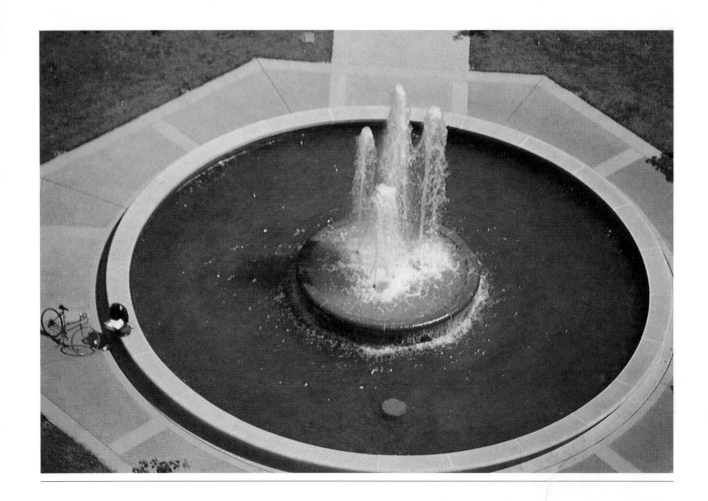

were intense, Jill managed to "wait them out" by isolating herself. At times she felt she was going crazy and, therefore, did not want anyone to know. Her attacks sometimes happened many times a week, often occurring several times a day. The frequency and uncertainty of onset caused Jill to become chronically tense, restless and unable to concentrate. She began to think about dropping out of school. Her medical workup was negative and Jill was given a tentative diagnosis of panic disorder. Through medication and behavioral therapy, Jill experienced a dramatic decrease in her symptoms and was able to continue in school.

Most college students cope fairly well with the pressure of everyday college living. They adapt in a constructive way—changing habits, behaviors and attitudes. These students grow and change to accommodate to their new environment and experiences. However, some students become overwhelmed and develop painful symptoms of anxiety disorders.

Mental Fitness

CHAPTER 3

58

Generalized Anxiety Disorder

This condition, also called free-floating anxiety, is characterized by persistent and chronic unrealistic worry. This disorder is most commonly seen in late adolescence and early adulthood. An individual lives in a constant state of tension and diffuse uneasiness. He or she is overly sensitive to interpersonal relationships and frequently feels inadequate and depressed. Symptoms include

- Trembling, shaking
- Muscle tension
- Fatigue
- "Keyed up," on edge
- Difficulty sleeping
- Difficulty concentrating
- Moodiness/irritability
- Shortness of breath
- Repeated anxious dreams (such as falling from high places)
- Excessive use of tranquilizers, sleeping pills and alcohol to decrease the painful symptoms
- Rapid pulse
- Sweaty hands
- Dry mouth
- Lightheadedness
- Nausea, diarrhea
- Hot flashes or chills
- Frequent urination
- Difficulty swallowing
- Gloomy outlook

Any of these symptoms may be triggered by an event you perceive as threatening. For some students, an impending blind date might initiate feelings of inadequacy or rejection that trigger an anxiety attack. Many people with generalized anxiety have a particular "fantasy of harm" that causes increased anxiety whenever they encounter that specific stimulus.

When should you seek professional help? When anxiety increases, especially if it becomes immobilizing, it is time to seek professional assistance.

Panic Disorder

This is broadly defined as a chronic condition manifested by attacks of high-level acute anxiety, usually occurring in the absence of fear-provoking situations. Panic attacks are linked not only to psychological factors, such as stress and low self-esteem, but also to biological factors. Research also shows that body chemistry changes can result in panic attacks.

Panic disorders tend to run in families, may be inherited, and occur more in college-age females than in the general population. Two to five percent of the population suffer from panic attacks, women twice as often as men.

Dr. Rifkin of the Mt. Sinai Medical Center in New York City states that one quarter to one half of panic disorder patients have a cardiac abnormality called mitral valve prolapse. The heart valve fails to close properly and palpitations occur, triggering a panic attack. Yale University psychiatrists found panic victims are far more sensitive to caffeine than healthy subjects. Caffeine produced panic-like symptoms in 71 percent of study participants with panic disorders.

A panic attack usually begins suddenly, sometimes in public and sometimes in private. The person experiences an intense fear, dread or foreboding; common feelings experienced are a sense of unreality or fear of dying, going crazy or having a heart attack. Specific phobias, such as agoraphobia (discussed a little later in this section), may trigger panic attacks. As fear builds, physical symptoms of severe anxiety that may appear are

- Dizziness
- Chest pain
- Palpitations
- Hyperventilation

Attacks can vary in intensity, frequency and duration. Occurring from once a week to several times a day, they may last from several minutes to several hours. Because of the intensity of the symptoms, people who experience panic attacks usually seek medical attention. Even if you experience only a mild panic attack, seek professional help. Without help, panic attacks may increase in intensity or frequency and become debilitating.

Phobias

A phobia is a persistent fear of some specific object or situation that presents no actual danger to the person. The danger is magnified out of proportion to the actual situation. The individual perceives the situation as a threat to survival and experiences high levels of anxiety, perhaps even a panic attack if escape from the situation is impossible. Phobias are divided into three areas: agoraphobia, simple phobia and social phobia.

Agoraphobia is the fear of being in places or situations from which escape would be physically impossible or help unavailable. It is frequently a complication of panic disorder. Agoraphobia is derived from the Greek word agora, or "meeting place." Many agoraphobics are fearful of open places, shopping malls, concerts, and so forth. Whenever the person is exposed to that environment, he or she may experience an intense fear reaction. Agoraphobia accounts for two-thirds of panic sufferers.

Simple phobias are irrational, exaggerated fear of those things that many of us fear, including snakes, heights, fires, spiders, and darkness. These reactions can vary from mild to extreme; for example, quitting college because you found a spider in the shower is an irrationally extreme reaction to fear.

Social phobia is manifested by a fear of exposure to focused scrutiny by others and/or the fear that you might do something to embarrass or humiliate yourself. Stage fright is the most common example of this condition. Social phobia is easily treated and the outcome is generally very good. Most of us live with our phobias and they don't disrupt our lives. If, however, the phobia begins to take over your life and interferes with functioning, seek professional help.

Obsessive-Compulsive Disorder

Obsession means a persistent thought, feeling or idea; compulsion is an impulse experienced as irresistible. A person with an obsessive-compulsive disorder feels compelled to think about something they do not want to think about or carry out some action against their will. The obsessive thoughts are unpleasant and create anxiety. The person defuses this anxiety by performing particular repetitive actions. Most of us have experienced a persistent thought about an assignment, romantic interest or song. Have you ever worried about an important appointment and awakened several times during the night to check the clock? As a child, you probably played "step on a crack, break your mother's back." This is a minor form of obsessive-compulsive behavior.

As an obsession builds, a person develops ritualistic behavior patterns. He or she may have to walk around the campus three times before a test, always wear the same clothes, and use the same No. 2 pencil. If anything interferes with this process, the person becomes agitated, anxious and is unable to continue until completing the ritual. The person may be considered excessively perfectionistic.

Mild compulsive behavior is common for many people. As long as the behavior is not extreme, injurious to your health, or overpowering, you may choose to live with the compulsive ritual. However, if it begins to take over your life and interfere with daily functioning, seek professional help.

Test Anxiety

Many college students experience some test anxiety. When you have test anxiety, you may have nightmares about a test, draw a blank on the first few questions, or develop the symptoms of moderate anxiety. The **Stress** chapter discusses test anxiety in detail. If the level of your test anxiety significantly interferes with your academic performance, sleeping patterns or other parts of your life, contact the counseling center at your college. Most colleges have effective short-term programs for test anxiety.

Coping with Anxiety

"An ounce of prevention is worth a pound of cure." This is especially true in coping with anxiety. The **Stress** chapter includes several important approaches to lowering your overall stress level at college. These techniques

---

The Lemon Test of Inner Power

If you have trouble feeling inner authority, try visualization. Visualizing is imaging or fantasizing. Your mind does not distinguish between fantasy and reality. To test the idea, try this:

Close your eyes and imagine (or visualize) a lemon. See its color and shape and texture. Now imagine yourself slicing into the lemon—smell the juice as it squirts out from your knife; listen to the "skwitch" sound as the knife cuts though; try to involve all your senses. Now, pick up half the lemon, bring it to your mouth and take a big bite. Can you feel your mouth puckering and your saliva accumulating in expectation?

Yet it is just an imaginary lemon, and you've not taken a bite—you've only visualized it. But, your brain doesn't know the difference! This power of visualization can be applied to any skill, goal or desire. Make your visualization as vivid as possible and repeat it until it becomes reality for you.

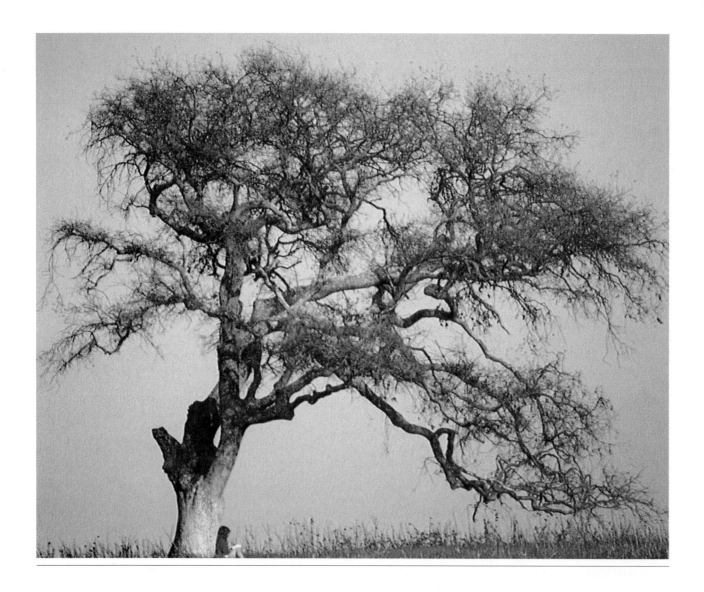

will also help decrease your anxiety level as well as improve the feeling of control over yourself and your situation. These methods include

- Control of the environment
- Physical exercise
- Relaxation methods
- Balanced diet
- Positive attitude
- Humor
- Music
- Calming colors and mood

Mental Fitness

CHAPTER 3

If you have high or uncomfortable levels of anxiety, you will need to take additional steps to relieve your discomfort. The following are suggestions for accomplishing this.

- Immediately remove yourself from the anxiety-provoking situation, at least temporarily. Forcing yourself to stay and "tough it out" while the anxiety level builds only tends to reinforce the anxiety. Leave, calm down and then return. If the situation continues, seek professional advice.
- Reach out! When you begin to feel immobilized, seek the help of a friend or classmate. Many people deny or feel embarrassed by their feelings. Other people want to help you; it is your reluctance that prevents you from reaching out. If you cannot talk to a friend, go to the student health center and talk with a professional. If you are acutely anxious, call a crisis phone number. Remaining alone only tends to reinforce the fear and anxiety and the idea that you are abnormal or crazy.
- Seek professional help. The prognosis for anxiety-related problems is very good. There is no need to suffer. The first step is to have a thorough physical examination and explain your symptoms honestly to a health professional. You are not crazy, but maybe you do need help. Several professional counseling methods are effective for treating anxiety problems.

General Psychotherapy   The purpose of psychotherapy is to alter your perception of a threat by exploring your thoughts, feelings and experiences to determine the underlying cause of the anxiety. Emphasis is on the relationship between the therapist and the client. Therapy is usually long-term, and choosing a therapist who is right for you is important. If you feel comfortable with the therapist and get some immediate relief from your symptoms, you know you are on the right track. The goal of psychotherapy is to give you insight into your feelings and how these feelings contribute to the present problems.

Rational-Emotive Therapy   The goal of rational-emotive therapy (RET) is to convince you that your unhealthy anxiety is caused by faulty perceptions or irrational beliefs about the stressor. The following is an example of irrational thoughts.

Facts and events—you receive a failing grade on your first English exam.

Irrational self-talk—"I knew I'd never make it in college." "I ought to have taken something easier." "English was always my weak subject." "I'm just a failure."

Emotion—anxiety, resentment, anger, depression.

The therapist assists the person to deal with the feeling that, yes—getting a low grade is unfortunate, but it is not the end of the world. The therapist helps you explore realistic ways of dealing with your emotions.

> **Angels can fly because they take themselves lightly.**
>
> **Jean Cocteau**

Irrational Ideas

Irrational beliefs may add stress to already stressful situations, leading in turn to anxiety. Albert Ellis, the developer of rational-emotive therapy, suggests several basic irrational ideas that may have this effect and are listed below. If many of these opinions seem to reflect your point of view, you may benefit from talking with a counselor about these issues.

1. It is an absolute necessity for an adult to have love and approval from peers, family and friends.
2. You must be unfailingly competitive and almost perfect in all you undertake.
3. Certain people are evil, wicked and villainous, and should be punished.
4. It is horrible when people and things are not the way you would like them to be.
5. External events cause most human misery—people simply react as the event triggers their emotions.
6. You should feel fear or anxiety about anything that is unknown, uncertain or potentially dangerous.
7. It is easier to avoid than face life difficulties and responsibilities.
8. You need something other or stronger or greater than yourself to rely on.
9. The past has a lot to do with determining the present.
10. Happiness can be achieved by inaction, passivity and endless leisure.
11. It is bad or wrong to be selfish.
12. Your worth as a person depends on how much you achieve and produce.
13. If you don't go to great lengths to please others, they will abandon or reject you.
14. When people disapprove of you, it invariably means you are wrong or bad.
15. There is a perfect love and a perfect relationship.

At the root of all irrational thinking is the assumption that things are done to you; the RET therapist will help you recognize that events happen in the world and it is how you react to them that creates positive or negative emotions.

Cognitive-Behavioral Therapy Most of the variations of behavior therapy have a common goal: reduction of anxiety by exposure to the fear-inducing situation. Systematic desensitization is one type of therapy for which the person is taught deep relaxation and then asked to visualize the phobic/feared object or situation. Joseph Wolpe, a phobia expert, identifies the following steps to this approach.

1. Identify the fear-inducing stressors.
2. Grade them from the least fearful to the most fearful.
3. Imagine least fearful situation.
4. Combine the visualization with a pleasant experience—muscle relaxation.
5. As you visualize mildly anxiety-provoking situations, upgrade to visualizing the next most anxiety-producing situation, and so on.
6. Actually encounter the situation or object that you want to handle differently with the support of the therapist. (For example, go to a party to meet new people.)

This approach is very effective but it takes time and a great deal of involvement by the therapist. The person also needs to be motivated enough to practice between sessions.

Mental Fitness

Medication Therapy   Drugs prescribed for anxiety are called "minor tranquilizers"; they include Librium, Valium and Xanax. These drugs clearly help anxiety, though they do have undesirable side effects, including drowsiness, dry mouth, loss of effectiveness after several weeks, and probable drug dependency. Drugs help but rarely cure anxiety problems. Long-term usage should be monitored carefully by a physician, because these drugs may cause serious medical problems, such as seizures, if stopped suddenly. It is vital to remember that drugs may control the anxiety but they do not eliminate the cause. Two other drugs, Tofranil and Nardil, are prescribed for panic attacks and agoraphobia.

Group Therapy   This involves a goal-directed meeting of seven to ten people with similar problems which is led by one to two professionals. The purpose of the group is to support you, give you a safe environment in which to explore thoughts, feelings and experiences, get group feedback, and practice new reactions to identified problems. Support, interaction and feedback among group members is the key for a successful group. The advantage of groups is that you meet individuals who have problems similar to your own, and the support helps you feel less isolated. Groups are also less expensive than individual therapy. However, these sessions do not always give you enough personal time.

Self-Help Groups   Many communities and colleges have self-help groups organized by individuals who are dealing with their own anxiety. Agoraphobia groups have sprung up all over the country and have been highly successful in giving support and suggestions on how individual members have dealt or are dealing with their problem. A self-help group does not have a professional leader but is led by a member with leadership skills. These groups help people help themselves. The emphasis is on positive behaviors, empathy and building self-esteem.

Assertiveness Training Groups   Lack of assertiveness may be one of the problems underlying serious levels of anxiety. Assertiveness training classes assist you to identify your own personal human rights, to learn to identify your own needs and wants, how to get what you want without guilt, to learn to say no, and to express uncomfortable feelings, such as anger, in a constructive way. Most college campuses have assertiveness training classes. The classes are set up in a nonthreatening way and teach specific techniques and methods for behaving assertively. Even if you don't have a problem with anxiety, this training is extremely helpful in dealing with life situations and relationships.

   Although anxiety is painful, even overwhelming at times, it can be controlled. The message is to ask for help. Our vignette characters, Jill and John, can lead productive lives through varying methods of anxiety intervention. There is no reason to suffer. Help and support are available. You are not alone. Tremendous strides have been made in both the physiological and biological treatment of anxiety.

Seeking Professional Help

- If your low self-esteem leads you to depression or thoughts of suicide.
- If your sense of failure in a relationship influences other aspects of your life so that you begin to see yourself as a failure in everything.
- If your degree of shyness prevents you from making friends and you feel isolated from virtually everyone else.
- Stress is increasing in your life and you realize your coping mechanisms are not working adequately to control the stress.
- You are feeling isolated, even alienated, from mainstream college life.
- You read every assignment three times and don't know what you have read; you spend hours staring at your books and do not internalize or understand the assignments.
- You have recently developed many nonspecific, vague physical symptoms that do not seem to be related to a specific physical cause.
- Your feelings of anxiety are out of control—where they would decrease in a short time, now they are constantly present in your life and greatly interfere with your ability to function.

Beyond the Text

1. Your friend claims to suffer from test anxiety whenever faced with a midterm or final exam. What advice would you give?

2. Some people find and discuss the negative aspects of every situation and event. What does this say about their approach to life?

3. Your best friend feels no one really likes her and that she is dull and unattractive. How can you help?

4. Applicants for college admission undergo rigorous academic screening including SATs, high school grades, and teacher recommendations. Should candidates be required to undergo psychological testing as well? Why?

5. You suddenly develop frequent headaches, but the doctor finds no physical cause. What could be going on?

6. Respond to the following statement: College students are too young to experience a true panic attack.

7. Respond to the following statement: Stress and anxiety are the same thing.

Supplemental Readings

Life Without Fear: Anxiety and Its Cure by Joseph Wolpe, MD. New York: New Harbinger, 1988. How to control your anxiety reactions through a "systematic desensitization" program.

Mind Power: Getting What You Want Through Mental Training by Bernie Zilbergeld, PhD, and Arnold A. Lazarus, PhD. Boston: Little, Brown and Company, 1987. A step-by-step guide that will give you the tools of mental training—very useful.

One Minute for Myself by Spencer Johnson, MD. New York: William Morrow, 1985. One minute several times a day, according to the author, is enough for you to assess how you are doing. This helpful book will enable you to find better methods of taking care of yourself and raising your self-esteem.

Panic—Facing Fears, Phobias, and Anxiety by Stewart Aggras, MD. New York: W. H. Freeman and Co., 1985. An easy-to-understand book about the causes and cures for fears and phobias. Emphasizes drug-free approach.

Rapid Relief from Emotional Distress by Gary Emery, PhD, and James Campbell, PhD. New York: Fawcett, 1986. Written for the lay reader by two experts in the field of cognitive therapy; includes quick practical ways to overcome anxiety.

The Healing Heart. Antidotes to Panic and Helplessness by Norman Cousins. New York: W.W. Norton and Co., 1983. The author shares his experiences of recovering from a massive heart attack as well as his strategies for summoning the regenerative processes needed to overcome illness and reduce panic.

Key Terms Defined

agoraphobia fear of crowds or open spaces

anxiety troubled or apprehensive feeling; experiencing a sense of dread or fear

compulsion irresistible urge to repeat an act that must be carried out to avoid anxiety

hypnotic agent that induces sleep

obsession persistent, repetitive unwanted thought

obsessive-compulsive disorder compulsion to repetitively perform certain acts and rituals, thereby relieving anxiety

panic attack unexpected, unprovoked, emotionally intense experiences of extreme fear and terror

phobia persistent, irrational fear of a specific situation or object

premenstrual syndrome (PMS) disorder occurring prior to a woman's menstrual cycle; stimulated by neuro-endocrine factors and causing physical discomfort and psychological distress

psychotherapy any of a number of related techniques for treating mental illness by psychological methods

self-esteem sense of pride in oneself, or self-love

tranquilizers drugs that act to reduce tension and anxiety

Emotional Disorders

Emotional disorders are quite common in our society. They are prevalent in all age groups, cross all socio-economic levels, and affect all races. These illnesses are debilitating and potentially life-threatening. It is important to be able to recognize symptoms of an emotional problem in yourself, a friend, or a family member. Professional intervention could make a difference between recovery or a long-term psychological disability.

Everyone feels down sometimes, and college students are no exception. Because you face so many stressors, you may be at risk for a serious negative state of mind, including depression, thoughts of suicide, or losing touch with reality. If you experience depression, this chapter may help you explore your feelings, identify when such feelings pose a danger, and help yourself (or a friend) feel better. The major emotional disorders—depression, manic behavior, and schizophrenia—are described in this chapter.

Contents

Key Terms

Aberrant behavior
Delusions
Depression
Hallucination
Lithium
Manic behavior

Manic-depressive illness
Paranoia
Psychosis
Schizophrenia
Suicide
Tangential speech

Depression Can Be Healthy

Dr. M. Scott Peck in his book *The Road Less Traveled*, asks you to view depression as a healthy phenomenon, especially if you have recently left home and are on your own for the first time. He suggests that any period of intense growth involves giving up parts of "the Old Self." Feelings associated with this letting go of some part of yourself may indeed be feelings of depression. In this view, depression is a healthy process of growth and letting go. The problem, however, is that you may only be aware of the process—just the feelings of depression. For instance, you may be depressed that your parents let you down, but also be in the process of taking responsibility for your own emotional well-being. Or, you may be feeling depressed about breaking up with your romantic partner but also be in the process of learning more about the type of person with whom you really fit.

Feeling Depressed

"I don't know if it is worth it—life I mean. Every day I can barely get out of bed. I'm not interested in my classes, and I don't really have any fun anymore. Just more of the same. Oh, I have a couple of so-so friends, but they aren't really interested in me. I feel lonely most of the time. College sure isn't what I thought it would be. I feel sort of down all the time, and I can't see that it is ever going to change."

Depression is a fact of life on college campuses and in the young adult population in general. Young adults often express alienation from society, friends and family; they feel overwhelmed by hopelessness; they see themselves as unloved, unwanted and lonely. Two thirds of those who attempt suicide are suffering from depression. If you are experiencing feelings like this, you also may be thinking about suicide. Even if you don't really want to end your life, you may be thinking of suicide as the only way to get rid of your pain. If you are feeling depressed, perhaps just reading about depression, what leads up to depression, its danger, and ways to relieve depression may encourage you to seek help.

At Risk for Depression at College

Life stress in college sometimes precipitates depression. Studies have found three psychosocial factors significantly related to depression: a family history of members who have experienced severe psychiatric illness; ongoing stressful life events, and a lack of social support. These risks show up in special ways among college students. You may not have any friends or confidants with whom you feel close. You may have to continually juggle academics, social life, and financial obligations.

Even with such stresses, you may have sufficient skills to maintain a fairly positive attitude. But stress can be cumulative. You might change residences, switch roommates, break up with a romantic partner, or face an unexpectedly heavy course load. Adding this new stress to your already burdened life could increase your stress to the point where the coping behaviors that once worked for you no longer are adequate—and depression results.

Just being at college can increase your risk for depression. College is a time of new beginnings as an independent adult directing your own life, and a time of completing childhood dependency on your parents. You are moving from the known to the unknown. You may find such shifts both exhilarating and frightening.

Away from home and separated from the security of loved ones, you may feel more alone and isolated than ever before. With change comes anxiety, and with anxiety comes fear of loss of control. You may not yet have developed appropriate coping skills for your new roles and social situations. When you feel unable to cope, you may experience depression and even entertain ideas of death as a solution.

Emotional Disorders

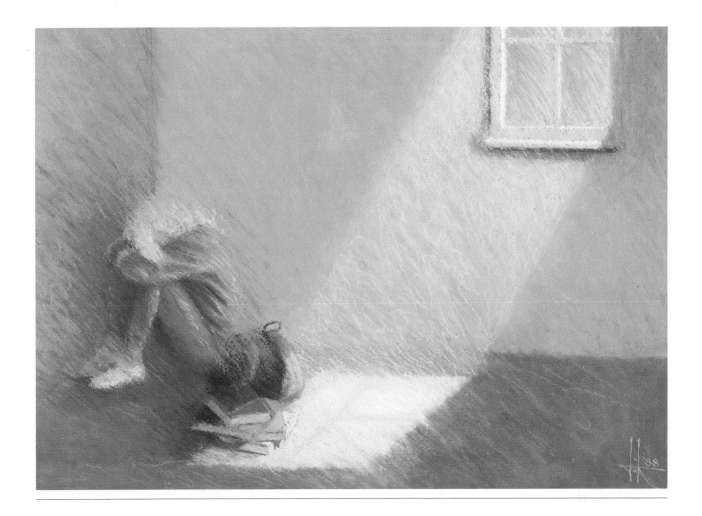

What Causes Depression

True depression is a deeply painful experience; one that envelops your total existence—physical, emotional and social. You may experience acute depression, which has a rapid onset and intense emotional pain that lasts a few days to weeks. Or you may feel chronic depression, a gradual sense of being immobilized, with limited response patterns and a pervasive gloomy attitude about yourself and life in general.

Depression may stem from a chemical imbalance, physical causes, emotional problems, stress, or an unrecognized source. Depression may relate to a particular life experience, or it may start as a general feeling of sadness. Sad feelings are frequently related to a sense of loss. This can be loss of a relationship, loss of confidence in yourself, or even loss of self-esteem. You may feel sad without recognizing a source for that feeling.

Depression is on one end of the continuum. At the other end is an affective disorder called mania. This illness involves mood swings of elation, euphoria and grandiose behavior. A mild form of mania is expressed by increased motor activity, little sleep, rapid thoughts, confidence, and noninhibition. Those who experience this disorder usually like the euphoria, happy feelings and fast pace. While it may appear to be fun, manic behavior usually evolves into a dangerous state. Exhaustion from extreme hyperactivity, flight of ideas, poor judgment, and distractability are common symptoms. Professional help is imperative before delirium, delusions and disorientation occur and physical health is impaired.

Manic episodes, or swings from depression to mania, can now be controlled with a miracle drug, lithium. A natural metallic salt, lithium has a dramatic effect on one's mood. It restores the chemical balance and brings behavior back into normal range. Individuals taking lithium need to be aware of guidelines for safe drug use: adequate fluid and salt intake to maintain a therapeutic lithium level in the blood; restriction of exercise for long periods in the heat or sun—increased fluid loss may bring lithium level to toxic range; and caution regarding use of other drugs including alcohol because the synergistic effect may be dangerous. Good judgment enables a person on lithium to live a normal lifestyle without extreme variations in mood swings or behavior.

Lithium can be toxic, so anyone taking it must consistently have blood levels of the drug measured at a laboratory. When the blood level exceeds a certain range, symptoms of nausea, vomiting, drowsiness, tremors, and slurred speech indicate toxicity. Since the central nervous system is the primary target, it is dangerous to continue the drug. Toxic symptoms indicate that medical treatment is critical. If you suffer from manic disorder and are taking lithium, pay attention to how your body feels, and at the first sign of drug toxicity, seek professional help.

Depression may be your reaction to accumulated stressors. Perhaps you have been having trouble with your grades (academic stressors), you can't seem to keep friends and your romantic life is non-existent or falling apart (emotional stressors), or you feel tired all the time, lacking the "get up and go" you used to have (physical stressors). Put all these stressors together, and the result may be depression.

Are You Sad or Are You Depressed?

People often confuse depression with transient sadness or unhappiness. "Down" feelings like gloom, hopelessness and discontent characterize depression. When you experience sadness, such feelings are of short duration; they do not totally take over your personality or affect all your perceptions, actions and behavior. Sadness usually stems from specific feelings of loss, such as loss of self-esteem, a relationship, or even losing a special object.

If a pervasive pain that permeates your whole being accompanies your feelings of sadness, and your life seems to take more effort than feels worthwhile, this sadness is labeled depression. In this state, your coping abilities are not meeting your emotional needs. Unless you help yourself

Emotional Disorders

Symptoms of Depression

Symptoms you may recognize as depression:

- You don't feel pleasure in anything—you don't enjoy doing the things you used to do.
- You don't have the energy to complete tasks, do your homework, dress well, or get involved in any activities.
- You frequently cry or have crying jags for no real reason.
- You don't feel good about yourself and often don't even like yourself.
- You feel isolated or apart from others, both physically and emotionally. You are very lonely.
- You feel unloved and unwanted by your friends and even your family.

You may also be depressed and not realize it if you experience many of these symptoms:

- You are irritable most of the time.
- You have trouble sleeping and wake up unrested.
- You have difficulty concentrating and your mind often wanders—nowhere.
- You feel an underlying anxiety.
- You have no appetite and get no enjoyment from eating—even the pizza and other snacks you used to love.
- You have other physical complaints like stomachaches and constipation.

If you are experiencing a combination of any of these symptoms and they have lasted for two weeks or more, ask for professional help. You may be experiencing depression; get help now before the depression increases and becomes dangerous.

or get help, you move deeper and deeper into depression and despair. Despair is the feeling that it is never going to change—never get better. To figure out whether you are experiencing depression, see the accompanying box on symptoms of depression.

Costs of Depression

The greatest cost of depression is suicide—loss of life is irreversible. With suicide, you give up your chance to enjoy anything that life has to offer. Even without suicide, depression has costs because depression distorts all your feelings, perceptions and interactions; it takes away from your potential for positive experiences. In the reinforcing negative cycle of depression, you feel bad so you avoid or relate poorly with other people and activities, and thus cut yourself off even more from any possible comfort and joy. To minimize strained relationships and missed opportunities, you must break this downward spiral as soon as possible.

One college student who was very depressed said to herself, "Well, I can always choose to kill myself; I might as well try talking to someone and see if it helps at all." It did, and this young woman went on to write about how helpful a counselor can be. She says to others, "Try talking to a counselor first, and perhaps you will begin to feel better as I did."

Depression is often the source of various physical complaints, such as stomachaches, constipation, headaches, and, of course, persistent fatigue, lethargy and very low energy or enthusiasm.

How to Relieve Depression

Depression is not a "forever" state. Over time it gets better, or it gets worse. Depending on what you do once you realize you're depressed, you could feel worse or better. You'll never feel better through thoughts of suicide, ignoring your feelings, or alcohol. Depending on the severity of your depression, you can feel better on your own or through talking with a counselor. Many times, depression improves only, or more thoroughly, through professional intervention.

Self-Help Measures *If* you're feeling down but can still carry on daily activities, and *if* you've been feeling this way for only a short time, you may be able to lift your depression through your own actions. See how you feel after trying these suggestions:

- Get proper sleep.
- Avoid alcohol and other drugs (if you need help with this, get professional counseling).
- Pay attention to eating a well-balanced and adequate diet. Particularly, avoid sugar and emphasize complex carbohydrates and fresh fruits and vegetables. Consider vitamin and mineral supplements.
- Increase your frequency of vigorous physical exercise. Such workouts release endorphins, brain chemicals that make you feel better.
- Simplify your life through stress management and time management. Use relaxation techniques such as meditation and extra time outdoors.
- Try to become aware of what is really bothering you, and work to resolve that issue directly. If what's upsetting you involves another person, consider that you cannot change someone else—only yourself and your attitudes.
- Find someone you can really talk to about your feelings—a therapist, counselor, minister or rabbi, or friend. Don't just complain. Try to brainstorm ideas for how you can get your life back on a more positive track.

Professional Assistance If you decide that you are truly depressed—if your down feelings envelop your life or if gradually over a period of weeks you have been feeling down, hopeless, useless—then this is the time to find professional assistance. Many who have come out of a depressive episode wonder how they got so turned off on life. Looking back, they wonder why they didn't seek help sooner. A recent study noted that even though many college students experience depression severe enough to justify professional help, few of them seek assistance. You may be hesitant to seek help. Somehow, admitting that you aren't able to cope with life right now is really difficult. But do you really want to continue to feel so terrible?

Talking to a Friend Who Is Depressed

Showing that you care by taking the time to talk to a depressed friend is really important. This kind of conversation can be uncomfortable and draining for you, especially if you feel uneasy talking about feelings. Here are some general interventions that may make your job of being a friend easier.

- Allow your friend to really express feelings. Don't cut him or her off or try to minimize the depth of the feeling. Just be there, in word and body language, so that your friend feels safe to talk. You may be providing a psychological lifeline.

- Acknowledge your friend's distress. Perhaps this validation of how terrible and painful life is will help your friend avoid making the point by trying to kill himself or herself.
- Reinforce positive thinking or responses. If your friend mentions any positive thought or action, talk about it. Any hopeful thought is the beginning of a positive trend in thinking.
- Don't play amateur psychiatrist. For example, don't reflect back what your friend says or why he feels this way. Just being present and really listening is enough. If possible, discuss the reality of the problem and possible solutions.

- One of the most effective and therapeutic actions on your part would be to suggest that you and your friend do something. Help change the pattern of immobilization and get your friend moving. Go to dinner or the movies; better yet, exercise or get outside. Any physical action will help lift the depression.
- Don't become depressed yourself. You can only do what you can do—set limits on your own time and energy, then seek outside assistance.

Don't expect people—either a counselor or your friends—to read your mind. If you can just tell a health counselor that you need to talk with someone about feeling depressed, you have taken a great first step toward feeling better. If you don't feel comfortable going to the health service, tell a friend, teacher, your RA, or anyone you feel close to—tell someone. Feelings of depression are not to be minimized—they can lead you directly to considering suicide as an option. Please find someone to talk to before this happens.

When you contact your health service, they can help you find a skilled professional who will determine the appropriate method of treatment for you. A physical exam may help determine whether some underlying ill-

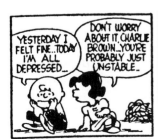 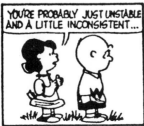 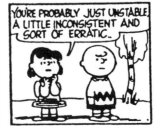 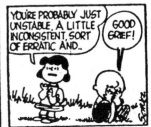

You can view depression as an exaggeration of your negative attitudes. Allowing a negative thought ("Nobody loves me" or "I'll never be successful") to run through your mind again and again can result in a depressed mood. To lift this depression:

- Recognize your negative thought.
- Choose to give it up.
- Focus on a positive thought.
- Experience your mood lifting.
- Repeat these steps as often as necessary until the negative thought fades.

ness or other imbalance has caused or been contributing to your depression. If no physical cause is found, treatment may include psychological counseling, medication or (more likely) both. Sometimes a short counseling intervention is all that is required. Give a few sessions a try; if you click with the counselor, great. If not, visit another counselor. Keep trying until you find someone who really understands you and facilitates insight you can relate to.

In addition to talking with someone, you may be given one of a variety of prescription drugs that really do help many people feel better. These "mood elevators" do just that—lift your mood. These medications can make a tremendous difference in how you view life. You won't have to be on medication forever—just for a period of time until the depression passes. However, avoid taking medication (including alcohol or other drugs) without medical supervision. Such substances change your body and mind chemistry; these changes can be particularly dangerous if you are already depressed.

Your treatment plan may also include supplements to correct vitamin or mineral deficiencies, dietary and exercise plans, and stress management training.

Considering Suicide

One of the most difficult subjects to talk about is suicide. Suicide is a deliberate action to take one's life. It is the seventh most common cause of death in the United States today and the second highest cause of death among college-age adults. These statistics are probably low, because many suicides may be disguised; for example, some car "accidents" are actually suicides. For every successful suicide, five to ten people attempt to take their life. As this indicates, the potential for committing suicide is approaching staggering proportions.

Contributing Factors

Several factors can contribute to a person's thoughts of suicide. The single most common cause of suicide is depression, which has just been discussed. Alcohol abuse and dependence is the second most common contributing factor. Since alcohol problems are reaching epidemic proportions on college campuses today, this issue is of particular concern. Other drugs besides alcohol may also play a role in suicide, particularly other depressants (tranquilizers, barbiturates), PCP and hallucinogens. The **Alcohol and Other Drugs** chapter gives information on how to recognize and treat problems relating to these substances. If you are depressed, or drink or do drugs a lot and feel depressed before or after drinking or doing drugs, walk to your health service, ask to speak with a counselor, and tell them what's going on in your life. Be specific and direct so they really get the picture.

A third factor is the feeling of being overwhelmed or in a crisis. You always had A's in high school, often without really working very hard; now you're competing with hundreds of classmates, most of whom were also A students in high school, and you're ashamed to tell your parents that you're not at the top of your class any more. You were popular in high school and had lots of friends; in college, finding compatible people, who feel the way you do and like the same activities you do, doesn't seem so easy. You worry about dates—getting them and how to act on them. You feel lonely a lot of the time or unlovable or unworthy. Maybe money is a major stressor—in high school, you could hold a job without much strain, but now trying to keep up with work as well as your academic load seems like too much pressure. And if your friends have more money than you do, you may feel deprived a lot of the time. These feelings are important, and you do need to handle them, but coping on your own can be difficult. If you have feelings of heavy depression or being overwhelmed by life and are considering suicide as a solution, find a professional counselor to talk with.

The fourth cause of suicide is using suicide-oriented expressions and actions in an attempt to psychologically manipulate someone else. For example, your ex-lover may say, "If you don't marry me, I'll kill myself." The intent of such individuals is to get their own way, not to actually kill themselves, but sometimes they miscalculate and wind up dead.

Facts about Suicide in College

Every year, 100,000 young people in the United States between the ages of 15 and 24 attempt suicide; over 5,000 actually succeed. Of these, 1,000 are college students. Statistics show that the greatest increase in suicide attempts in recent years has been in this young adult age group.

Approximately three times as many females as males make attempts at suicide, but more males succeed. This trend seems to be changing; more females are completing their suicide attempts than in the past. These statistics cannot begin to tell the story of the disastrous loss these deaths and attempted deaths take.

Contemplating Suicide

Death imaging is not unusual when a person experiences intense change and moves through a transitional period in life. College can be a time of questioning. "What is the real meaning of life?" "Why am I here?" "Why did I make it into this college but not the one I most wanted to go to?" "Is this all there is to life?" "Will things really change?" Such questions can initiate an attitude of ambivalence about life.

This contemplation of the meaning of life can help you begin a journey of self-discovery. This journey could lead to affirming that you are a valuable, worthy and important "self" whom you know and like; conversely, it could lead to concluding that you don't have a clear identity, direction or reason to live. If the latter is closer to your ideas about the meaning of your life, you may see suicide as a possible solution.

Perhaps it is a little soon to come to this conclusion. You and you alone have a choice—a choice to live or die—but why exercise it right now? Give the alternatives another try. The path of self-exploration can be truly exciting, challenging and rewarding. With expert guidance, this may in fact be the most important journey you will ever make. So, if you are contemplating suicide, find a therapist you can relate to and talk to right now.

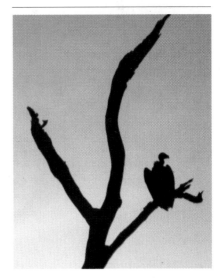

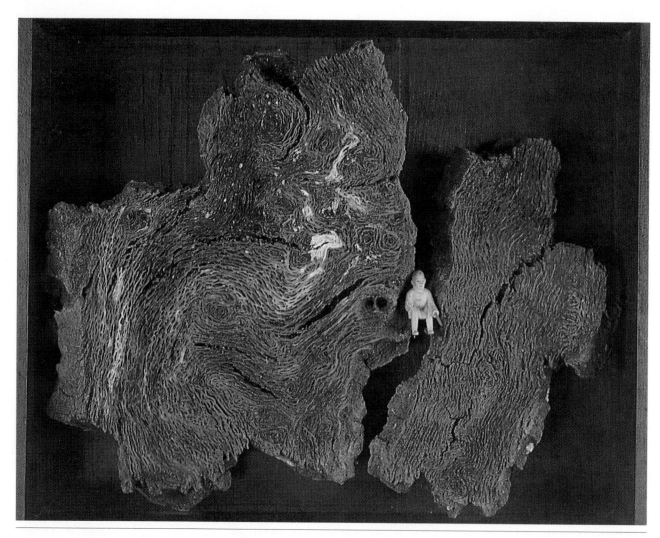

Lost in the Vastness of It All

Warning Signals for Suicide

Over 1,000 college students commit suicide every year. The incidence is two times higher in college students than in the normal population. Eight out of ten people who commit suicide give overt or covert warnings that they are considering suicide. Pay attention to these warning signals.

Depression Seems Better   A depression that has been deep but is now beginning to lift may signal an extremely dangerous time. Now an individual has the energy to formulate a suicide plan and carry it out. A person may appear relieved (as if a decision has been made) and act and feel less depressed, even satisfied with life at the moment, saying things like,

"Everything is working out," or "Everything is falling into place." Such expressions and actions may be covert, or hidden, signs that a person has decided to end the pain by suicide; someone who makes this decision does feel relieved. You may also see overt signs, such as saying good-by, giving away possessions, or asking to see family members.

Verbal Expression Centered Around Depressing Thoughts   Listen to the words your friend says. If he or she is making comments like, "People would be better off without me" or "I wonder if life is worth living," and these words illustrate his or her entire way of thinking, suicide is a definite possibility.

Withdrawal   The person lacks contact with friends and demonstrates little or no participation in activities or interaction.

Isolation   In isolation, the final stage of withdrawal, the person appears totally apart from everyone, even family.

Loss of Interest   The person evidences no real interest in others, their joys or problems, or in activities—all things this person used to participate in and enjoy.

No Experience of Joy or Fun   Life is a drag. You never observe the person laughing, clowning around, or having fun. They constantly appear down and gloomy and never initiate fun activities.

Neglect of Personal Hygiene   You notice that the person is not keeping themselves up; they wear dirty or grubby clothes and don't seem to care how they look.

Loss of Appetite   Food is not appealing, and even the thought of eating is not anticipated. This person stops coming to meals, isn't interested in sharing a pizza, and never seems to enjoy thinking about food or eating it.

Alternatives to Suicide

If you notice that a friend is experiencing one or more of these signals, please plan to intervene promptly. The accompanying material gives suggestions on how to help if a friend is considering suicide. At this stage of depression, your friend may not be able to recognize the danger or ask for help. You can talk the situation over with a counselor who will help you to make decisions—ones that may be life-saving for your friend.

Intervention is usually effective. If your friend gets treatment, even temporarily, he or she may be able to move away from suicidal thoughts. Sometimes, only one set of circumstances combine to place a person at risk for suicide. If suicide is prevented for a while, these circumstances change, and the danger period passes. Of all those who attempt suicide,

Suicide Threats Are Serious

Any suicide threat—whether obvious or covert—presents real danger. Take this threat seriously. Report it to someone who can make a decision. Intervention now can save someone's life.

> **'Tis more brave to live than to die.**
>
> **Meredith**

Emotional Disorders

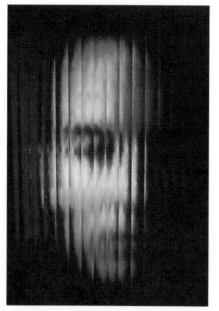

at least half are ambivalent about the choice. With help and an intervention, most of these severely painful emotional crises and deaths may be avoided. Remember, however, you may not always be able to reach your friend or intervene effectively. If tragedy occurs, do not blame yourself or others. Ultimately, the decision to take one's life is an individual choice.

Schizophrenia—Losing Touch with Reality

A patient asked her doctor if he felt she was crazy. The response was, "It depends on your definition of crazy." Though not really a therapeutic answer, the doctor's comment does illuminate the fact that a wide range of behaviors may or may not be labeled as "crazy." Our society has an entire anthology of aberrant behaviors with psychiatric names, but not one is specifically defined as crazy. You can behave in many unusual ways, act loose around the edges, a little weird, even paranoid, and still not achieve the label of crazy. The term "losing touch with reality" may be more useful than the label "crazy." Mental health professionals may call such mental states schizophrenia or psychosis, terms that have very negative con-

Signs of Schizophrenia

Aspect of Life	Typical Symptoms
Emotions	Inappropriate responses to stimuli
	Blunted or flat emotions
	Fear of warmth or closeness
	Erratic and negative feelings
Thought	Cannot tell real from unreal
	Delusions and hallucinations
	Disorganized and confused thoughts
	Tangential or circumstantial conversation
	Bizarre ideas and language
Interpersonal Relationships	Thoughts only of self, autistic
	Unpredictable responses when approached
	Socially isolated
	Mute and unresponsive, withdrawn
	Impaired role functioning
Behavior	Deteriorated level of functioning, immobilized
	Inability to make decisions
	Poor judgment
	Bizarre or peculiar behavior
	Lethargic, loss of initiative
	Poor personal hygiene and grooming

A Recipe for Mental Health

The recipe for mental health is complicated and different for every individual. Dr. Jerome Frank, a professor of medicine at Johns Hopkins University, defines mental health as "a sense that life has meaning, a feeling of personal security, the capacity to utilize opportunities for enjoyment, and to accept and surmount the inevitable suffering that life brings." Dr. Frank also includes in his definition the ability to initiate and maintain healthy relationships with others and to adapt to change successfully.

notations. To distinguish such problems from depression, remember that depression principally disrupts a person's *mood* level. With a psychosis such as schizophrenia or paranoia, the main problem seems to be a dysfunction of the *thought* and *behavior* processes.

No one theory explains the roots of schizophrenia, although several hypotheses suggest that genetic predisposition, a chemical imbalance, or a combination of family and environmental influences play roles. What is understood is that when a person suffers from this disorder, it is a major psychological breakdown and the person ceases to function as a rational, logical individual. A primary manifestation of this illness is the inability to distinguish real from unreal. Delusions of persecution are common, as are hallucinations and hearing voices. To an affected individual, these belief systems (I am the President of the United States) are real, and the voices that direct every thought and action are also very real. Losing touch with reality can be frightening and requires immediate intervention.

When we talk to God, we're praying. When God talks to us, we're schizophrenic.

Lily Tomlin

Signs of Losing Touch

This disorder is not common on college campuses, but it does occur, often in relation to extreme stress. One college student, after a very stressful semester and just before final exams, began lecturing to others in the quad. She told students she was the archangel incarnated and she was sent by Jesus to help them repent. This stressed student had suffered a mental breakdown or, technically, a schizophrenic break.

People who are no longer able to cope with a myriad of stressors may resort to entering their own world, one that is not real to the rest of us. If this breakdown of ego boundaries does occur, it requires professional help immediately. They are vulnerable to false ideas (delusions), voices, seeing visions, and other sensory misperceptions (hallucinations).

Other manifestations of this disorder are confused and disorganized thoughts in which conversations are tangential, inappropriate, unclear, or even a "word salad." You may also observe inappropriate mood or emotional reactions in which the affect, or emotional content, seems flat or blunted. These people may exhibit very inappropriate, negative, bizarre, or apathetic behavior. Finally, the quality of their interpersonal relationships diminish to the point of having great difficulty in relating to others. They may become mute and withdrawn. If you observe any of these symptoms in a friend or acquaintance, realize that this person should receive professional help immediately.

Paranoia and What To Do About It

Another disorder that you might observe is paranoid thinking. This may be a part of a schizophrenic breakdown or it may occur separately. In either instance, the person needs professional help. Paranoid ideation is manifested by extreme suspiciousness, leading to delusions of persecution. The person's responses seem unduly angry, resentful and unpredictable. Though at first the paranoid thinking seems quite rational (in this day, the CIA could be tapping the phone and following him), this thinking becomes more and more illogical and unrealistic. Do not attempt to argue or disagree with this kind of thinking; it is part of the disease pathology and will last until the personality is reintegrated. Refer or take this person for help.

Beyond the Text

1. Your friend has been depressed for weeks but has suddenly snapped out of it and talks about things improving. What would you do?

2. Your boyfriend is depressed and talking about dropping out of school because he has failed two math tests. What would you do?

3. Your friend has started "sleeping around" inappropriately, she has given away most of her best clothes and stereo, and sleeps only about two hours a night. What would you do?

4. Respond to the following statement: Young, talented, good-looking people have no reason to commit suicide.

5. Your neighbor exhibits bizarre behaviors but claims that everyone does weird things. How would you respond?

6. A classmate believes the CIA is following him and has a tap on his phone line. What advice would you give him?

Supplemental Readings

I Never Promised You a Rose Garden by Hannah Green. New York: Holt, Rinehart and Winston, 1964. A classic book on schizophrenia that relates the tortuous journey of a young woman from madness to sanity.

Sanity, Insanity, and Common Sense by Rick Suarez, PhD, Roger C. Mills, PhD, and Darlene Stewart, MS. New York: Fawcett, 1987. An incredibly useful book for both therapists and lay people that covers the psychology of the mind—including feelings, perceptions, thoughts, and behaviors.

The Feeling Good Handbook by David Burns, MD. New York: William Morrow, 1989. Especially helpful for people experiencing anxiety, depression, and relationship problems; written in lively style, provides helpful step-by-step guidelines.

The Healer Within: The New Medicine of Mind and Body by Steven Locke, MD, and Douglas Colligan. New York: E. P. Dutton, 1986. Discuss the evidence showing that the mind and body are intimately connected.

The Right to Feel Bad: Coming to Terms with Normal Depression by Lesley Hazelton. New York: Doubleday and Co., 1984. The author argues that depression is a normal reaction to certain experiences and need not be treated like a disease. Offers ways to cope with depression.

Too Young to Die. Youth and Suicide by Francine Klagsbrun. New York: Pocket Books, 1981. The author draws on interviews with young people who have tried to kill themselves to help you recognize danger signals and show you how you can intervene to save a life.

Key Terms Defined

aberrant behavior deviating from what is accepted as normal

delusions false belief maintained in spite of facts or evidence to the contrary

depression unshakable feeling of sadness accompanied by feelings of hopelessness, worthlessness, and despair about the future

hallucination false sensory perception that is not based on reality and is not accounted for by external stimuli

Lithium natural metallic salt (medication) that restores chemical balance in the body and reverses mania

manic behavior mood swing of euphoria, elation, and grandiose thinking; thought to be caused by a chemical imbalance in the body

manic-depressive illness form of disorder characterized by mood swings from euphoria and grandiose behavior to depression

paranoia feelings of suspicion and persecution; unconscious mechanism of projection in which the person projects his own thoughts upon others

psychosis major impairment of ego functioning, especially reality testing; grave maladjustment to everyday life, common symptoms of delusions and hallucinations

schizophrenia form of psychotic disorder that is manifested by the person losing touch with reality, becoming withdrawn, acting inappropriately and displaying a disordered thought process

suicide deliberate action to take one's life

tangential speech manner of speaking that is off target or off the original point

Eating and Sleep Disorders

Today's college students face high expectations regarding how they should look, act, and perform. If these high expectations cannot be met, disappointment, frustration, and anxiety may result. It makes no difference whether the expectations come from one's parents, friends, or oneself: the effect is still the same. Sometimes the pressure is so extreme that eating and sleeping disorders develop. The effects of these pressures and the accompanying stress often result in behavioral problems, such as eating and sleep disorders.

Our culture seems preoccupied with slimness. This message is so pervasive and compelling that dieting, weight control, and fitness have become national obsessions. It is easy to understand how this compulsion can generate an epidemic of eating disorders among young people, many of whom are high school or college students.

Another group of stress-related conditions is described as "sleep disorders." Researchers have concluded that sleep disorders are mainly symptoms of underlying problems; some psychological, others physiological. Sleep disorders are not limited to college students, but the stress associated with college life frequently causes sleep-related problems.

This chapter provides you with background information on eating and sleep disorders so that you can more fully understand their characteristics and underlying causes. Self-assessment guidelines and suggestions are included for you to apply to yourself or when helping (or understanding) a friend.

Contents

Key Terms

Amenorrhea	Eating disorders
Anorexia nervosa	Insomnia
Bulimia	Laxative
Circadian rhythm	Narcolepsy
Dehydration	Parasomnia
Depression	REM
Diet	Sleep apnea
Diuretic	Starvation

Eating Disorders

■ *Annie had been studying ballet since she was seven. She had never wanted to be anything other than a ballet dancer, and had never considered any other career for herself. Oberlin College had awarded her a full scholarship to study. At age seventeen, her teachers began to notice her changing hips and thighs. The director of the school called her into his office and told her not to jeopardize her future. "If your weight becomes a problem, there's not a company in the world that will take you," he said.*

Annie reduced her already insufficient caloric intake from 1,200 to 600 calories per day, measuring and mentally recording every bite and spoonful of food. She added an evening ballet class, making a total of six classes a day.

Her weight dropped from 117 on her 5'6" frame to 99 pounds. She stopped menstruating, her hair lost its luster, and she was cold all the time. She was on her way to becoming anorexic. Her teachers told her she looked "just right." Her dance friends, all of whom were thin themselves, were not alarmed by her developing emaciation—they envied her.

■ *Janet's parents were flying to the Bahamas over Christmas vacation, so she was left to entertain herself at the University of Wisconsin during the holidays. Her close friend DeeDee asked her to come home with her for Christmas dinner and stay a few days, to which Janet happily consented.*

The dinner was long and excellent. DeeDee and Janet were encouraged to eat to excess, and they did. After the meal, DeeDee asked Janet to come upstairs with her to listen to some music in her room. When they got there DeeDee said, "OK, I've eaten too much Christmas dinner as usual. I don't want it to turn to fat. I'm going to vomit. Do you want to come with me?"

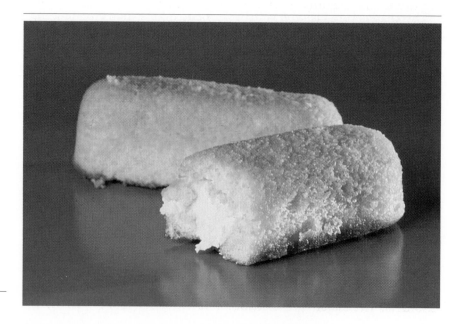

Eating and Sleep Disorders

Each drank warm water with salt, stuck a finger down her throat and forced herself to vomit. After brushing their teeth, they waited ten minutes, and went back downstairs to join the family.

- *Sarah began binging and purging in her freshman year at college after she gained ten pounds from dorm food. At first she was depressed about her weight, then she became desperate and panic-stricken. If she couldn't control her eating, she thought she could at least control the amount of calories her body was absorbing by vomiting and taking laxatives.*

   For two years she has been on a binge-purge cycle. She knows her behavior has a name—bulimia—but she is too ashamed to talk about it to anyone.

- *In addition to being a heartthrob and a good student, Gary was captain of the wrestling team. Sometimes before matches Gary would have to drop two or three pounds quickly to "make weight." He had difficulty reducing his food intake and hated any sensations of hunger. Like many other athletes whose sport depends on maintaining a specific weight, Gary discovered that vomiting enables him to have it all: he can eat what he wants and still "make weight."*

Annie's anorexia and Sarah's bulimia are extreme manifestations of disturbed eating habits, but these college students are not alone. In studies at the University of Chicago over 25 percent of entering freshmen report vomiting sometimes to lose weight. However, one incident of vomiting doesn't mean you are bulimic. One fasting diet doesn't make you anorexic. Eating when you're depressed or stressed doesn't mean you have an eating disorder. What differentiates the individual with a true eating disorder—anorexia, bulimia, or compulsive eating—is that such actions are a pattern of behavior over time that has both physical symptoms and significant emotional meaning for the individual. According to the vast majority of therapists and researchers, the causes (and cures) of eating disorders have less to do with food than with one's attude toward self. In *The Slender Balance*, Susan Squire states, "Our cultural obsession with weight has blurred and in many cases erased the line between simple dieting and having an 'eating disorder'—a distorted pattern of thinking about and behaving around food."

The following material can help you understand what eating disorders are, their causes and effects, and how you can help a friend, family member or yourself find effective help to overcome an eating disorder. Each type of eating problem has specific physical and behavioral signs. Consider whether you recognize yourself or a friend when you read the descriptions that follow.

Anorexia Nervosa: The Consequences May Be Fatal

The term anorexia is a misnomer because loss of appetite is rare. This disorder is related as much to social and psychological problems as to eating and body weight symptoms. It is complicated by serious physiological disorders. The major characteristics of anorexia nervosa have been es-

Anorexia Nervosa—Patient Recovery

Recent studies indicate that half of all patients recover within 4 to 6 years, and three-quarters within 12 years. Recovery after this appears to be rare. About 1 in 30 patients die.

Source: *British Medical Journal*, July, 1989

tablished by the American Psychiatric Association. They are presented as diagnostic criteria adapted from the DSM-III-R, 1987.

- Distorted body image (such as seeing self as fat even though body is excessively thin; person will say they "feel fat")
- Intense fear of gaining weight or becoming fat, even though underweight and weight loss is progressing
- Refusal to maintain body weight over a minimal normal weight for age and height
- Weight loss of at least 25 percent of original body weight; also, weighing less than 85 percent of expected weight
- Amenorrhea in females; three or more consecutive menstrual periods missed

Examples of other peculiar behaviors and symptoms that you may observe in persons suffering from anorexia are

- Overinvolved or fixated with food; may prepare elaborate meals for others but severely limit themselves to a few selections
- Hoarding, concealing or throwing food away
- Diet may be extreme and not well-balanced; follows food fads
- Shows obvious signs of tension at mealtimes
- Exercises compulsively; walks or runs whenever possible; stands rather than sits
- May have fine, downy hair on body due to suppressed female hormones

The physiological problems that occur as a result of severe weight loss include metabolic dysfunction, low blood sugar levels, heart irregularities, serious endocrine or hormonal abnormalities, and emotional disturbances. This disorder is usually not self-limiting; that is, unless there is appropriate intervention, the course of anorexia may be unremitting until death. This is because most people with anorexia deny or minimize the severity of the illness and are resistant to therapy. There are, however, instances when anorexia is episodic or one single episode will occur followed by a return to normal weight. Since there is no way of predicting whether the anorexia you are observing in yourself or a friend is a single episode or will continue as a constant pattern, intervention with professional help is suggested. The consequences of remaining on the anorexia path may be fatal. Severe weight loss may necessitate hospitalization to prevent death from starvation; 15 to 21 percent of those suffering from this disorder die.

"I wish I had anorexia," a moderately overweight woman said to her companion when a strikingly thin young woman walked by. This woman's glib remark about anorexia indicates her ignorance of the pernicious nature of eating disorders. She completely misinterprets the seriousness of the health and the emotional problems anorexics (and bulimics) suffer. Unfortunately, she, like many people, confuses thinness with happiness and starvation with glamour.

According to the American College Health Association, the psychological effects of anorexia may include depression, mood disturbances, feelings of chronic low self-esteem, insomnia, or other disruptions of regular sleeping patterns. Many anorexics become socially isolated. Their minds are never free from harsh, perfectionistic recriminations. Calorie-counting and body weight form the sum total of their thoughts. One said, "I withdrew from my friends. They were glad to see me go because I'd become so distant and preoccupied."

Bulimia: A Potentially Harmful Practice

College is filled with tempting foods, and many of us succumb. However, not everyone who occasionally overindulges is bulimic or a compulsive eater. In one survey, 32 percent of women among 1500 college students reported binging at least twice a month, but only 1.3 percent met the medical criteria for bulimia, which include

- Recurrent episodes of binge eating—rapid consumption of a large amount of food in a short period of time
- Awareness that the eating pattern is abnormal and fear of not being able to stop eating voluntarily—feeling a lack of control over eating patterns
- Regular episodes of self-induced vomiting, use of laxatives or diuretics, strict dieting or fasting or vigorous exercise to prevent weight gain
- Minimum average of two binge eating episodes a week for at least three months
- Constant overconcern with body shape and weight

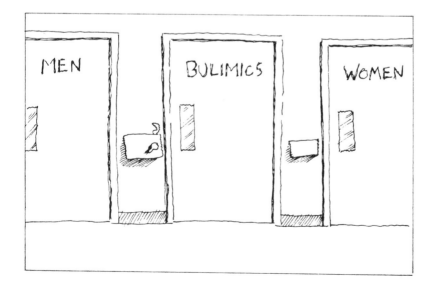

> ### Family Pattern?
>
> A recent UCLA study has found a substantially increased rate of anorexia and bulimia among relatives of patients with eating disorders. Researchers are continuing to investigate more thoroughly the extent to which eating disorders correlate with family background and possible causes of this pattern.

Eating and Sleep Disorders

CHAPTER 5

In addition to the diagnostic criteria presented by the DSM-III-R, other associated features of this disorder that you may observe in a friend or recognize in yourself are

- Depressed mood and self-deprecating thoughts following the eating binges
- Consumption of high-calorie, sweet and easily digested foods during a binge
- Inconspicuous eating during a binge
- Frequent weight fluctuations greater than ten pounds due to alternating binges and fasts
- Expressions of great concern about weight and weight gain

Bulimia can have serious consequences. First of all, binging can stress the digestive system. Starvation, laxative abuse, vomiting, and binging cause a complete disruption in homeostasis; the results are severe electrolyte imbalance. Using laxatives and diuretics can contribute to heart and kidney damage and to seizures. Vomiting can lead to weakness (because insufficient nutrients are consumed), dehydration, gastric ulcers, and internal bleeding. Loss of serum potassium by vomiting can lead to heart or kidney failure. Teeth and gums often become eroded and infected from the frequent presence of acid vomitus in the mouth.

Like anorexics, bulimics often display a low sense of self-worth, but generally maintain social contacts. Susan and Wayne Wooley, cofounders of the Eating Disorders Clinic of the University of Cincinnati Medical College, describe bulimics as "outwardly friendly, competent and in control. But beneath that facade, they are angry, hurt, lonely, needy."

Compulsive Eating: Binging Without Purging

Many of the signs of compulsive eating are the same as those for binge eating, without purging. Someone with an untreated compulsive eating problem may be significantly overweight or even obese, but extreme excess weight is not a necessary criterion. The telling element is compulsive behavior about food, such as

- Consumption of high calorie, easily ingested food during a binge
- Eating strange foods (for instance, dry cake mix) or combinations of foods
- Inconspicuous eating during a binge (may hoard food or lie about intake)
- Termination of such eating episodes by abdominal pain, sleep or social interruption

Compulsive eating can lead to obesity if not treated. Obesity has been linked to coronary heart disease, high blood pressure, and diabetes. Obese individuals also have higher rates of respiratory infections, bone and joint problems, hernias, and gall bladder disease. And, as with bulimia, binging can directly damage digestive organs.

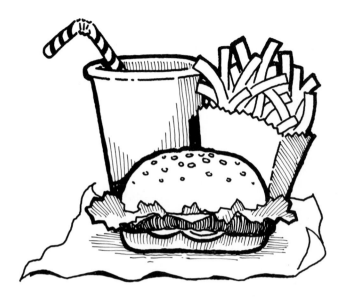

The dysfunctional aspects of an eating disorder may manifest themselves in all your relationships—with family, friends and potential romantic partners. Low self-esteem, compulsive thoughts and behaviors, and inability to deal directly with problems, strain the emotional resources of people who really care.

Why Does She Do It?

Although considerable research has been done on eating disorders in the last ten years, the causes of anorexia and bulimia remain unclear. Most theories have a psychological base; a few have physiological components. Social and family problems seem to be a major factor. In general, genetic causes or even a genetic predisposition does not seem to be a popular explanation for eating disorders. Perhaps a metabolic or hormonal imbalance is not only a result, but a contributory cause of the problem. One researcher at Yale is exploring the connection between bulimia and insulin—that the taste or thought of sugar raises blood insulin levels, which in turn creates the hunger sensation. As one compulsive eater described it, "Food is just too stimulating and compelling."

Anorexia and bulimia are primarily, though not exclusively, found among women in mid to late adolescence (only five percent of victims are male). To women in this age group, thinness often symbolizes social and professional success. Young women faced with aspirations to achieve popularity or gain positions of power often overreact. Most sufferers have been concerned about weight for long time, and have dieted many times. One anorexic said, "I began to worry about my weight when I was only eight. My older sister was obese and my mother was always dieting. I knew it was terrible to be overweight."

Most therapists emphasize the role of the family in the development of eating disorders. Anorexics often come from overprotective families in which the anorexic has the "good girl" role; an anorexic's struggle for control over her own food consumption serves as a symbolic fight for identity and independence from parental control. At first, becoming slender may inspire praise from family and friends (before they become worried about excessive weight loss).

Bulimics often have "traditional" families in which the mother neither works outside the home, nor has a "career." The father has a strong personality but is emotionally detached. In an attempt to respond to the pressure to be a "superwoman"—attract a mate and create a home and family as her mother has done, and build a significant career as her father has done—a young woman may alternate between wanting to feed her emotional self and wanting to purge herself of vulnerability. Some bulimics seem to be trying to help their mother (and all women) become more powerful. One bulimic said, "Every time I lose a pound, I lose a pound for my mother. Every time I vomit, I vomit for my mother."

Who Is at Risk

Many young women are particularly at risk for eating disorders at college. Increased pressure and competition for academic and social success can reinforce perfectionist goals. Food cues are almost omnipresent, and with fewer external controls than at home. Students who engage in certain competitive sports and dance activities scrutinize every ounce of their body weight.

Higher incidences of the disorders cluster around geographical areas where stress runs high and residents are concerned about wealth, status and high achievement. Because most college girls come from families who value achievement and status, and because the pressures to achieve during college increase, they are highly susceptible.

How the Disorder Begins

Separation from family is a frequent trigger for eating disorders. Coupling this with heightened academic and social stress, pressure to look good, or confusion about dating and social situations creates a perfect host. Says Debbie Smith, head nurse at the inpatient Eating Disorders unit at Children's Hospital at Stanford, "College is a vulnerable time for many students. They are under a lot of pressure. If vomiting relieves that one stress about looking good, it makes it that much easier for them."

Eating disorders often start slowly, without being noticed. A high-school teenager who diets just like her friends (and perhaps her mother) may, during the pressures of college, gradually develop more rigid limits for herself. In the process she can lose a dangerous amount of weight. A perpetually overweight teenager may have had food portions controlled by her parents; at college she binges more often and becomes obese.

Many college students put on the "freshman fifteen" during their first term. Often an innocuous, humorous or thoughtless remark, such as, "Sweetheart, you're beginning to put on a little weight—maybe you should start a diet," triggers an eating disorder. A few slightly critical comments about weight may be all that is necessary to propel a vulnerable and uncertain individual into a cycle of exercise, dieting and obsessional thinking about one's body. Dr. Hans Steiner states that the precipitating event can also be "separation from the family of origin (this applies particularly to college freshmen) or a sexual experience." Almost half the bulimia patients at the Eating Disorders Clinic of the University of Cincinnati Medical College had suffered sexual abuse.

How To Help a Friend

Eating disorders may be deceptive. If you haven't already been "let in on the secret" that your friend has an eating disorder, you would have to be exceptionally perceptive to figure it out by yourself.

Anorexics and bulimics do not like to leave clues. By and large, eating disorders, especially bulimia, are closet illnesses. Also, for many years bulimia doesn't "show"; it is primarily a disease of the internal organs. Girls with bulimia are well-dressed, engaging, very attractive, and sporty. Their social selves are carefully and elaborately constructed disguises; they must do this to protect themselves, to camouflage their disorder from the public eye.

Anorexics, too, like to shield their illness from public scrutiny. They bury themselves in baggy or excessive clothing, obscuring the true degree of their emaciation. Their excessive thinness may elude disguise only after the illness has already progressed to a serious stage.

Some anorexics and bulimics use compulsive exercise as another weight-controlling mechanism. By themselves, daily jogging or poor eating habits don't indicate an eating disorder. To possibly determine whether someone you know has an eating disorder, review the signs mentioned on the preceding pages, and consider how your friend would answer the questions in the self-test in the accompanying box.

It is difficult to balance your desire to help a friend against the possibility of destroying the friendship if you give unsolicited attention to her problem. Since most anorexics and bulimics don't want others lecturing them about weight loss or telling them what they should or shouldn't do, making your concerns known to them can be tricky.

The best initial step is to be forthright about your knowledge of their disorder and be open about your concern for them. Let them know you wouldn't have violated their privacy unless you were very worried. As a friend, the most helpful thing you can do is acknowledge that they have a problem and that you are there to help them if they need it.

If your friend is ill and her life is in danger, alerting a professional may be imperative. Consider informing your campus health center or your friend's parents. If your community has a highly respected eating disorder clinic, perhaps you and your friend could call for an appointment. Medical institutions are bound to confidentiality when treating a patient, so you do not need to be concerned that you would be forcing your friend to expose a secret to someone other than a medical professional. These are difficult actions to take, but they are preferable to silently watching a friend starve or self-destruct.

Actually, It's Not My Friend . . . It's Me

If you have an eating disorder, the first step toward freedom is to break the denial. Tell yourself the truth: that you are anorexic or bulimic. The next step is to seek help. Remember, these disorders are insidious; what begins as a mere diet or flirtation with vomiting often develops into months or years of debilitating illness. Early recognition gives you the best chance for a cure. Dr. Steiner states, "Early identification and aggressive treatment are the only hope for preventing chronicity."

When they have been treated and cured, recovered anorexics and bulimics feel that they were confined to a nightmare. Jane Fonda says of her own struggle with bulimia, "Yes, I was bulimic—on the binge-and-vomit treadmill—for more than fifteen years. It just about ruined my life. The bulimic or anorexic needs help, understanding and support."

Don't feel you have failed if your friend still refuses to acknowledge and get help for her problem. Many bulimics take five years to recognize their illness and seek help. Let your friend know you are ready to be supportive if and when she does want to talk.

Treatment Options

Though cures are seldom easy, eating disorders can be corrected. As with recovery from dependence on alcohol or other drugs, the victim must not only avoid problem situations but change patterns of social interaction.

Very few sufferers resolve the condition on their own. A combination of medical and psychological support is crucial to treat eating disorders. If you are medically stable, your electrolytes, vital signs, weight, and blood chemistry will be monitored; this will be in conjunction with either group or individual therapy. If you are medically unstable, more aggressive medical intervention will be necessary until you are out of danger.

You should never be without physical and psychological help. Dr. Steiner states, "Complexity of medical and psychiatric symptoms dictate a collaborative effort of two specialties." Treatment of only one aspect of the disease usually fails. According to a recent report by Dr. Stewart Agras, professor of psychiatry and behavioral science at Stanford University, about 60 percent of bulimics can be cured through either antidepressant drugs or cognitive behavior therapy; virtually none of the bulimics make progress without treatment. Dr. Agras is currently studying whether combining both drug and behavioral therapy has an even higher cure rate.

Behavioral techniques include learning to eat three nutritionally balanced and adequate meals daily (particularly a meal early in the day), coping with types of situations that have triggered binging and purging, and correcting the body image. The goal is not simply to get the anorexic to eat, the bulimic to stop vomiting, and the obese person to lose weight, but to have each individual develop a less intense relationship with food and a healthier attitude toward his or her own value as a person.

Sometimes the best advice is not what you want to hear. The truth is that abandoning dieting is the most successful treatment for eating disorders. Eating disorders begin with dieting; restriction is inexorably the precursor to binging. So rather than tighten up on yourself, learn to ease up a little. Susan Squire states, "First you must give up the idea of rigid dieting, or you will always be stuck on your personal weight see-saw. The sci-

Seeking Professional Help

If you suspect that a friend, family member, or you may suffer from an eating disorder, health professionals and support groups can provide essential help. Seek help if you or someone else

- Has several of the signs of anorexia, bulimia or compulsive eating listed earlier in this section
- Has a body weight 10 percent below ideal body weight and frequently fasts or consumes a minimal diet
- Has missed three or more menstrual periods
- Binges and purges more often than once a month

Even if problems are not yet serious, early intervention can prevent severe damage and make the cure easier. If you attend a major university, your university hospital clinic will have inpatient and outpatient services. If not, your student health center, school nurse or dean's office can recommend doctors in the area who are knowledgeable in treating eating disorders. The National Association of Anorexia Nervosa and Associated Disorders (ANAD) offers international referrals and information; all their services are free. Many colleges offer support groups led by trained therapists. Campus support groups of other students who have suffered eating disorders may be a good place, not only for ongoing support, but for someone hesitant about professional help to start talking about their concerns. Overeaters Anonymous is a nationwide self-help organization for compulsive eaters, fashioned after Alcoholics Anonymous. It operates local support groups in many communities.

However, in searching for treatment, remember one caveat— not every "eating disorders clinic" you hear about through radio, advertising and TV is what it ought to be. A professional advises, "See what the programs offer. Don't just pick one assuming that if they have a program they know what they are doing. One therapist told his clients to make a video tape or audio cassette of themselves vomiting so they would see how gross they were. Naturally, they found that antitherapeutic. Also, if they say they can cure you in X amount of weeks, it's bogus."

entific evidence is formidable and growing that the more restricted your weight-loss diet, the more likely you are to become bulimic, though you may have started out a simple nosher."

Substitute new values and new achievements for those relating to weight and food. When you're around someone with an eating disorder, stay away from talk about food, recipes, weight and eating disorders; involve yourself and your friend in the arts, nature, academics, or other campus activities. Recognize your friend's talents in other areas.

Physical and emotional setbacks along the way are normal. Recovering bulimics experience digestive upsets, bloating and hunger. Anorexics must struggle, often through therapy, to accept a new body shape. Compulsive eaters often must work against a metabolism that fights against fat loss. Rather than hoping to change your life overnight, the best approach is to set your sights at moderation and don't try to rush success. Even if you feel that conquering your eating disorder is overwhelming—that you are like an inchworm about to climb a mountain—it is important to take that first step, until, inch by inch, you are moving back towards health.

Sleep Disorders

Sleep is a precious commodity at college, invariably in short supply. Academic requirements, social attractions, personal needs, and, for many, employment hours all compete for your time. With too many activities and too few hours, sleep often comes out on the short end of time allotments. You can recover quite easily from an occasional late night or early morning stint. What concerns many health educators are the illnesses that creep up on students who endure chronic sleep deprivation. Some students chronically depend on caffeine and other stimulants to stay awake; some habitually use alcohol, sleeping pills or other depressants to get to sleep. High nighttime noise levels in some college residential situations disturb sleep further. Amid the stress, confusion and chemical imbalances experienced by college students, sleep therapists are diagnosing a growing number of sleep disorders. Experienced researchers compare sleep to sex: quality counts more than quantity.

This section describes sleep and its importance to your health and wellness. It includes a brief summary of sleep disorders, along with recommendations on how to recognize the need for professional counseling. Whether you've recently been having insomnia or other sleep problems, you'll get tips on how to experience more restful, efficient sleep.

Sleep and Our Biological Rhythms

Of all the biological rhythms, sleep is probably the most studied and yet least understood. It is both relentless (nobody lives without it) and flexible (which tempts us to abuse it). Sleep deprivation studies in humans invariably end because the subjects simply cannot, after about a week, stay awake. And yet, after a couple of days of recovery sleep, no permanent ill effects can be detected. Some recent animal experiments, however, suggest that prolonged sleep deprivation may have serious effects when carried to the extreme.

The body seems to be "at rest" and the brain "switched off" during sleep, but, in reality, while our body remains immobile, nearly every organ and system is undergoing measurable changes, some of them drastic, during sleep. And while the brain seems nonreactive to outside

The Stages of Sleep

To the casual observer, sleep is little more than "not waking," a dormant period of inactivity and unresponsiveness. A closer look, however, even without sophisticated instruments, discloses that quiet sleep alternates with periods of restive twitching, erratic breathing and rapid eye movements beneath closed lids. Recognizing these alternating periods as distinct psychophysiological states, scientists in the mid-1950s dubbed them rapid eye movement (REM) and nonrapid eye movement (NREM) sleep.

Further investigations, using electroencephalography (EEG) and other physiological measuring techniques, revealed that NREM sleep could be subdivided into four stages. It was also determined that REM sleep was associated with the subjective experience of dreaming.

NREM stage 1 is a transition between wakefulness and sleep. Most people spend very little time in this stage as they pass into deeper sleep, but some pathological conditions may cause a person to spend a significant portion of the night in stage 1.

Stage 2 constitutes the majority of an adult's night of sleep. It has characteristic EEG patterns and is distributed across the night.

Stages 3 and 4 sleep are the deepest sleep stages and are defined by slow, coma-like EEG waves. Most slow-wave sleep occurs in the first half of the night. In young adults, these stages constitute about 15 percent of total sleep time but decrease over the years; in old age they may disappear entirely.

The rapid eye movements from which REM sleep derives its name are only one of a multitude of the physical manifestations of this sleep stage. During REM, the nervous system shows widespread instability and nearly every measurable physiological variable exhibits some change. Infants spend nearly half of their sleep in REM, while adults spend about 25 percent. REM occurs at 90-minute intervals during the night, and most people awakened from a REM period report a dream.

Typical Sleep Pattern of a Young Human Adult

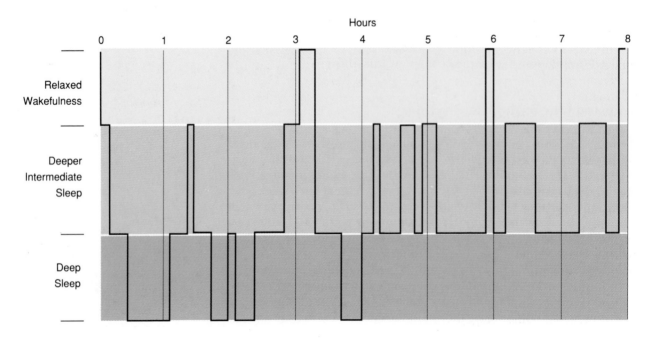

stimuli, it is still processing and filtering sensory information from the outside and is as active (albeit in different ways) as the awake brain.

Many hypotheses have been advanced to explain the function of sleep. Even without an all-encompassing and generally accepted theory, scientists have discovered some principles that can inform and guide you toward healthy sleep. As sleep deprivation studies show, humans have no absolute daily requirement for sleep in the short term. In general, you should sleep enough to maintain optimal alertness during the following day. But how much is that? There is no simple answer. For a typical college student, age 18 to 25, the normal range would be from 6 to 10 hours per night.

Why do some people need to sleep longer than others? Perhaps for the same reason that some people are taller than others, or run faster: a mixture of genetic and lifestyle factors. Some studies have shown that short sleepers tend to be characterized as action-oriented on personality tests and long sleepers tend to appear more introspective and brooding. Abnormal sleep length may also be a sign of illness.

Circadian Rhythms Clash with Twentieth Century Lifestyle

We are familiar with all kinds of clocks: primitive sundials that stand in a garden, clocks on towers, clocks on dashboards, clocks on our wrists, or on our radios. We carry around in our brains a more subtle, intricate system of biological clocks that dictates our physiology and behavior as powerfully and regularly as a digital watch or an electronic clock radio.

Because our internal clocks are usually well synchronized with each other and with the external clocks that we have come to accept in society, we may remain blissfully unaware of their existence. But when they go wrong, as we try to adapt a biological system that has evolved over millions of years to a twentieth century lifestyle that increasingly ignores the boundaries of day and night, these biological timekeepers become unmasked and assert themselves in sometimes unpleasant ways. Scientists are attempting to understand how our biological rhythms can be protected to insure optimum health and performance.

Circadian rhythms are cycles of biological functions regulated by your internal clock. These cycles, which run for a period of about 24 hours, are also known as biological rhythms. Scientists have discovered that each gland and organ has its own activity rhythm and that they behave in a synchronized manner.

Circadian rhythms have been discovered in most biological functions. The best example of an internal circadian rhythm is the rhythm of body temperature. It has a daily peak in the afternoon and a minimum level in the middle of the night. When you stay awake to study for an entire night, you experience the ebb of energy and performance that marks this minimum, usually around 4 AM. In fact, at 4 AM the likelihood of making an error, whether simple attention lapse or falling asleep at the wheel, is 60 percent higher than average.

Dealing with Jet Lag

- Avoid alcohol and caffeine during the flight.
- Drink water (not carbonated drinks) to avoid dehydration.
- Adopt the new time schedule for meal and sleep times as soon as possible, even before you leave on your trip.
- Avoid taking naps in the new time zone.
- Consider using short-acting sleeping pills only with your physician's advice.
- Try 1 gram/night of L-tryptophan (a natural amino acid) to encourage sleep while adapting to the new time zone.

When You've Just Pulled an All-nighter

When dawn arrives and you've not slept yet, your best strategy is to keep going and go to sleep early that night. A nap in the morning or afternoon will disrupt your internal systems. A few hours of daytime sleep will probably result in a sleep hangover anyway. You'll feel worse with a little sleep rather than none.

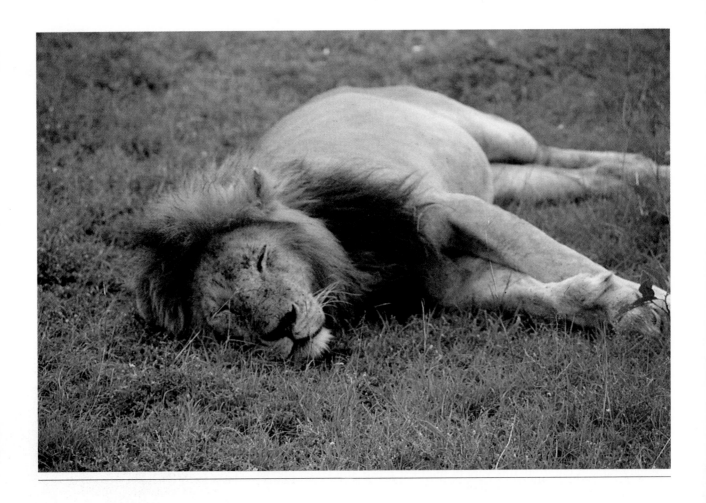

Many rhythms have a relationship not only to clock time but also to each other. The secretion of growth hormone is keyed to the sleep rhythm. The daily growth hormone secretion peak occurs about an hour after you fall asleep, even if sleep onset is delayed.

However, our natural internal rhythms can become desynchronized when disturbed by such stressors as flying across several time zones (jet lag) or erratic sleeping and waking habits. College students frequently experience the latter condition.

Once your biological rhythms are out of phase with one another, you are more prone to feel stress in the form of irritability, exhaustion and perhaps even lowered resistance to illness. When you become aware of your rhythms, you are more prepared to understand and deal with your ups and downs. You are also more realistic when allocating your time for work, play and sleep.

Predators and Prey

In the animal kingdom, long sleepers such as lions tend to be predators. Short sleepers like gazelles tend to be prey. Think about it—which are you?

Sleep Disorders

Sleep disorders are a growing medical subspecialty. A decade ago only three clinics specialized in these disorders; today there are scores, and hundreds of hospitals perform at least some sleep-related tests.

Some sleep disorders are serious medical conditions—even life-threatening; others are amenable to self-help. Sleep disorder specialists treat insomnia, excessive sleep, nightmares, sleepwalking, circadian rhythm disorders, and other conditions.

Insomnia

Insomnia is probably the most common sleep-related complaint. Insomnia, like fever, is not a disease in itself but a symptom. Also, like fever, it can have many different causes. To treat insomnia effectively, one must discover its source.

Transient and situational insomnia affects nearly everyone at some point. Psychological stress, pain, environmental factors (noise, heat, cold), or anxiety about a big presentation or exam can cause nearly anyone to have difficulty falling asleep or staying asleep. Without treatment, this type of insomnia usually disappears when the stress subsides. Persistent psychophysiological insomnia occurs when sleep habits fail to return to normal (sometimes not for decades!) after a period of situational insomnia.

If you have bouts of situational insomnia, you can usually improve sleep by resolving or reducing worrisome stressors. If you just can't sleep well because you're worrying about certain term papers or exams, expect your sleep to return to normal when those challenges have passed. Social isolation, boredom, and self-preoccupation also contribute to situation insomnia.

Psychiatric disorders, especially depression, are often associated with insomnia. There is a highly typical sleep pattern in endogenous (biological) depression. Depressives typically have some difficulty falling asleep, but are also plagued by early morning awakenings from which they cannot return to sleep. Manic-depressives may be unable to sleep during their manic episodes and unable to stay awake during the depressive phase of their illness. The disturbed timing and distribution of sleep stages is also a hallmark of depression.

Irregular breathing and periodic leg movements during sleep, though more commonly associated with excessive sleepiness, may also be causes of insomnia complaints because they disturb sleep.

Persistent psychophysiological insomnia usually will not get better on its own, and treatment must be tailored to the individual. Insomniacs with anxiety that results in muscle tension may benefit from biofeedback or relaxation training; those with problems rooted in learned behaviors (those who can, for example, sleep on the sofa but not in the bedroom)

What does the swallow know of the owl's insomnia?

Rafael Alberti

Laboratory testing shows that insomniacs average only 30 minutes less sleep a night than normal sleepers and that they usually fall asleep within 15 minutes after going to bed. But they think they're missing a lot more sleep than that.

Source: *Staying Well Newsletter*

Eating and Sleep Disorders

CHAPTER 5

99

may need therapy aimed at changing maladaptive behaviors. Still others who have had problems sleeping since childhood may have intrinsically weak sleep habits and may benefit from drugs, such as the antidepressant drug Elavil, or special biofeedback techniques.

Professional therapy for insomnia addresses the underlying cause, yet sleeping medications (hypnotics) are a billion-dollar-a-year industry and are widely prescribed by nonspecialists for all types of insomnia complaints. The most widely prescribed sleeping medications are the benzodiazepines, relatives of the tranquilizer Valium, which is sometimes prescribed for sleep but is not, strictly speaking, a sleeping pill. Dalmane, the most widely prescribed sleeping pill for years, and a very effective hypnotic, is gradually being superceded by a new generation of shorter-acting benzodiazepines (for instance, Halcion). These drugs remain effective for only a few hours and eliminate the "hangover" some people experience with other sleeping medications.

Though sleeping pills may work well for a few nights, if used chronically they may actually make sleep worse and induce an insomnia "rebound" when withdrawn. Sleep is more difficult than before starting the medication. Still, for some people, sleeping medication may be effective for an occasional bout of insomnia. Research indicates that alcohol is the most frequently selected sleep medication by college students. This is not an effective sleep enhancer, because alcohol affects brain function and, therefore, sleep patterns. Also, when alcohol and sleeping pills are mixed, the result can be lethal.

Excessive Sleep

People who are chronically sleepy or have uncontrollable attacks of sleepiness are often considered lazy and become the objects of ridicule or derision. Though insomnia may often be a sign of psychopathology, excessive sleepiness is almost always a sign of a medical illness, sometimes a very serious one.

To diagnose excessive sleepiness, sleep specialists use a special daytime nap test in a sleep lab. Normal individuals may have abnormal test results if their sleep is restricted or disturbed, but excessively sleepy people are sleepy despite a normal amount of sleep at night. The two most common causes of excessive daytime sleepiness are narcolepsy and obstructive sleep apnea syndrome.

Narcolepsy   This is an inherited condition that causes excessive daytime sleepiness, uncontrollable sleep attacks and cataplexy (a sudden loss of voluntary muscle control). Symptoms of this disorder frequently surface when the person is from 13 to 22 years of age. Sometimes the condition does not occur until the individual reaches college age or even later in life. When masked by many other environmental and behavioral factors, narcolepsy may be difficult to recognize.

Eating and Sleep Disorders

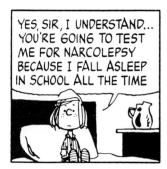 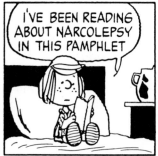 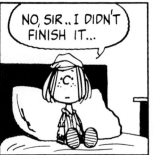 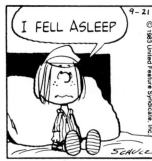

In normal adults, REM sleep occurs about 90 minutes after sleep onset and again at 90-minute intervals throughout the night. It rarely occurs at all during short daytime naps. Narcoleptics go very quickly—sometimes directly—into REM sleep at night and during daytime naps or sleep attacks. In addition to sleepiness, narcoleptics experience cataplexy, a sudden loss of muscle tone that can make the head droop, the extremities weak, and may make the narcoleptic fall to the floor in what is often mistaken for a seizure, although narcolepsy and epilepsy are unrelated.

Sleep labs use brain-wave recordings to diagnose or rule out narcolepsy in individuals with a complaint of excessive sleepiness. There is no cure for narcolepsy. In addition to being hereditary, narcolepsy is associated with a blood group that is often a marker of autoimmune diseases.

Treatments of narcolepsy are of two types, stimulants such as Ritalin or amphetamines are used to control daytime sleepiness, and drugs such as tricyclic antidepressants (which suppress REM sleep) are used to control cataplexy. These drugs may become ineffective over time and can have many unpleasant side effects. New treatments for this chronic illness are being sought. Many narcoleptics are able to function normally, but others are totally disabled.

Obstructive Sleep Apnea   Snoring, a favorite target of cartoonists and comedians, has only recently been recognized as anything but funny. In its early, mild, and relatively benign form, it is a nuisance to bed partners. When it is more persistent and severe it is a prime symptom of obstructive sleep apnea syndrome (OSAS), a disorder in which the soft tissue of the upper airway collapses on itself during sleep, breathing stops for seconds or even minutes, the airway abruptly and noisily opens, and breathing resumes. Because of the frequent arousals and sleep disturbances, one of the prime symptoms of OSAS is excessive sleepiness.

OSAS can occur at any age and affect either sex, but most sleep apneics are obese middle-aged males. OSAS increases in severity with increasing age, and hypertension and cardiovascular problems are common. Though research continues, researchers currently predict that most

Eating and Sleep Disorders

Stop Snoring!

If your doctor determines that your snoring does not stem from apnea or another serious condition, you may still want to snore less, just so your roommate or lover doesn't kick you out of the room in the middle of the night. Try these suggestions from *Stop Snoring Now*, by Dan Carlinsky.

- If you're fat, lose weight.
- For at least two or three hours before bedtime, don't drink alcohol or take sleeping pills, antihistamines or tranquilizers. They depress the central nervous system and make your tongue floppy and your throat muscles loose.
- Add some humidity to your bedroom. A dry throat will tend to vibrate more than one that's moist. A container of water near the radiator could do the trick.

- Whether you sleep on your back or your side, extra height under your head will align your airway.
- Don't eat carbohydrates or dairy products just before bedtime; they cause a build-up of mucus that can interfere with breathing.
- Try taking honey (chew honeycomb or swallow a couple of spoonfuls of liquid) daily for a few weeks. Clears up the breathing, some folks say.
- The face-up position is the most likely to produce snoring. As many as four out of five people who snore do so only on their backs. The solution is to get them to roll onto one side or the other.

Now, some ideas for the one who does the listening. Since you never know what may work, why not try these.

- Affix something uncomfortable to the back of the pajamas to prevent them from sleeping on their back.
- Consider earplugs or a sleep-inducing machine.
- Whistle near the offender's ear—not a loud wake-up whistle, just a few little chirps.
- Lean in close and whisper softly, "Please stop snoring."
- And here's perhaps the best tested, most surefire method known, its only drawback being the need for endless repetition: Belt him one and yell, "SHUT UP!"

Source: Dan Carlinsky, *Stop Snoring Now*

heavy snorers will develop sleep apnea as they grow older. Treatments include surgery, antisnoring devices and drugs. However, nearly every person with sleep apnea can benefit from weight loss. If you snore heavily, have a sleep evaluation if you develop excessive sleepiness, morning headaches or high blood pressure.

Periodic Leg Movements   These are rhythmic involuntary leg muscle jerks, typically occurring two or three times a minute over extended periods. Usually a bed partner is the first to notice that an individual has PLM. Many PLM sufferers also have restless legs, an uncomfortable sensation in the legs that makes it difficult for them to remain asleep or even in bed. The disturbed nocturnal sleep makes many people with PLM sleepy during the daytime. Some pharmaceutical treatments are available, but science does not yet have a satisfactory explanation or real cure.

Parasomnias

A number of sleep disorders of various origins are lumped together into the category of parasomnias. Because they remain for the most part difficult to study in the sleep lab, they remain somewhat mysterious. However, they tend to run in families and appear more frequently under conditions of stress.

Nightmares Bad dreams or nightmares come during REM sleep, and the dreamer can usually recount some sort of vivid story with frightening content (being chased by a monster or falling from a great height). There are many theories about the causes of nightmares. Psychotherapy and lucid dreaming are often helpful treatments.

Night Terrors Fairly common in small children, night terror involves an awakening from deep sleep, usually in the first half of the night. They are manifested by extreme anxiety and agitation without the ability to recall an actual dream.

Sleepwalking This condition often occurs in the same individuals who report night terrors, and at around the same time of night, suggesting that they share a common cause, both being disorders of arousal. Sleepwalkers, counter to folklore, may be awakened without ill effects (although they usually resist such attempts) and do not have any special sensibility that protects them from harm. Each year people are injured or killed by sleepwalking, and steps must be taken to insure that sleepwalkers do not harm themselves or others. Most children grow out of this disorder, but when it continues into adulthood, psychotherapy or drugs may be indicated.

Circadian Rhythm Disorders

Certain types of sleep problems occur when your internal clock malfunctions. Here are brief descriptions of such problems that may occur to college students.

Free Running In the absence of daily commitments, some people behave as if they were in time isolation, adopting a 25-hour day. This means that if on Monday night, you go to bed at 10 PM and awaken at 8 AM, on Tuesday you go to bed at 11 PM and awaken at 9 AM. If this continues, by the following Monday, you will be going to bed at 5 AM and getting up at 3 PM and so on. If you have no daily commitments you may be able to adapt to such a schedule, but intermittent work or social demands may fall at the wrong time of the cycle and be unpleasant or even dangerous.

Phase Advance/Phase Delay Many individuals cannot adapt their sleep schedules to the schedule they would like. Some cannot fall asleep until early morning, although they wish to go to sleep near midnight. Once asleep they sleep normally. Others, though more rare, fall asleep consistently earlier in the evening than they wish and wake up too early. A treatment for phase delay called chronotherapy calls for allowing the

The All-night Cram Session

When facing a crucial midterm or final exam, you may feel that your only recourse is an all-night study effort. Research indicates that you risk little taking a memory-type exam after an all-night session. However, you cannot expect to perform well on exams requiring you to analyze and synthesize material. Results on essay tests and those testing your logical mind may suffer as a result of sleep deprivation.

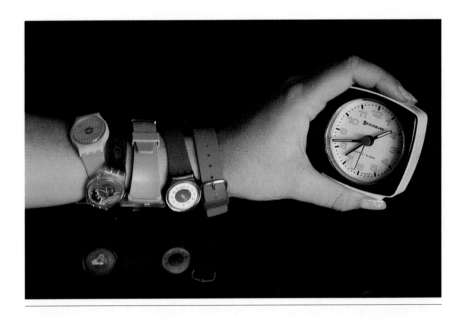

rhythm to free run forward until the desired sleep time is reached, then rigidly enforcing wake-up times to avoid recurrence of the delay.

Desynchronization   In the above disorders, and in normal functioning, most bodily rhythms stay coupled to each other, or at least cluster in groups. In desynchronization, rhythms lose their normal relationship to one another. Desynchronization may also occur transiently, as during jet lag when different rhythms require different lengths of time to adapt to a new time zone.

Getting the Most Out of Your Sleep

Most of us at some time suffer from insomnia, difficulty falling asleep or other mild sleep disturbances. You can usually improve the quality of

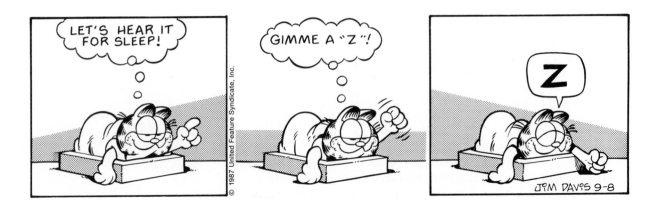

Lucid Dreaming

Most people who remember their dreams can recall at least a few occasions when they were aware that they were dreaming. For most of us, this is a rare, fleeting experience, but some people experience lucid dreaming regularly and at will.

You can use lucid dreaming for creative self-exploration, problem solving, therapy, or just fun. Using particular techniques, scientists have been able to study individuals who have native talent for lucid dreaming and help others who want to learn the technique.

- Remember your dreams. Practically everyone has several REM periods each night, but many people would say that they seldom, if ever, dream. In fact, "failure to dream" is almost

always a failure to recall dreams. You recall your dreams best when you awaken directly from a REM period. Because REM periods are longer in the morning hours, you more frequently remember dreams in the morning than when you awaken in the middle of the night. Setting the alarm for half an hour earlier than usual may allow you to harvest more dreams. Motivation is another big factor in dream recall. Keeping a dream diary and pen near the bed and remembering the intention to recall your dreams just before retiring are simple techniques that often stimulate a startling increase in dream recall.
- Be aware of your mind state. You can practice questioning yourself to discover whether

you are dreaming even while you are awake. Several times a day, ask yourself, "Is this a dream?" Not only will the habit spill over into your dream state, but you will become better at quickly detecting those dream features that clue you in to the fact that you are dreaming.
- Hang in there! Being conscious in your dream state may at first be so exciting that you immediately wake up. With practice, you can learn to sustain the lucidity. With more practice, you can learn to sustain the lucidity and sleep simultaneously.

---

your sleep considerably by changing certain behaviors that affect sleep. Though the study of sleep is still quite new, researchers and clinicians generally agree on several principles that enable you to benefit from your sleeping hours. The following suggestions may help you, but if you are having serious sleep problems, you'll want to consult with your health care provider and perhaps a sleep specialist.

Maintain a regular sleep schedule. Get up at the same time every day. This is key because your internal clock is synchronized with daylight hours; variations in the time you start the day throw off your body processes. Regulate the amount of sleep you attain by changing the time you go to bed. Feeling sleepy is by far the best indicator of when to go to bed. You can't force yourself to go to sleep, so if you don't feel sleepy, you're better off staying up. Getting up at the same time every day is not entirely realistic for typical college students. However, sleep researchers recommend that you do not sleep excessively late on weekends or on other days when you do not have morning classes.

Incorporate decompression time and presleep rituals into your life. Such techniques have proven effective for students who experience busy, high-pressure days. Reading an adventure or mystery book, watching TV, or listening to music can take your mind off today's experiences and tomorrow's problems. Nightly rituals such as opening your window, brushing your teeth, organizing your notebooks and textbooks for tomorrow's classes, setting the clock radio, and so forth can orient your mind and body toward the relaxation phase of sleep.

Sleep in a dark, quiet room. Don't spend waking hours in bed. For example, don't study in bed and don't conduct such anxiety-producing activities as balancing your checkbook or discussing family or dating problems while in bed.

Sleep only at night. Don't take daytime naps to catch up, especially in the late afternoon or evening. Getting just enough sleep to barely make it through the day may be insufficient for safe driving, safe use of laboratory equipment, or concentrated study. Consistent sleep deprivation affects your productivity, stress-coping stamina and perhaps, your immune system. When you become run down and vulnerable to colds and other illnesses, you may be suffering from lack of sleep.

Use your body, not someone else's behavior, as the guide for your sleep needs. What you need in the way of sleep may differ greatly from your friends or your roommates. For instance, just because someone else gets up for eight o'clock classes, don't consider yourself lazy if you can't. Roommate disagreements on sleeping hours and conditions (such as open versus closed windows, lights, noise, and so forth) can create stressful conditions. Sleep is basic to health and performance, so do not hesitate to talk openly about any sleep-related conflicts. Work on compromises, but if you cannot reach agreements that allow you to get the kind of sleep you need, you may want to consider changing rooms.

Avoid caffeine and other stimulants near bedtime. Caffeine taken within three or four hours of bedtime disturbs sleep patterns. Caffeine is present not only in coffee but in many teas and sodas and even over-the-counter medications.

Give up cigarettes. The nicotine in cigarettes (as much a stimulant as caffeine) impairs your sleep. In one study, nonsmokers fell asleep after about 30 minutes, while smokers needed an average of 44 minutes.

Avoid alcohol near bedtime. A drink may make you feel sleepy, but alcohol actually disrupts sleep. It exacerbates any existing breathing disorder. After a long evening of drinking alcohol, you may wake up frequently with withdrawal symptoms (such as headache or thirst) that make further sleep difficult.

Avoid excessive liquid intake during the evening. Such intake results in a full bladder and the urge (or need) to get up and empty your bladder.

Avoid sleeping pills. Over-the-counter sleeping aids merely make you groggy. They do not induce sleep. Prescription hypnotics should be used only occasionally and under the supervision of a physician. This type of medication is addictive; if you become dependent, your system may revert to insomnia when you withdraw from the medication. Though most modern sleeping pills are safe, death from an overdose of sleeping pills or due to mixing sleep or pain relief medication with alcohol is not uncommon.

Refrain from vigorous physical exercise just prior to bedtime. Exercise raises your metabolism and temperature as well as awakening all your bodily systems. To become sleepy, you want the opposite effect, a general slowing down. However, exercise earlier in the day can have a very positive influence on sleep quality.

Avoid heavy meals near bedtime. Because fats and gas-producing foods are difficult to digest, they disrupt sleep when ingested too close to bedtime. If hungry, try a light snack. If you are bothered by hunger pangs late in the evening, a light snack may help you get to sleep. Breakfast cereals, a light sandwich, and warm non-fat or low-fat milk are considered helpful.

Beyond the Text

1. Respond to the following statement: Anorexia nervosa and bulimia are women's diseases?

2. Your food is always missing from the refrigerator. You suspect your roommate, but he/she denies taking it. What should you do?

3. You notice that one of your friends disappears into the bathroom after every meal. She's quite thin and you suspect she may have an eating disorder. What should you do?

4. Your roommate stays up studying until 3:00–4:00 a.m., sleeps until 8:00 a.m., goes to classes from 9:00 a.m. to noon, and then sleeps for 2 to 4 hours in the afternoon. Is this an unhealthy schedule? Why?

5. You have trouble getting to sleep, especially during busy periods (just when you really need your sleep). What could account for this situation and what can you do about it?

Supplemental Readings

Breaking Free From Compulsive Eating by Geneen Roth. New York: New American Library, 1984. Supportive guide to developing new eating habits and breaking away from obsessive eating problems.

Bulimia: A Guide to Recovery by Lindsay Holl and Leigh Cohn. Santa Barbara, CA: Gürze Books, 1989. Answers the 20 questions most commonly asked about bulimia and provides suggestions on how to break this behavior pattern, including case histories of what has worked for others.

Dreams: God's Forgotten Language by John A. Sanford. New York: Harper & Row, 1989. Explores the psychological and spiritual significance of dreams; shows how dreams can help us find healing and wholeness.

Dying to be Thin, Understanding and Defeating Anorexia Nervosa and Bulimia—A Practical, Lifesaving Guide by Ira Sacker, MD, and Marc Zimmer, PhD. New York: Warner Books, 1987. Detailed explanation of the causes and symptoms of bulimia and anorexia nervosa and how and where to find help.

Eating Disorders by Hilde Bruch. New York: Basic Books, 1973. A complete treatise describing anorexia nervosa, bulimia, and other eating disorders.

Treating and Overcoming Anorexia Nervosa by Steven Levenkron. New York: Warner Books, 1982. If you struggle with this disorder or have a friend who does, this book presents a knowledgeable, proven approach to breaking the pattern of this critical and potentially life-threatening disorder.

Key Terms Defined

amenorrhea absence of menses; can be brought about by anorexia nervosa

anorexia nervosa eating disorder characterized by refusal to eat or aberration in eating patterns due to emotional states

bulimia eating disorder characterized by episodic binge eating followed by purging or vomiting

circadian rhythm regular recurrence of biological activities within cycles of approximately 24 hours

dehydration condition resulting from excessive loss of body fluids

depression illness characterized by sadness, hopelessness, and despair

diet customary amount and kind of food taken in by a person from day to day

diuretic agent that promotes urine secretion

eating disorders group of disorders, primarily psychiatric in nature, resulting from distorted beliefs about the relationship of food intake to body image; can become life threatening

insomnia inability to fall or remain asleep during the night

laxative medicine that promotes evacuation of bowel contents

narcolepsy recurrent, uncontrolled, brief episodes of sleep during waking hours

parasomnia grouping of sleep disorders, including sleepwalking, nightmares, and night terrors

REM stage of sleep in which dreams occur characterized by rapid eye movements. NREM is nonrapid eye movement sleep and is subdivided into four stages

sleep apnea episodes during sleep in which breathing stops

starvation long period of food deprivation

Time Management

Time and how you use it play an important role in college. You have many options for spending your time: to explore and master new areas of knowledge, prepare for a future career, discover more about your own personality, develop new friends and relationships, attend exciting social events, and express your independence.

Paul A. Grayson, PhD, of Wesleyan University, states that "no other environment—not high school beforehand or the conventional work-place or even graduate school afterwards—poses quite the same challenging set of time conditions as the undergraduate experience. What makes this period so challenging, demanding and stressful are two factors: (1) unstructured time and (2) lack of time management skills." Colleges and universities expect students to demonstrate a skill for which they typically have not been prepared by previous school experiences, the skill of budgeting time.

This chapter identifies many of the competing demands for your college time and presents methods of developing your own time management programs. Finally, tips for avoiding many common time wasting activities are suggested.

Contents

Key Terms

Brinksmanship

Circadian rhythm

Maladaptive response

Perfectionism

Procrastination

Time management

Type A personality

Type B personality

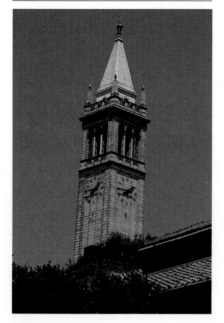

The Dilemma of College Time

Attending classes, studying for tests, writing papers, and pursuing related academic interests require the bulk of your time and attention. But other demands, such as the need to earn money, may confront you as well. Social life is a major aspect of college life, the dominant focus for some students. Faced with the dilemma of too many demands with too little time, common student reactions include the following:

Behavioral Problems Students frequently display maladaptive responses to their new-found freedom of daily college time. These include procrastination, learning problems, sleep disturbances, eating disorders, mismanagement of money, alcohol and drug abuse, and overemphasis on social and recreational activities. Though not the only cause, a contributing factor to these problems is the absence of an externally imposed schedule of daily activity. The stress and anxiety associated with unstructured time may result in your becoming even more inefficient. At this point it may be appropriate to seek counsel from the college health service or dean's office. Additional information is presented in **Seeking Professional Help** later in this chapter.

Compromise Students who compromise academic assignments in order to participate in more social activities may receive low if not failing grades. Giving up important segments of college life, such as social relationships, should not be necessary. Some trade-offs are expected and appropriate. If you work part-time or full-time while attending college, you may require five years or more to fulfill all your academic requirements. Compromise is positive when it contributes to a greater balance among all the important demands on your time.

Increased Productivity Covering more material in less time is a valuable skill. You can increase your productivity by completing a speed reading course, learning to organize written assignments more quickly, or using a personal computer effectively. Word processing software can save you considerable time and reduce the stress associated with completing term papers on schedule.

Time Management You can't literally manage time, because time will continue to move at the same rate tomorrow as it did yesterday. What you can manage, however, is yourself. The common descriptive term for this process is "time management." A time management program is a helpful tool throughout your college career. It does not require as much discipline as you might imagine. The rewards of developing and implementing a program include (1) making better use of your time, (2) reducing academic stress, and (3) identifying blocks of time that can be used for activities you thought you couldn't fit into your life, such as physical fitness, music, campus organizations, community service, and so forth.

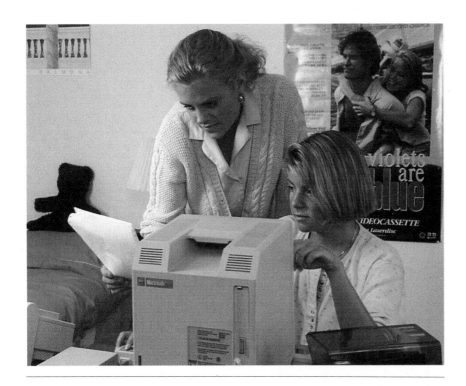

Personality Traits and Your Attitude About Time

Researchers on the relationship between time and personality agree that your actual use of time is a reasonably accurate reflection of your personality. The Type A personality normally is concerned about deadlines, course loads, and lack of time. The Type B personality is more relaxed about the work loads and deadlines. Either type can accurately estimate the amount of work that must be accomplished and how long it will take. In modest amounts, anxiety mobilizes the Type A to action. However, excessive anxiety can result in paralyzing tension. Speculative worry wastes valuable time and energy that would be better applied to more constructive work.

Some Type B individuals play the brinkmanship game. Until brought to the very edge of disaster, they may postpone studying for mid-terms or beginning research papers. Suddenly mobilized to action, such a student pulls an all-nighter in a mad dash to make it just under the wire. Worked to perfection, this can be an exciting way to live. However, miscalculations can result in missed deadlines, poor grades, and disappointing academic performance. When faced with failure, this Type B often pretends not to care, but may actually experience anxiety, guilt and depression.

Time Management

Daily Energy Cycles

Lisa hates to get up in the morning. She picks up speed as the day progresses and her most productive study time is 8:00 PM to midnight. In contrast, Ben prefers to work on difficult assignments from 7:00 AM to mid-morning. At 10:00 PM Ben is sound asleep, just when Lisa is grinding away on her assignments. Why would these two students have such different styles?

Each person has a habitual energy cycle that repeats quite closely from day to day. It is helpful to identify your energy cycle. Then, plan your study time, especially heavy reading, writing, calculating, and other assignments requiring intense concentration to coincide with periods of *your* highest energy. It may be difficult to obtain a class schedule that coincides with your high energy cycle. But, you should be aware of potential difficulties if you are a "night person" who signs up for a particularly difficult course offered at 8:00 AM. Schedule activities such as socializing, shopping, watching TV, doing your laundry, telephoning, and cleaning your room for periods of lower energy levels. Then, if your energy is totally dissipated before you can clean up your room, you'll have a good excuse.

Your answers to the following questions will indicate your attitude about time:

		Yes	No
1.	I almost always feel rushed.	☐	☐
2.	When someone is late, I get very angry.	☐	☐
3.	I'm so busy handling crises, I never seem to get anything else done.	☐	☐
4.	At times I feel almost totally overwhelmed by time deadlines.	☐	☐
5.	I try to do everything myself.	☐	☐
6.	Usually I say yes to requests or demands made by others.	☐	☐
7.	I feel guilty if I'm not busy all the time.	☐	☐
8.	I rarely set priorities for my activities.	☐	☐
9.	I spend a lot of effort making every minute count.	☐	☐
10.	It really annoys me to see other people wasting time.	☐	☐

If you answered yes to the majority of the questions, you are displaying attitudes typical of a Type A personality. For each of the preceding questions, ask yourself, "Why did I answer yes or why did I answer no?" This will give you clues about your overall attitude concerning time. We develop lifestyle habits regarding time. Most people don't consider how or why they follow a certain routine, nor do they assess their attitude toward time and its value. If time is a stressor for you now, it probably will become a much greater source of stress during college unless you develop a workable time management program.

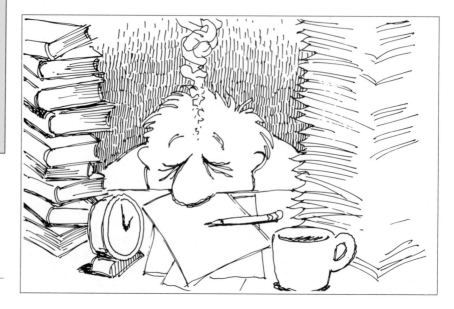

Developing Your Own Time Management Program

The one major characteristic that distinguishes a person who succeeds in getting things done from one who doesn't is time management. It is important to know, however, that while time management is a skill and a specific activity that can help you get things done, it is only a vehicle. Indeed, time management is the car; the motor is goals. If you want to get good grades, be involved in extracurricular activities, and have a fulfilling personal and social life, you need to do more than simply write down certain activities at certain times on a piece of paper. Perhaps you have tried that before, with the best of intentions, and wondered why those activities still didn't get done. The act of managing your time depends on a very important first step—setting specific and personal goals.

Setting Goals

The motor that students need to successfully drive their time management vehicle is a solid set of well-thought-out and consistently reviewed goals. **Good time managers are good goal setters.**

So the very important first step in managing your time is to set some goals. There are lots of ways of thinking about and establishing goals, but the easiest way is to start from scratch. It is crucial that you define your own goals, not objectives influenced by expectations of parents, siblings, peers, or others. First, define *your* overall goal in attending college. Then, list four or five goals that you can set for the current academic year.

This goal-setting exercise may have been easy or difficult, depending on how much you have already thought about why you are in college and what you intend to get out of it. The important point to remember is that you won't be as likely to achieve or accomplish very much if you don't have a clear idea what it is you want to achieve or accomplish. Your college education is like a ship. It requires a rudder and a port of destination. Otherwise, it will drift aimlessly and be captive to any wind or storm that comes along.

Having written some goals, the second important step in goal setting is to evaluate them. Use this guide to make sure your goals are adequate and helpful. And, by all means, change your goals when necessary to make them help you be a better time manager.

List your goals in order of importance. Clearly, your academic goals should be first. If they aren't and you are unwilling to change them, talk to friends, family, deans, counselors, and instructors about your college and life goals.

Make your goals as concrete as possible. It is hard to work toward your objectives when they are vague, or to know if you have achieved them. Intangible goals, such as "to be a good person" or "to do well academically," are certainly a good place to begin, but translate them into more specific,

Managing Your Time

1. Assess your attitude about time and analyze how you now utilize it.
2. Determine the parts of your schedule you can control and the ones you can't.
3. Define your goals and establish priorities that match your personal aspirations.
4. Plan the important segments of your life to make efficient use of your time and energy.
5. Neutralize time-wasting activities that threaten to undermine your program.
6. Monitor your progress, reevaluate your goals, and modify your program.

Time Management

CHAPTER 6

measurable goals. "Become the school newspaper editor" and "achieve a B average in all my courses" are more specific, and you'll clearly know whether or not you are achieving or have achieved them.

Set realistic goals.　Think seriously about what you really are capable of doing. Set targets that will challenge but not defeat you. If you know that you are not a good science student, rethink your goal of being a doctor. Many other rewarding careers in the health care professions do not require as many years of rigorous scientific learning.

Choose goals that reflect a balance between academic and personal life.　If your academic goals are at the top of the list (where they should be as long as you are in college), your other goals should include extracurricular activities, physical fitness, hobbies, clubs, personal time, and so forth.

Include both short-term and long-term goals.　Simply put, your very specific short-term goals help you to accomplish your specific long-term goals. For example, the short-term goal of achieving a B average in the fall semester will help you achieve your long-term goal of having a B+ average when you graduate next year.

Failing to plan is planning to fail.

Here are some examples of specific goals a college student might have.

Example A:　Goals for Fall Semester

1. Obtain a B in every course (B+ average by the end of the year)
2. Hand all papers in on time
3. Join debating club
4. Begin to learn how to play the guitar
5. Write one letter to a friend every week

Example B:　Goals for Spring Term

1. Attend almost every class and complete all reading assignments on time
2. Pick a major by the end of the term
3. Exercise Monday, Wednesday, Friday (run or lift weights)
4. Read for pleasure several hours every week (before dinner or on weekends)
5. Volunteer as a student health counselor

Setting goals should not be a one-time activity. At the very least, review your goals every month. You may find that once you are on your way to achieving your objectives, some become more important or you develop new ones. As long as you are a student, however, learning and doing well academically should be your primary and most important goal.

Managing Your Time to Achieve Your Goals

Once you have established goals, learning how to manage your time becomes a step-by-step process.

Developing Your Term and Weekly Schedules   Making a graphic representation of your time is an essential step in successfully managing your time. You need to see your plans and commitments on paper, prominently posted on your wall or in your notebook. Good time managers commit their schedules to paper; they don't depend on having them in their heads.

Two types of master schedules are helpful. The first is a **year or term calendar** that represents the whole academic year or at least the entire semester or quarter. The bigger the calendar the better! Large wall or desk blotter calendars are available at most bookstores. They are also easy to make. Post one on your wall, near your desk or bureau. Make a point of looking at it once or twice a day to keep track of how much time you have before the next major event. Don't fill this schedule with too many items, just the most important ones, especially those related to your academic goals. Then, in one glance, you can see and keep track of important events such as:

First and last day of classes

Quizzes, exams and projects

Term papers and other assignments

Holidays and vacations

The second type of master schedule is the **weekly master schedule**. Use the accompanying model to create a weekly master schedule that fits the classroom hour system your college uses. Create your weekly master schedule by recording only those structured or required events that occur every week, for example, classes, labs, meals, exercise or sports, extra-curricular activities, meetings.

Perhaps the most important reason for creating a weekly master schedule is that it quickly reveals where your available time is during the week. Most students know intuitively that there is usually quite a bit of free time in the evening after dinner, and that is when they tend to study. But many students don't realize, until they make a master weekly schedule, where else they have available and valuable time—in the afternoon, in the morning, and between classes. The good time manager makes use of these other times to study, learn and write papers.

Having created a master weekly schedule for the semester, make several copies—one for each week. Post the original on your bulletin board, by your desk or bureau, or on the outside of your notebook. Place it in some prominent place so it can serve as a constant reminder that (1) you do have time available to you and (2) where that available time is each day.

> **Even if you're on the right track, you'll get run over if you just sit there.**
>
> Will Rogers

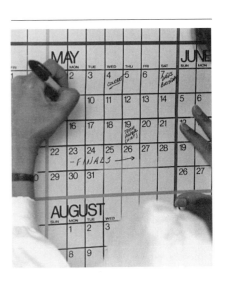

115

Weekly Planning Worksheet

FALL QUARTER

Time	Monday	Tuesday	Wednesday	Thursday	Friday	Saturday	Sunday
9:00	Calc.		Calc.		Calc.		
10:00	Am. Lit.		Am. Lit.		Am. Lit.		
11:00	Hist.	Hist.	Hist.	Hist.			
1:15 – 2:45		French ↓		French ↓			
3:00		Am. Lit. section ↓					
Evening							
Telephone Calls							
Errands							

Time	Monday	Tuesday	Wednesday	Thursday	Friday	Saturday	Sunday
9:00	Calc.	review for quiz ↓	Calc.	8:00 Run w/ Jack	Calc.	clean room	Church
10:00	Am. Lit.		Am. Lit.		Am. Lit. (paper due)		
11:00	Hist.	Hist. (QUIZ)	Hist.	Hist.		Study	Brunch w/ Mary
1:15 – 2:45	Prep. for section	French	French Lang. Lab	French	(run errands)	Football Game	
3:00	Am. Lit. section	Meet w/ calc. T.A.		Finish Am Lit paper			Study ↓
4:00			I.M. V'ball		I.M. V'ball	Dorm Party	
Evening	Study @ Library	Am. Lit paper	Study (in room) 10 pm. Hall Study Break	↓	Movie		(Break for dinner)
Telephone Calls	Dr. Porter 964·3731 (contact lenses ready?)		Jack (running Thurs.)				Eve. Parents
Errands		Pick up contacts (Late aft.)	Bookstore	NONE– paper due Fri.	Make advisor appt. for next week		Laundry!

Working for Success

The secret of success is the constancy of purpose.

Benjamin Disraeli, 1804–1881

Accomplishing your academic goals requires that you define long-term goals and back them up with shorter range, down-to-earth objectives. A key resource that you need to manage efficiently is your time. Nearly all successful people, regardless of their chosen career, emphasize the importance of setting goals and of effectively using one's time when striving for them. Attitude is a very important success factor because a positive attitude gives you more enthusiasm and energy to continue working in the face of obstacles.

How do you work for success in a college environment which is characterized by competition and stress? First, analyze your classroom and study experience and take responsibility for your choices, decisions, and lifestyle habits. Use your energy to determine *how* you will accomplish each task. Visualize yourself as succeeding by completing each specific step along the way to finishing the whole task.

- *Unwavering commitment to success.* Be consistent in your thoughts about your ability to succeed. Thinking about possible events that could prevent achievement will drain energy that can be more effectively used to create the results you desire.

  You may find it helpful to write down your goals and planned activities on a file card and keep the card where you can often review your pathway to success. A study of the most successful CEO's of major corporations revealed that the majority of these successful leaders had their personal goals written down—specifically—and often referred to them during hectic times that required major executive decisions. Reinforce your commitment to success by thinking specifically about what you must do to stay on target.

- *Unfaltering concentration on essentials.* Do you feel overwhelmed by the many requirements that place demands on your time? Term papers, midterm exams, write-ups for laboratory courses, and oral reports are often all due within a short time period. Professors seldom change due dates. Success in completing the required work rests on your ability to alter the way you think about the large amount of work and devise your study strategies accordingly. Success can be more easily accomplished by focusing on one requirement to the exclusion of all the others. Isolate each job. Even if you focus on one topic or assignment for a period of several hours, you will have completed a specific target assignment. Create one success for yourself and you will exert more control over your work and be better able to create further successes.

  Success is built on making very careful choices. For example, treat your highlight marker as if you will own only that one during your entire college experience. Be very particular about the content of a book that you think is worthy of the color of that pen and give yourself the advantage of needing to review only the essentials, the bare framework of information.

- *Teaming up for success.* Athletes in team sports and their coaches know the power that comes with mutual effort and support when working for success. You can use strategies similar to those used in sports for academic success. You might find other students in a particular class who are interested in a commitment to success and arrange to work together as a study group. Responsibility for large amounts of assigned readings might be divided, with each student taking responsibility for outlining a section and teaching the other members of the study group. Actively practice complimenting members of the group for work well done and for achievements earned as the result of working together. You will feel good sharing your success and sharing in the success of others with whom you work.

So much of college stress is based on a perceived lack of time, especially if you work while attending school. Time management techniques can help you maximize your time, relieve considerable stress, and achieve your personal goals.

Lida Chase, PhD

Each weekend, plan the upcoming week by filling in a new copy of your weekly master schedule. You already have the structured weekly events listed on it (classes, labs, and so forth). Decide specifically when you are going to do the things that will help you accomplish your goals. Fill in the open time slots to plan your day-by-day activities for the next week.

Another helpful time management tool is a small (3¼″ × 5″) spiral notebook. Easily carried in a pocket, purse or backpack, this notebook contains your running list of errands, phone calls, items to purchase, and other "things to do today." Blank pages become convenient space for need-to-remember phone numbers and paper on which you can give your phone number to someone else.

How to Make Good Use of Your Time

- As a helpful general rule, schedule some time for study on every one of your classes every day or every other day. If the course is difficult (math, language, physics), spend at least an hour on it every day. Research on learning has shown that more learning occurs when a student studies one hour every day for five straight days rather than eight hours all on Saturday or Sunday. The human mind processes more efficiently and retains information longer if it is exposed to information in regular periods of time (one to two hours) instead of in one cramming session.

- Use the time (even five to ten minutes) between classes to review for the next class, or go over the notes you just took. Many students don't realize that a lot of learning can occur in five to fifteen minutes.

- Make every attempt to do some studying before going to dinner. A good idea is to study your most difficult or demanding course during the day. Daylight hours are generally more productive than evening hours for most students. Also, you will be more motivated to work on your other courses because you have your most difficult course already completed.

- Do your reading either during the day or early in the evening. Academic reading should not be seen as a relaxing activity, done on your bed or in an easy chair. Rather, effective and efficient textbook reading should be an intense activity. Good readers concentrate on pulling out and recording the key ideas, facts and organization.

- Schedule regular review of your class notes and reading assignments. Regularly reviewing your notes and readings is the most powerful way to learn, especially if you practice reciting the facts or explaining the concepts out loud. Devote some portion (five to twenty minutes) of each study period reviewing previous notes and readings. Regular review throughout the term is the best method of exam preparation.

- Schedule hourly breaks when reading, taking notes or writing. When memorizing facts, formulas or other detailed materials, breaks should be at half-hour intervals. Between subjects, take a complete five-to-ten minute break. Movement such as stretching and walking is helpful dur-

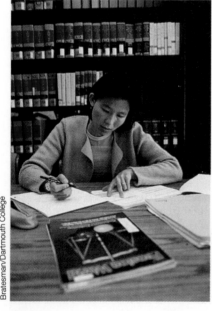

ing such breaks. This will release tension that has built up in your body and will allow your mind to make the transition from one subject to another.

Here are some additional tips for developing an effective weekly schedule:

- Eat breakfast every day. This simple activity puts some structure into your day and gets you ready for the day ahead. Rolling out of bed and walking sleepily into class on an empty stomach is not conducive to learning. Breakfast is a valuable meal for sustaining energy throughout the day. Also, breakfast time can be spent planning your day and the tasks you want to accomplish.
- Establish a regular sleep schedule. Research shows that the body has an internal clock. If you go to bed and wake up at regular times, you set that internal clock and your sleep will be more restful, allowing you to be more awake and alert the next day. Also, know how much sleep you, as an individual, need. Some students need to sleep eight hours, others only six.
- Schedule some kind of active exercise at least three times a week. Running, aerobics, swimming, weight lifting, tennis, squash, and walking are all good forms of exercise. Regular exercise structures your day and week. You can plan to study before and after exercise. Exercise not only

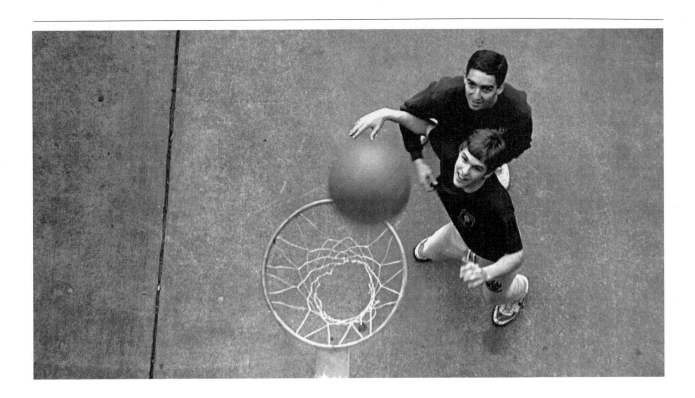

keeps you in good physical shape but also builds your self-esteem and helps you to concentrate and learn.

- Schedule some time just for yourself every day or on some regular basis. This time can be used to relax, visit with friends, do laundry, go shopping, write letters, listen to music, watch TV, take a nap.
- Learn to say no. Saying no to requests and invitations is very difficult, but you can't do everything—for yourself, much less for your friends and classmates. Your specific short- and long-term goals can help you decide when to say yes and when to say no. It sounds selfish, but your goals should come first. On the other hand, managing your time effectively can help you find more time to help and be with others.

Effective planning is both flexible and continuous. As assignments and social schedules change, adjust your plans accordingly. One assignment may take less time than you predicted, while another one involves more time-consuming research than you imagined. Your weekly plan will help you develop a routine of predictable blocks of study time. Two open periods three mornings per week may present ideal library research or study sessions. As the week advances, monitor your progress and results. Modify your plans accordingly. Toward the week's end, begin listing special events or important deadlines that will come up next week.

Estimating Your Peak Load Periods

Since each quarter or semester builds momentum toward mid-terms and final exams, expect two peak demands on your time. Plan your time and start on your assigned material early in the term. You will minimize the last minute all-nighters and reduce some of the stress on your body caused by pressure and fatigue. And, as research has documented, your study efficiency and recall skills diminish as the fatigue factor increases.

A major task is to estimate how much of each course's reading you can realistically cover and how much time your papers will require for research, organization and drafting. By starting with your deadlines and working backwards, you can arrive at the strategic point for starting each critical project. At first, you will experience some difficulty estimating how much time is required for certain tasks such as reading, research and writing. Your high school experiences will be helpful, but the complexity and amount of reading in college may stagger you at first.

By keeping track of your reading speed on both complex and straightforward material, you will be able to estimate hours required on future assignments. Few college students are able to complete all assigned readings. As you develop the technique of surveying and highlighting required readings, your efficiency will increase. Professors and TA's often give clues regarding what is essential to read. Lecture content may repeat material in a certain textbook. By taking complete lecture notes, you may be able to skim the textbook and allocate the time you saved to other more demanding assignments.

There is no way to save time. All you can do is spend time.

Where You Study Is Important, Too

One final important point about time management is where you study. For most students, the residence hall, dorm, home, fraternity, or sorority is the worst place to study, especially in the evening. Any or all of the following will disrupt and interfere with learning: phone, TV, stereo, bed, magazines, noisy roommates, and friends.

The best place to study is some place where it is quiet and free from distractions, not the local coffee house. Your concentration, motivation and efficiency will increase. In other words, more work will get done in less time. Locate a comfortable study place in the main library, an empty classroom, a departmental library, or any other location that provides uninterrupted and quiet surroundings. Be creative; spend some time searching out a special and convenient study site. Once you have found it, go there consistently. You can actually increase your ability to study by going to one place that is only for studying, whether it's for half an hour or for three hours.

Wasting Time: It's Easy, Fun and Devastating

Everyone knows how to waste time. It's easy and fun, but wasted time can neutralize all the time you gain through planning and conscientious follow-up. It is common to blame someone or something outside of yourself as the cause of your wasted time. Check off the "self-generated" versus the "external" time wasters that you've experienced lately. You may surprise yourself.

> **The best laid plans of mice and men are often led astray.**
> **Robert Burns**

Self-Generated Time Wasters
- ☐ Lack of organization
- ☐ Procrastination
- ☐ Inability to say no
- ☐ Lack of interest
- ☐ Fatigue
- ☐ Idle socializing
- ☐ Unnecessary perfectionism

External Time Wasters
- ☐ Unexpected visitors
- ☐ Telephone calls
- ☐ Waiting for someone
- ☐ Excessive noise
- ☐ Waiting in lines
- ☐ Traffic/parking congestion

Self-Generated Time Wasters

A few thoughts about self-generated time wasters will help focus your attention on easily overlooked common causes, and how to solve them.

Lack of Organization With many books, lecture notes, assignment sheets, syllabi, and so forth to keep track of in relatively little workspace, it's a wonder that the average student ever finds anything. However, close monitoring of your assignments, classroom and reading notes,

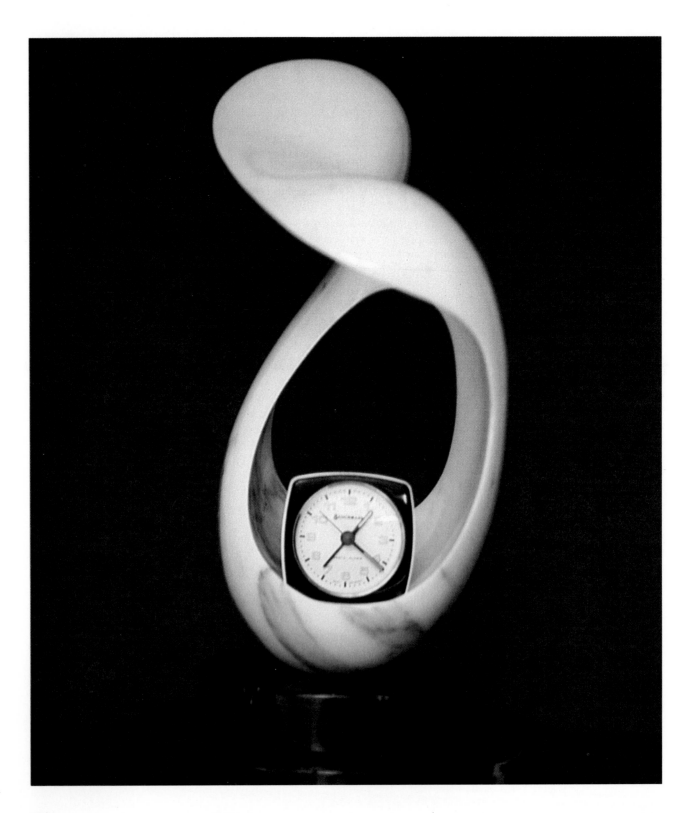

calendar, and books (purchased and borrowed) is essential. Setting up a filing system may sound alien, but it will prove to be a major time saver. A well-organized workspace helps you focus on your studies with minimal distraction. Keep your master calendar for the term and your weekly calendar within sight.

Procrastination   This is *not* the same as meditation. Meditation can be a technique for relaxation, while procrastination is closer to a form of vegetation. Procrastination often is the response to tasks that are boring, unpleasant or too difficult. For some students procrastination becomes a way of life with an endless stream of diversions and excuses. How do you deal with this dilemma?

- Set deadlines for yourself. Complete a reading assignment by a certain date; rough draft by another date.
- Divide a project into subtasks: research, outline, rough draft, final draft.
- Establish a series of rewards. Work for so many hours, then go for a short walk, have a snack.
- Start early and try to get the most burdensome aspects out of the way first.

Inability to Say No   College life offers many activities day and night. There's someone ready to attend any event, or if things are dull, to create an event. People who go along are always asked. Friends who do favors are targets for more requests. You can gracefully decline when your priorities commit you to study. Your true friends will respect your priorities and leave you alone.

Lack of Interest   It is difficult to concentrate on subjects or assignments that do not interest you. The actual course may not match the course catalog description, or the professor may prove to be less than entertaining. Changing or dropping a course can reduce your boredom and reduce your losses. Perhaps you can find another subject that fulfills the same prerequisite. If the course is an absolute prerequisite, you may have no alternative.

Idle Socializing   Developing social relationships is one of college life's most valuable and interesting rewards. However, idle socializing is a time waster when you allow it to interrupt your concentrated study. You may have sufficient self-discipline to continue with your work, but others may approach you for conversation. Develop the knack for rejecting social invitations during study periods unless you are ready for a break. Then socializing becomes a helpful method of relaxation.

Unnecessary Perfectionism   After investing many sessions into writing a paper, you may want to make it even better. You've studied for an exam but feel that you should put in more time. Revising, retyping and continued study might enhance your project slightly, but perfectionism di-

> **You can't escape the responsibility of tomorrow by evading it today.**
>
> Abraham Lincoln

verts you from other tasks and deadlines. If you are dealing with concurrent deadlines, you may jeopardize your overall results by concentrating too much time and energy on perfecting only one project.

External Time Wasters

Visitors   Study in your room? Study in the library? Where can you hide without visitors? Someone is always willing to talk and invite you to interrupt your work. After you tactfully decline, frequent visitors will call on others who are more receptive to interruptions. Perhaps you can suggest another time for getting together.

Telephone Calls   While studying in your room, you can repel visitors, but avoiding phone interruptions is more difficult. Unplugging the phone or using an answering device are two alternatives. When you receive an interruptive phone call, explain your situation and offer to call back later.

Waiting   College life involves waiting—for professors, friends, meals, tickets, and so forth. You can minimize the time-wasting effects of waiting by planning to "beat the rush," carrying light reading, or using the phone when a personal appearance is unnecessary. Sometimes you can trade off with roommates or friends to run errands for each other.

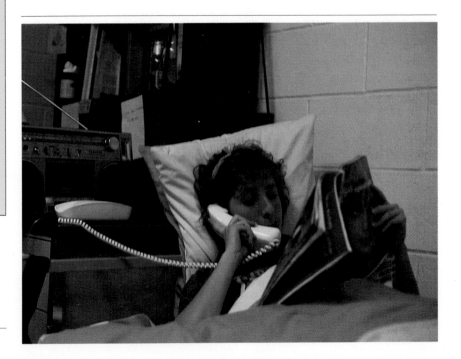

Unproductive Study Sessions with Others   Some courses involve group discussions, case histories, or team reports. To make the most of such interactions, all members of the group should be on time and prepared for a given session. Peer pressure pays dividends in these situations when the majority are truly motivated to accomplish something positive. If you conclude there's no hope for tangible progress, get a group consensus that the meeting is futile and schedule another session.

Space Management

Managing your space is nearly as important as managing your time. Though you may accomplish much of your studying at a library, study lounge, or computer center, you still need a space in your room that serves as your work center. A well-lit writing surface and appropriate chair are essential. Good posture and lighting can minimize the physical stress caused by prolonged study periods. Your work area should include space for storing your textbooks, notebooks and references (dictionary, thesaurus). Being unable to find the book you need wastes precious time. If you use a personal computer, you need additional space for printer paper as well as the monitor, keyboard, disk drive, and printer. Your study supplies (note paper, pens, pencils, highlighters, calculator, and so forth) should be stored in predictable locations so they are readily available.

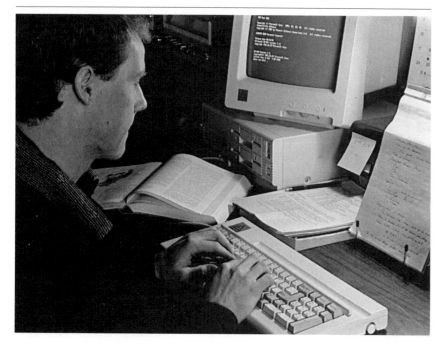

Time Management

Beyond the Text

1. At your parents' request, you joined the French Club, and at your friend's request you joined the soccer team. You also got a part in a play and a D on your midterm in geology, your major. What do you do?

2. You have an important test the next day, but your boyfriend is insisting you go to the basketball game with him. What do you do?

3. "I never have enough time" is a common complaint from college students. What steps can you take to "gain" time when there are only 24 hours in the day?

4. What is the difference between wasting time and taking time for personal relaxation?

5. Suggest strategies that you can use to balance competing demands on your time?

6. Many very successful individuals write down their goals, refer to them often, and revise them periodically. Define four or five goals for yourself that are ralistic and can be achieved within six months.

Supplemental Readings

How to Get Control of Your Time and Your Life by Alan Lakein. New York: Signet, 1973. A classic step-by-step orientation to time management.

Make the Most of Your Mind by Tony Buzan. New York: Linden Press, 1984. Introduction to memory enhancement, speed reading, numerical skill, creativity, and analysis.

Manage Your Time, Manage Your Work, Manage Yourself by Mervill Douglass and Donna Douglass. New York: American Management Association, 1980. Describes how time management is really self-management; topics include time and personality, clarifying your objectives, and eliminating time wasters.

Personal Time Management by Marion E. Haynes. Los Altos, CA: Crisp Publishing, 1987. Describes how to deal with the dilemma of limited time by sorting out the important from the urgent; a concise, practical presentation with worksheets.

Student Success Secrets by Eric Jensen. New York: Barron's Educational Series, Inc., 1982. Presents study skills, test-taking strategies, and reading and writing techniques to assist the reader to develop positive habits and achieve academic success.

Key Terms Defined

brinksmanship practice of creating the impression that one is willing and able to pass the brink (edge of a cliff) of total warfare rather than concede

circadian rhythm regular recurrence of biological activities within cycles of approximately 24 hours

maladaptive response reaction in which one fails to adapt to the situation; an inappropriate reaction

perfectionism disposition to regard anything short of perfection as unacceptable

procrastination to intentionally put off things that need to be done

time management process of planning and carrying out one's activities in relation to available time, tasks to be performed, and prearranged deadlines

Type A personality characterized by impatient, aggressive, and fast-paced lifestyle; associated with heart disease

Type B personality characterized by patient, unhurried, relaxed attitude

126

Nutrition Awareness

Your eating habits affect almost every aspect of your life: appearance, energy, stamina, resistance to illness, mental outlook, stress level, susceptibility to substance abuse, even academic and social success. The relationship between what you eat and your health and behavior is so subtle that you may be overlooking connections that could change your life for the better.

Healthy eating is a choice, but in order to make good choices you need the right information. Understanding nutrition, the science of food, can help you learn how to eat for maximum health. This chapter examines the nutritional value of food, explains how the body converts the food you eat, and teaches you how to recognize and respond to the full range of eating choices you encounter at college. In addition, this chapter gives you practical advice on how to design and carry out your own plan for healthy eating—in any setting.

Key Terms

Additive

Basal metabolic rate

Carbohydrate

Cholesterol

Complementary proteins

Complete proteins

Complex carbohydrates

Fat

Glucose

High-density lipoproteins

Insulin

Low-density lipoproteins

Nutrient

Nutrition

Protein

Contents

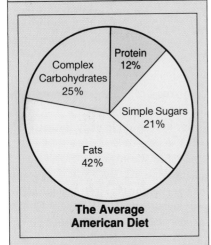

**The Average
American Diet**

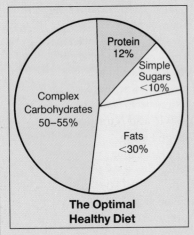

**The Optimal
Healthy Diet**

Understanding Healthy Eating

Nutrition is the science that deals with food. Food furnishes your body with chemical substances called nutrients, essential for life. These nutrients are necessary for building, repairing and maintaining cells and body tissues, regulating body processes, and providing energy. We all must eat a certain amount of essential nutrients for survival. And, while we all require the same nutrients, we do so in varying amounts. For example, the larger you are, the more nutrients your body needs. Children need more energy than their size would indicate, because they are growing. The elderly require less energy because they are more sedentary.

The energy in food is measured by calories. A food calorie is the amount of energy required to raise the temperature of 1,000 grams of water one degree Celsius.

The sources of energy or calories in the diet are carbohydrates (four calories per gram of CHO), proteins (also four calories per gram of protein), and fats (more than double, at nine calories per gram of fat). The only other substance that is a source of calories is alcohol, providing seven calories per gram. Nutrients are comprised of carbohydrates, proteins, and fats as well as vitamins and minerals. Water, while not directly a nutrient, is necessary for life.

If your diet is typical, 40 percent of your calories come from fat; 45 percent are from carbohydrates (of which only 6 percent are from complex, unrefined carbohydrates); and 15 percent are from protein. Compare the average American diet on the accompanying chart to the Optimal Healthy Diet.

Carbohydrates—A Part of Life That Should Be "Complex"

Carbohydrates, the starches and sugars in food, are your chief source of energy. As your body metabolizes carbohydrates, it forms glucose. Glucose is measured in the body as blood sugar and is "burned" as fuel by the tissues. Some glucose is converted to glycogen and stored by the liver for later use.

The primary types of carbohydrates are simple and complex. Simple sugars include cane and beet sugar (what we usually think of as table sugar), dextrose (often listed on packaged foods), and the sugars found in fruits and in milk. Fruit and milk are healthier sources of simple sugars than are the other items, because fruit and milk also contain essential vitamins and minerals, and fruit contains fiber.

Starches are complex carbohydrates, so called because of their more elaborate chemical structures. Complex carbohydrates include bread, pasta, potatoes, rice, grains, breakfast cereals, and beans.

Jean Flatt, of the University of Massachusetts Medical School, has been studying carbohydrates and their conversion to fat. He and his co-workers suggest that our bodies are reluctant to convert carbohydrates to fat. He fed healthy young people 2,800 calories (700 grams of carbohy-

Good Food and What It Does

Protein	*Health maintenance*: Build and repair tissue, help with body growth, maintain immune system, provide zinc and iron 2 servings	Beef, chicken, pork, fish, eggs, legumes, beans (including tofu), nuts
Complex Carbohydrates 	*Energy*: Provide energy for activity, thinking, normal bodily functions 6 servings	Grains (wheat, corn, rice, millet, oats; often in products like bread, cereal, pasta), beans, potatoes, nuts
Fruits and Vegetables	*Protective*: Provide vitamins and minerals for bone growth, brain function, operation of other bodily systems 5 servings	Apples, bananas, oranges, pears, broccoli, green beans, carrots, lettuce, tomatoes, spinach
Dairy Products	*Bone maintenance*: Provide calcium and Vitamin D 2 servings	Skim and low-fat milk, reduced-fat cheese, cottage cheese, ricotta cheese, yogurt

drates) and the whole amount "was accommodated as glycogen (carbohydrate) storage." Thus, he concluded, only when you eat massive amounts of carbohydrates will they convert to fat. The more carbohydrates you eat, the more you burn, and the more you store.

Keep in mind when you are planning or evaluating your diet that refined carbohydrates (white bread, cookies, cake, candy, and so forth) are really not healthy; for example, when wheat is turned into white flour, up to 80 percent of its trace nutrients are lost. "Enrichment" may replace some of the vitamins and minerals, but not all—and not the fiber. Why choose complex carbohydrates? They are an important source of nutrients, fiber, and calories.

Nutritional Value Complex carbohydrates are more likely to be found in foods with more protein, vitamins and minerals than are simple carbohydrates.

Fiber Complex carbohydrates are more often found in foods that provide significant amounts of fiber. Fiber aids in digestion, may protect you against disease, and may even help you lose weight.

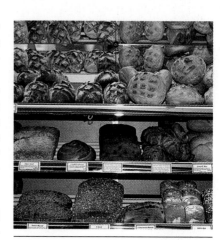

Nutrition Awareness

CHAPTER 7

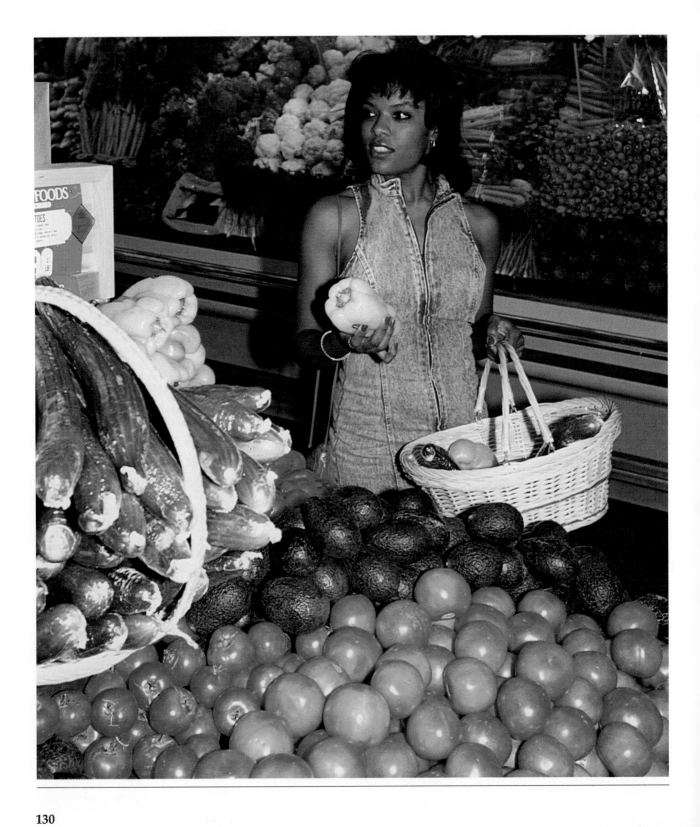

Calories Complex carbohydrate foods contain a lower concentration of sugars and fat; thus, they do not provide more calories than you need. When your system does not burn as fuel all available calories, your body stores the excess as fat.

Too few carbohydrates may lead to fatigue, depression and a breakdown of body protein for energy. On the other hand, ingesting too many carbohydrates does not leave you room for foods that contain other nutrients necessary for health. The Select Subcommittee on Nutrition and Human Needs of the U.S. Senate recommends that you get about 55 to 60 percent of your calories from complex carbohydrates. This means that at least half of every meal and snack should be complex carbohydrate foods. While Americans already eat a lot of complex carbohydrates (for example, the average American eats 15 pounds of cereal every year), we just do not eat enough.

A few tips for getting the most health and enjoyment out of carbohydrates:

- Choose whole grain breads instead of white, enriched grain products. Remember, enriching the flour does not restore valuable minerals and vitamins, or fiber.
- Reduce or eliminate your use of high-fat condiments with your carbohydrates. This includes butter, margarine, sour cream, cream sauces, most salad dressings, and gravy. The carbohydrates themselves are low in calories; it is what you put on them that adds to your waistline.
- Reduce intake of simple sugars, alcohol, and other processed foods with high sugar content. They add no nutrients to your body, only calories. A cookie after a wholesome lunch is fine; cookies for lunch is not.

Fats Can Make You Fat

If you are watching your weight, you are probably trying to avoid sweets and starchy foods. But take a hard look at fatty foods, like hamburgers, french fries, and ice cream. They may be your dietary downfall. According to Jane Brody, nutrition writer for the *New York Times* and author of several health and nutrition books, "We could fully satisfy our nutritional requirement for fat by consuming the equivalent of one tablespoon of vegetable oil each day. But the average American consumes eight times that amount—the fat equivalent of one stick of butter a day—and in the process packs in a load of extra calories. . . . Fat makes a far greater contribution to the weight problems of Americans than does sugar." Fat contains more than twice as many calories for its weight as any other ingredient in a food. An ounce of fat has 255 calories; an ounce of protein has only 113. As you can see, ounce for ounce, fat has more than twice as many calories as lean meat.

Fat occurs in different forms, the most prevalent of which is triglycerides. Triglycerides, the chemical name for fats, appear in two forms, saturated and unsaturated fats. Most triglycerides contain more than one kind

Reduced-Calorie versus Low-Calorie

Reduced-calorie means the product must contain at least one-third fewer calories than a similar food that is not reduced, but it must be equal nutritionally to the food for which it is a substitute. **Low-calorie** means that the food contains no more than 40 calories per serving.

Fat Savings Chart

By making just a few shifts in food selections, you can considerably reduce the amount of fat you consume. Here are some suggestions.

In Place of . . .	Fat (Grams)	Substitute . . .	Fat (Grams)	You'll Save Fat (Grams)
Potato chips, 1 oz.	10	Pretzels	1	9
Peanuts, ¼ c.	18	Popcorn, plain, 1 cup	0	18
Wheat thins, 16	6	Ry-Krisp, 4½	0	6
Sausage pizza, ¼	17	Cheese pizza, ¼	4	13
Whole milk, 1 c.	8	Non-fat milk, 1 c.	0	8
Low-fat milk, 1 c.	5	Non-fat milk, 1 c.	0	5
Ice cream, vanilla, ½ c.	7	Ice milk, vanilla, ½ c.	2	5
Milk chocolate bar	10	Granola bar, cinnamon	4	6
Beef hot dog	13.5	Turkey hot dog	8	5.5
Chicken, 3 oz. dark with skin	13	Chicken, 3 oz. dark without skin	8	5
Tuna in oil, 3 oz. drained	10	Tuna in water, 3 oz. drained	1	9
Cream of mushroom soup, 10 oz.	11	Tomato soup, 10 oz.	2	9
Bologna, 2 oz.	17	Turkey breast, 2 oz.	2	15
Mayo (Hellman's) 1 Tb.	11	Spin Blend salad dressing (Hellman's) 1 Tb.	5	6
Italian dressing (Kraft) 1 Tb.	8	Italian dressing, reduced calorie (Kraft) 1 Tb.	0	8
Swiss cheese, 2 oz.	16	Swiss cheese, 1 oz.	8	8

Source: "Ferreting Fat from Your Diet," *Nutrition Action*

of fatty acid and most food fats are combinations of different triglycerides. Saturated fats, so named because they contain no double bonds between the carbon atoms, include any fat that becomes solid at room temperature. These fats (often called visible fats) include all animal fats, such as butter, fat on meat, lard, as well as palm and coconut oils and hydrogenated vegetable oils. Unsaturated fats are those that contain one, two, or more double bonds between carbon atoms. They are monounsaturated fatty acids, found in olive, peanut, cottonseed and avocado oils, or polyunsaturated fatty acids (PUFA) found in corn, soybean, safflower, sunflower, or flaxseed oils. PUFA's, containing two or more double bonds, are more susceptible to oxidation because the more double bonds a fatty acid contains, the quicker oxidation and spoilage occur. The food industry often will hydrogenate this type of fatty acid to prevent rancidity. Hydrogenation of PUFA may produce either monounsaturated or saturated fatty acids. Partially hydrogenated vegetable oil means that the product contains more saturated fat than if it were made with just plain vegetable oil. Fat modified products are not necessarily low-fat or low-calorie. Experts recommend that less than 10 percent of our fat allowance come from saturated fats, less than 10 percent come from polyunsaturated fats, and the remainder come from monounsaturated fats.

Cholesterol   Cholesterol is an essential compound in your body. It is a fat-like substance, a blood lipid, that your liver synthesizes in amounts sufficient to meet the body's demands. Cholesterol is a component of hormones and cell membranes and helps control their permeability. Animal products are the only food substances that naturally contain cholesterol. Cholesterol is often confused with saturated fats found not only in animal and dairy products, but also in vegetable sources such as coconut and palm oils. Although saturated fats do not contain cholesterol, they en-

"Fake Fats"

In January 1988, NutraSweet Company announced plans to market a low-calorie, low-cholesterol fat substitute, trade named Simplesse. The U.S. Food and Drug Administration is currently investigating the claims and safety of this product. NutraSweet claims that because Simplesse is made from egg white protein or milk protein, it is a natural product that does not require government approval.

Simplesse has 1.3 calories per gram, compared with 9 calories per gram of fat. Simplesse is designed for dairy desserts and salad dressings; Procter and Gamble has been working on a fake fat for frying and baking, tradenamed Olestra. If such products become available and you try them, follow these precautions: use them only in moderation, don't expect them to solve weight problems, and keep yourself informed about consumer and scientific reports on health issues related to these products.

Choose "Skinny Dips" to Decrease Party Fat Intake

	Calories	% Calories from Fat
Light cream cheese, 1 tbsp. instead of	30	75%
Cream cheese, 1 tbsp.	50	90%
Light sour cream, ¼ cup instead of	90	60%
Sour cream, ¼ cup	123	86%
Low-fat yogurt, ¼ cup instead of	35	22%
Yogurt, ¼ cup	58	36%

Saturated Fats and Cholesterol

Food	Saturated Fat (g)	Cholesterol (mg)
Hotdog	9.0	50
Beef Liver, 3 oz.	2.5	372
Bacon, 1 strip	0.9	5
Egg, 1 medium	2.0	253
Shellfish, 1 oz.	0.6	45
Cheese, 1 oz. cheddar	6.0	30
Chicken, 3 oz.	1.2	76
Salmon or Tuna, 2 oz.	1.4	—
Cottage Cheese (1% fat), 2 oz.	1.0	10
Coconut Oil, 1 tsp.	4.4	—
Mayonnaise, 1 tsp.	0.7	8
Safflower Oil, 1 tsp.	0.4	—
Butter, 1 tbsp.	7.1	31
Whole Milk, 1 cup	5.1	33
Skim Milk, 1 cup	0.3	4
Ice Cream, 4 oz.	5.0	43

Fat Intake for Children

Health experts all agree that children younger than age two should have no dietary restrictions (including fat) for the purpose of preventing heart disease. Older children can thrive on moderated fat intake. So, from age 2 to 92 we would all be healthier if we reduced our fat intake to 30 percent of our daily calories.

Source: *Tufts University Diet and Nutrition Letter*, April, 1989

hance the absorption of it into your blood stream. Saturated more than unsaturated fats increase this absorption process.

The medical and media groups have recently promoted diets low in cholesterol. While this is certainly healthy, it is important to be aware of all the facts. As far as is known, there is an indirect, not a direct, relationship between the cholesterol you eat and the amount of cholesterol that forms deposits along your arteries. For example, studies indicate if your diet is high in cholesterol (you eat great quantities of animal products), but you do not consume saturated fats, your blood cholesterol level may not be abnormally high. Additionally, studies indicate that dietary intake is only one of several factors influencing serum level of cholesterol. Other factors may influence whether your body retains or cleanses itself of excess cholesterol, such as physical exercise, Vitamin C intake, ingestion of rancid fats, whether cholesterol-containing foods are fresh or packaged, and the frequency of consumption of cholesterol-containing foods. For example, one study found that men who eat one egg every day experienced elevated cholesterol levels, but men who ate two eggs every other day did not.

Cholesterol is carried in the blood by three different lipoproteins, referred to as low-density lipoproteins (LDL), very low-density lipoproteins (VLDL), and high-density lipoproteins (HDL). Physicians speak of "good" and "bad" cholesterol. These labels refer to excess cholesterol that adheres to the walls of coronary arteries as LDLs or "bad cholesterol," and to the form of lipoproteins that pick up the excess cholesterol in the blood and carry it back to the liver for removal from the body as "good cholesterol" or HDLs. Currently, researchers are concluding that the ratio of HDLs to LDLs is the most important determinant in whether or not you develop coronary heart disease.

In 1989, the National Research Council reported evidence of a direct relationship between dietary fat intake and the risk of cardiovascular disease and certain types of cancer. In light of the latest research findings, public health educators recommend that Americans should eat less fat, especially saturated fats. The most common sources of saturated fat are cheese, milk, and animal meats. If intake of saturated fats is reduced, your cholesterol level will also decrease—but only if you reduce intake of animal products in your diet. Cholesterol-related health risks are a growing problem not only for the middle-aged and elderly, but also increasing numbers of young people in the United States are showing arterial cholesterol build-up. Even in your twenties, when you may feel too young to worry about such long-term effects of cholesterol as heart disease and cancer, it is important to have your cholesterol level checked. A serum cholesterol level of over 200 milligrams per deciliter (mg/dL), regardless of your age, indicates the need for some dietary alterations. This is especially applicable if you or family members have a history of heart disease or cancer. For a more technical discussion of the relationship of cholesterol to these diseases, refer to the chapter on **Cardiovascular Disease and Cancer**.

To be healthier today and limit your long-term risk of developing coronary heart disease, cancer, obesity, high blood pressure, and stroke by 20 percent

- Limit fats to 30 percent of your daily calories.
- Keep saturated fats to less than 10 percent of your daily calorie intake.
- Keep cholesterol below 300 mg daily intake (limit animal fats, eat low-fat dairy products, cut down on fried foods, pastries, egg yolks, cert shellfish, and organ meats).

Nutrition experts and medical researchers agree that our di be much healthier if we limited fat to between 25 and 30 perce calories—not much more than half the current American averag each tablespoon of fat contains 100 calories, all ready for your body to store very efficiently as fat.

Where is the fat in your diet? Most fat comes from protein foods—either directly from animal meat and dairy products, or from nuts and seeds. Pure fats are easy to see: butter, margarine, oil, mayonnaise. But according to the Department of Health and Human Services, only about 15 percent of fat intake comes from pure fat sources and other very fatty foods, such as bacon, cream cheese, and peanut butter. The USDA estimates

Great Cholesterol Fighters

Philadelphia agriculture department researchers, Peter Hoaglund and Philip Pfeffer, suggest we eat carrots if we want to lower our cholesterol level. They found that eating two medium-sized carrots a day for three weeks lowered blood cholesterol an average of 11 percent in healthy volunteers. Similar results were also found with broccoli, cabbage, onions, apples, grapefruit, and oats and bean fiber. The key ingredient appears to be calcium pectate which binds with bile acids to decrease cholesterol assimilated into the blood stream.

Source: *Staying Well Newsletter*, June, 1988.

Cholesterol Sources

Cholesterol is only found in animal products, but only one of every three

Nutrition Awareness

CHAPTER 7

135

that 40 percent of fat comes from meats. Dairy products such as milk, ice cream and cheese provide about 20 percent.

With that in mind, here are tips for limiting the fat you eat:

- Choose low-fat alternatives instead of high-fat foods, as shown on the accompanying Fat Savings chart.
- Choose low-fat protein foods, (water-packed tuna, low-fat cottage cheese) rather than red meat, dairy, or nuts.
- Eat fish and chicken more often instead of red meat. Avoid the skin of chicken (it is pure fat). When you do eat red meat, choose pieces with as little fat as possible and trim off the fat before cooking.
- Eat cheese (including cream cheese) only in small quantities and infrequently. Choose low-fat varieties of cheese, cream cheese, yogurt, and cottage cheese.
- Choose low-fat or nonfat milk instead of whole milk.
- Avoid fried foods and processed foods. If you do fry, use canola oil or olive oil.
- Use monounsaturated fats for salad dressings, sauteing, or cooking.
- Avoid or use less of the fatty condiments—butter, mayonnaise, sour cream, gravy. For example, instead of sour cream, use a combination of low-fat yogurt, cottage cheese, and lemon.
- Select sweet desserts only when you cannot resist them.
- Make careful selections when you are eating out. A Big Mac, french fries and milk shake contain 53 grams of fat, more than the fat intake recommended for many people for an entire day.

Protein—Getting the Right Amount and the Right Kinds

Protein is necessary for growth and repair of body tissues, including muscles, blood, skin, internal organs, hormones, and enzymes. Protein also becomes a source of energy when your diet lacks sufficient carbohydrates or fats, or when you eat more protein than your body needs.

A healthy body needs 22 amino acids; though your body synthesizes 13 of these naturally, you must obtain the remaining 9 through food intake. Foods that contain the essential amino acids—meats and dairy products—are known as complete proteins. Incomplete proteins—grains and vegetables—contain fewer than the essential nine. Various incomplete proteins can be combined to form complete proteins—rice and beans, for instance. If you eat a variety of vegetables, grains, and beans on the same day, your body will create complete proteins because we have internal reserves of amino acids.

Many Americans have been raised to believe that a meal is complete only if it has meat, cheese, or eggs—and dinner especially requires red meat, or at least fish or chicken. Today, we know that this is not necessary. However, to ensure your daily need for iron, zinc, and other minerals packaged in protein foods, it is recommended that you have two servings, 2 to 3 ounces each, of protein foods every day. It is best to mix and

What's in Fast Food?

Food Item	Calories	Fat (tsp)
Fish		
Whaler sandwich (Burger King)	540	5
Filet-o-Fish (McDonald's)	435	6
Potatoes		
Home fries (Wendy's)	360	5
Fries, regular (McDonald's)	220	3
Chicken		
Chicken sandwich, multi-grain bun (Wendy's)	320	2
Chicken McNuggets (6) (McDonald's)	323	5
Original Recipe (thigh) (Kentucky Fried Chicken)	257	4
Specialty chicken sandwich (Burger King)	690	10
Burgers		
Hamburger (McDonald's)	263	3
Hamburger (Burger King)	310	3
Cheeseburger (McDonald's)	318	4
Jumbo Jack (Jack-in-the-Box)	485	6
Big Mac (McDonald's)	570	8
Whopper w/cheese (Burger King)	760	10
Shakes		
Milk shake, average (McDonald's)	367	2
Shakes, regular size (Carl's Jr.)	490	2
Breakfast Items		
Egg McMuffin (McDonald's)	340	4
Sunrise sandwich w/bacon (Carl's Jr.)	410	5
Sausage McMuffin w/egg (McDonald's)	517	7
Sausage crescent (Jack-in-the-Box)	584	10

Source: Center for Science in the Public Interest

Protein Content of Selected Foods

The foods below are all good sources of protein. The listed protein amounts are averages. You can use these figures to estimate your normal protein intake. The RDA for protein for college-age men is 56 grams; for college-age women, 44 grams.

Food	Protein (grams)	Food	Protein (grams)
Dairy and Eggs		*Grains*	
Cottage cheese, ½ cup*	14.0	Whole-wheat flour, ½ cup	8.0
Milk, 1 cup*	8.5	Spaghetti, 1 cup cooked	6.0
Cheddar cheese, 1 oz.*	7.1	Bagel, 1	6.0
Egg, 1 medium	6.1	Cornmeal, ½ cup	5.5
Ice cream, ½ cup	2.4	Rice, brown, 1 cup cooked	5.0
		Rice, white, 1 cup cooked	4.0
Meat and Fish		Enriched bread, 1 slice	2.0
		Whole wheat bread, 1 slice	2.5
Tuna, canned, drained, 4 oz.	32.0		
Chicken, 4 oz. cooked	31.2	*Legumes*	
Hamburger, 4 oz. cooked	30.7	Soybeans, ½ cup cooked	12.0
Sirloin steak, 4 oz. cooked	26.7	Peanut butter, 1 oz.	7.1
		Cashews, 1 oz.	4.8

*Low-fat dairy products often contain added milk solids, which increase the protein content slightly.
Source: *UC Berkeley Wellness Letter*; with additional data from *Bowes and Church's Food Values of Portions Commonly Used*

match animal and vegetable protein foods, because animal protein intake is highly correlated with the intake of saturated fat. Dairy products will also provide you with protein and many other essential nutrients. But if your diet includes too much dairy and meat, you are probably consuming too much protein.

It is important to find a balance for your protein intake. The recommended daily allowance is 0.8 grams per kg of ideal body weight for adults. You should not exceed 1.6 grams per kg of weight (or double the suggested amount). This translates to a daily 5½-ounce hamburger for a 120-pound woman or an 8¼-ounce patty for a 180-pound man. Too little protein will not provide your body with the body-building nutrients it requires. Excess protein may burden your body in several ways. Most Americans get 12 to 15 percent of their calories from protein—they need 8 percent for health. Too much may cause stress on your liver and kidneys. Protein processing uses up some of your calcium reserves and can lead to dehydration, a particular problem with athletes who eat more steak than potatoes. Also, many animal protein sources have a high fat content so you may be eating much more fat (and the calories associated

Cutting Out the Fat in Protein

Very High-Fat Protein Sources (75% or more of calories from fat, unless noted)	Moderate- to High-Fat Protein Sources (30–40% of calories from fat)	Low-Fat Protein Sources (30% or fewer calories from fat)
Pork (including bacon and ham)	Chicken without skin	Fish, broiled
Regular hamburger	Pot roast	Beans
Cold cuts	Turkey, dark meat	Turkey, white meat
Cheese (50–75%); cream cheese	Yogurt, low fat	Cottage cheese, uncreamed
Hot dogs	Pizza	Tuna in water
Nuts and seeds	Granola	Shellfish

Source: *Jane Brody's Nutrition Book*

with fat) than you need. Check the examples of high-fat animal protein foods and low-fat alternatives in the accompanying box. To have an adequate protein intake without overdoing or underdoing, try one of the following approaches:

- Eat portions of animal protein about the size of your palm—two servings/day.
- Eat animal protein less often.
- Use the meat portion of your meals as a condiment rather than the main course. (Ethnic foods often feature this approach—such as oriental stir-fry dishes, Italian pasta sauces, and Mexican enchiladas and tacos.)
- Eat meatless (and cheeseless) meals a few times each week. Rice, beans, pasta, bread, and even many vegetables have plenty of protein if eaten in amounts and combinations appropriate for meeting other nutritional needs.

Eliminating most or all protein from your diet can be dangerous. Many young people today, especially females, cut down on protein as a way of losing weight or saving money. Protein deficiency affects your entire body—tissues, skin, and muscles, as well as body processes. Being protein-deficient impairs your ability to function, cope with stress, and fight infection. It may also lead to an inadequate intake of iron and zinc.

Vitamins and Minerals—Abundant in Fruits and Vegetables

Vitamins are organic food substances that have no caloric value and provide no energy; they are, however, essential in small amounts to convert food into energy for growth, maintenance, and the functioning of body processes. Vitamins are found only in living things—plants and animals—and usually cannot be synthesized by the human body. Vitamins D, K,

Sources of Protein in the American Diet

The latest USDA Nationwide Food Consumption Survey indicates that Americans obtain 40 percent of their protein from meats, poultry, and fish; 18 percent from dairy products; 4 percent from eggs; 18 percent from legumes and cereal products; and 7 to 8 percent from fruit and vegetables.

and some B vitamins are manufactured by the body but must also be obtained from food.

Minerals are inorganic substances, widely prevalent in nature and essential for metabolic processes. Major minerals include calcium, manganese, cobalt, zinc, and molybdenum. Minerals act as catalysts for major body processes, and their actions are interrelated. A deficiency in one mineral affects the action of others. It is essential to consume foods having adequate mineral values because a mineral deficiency can result in severe illness. However, excessive amounts of minerals can throw the body out of balance and create a deficiency of another mineral.

Your body's major sources of most vitamins and minerals are fruits and vegetables, meats and whole grains. Fruits and vegetables are also a good source of fiber, particularly raw vegetables and whole fruit (as opposed to juice). Fiber aids in digestion, weight management, and disease prevention. All fresh fruits and vegetables also provide water to help hydrate the body.

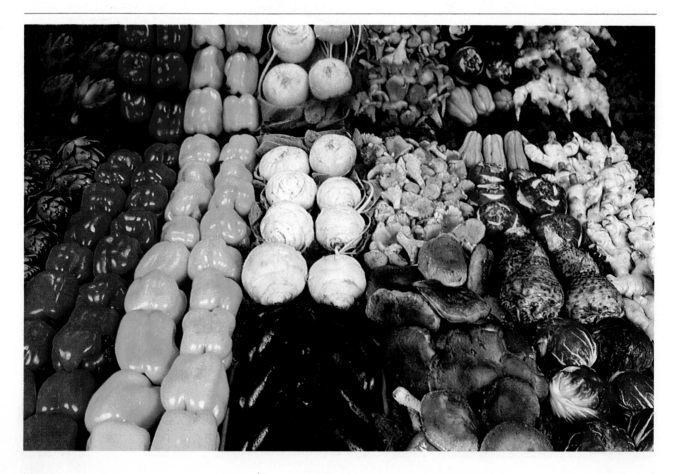

To get vitamins and minerals from fruits and vegetables, every day eat at least

- One citrus fruit or one serving of potato, tomato, broccoli, cauliflower, or strawberries.
- One fresh yellow vegetable or fruit and one green one, the darker in color the better.

Several nutritional studies reveal that over 60 percent of the U.S. population is deficient in one or more vitamins and minerals. Many people lack adequate Vitamin A and Vitamin C in their diets—exactly what you'll find in dark yellow and green fruits and vegetables. The carrots your parents encouraged you to eat are still good for you, but so are cantaloupes, apricots, strawberries, tomatoes, fresh spinach leaves, bell peppers, and asparagus.

Should You Take Vitamin or Mineral Supplements?

Vitamins and minerals are the tiny keys that allow your body to effectively use the protein, carbohydrates, fats, and other nutrients you consume. If you eat a well-balanced diet that includes plenty of whole foods (whole-grain breads, fresh fruits and vegetables), you're probably getting most of the vitamins and minerals you need. Eating well is the best way for your body to maintain its efficiency at extracting nutrients from what you eat.

Nutritionally, the most perfect foods are often home-grown, served fresh or lightly steamed. If you don't eat that way (and few college students do), you may want to take the time to plan your diet, shop at markets that carry organic produce, and balance the four food groups in your daily food intake.

An analysis of the diets of 212 college students who selected their meals from the four food groups revealed that a full two-thirds of them came up short of the RDA for Vitamin E, Vitamin B_6, iron, and zinc. Only two-thirds met the RDA for folate (a B vitamin) and magnesium.

In fact, Janet King, a professor at the University of California at Berkeley, analyzed foods in the American diet and concluded that an individual must eat 2,000 perfectly balanced calories per day to get the RDA for every vitamin and mineral. Probably not even many nutritionists manage that. Moreover, some nutrition experts consider the RDA low for many vitamins and minerals.

A well-balanced daily vitamin supplement can provide nutrients your diet lacks. Pills and capsules should not take the place of eating well—their purpose is to supplement your diet. Before taking any supplements, consult the chart at the end of this chapter, which lists dietary sources for each vitamin and mineral, recommended dosage ranges, and signs of deficiency or toxicity. As this chart details, certain vitamins and minerals can be harmful if taken in doses greater than your body can handle. If you do take vitamin or mineral supplements, take them with meals so that they

How to Be a Healthy Vegetarian

Ten or twenty years ago, most nutritionists felt that balancing vegetable proteins to achieve healthy nutrition was difficult. Health-conscious vegetarians tried to figure exactly the right number of tortillas to eat with the right amount of beans at every meal to make a balanced protein. Today, we understand that being a healthy vegetarian is much easier than that. The amount of protein required to maintain health is less than nutritionists had previously believed. Moreover, the protein resources of most plant-source foods is greater than researchers had earlier estimated.

If you eat several kinds of complex carbohydrates and vegetables at each meal, your body will be able to manufacture the complete proteins from the amino acids in the various foods. For instance, combine Mexican rice and beans with corn tortillas. Or have a glass of milk when you have peanut butter on whole wheat toast.

Many vegetarians eat large amounts of eggs and cheese. Because these foods contain high levels of cholesterol and fat, vegetarians should limit consumption of them. If you eat no animal products, including no eggs or dairy products, you will probably get insufficient Vitamin B_{12}; nutritional yeast or possibly supplements are essential in such cases.

The resources list for this chapter includes several excellent books with good vegetarian nutritional information (and recipes).

will act synergistically with the nutrients in your food. Here are a few additional notes on nutrients particularly relevant to college students.

Calcium   If you are a woman, an athlete, or both, you should be concerned about calcium. Your body can only build and maintain bones strong enough to resist osteoporosis and breakage if it has sufficient calcium.

Calcium supplements are appropriate for some women and athletes. They are usually not necessary if you eat well. If you consume dairy products, you're probably getting your daily requirement of 1,000 mg. (One-and-a-half ounces of cheddar cheese supplies about 315 mg.) Some people are allergic to milk, and many are unable to digest the lactose it contains. If you are lactose-intolerant, you may be able to substitute cultured milk products such as buttermilk, kefir, and yogurt. You don't have to drink milk to get the calcium you need, but this is one of the most efficient ways. (One cup of low-fat milk supplies 298 mg of calcium.) Include deep green, leafy vegetables, soybeans, and fish in your diet. See the chart on the calcium scoreboard.

To metabolize calcium, the body requires other minerals as well. If you chronically ingest excessive amounts of calcium, you may develop deficiencies of iron, zinc, and magnesium (as well as constipation). Be sure to include magnesium with your calcium supplements.

There are actions you *can* take to maximize your body's calcium intake. Limit your consumption of alcohol, caffeine and sugar. To assist in assimilation, take calcium supplements with vitamin C, and take calcium

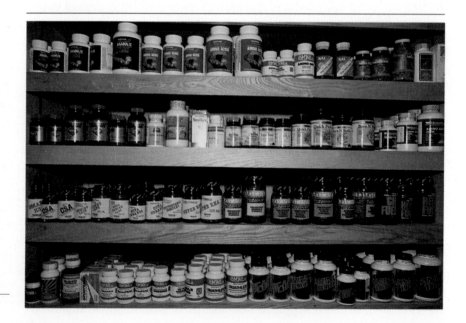

Sources of Calcium from the Calcium Cupboard

Food	Serving	Fat (g)	Calcium (mg)
Whole milk	1 cup	8.50	290
Skim milk	1 cup	.20	300
Low-fat milk	1 cup	2.60	298
Low-fat plain yogurt	1 cup	1.00	415
Frozen yogurt (2% fat)	1 cup	3.00	200
Ricotta cheese (part skim)	¼ cup	5.00	167
Low-fat cottage cheese	1 cup	4.00	160
Cheddar cheese	1 oz.	9.20	210
Tofu (calcium sulfate)	3½ oz.	4.20	139
Soy tempeh	3½ oz.	7.50	142
Shrimp	1 cup	3.00	147
Pinto beans, cooked	1 cup	1.00	130
Cornmeal tortillas	2	trace	120
Spinach, cooked	1 cup	0	86
Almonds	10 nuts	5.40	23
Garbanzo beans, raw	1 cup	9.60	300

Sources: USDA and *Laurel's Kitchen*

before going to bed. Studies show that you absorb one third more calcium when your body is resting.

Osteoporosis   Calcium deficiency can lead to osteoporosis, a loss of bone material that results in loss of bone mass. This porous bone condition afflicts 20 million Americans, the majority of whom are older women. Many factors appear to contribute to this disabling disease. Lack of exercise, especially in middle age, is one factor. A drop in estrogen due to menopause is another. Estrogen is the female sex hormone that is present from the time of menstruation to menopause. This hormone protects the system against bone loss. The body is constantly breaking down and rebuilding bone, but when a person has osteoporosis, the body cannot replace bone as fast as it is losing it. Women are especially at risk because of this drop in estrogen level. In addition, they increase the risk if they drink a lot of carbonated soft drinks because these sodas contain phosphoric acid, which carries away calcium in the urine. Women who smoke are also at risk. New findings indicate that female smokers exposed to cigarette smoke that contains cadmium have a significantly higher bone loss. While still young, it is unlikely that you will develop osteoporosis. But, as you age, if you smoke, if you do not replace the estrogen during

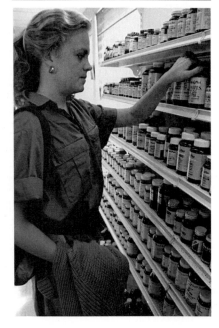

and after menopause, if you don't exercise regularly, and if you have been calcium-deficient, your risk will increase exponentially.

Maximum bone mass is achieved by 30 years of age and then it is maintained without much change until about 45 years. During the maintenance period, calcium intake can remain at the minimum RDA (1,200 mg/day); but at about age 45, when this bone mass begins to decline, more calcium may be necessary. It is important to build up your bone "bank balance" in the early years, because the more bone mass that is available before age-related loss begins, the less it is likely to decrease significantly.

Iron   If you are a woman, you may not be getting enough iron from your food, particularly if you menstruate heavily, often restrict your caloric intake, or don't eat meat. Also, just one cup of tea after you eat reduces your iron absorption from that meal by one half to two thirds. A study of college women at Cornell University concluded that "for most young women, the only feasible way to reach the (RDA) for iron is to use an iron supplement."

If you take supplemental iron, take it with vitamin C to double the iron absorption. Examine the accompanying chart to see whether you may have depleted iron stores. Because excess iron can cause problems, ask your health service to test you before taking any iron supplement greater than 100 percent of the RDA.

Zinc   Necessary for fighting virus infections and bacteria, zinc is an important nutrient for the immune system. Zinc facilitates the body's growth and muscle development. If you are a man, zinc may be particularly important because ejaculation depletes the body's zinc stores. Though the RDA is 15 mg, indications are clear that many people are zinc-deficient. Many protein foods, both animal and vegetable, contain zinc as well as iron. Good food sources of zinc are listed in the vitamin appendix at the end of this chapter.

Beta Carotene   This derivative of vitamin A is an important nutrient for your immune system. Because beta carotene is water soluble (unlike vitamin A), overdosing is not a major concern. To get sufficient beta carotene, eat lots of dark green, yellow and orange vegetables and fruits.

B Vitamins   If you drink coffee regularly, are under a lot of stress, and can't eat foods with high Vitamin B, you may want B vitamin supplements—the B complex vitamins are all important for stress and to build your immune system. Don't take them in the evening, as they may keep you awake.

Vitamin C   Many people believe Vitamin C helps prevent or treat colds and recommend 1,000 mg (1 gram) as a reasonable daily maintenance dose. The National Research Council recommends 60 mg as adequate for daily intake. If you consume two to three servings of both fruits (espe-

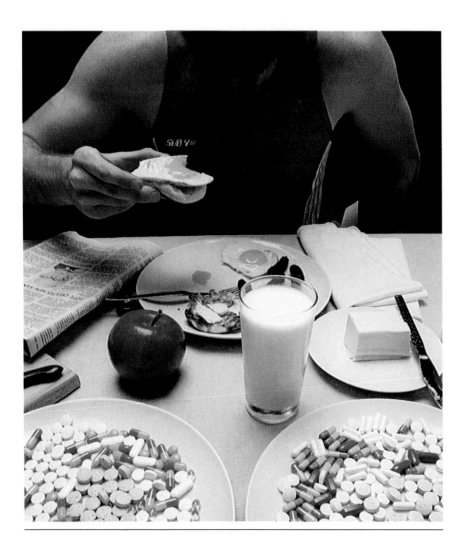

cially citrus) and vegetables, you will meet the daily requirement. If you do choose to take Vitamin C supplements, overdosing is rarely a problem because it is water soluble.

Water Is an Essential Nutrient

Your body contains between 40 and 50 quarts of water, making water your body's primary component. Your blood is primarily water, of course, but so are your cells, your muscles, and most body parts; even your brain is 74 percent water. Water is essential for nutrient digestion and distribution, waste disposal, body cooling, joint and membrane lubrication, and disease fighting.

You lose several quarts of fluid every day—through perspiration, elimination, mucus, and so forth. To perform effectively, you must keep

Eat More Fiber

The National Research Council advises that we all eat more fiber. Fiber is a plant food that has the capability of passing through the digestive system undigested. There are two kinds of fiber, soluble and insoluble. Beans (kidney and pinto), fruits, vegetables, and oats contain soluble fiber which lowers blood cholesterol and helps to control blood sugar in diabetics. Bran, whole-grain breads and cereals, popcorn, and dried beans contain insoluble fiber, which may help to prevent colon cancer and other digestive diseases. Eat a daily diet that contains four to six servings of whole-grain breads and cereals plus four to six servings of fruits and vegetables and you will have an adequate intake of fiber.

well hydrated. "A reduction of 4 to 5 percent in body water will result in a decline of 20 to 30 percent in work performance," points out University of Pennsylvania nutrition professional Dr. Helen A. Guthrie.

In normal weather, you should drink at least six cups of liquids per day; drink significantly more in hot weather or when you are physically working hard.

The best thirst quencher?—cool water. Avoid sweet drinks (sodas, juices, and alcohol, including beer) when you are thirsty or underhydrated; sugar reduces the amount of water in your bloodstream and body tissues by drawing fluid into the digestive tract. Caffeine and alcohol are diuretics and actually increase water loss. Also, when you are thirsty, do not drink through a straw—your mouth taste buds do not know they have been satisfied.

Fiber Is for Every Body

The average American eats 10 to 15 grams of dietary fiber per day, although the National Cancer Institute recommends 30 to 40 grams per day. Are you getting too little fiber? You probably are, if you are on a low-calorie diet (especially a low-carbohydrate diet), if you eat lots of fast foods, or if you eat primarily white bread and white rice instead of their whole grain, browner equivalents.

Do scientists recommend higher fiber intake just so people can avoid constipation? No, they have found even better reasons. High-fiber foods, such as whole grains, beans, seeds, and fresh, raw vegetables and fruits, can help you lose weight, keep your heart and gastrointestinal tract

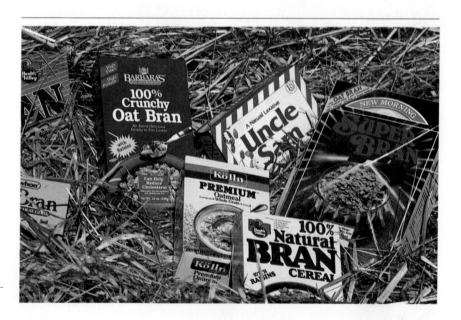

Choosing High-Fiber Foods

To maximize your health and lose weight more easily, emphasize high-fiber foods in your diet.

Low-Fiber Food	High-Fiber Food
Fruit juices	Whole fruit
White English muffins	Whole wheat English muffins
White or French bread	Whole wheat bread
Cooked, particularly overcooked, vegetables	Raw, or slightly steamed, vegetables—and salads
Cream of wheat	Oatmeal
Most sweetened cold cereals	Bran cereals, shredded wheat
Potato chips	Popcorn
Mashed potatoes	Peas
Salad bar bacon bits	Salad bar garbanzo beans

healthy, and reduce the risk of developing certain cancers and degenerative diseases. For example, nutrition experts recommend eating more vegetables from the cruciferous family, as they have been found to help prevent cancer. These foods include broccoli, brussels sprouts, cabbage, and cauliflower.

Fiber helps with weight management in several ways. Most high-fiber foods have low caloric density, which means you can eat a large amount of such foods yet consume fewer calories than with low-fiber foods. For instance, a cup of orange juice has the same number of calories as two oranges; yet eating the oranges means more fiber, takes longer, and is more filling.

Fiber slows down the rate of food digestion, leading to a smaller rise in blood sugar. When blood sugar level is low, your body burns calories as they are ingested, rather than storing some of that blood sugar as fat. High blood sugar triggers the excretion of insulin, which stimulates conversion of sugar to fatty acids—stored as fat in tissues or organs.

While the National Research Council (NRC) states that evidence for a protective role of dietary fiber is inconclusive, most nutrition experts believe that eating a high-fiber diet reduces your risk of heart disease and of some types of cancer. To take advantage of these properties of fiber, minimize your intake of fatty and cholesterol-laden foods. However, if you choose to eat a fried food, have a big salad with it. If you do eat buttered toast, make it whole wheat. You do not need to eat fiber as a separate element of your diet to get enough. Instead, select foods high in fiber. The nearby chart has a list of good choices.

Sodium, a Famous Electrolyte

In partnership with body fluids are substances called electrolytes, distributed throughout the body in both the extracellular and intracellular compartments. Electrolytes contain electrical charges; opposites combine with each other to form neutral compounds in the body. Sodium, a positive cation, and chloride, a negative anion, are combined to form sodium chloride, the most common source of table salt. These electrolytes are essential to the human body, but when our intake is too high, they may cause problems.

Americans eat a potentially dangerous amount of salt. According to the National Research Council we need less than six grams daily—about one teaspoon. In fact, we eat four times more salt than the pioneers consumed less than two hundred years ago. So where do we get our excess? The most common source of salt is cooked in food and added at the table. You also consume it in soy sauce and tamari, monosodium glutamate (MSG), baking powder, baking soda, and certain preservatives. Sodium abounds in fast foods, processed and cured foods.

The price we pay for constantly priming our salt taste buds may be increased rates of high blood pressure (which can lead to strokes, brain damage, and heart attacks), fluid retention, premenstrual syndrome (PMS), and kidney problems. Experimental data also indicate that a high salt intake can damage the stomach lining and cause severe gastritis.

Scientists have demonstrated that low-sodium diets often alleviate or improve these conditions. In fact, since none of us knows whether we will develop high blood pressure—about 15 to 20 percent of Americans do—medical experts recommend that everyone reduce sodium consumption.

Contrary to popular belief, when you exercise heavily and perspire, you usually do not need extra salt. You need additional potassium and, of course, more fluids. So, in case of heavy perspiration or heat exhaustion, try an orange instead of extra salt.

A few tips on how to limit your salt intake:

- Always taste your food before deciding whether to add salt.
- Reach for the salt shaker with decreasing frequency, until you finally do not reach for it at all, or at least only for a few special foods.
- If you cook, add little or no salt while preparing foods. Using other herbs for flavor reduces the amount of salt your taste buds crave.
- Substitute low-salt snacks for high-salt ones.

The nearby chart gives some suggestions for snack alternatives.

Sugar Does More Than Rot Your Teeth

As was mentioned earlier, sugar is a simple carbohydrate that gives you energy and satisfies hunger, but provides no nutrients. Whenever something sweet is offered to eat, it always disappears. Sugar tastes great to most of us; so good in fact that we want it more and more. Some of us even call ourselves "sugarholics."

As you will note in the Optimal Healthy Diet, you can consume 10 percent of your daily calories as simple sugars (and this includes cookies, cake, ice cream, frozen yogurt, cola drink and, of course, alcohol). If you can keep sugar to only 10 percent and meet the rest of the suggested guidelines, your diet will be considered healthy. If you are a heavy sugar consumer, what are some of the negative aspects of a high sugar intake?

Sugar (as well as all those other natural sweeteners, such as honey, molasses, and corn syrup) can cause dental problems, weight gain, and vitamin deficiency; sugar can influence your level of alcohol consumption and may contribute to development of depression and heart disease.

Ever since you gorged on your first bag of Halloween goodies, people have been warning you that sugar is not good for your teeth. Brushing and flossing after eating sugar helps to minimize the damage. Even chewing sugarless gum helps to clean sugar from your teeth and gums.

Sugar contributes to weight problems in more ways than just adding nutritionally empty calories. Sugary foods often contain large amounts of fat. Also, when you eat sugar, your insulin response causes the body to store as fat a high proportion of all the calories you eat.

Sugar lacks the vitamins and minerals you need to metabolize it. When you eat large quantities of sugar, your body's stores of B vitamins may be depleted, leaving you deficient of vitamins you need to fight stress, maintain a healthy nervous system, sleep well, and keep many other systems in balance.

Sugar Substitutes

Based upon a 1989 national survey conducted by the Calorie Control Council, 93 million Americans were consuming products containing sugar substitutes. The FDA-approved low-calorie sweeteners are saccharin, aspartame (marketed as Nutra-Sweet) and acesulfame potassium (marketed as Sunette). Three additional sweeteners are now being considered by the Food and Drug Administration.

Sugar substitutes enable you to avoid the 16 calories per teaspoon of table sugar, or sucrose, but all consumer reports on these products are not sweet. The FDA has received complaints of headaches, rashes, dizziness, convulsions, and depression all attributed to low-calorie sugar substitutes. While studies continue on their possible side effects, Stanford University nutritionist Laura Brainin-Rodriguez recommends that you limit your consumption to only one or two servings per day. If you suspect that you are reacting negatively to sugar substitutes, then give up all consumption of products containing these.

Yeast and Inner Ecology

Yeast isn't just for baking bread. Certain kinds of yeast live in your gastrointestinal tract, maintaining a delicate ecological balance with bacteria, fungi and other normal flora. Heavy use of broad-spectrum antibiotics reduces bacteria, allowing fungi and yeast to flourish, in some cases out of control. One yeast form that often thrives in such conditions is **Candida albicans** which thrives on a high sugar diet. Some segments of the medical community are now investigating an increase in Candida production as the cause of a wide range of symptoms. Although yeast problems manifest more clearly and commonly in women (as vaginal yeast infections), the classical symptoms of Candida can affect either men or women. These symptoms are:

- Intestinal gas
- Bloating after meal
- Fatigue
- Depression
- PMS
- Increased allergies

If you have any of the above symptoms, crave sugar and suspect a yeast problem, contact a physician who will test your yeast level and prescribe a treatment regimen.

Over the past 70 years, the proportion of sugars and starches we eat has changed. In the early 1900s, 68 percent of total carbohydrates came from starch, compared to 47 percent in 1980. Likewise, the contribution of sugars to our carbohydrate intake increased from 32 percent in 1909 to 53 percent in 1980.

In fact, since the mid-1800s consumption of sugar in the United States has increased from 40 pounds per person per year to over 120 pounds. The average American eats 77 pounds of refined sugar; add another 45 pounds from corn sugar sweeteners in processed foods and drinks, and this adds up to more than five ounces per day. During this time, heart disease and other degenerative diseases have also increased. Rare in the 1800s, heart disease today is responsible for one in every two deaths.

According to Nobel Prize winning chemist Dr. Linus Pauling, "It is the increase in the consumption of sugar that has brought on the pandemic of heart disease in the prosperous industrial countries of the world." While sugar is not now considered a major contributor to heart disease (fat is), it does give us something to consider. Especially for women, risk for heart disease is greatest among those who combine smoking, sugar, "junk food," and birth control pills.

The best response to frequent, high sugar consumption is to examine why you are eating so much—are you not getting enough complex carbohydrates, are you really hungry, or are you bored or depressed and feel that eating sugar, especially chocolate, makes you feel better? Do you deprive yourself of food all day, only to break down and binge on sugared foods? Try to solve these problems directly, rather than just masking their symptoms with sugar.

Here are some practical tips to help you reduce your sugar consumption:

- Become aware of the sugar content of foods you eat—jams, sodas, condiments (catsup is 50 percent sugar), desserts, ice cream, most yogurts, cocoa, packaged foods. Did you know that the average 12-ounce soft drink contains 8 to 12 teaspoons of sugar?
- If you feel the urge for sugar when you are studying, ask yourself what you really want—relaxation? escape? reward? Give yourself five minutes off to listen to music or read something fun instead.
- When you want sugar, do not reach for a candy bar—eat a complex carbohydrate or a piece of fruit.
- Reduce the amount of sugar you add to foods—your coffee or cereal, your toast or bagel, and so on. Eventually you may be able to cut down or even eliminate it entirely. Don't worry, you will still consume enough in processed foods, baked goods, and so forth.
- Substitute mineral waters, herbal teas, or even low-calorie sodas for sugared soft drinks.
- If you cannot totally give up sweet desserts and yogurts sweetened with sugar or honey, limit their frequency—for instance, have yogurts only on Mondays and Wednesdays, instead of every day.

Additives and Preservatives

American food manufacturers use thousands of artificial colorings, preservatives, flavorings, and emulsifiers in their products. Such additives make food less expensive, safe to eat, more visually appealing, and easier to store. Experts calculate that the average American consumes five to eight pounds of additives annually. Some may be safe, some are important in avoiding food poisoning, and others are not yet sufficiently tested. A few of these additives have been associated with allergic reactions and with a higher risk of cancer. Sulfite, for instance, may precipitate a life-threatening allergic reaction, especially for a person with asthma.

The National Research Council (NRC) (1989) reports that in the United States nearly 3,000 substances are intentionally added to foods during processing. Another estimated 12,000 chemicals are used in food packaging. In spite of these alarming figures (at least for anyone who wishes to eat natural, organic food), the council points out that individual exposure is very small.

Of the few food additives that have been found to be carcinogenic, all but saccharin have been taken off the market. The NRC says there is no evidence that nitrates cause cancer, and nitrites are probably not direct carcinogens. Some additives are necessary and not harmful, compared to the presence in foods of very dangerous organisms that cause spoilage. For example, nitrites in bacon might cause cancer if eaten in very large amounts; but, these substances also prevent the very fast and dangerous spoilage of this fragile product. Spoilage was responsible for many deaths (botulism, food poisoning) before additives were utilized. Clearly, as consumers we are protected by some of these products; but, we will be even healthier if we use products containing additives and preservatives judiciously.

In conclusion, the research council states that there is a shortage of data on the impact of nonnutritive substances in our diet, but the council believes that these are unlikely to present a cancer risk. If you wish to minimize your personal risks, then you will probably choose to ignore the "Don't worry about it" attitude and the well-financed advertising promoting certain processed foods. You will eliminate as many foods containing additives and preservatives as possible from your diet. Does that mean giving up all junk food? No, it only means cutting down, substituting high quality natural foods when possible, and gradually making your diet more healthy.

Minimize additives in the food you eat:

- When possible, choose simple, unprocessed foods. For instance, choose to make your own popcorn instead of microwave popcorn, and eat fresh meats instead of hot dogs or packaged cold meats.
- When you buy packaged foods, read the label. Choose foods having the shortest list of ingredients and those in which you recognize every ingredient.

What Are USRDA and RDA?

The nutrition label on a food package indicates the percentage of USRDA (U.S. Recommended Daily Allowance) that food provides. It gives the maximum RDA figure for a nutrient. RDA stands for Recommended Dietary Allowance and is age and sex specific. For many nutrients, the Food and Nutrition Board, a committee of the National Academy of Sciences, sets RDAs as "the levels of intake of essential nutrients considered . . . on the basis of available scientific knowledge, to be adequate to meet the needs of practically all healthy persons."

Nutrition Awareness

How to Read a Food Label

Reading the nutritional information on the side panel of packaged foods can help you make healthy choices whether you're buying yogurt, crackers, cereal, beverages, or other items. Nutritional panels usually have several parts: serving size, nutritional content, and ingredient list. Nutritional content includes the amount of calories, protein, carbohydrates, fat, and sodium per serving. To evaluate nutritional content, also look at serving size—if you're eating two portions of cereal, you're getting twice the listed amounts of calories and so forth. Remember, "carbohydrates" include both sugars and complex carbohydrates; you can judge complex carbohydrates independently only if the manufacturer includes a separate carbohydrate table that separates carbohydrates by type. Many cereals and other products that promote their fiber content include this information.

The ingredients list provides additional useful information:

- Order of ingredients: By law, ingredients must be listed in volume order; that is, "potatoes, meat" means that a soup has more potatotes than meat, while "meat, potatoes" means it has more meat.
- Sugar content: Manufacturers may use several kinds of sugars but list them separately, so sugar doesn't look like the largest ingredient, but your body knows they're all sugar. For instance, one bran-type cereal contains sugar, brown sugar syrup, cereal malt syrup, honey, and corn syrup. If a

NUTRITION INFORMATION PER SERVING		
SERVING SIZE: ⅔ Cup (1 ounce: 20.3g)		
SERVINGS PER BOX: 18		
SPOON SIZE Shredded Wheat Cereal	1 oz.	with ½ cup whole milk
Calories	110	190
Protein	3 g	7 g
Carbohydrate	23 g	29 g
Fat	1 g	5 g
Sodium	**	60 mg

**Not more than 10 mg/100 g
 Not more than 10 mg/1 ounce serving

PERCENTAGE OF U.S. RECOMMENDED DAILY ALLOWANCES (U.S. RDA)		
SPOON SIZE Shredded Wheat Cereal	1 oz.	with ½ cup whole milk
Protein	4	15
Vitamin A	*	2
Vitamin C	*	*
Thiamine	4	8
Riboflavin	*	10
Niacin	8	8
Calcium	*	15
Iron	6	6
Phosphorous	10	20
Magnesium	8	10
Zinc	4	8
Copper	6	8

*Contains less than 2% of the U.S. RDA of these nutrients.
INGREDIENTS: 100% natural whole wheat. To help preserve the natural wheat flavor, BHT is added to the packaging material.

product has little sugar, then most carbohydrates are probably complex.
- Artificial colors, flavorings, and preservatives.

- Ask the food service manager at your school to label foods that have these additives and to avoid buying food with potentially harmful additives whenever possible (foods without preservatives sometimes cost more, so your food service may only cooperate partially with such requests). Ask that the salad bar be sulfite free.
- Reduce intake of foods having the following additives:

Additive	Found in
Artificial coloring, especially butter yellow and sudan red; of the common food coloring agents (beta carotene is natural and safe)	Many foods, especially colored cherries
Brominated vegetable oil (BVO)	Citrus-flavored sodas
Butylated hydroxytoune (BHT)	Cereals, gum, potato chips, oils
EDTA and phosphates	Soft drinks, baked goods, other foods
Caffeine	Coffee, tea, cocoa, sodas
Quinine	Tonic water, sodas
Sodium nitrite, sodium nitrate	Hot dogs, sausage, processed meats, ham, bacon, other preserved meats
Sulfites	Salad bar, sprayed on salads, fruits

Lifestyle and Nutrition

For the most part your nutritional needs are the same in college as they will be for the rest of your adult life. A few special circumstances may apply. If you are still growing (true for many freshman and sophomore males), you need additional protein, calcium, and carbohydrates. Significant alcohol consumption reduces your nutritional health. So does stress. Your fitness activities or goals may also play a special role in considering your dietary needs.

Alcohol and Nutrition   Alcohol is addictive, habituating, diuretic, and significantly antinutritious. Metabolizing alcohol depletes your body's stores of B vitamins and folic acid. Over time, alcohol also inhibits absorption and increases excretion of other nutrients.

Alcohol is high in calories, so it often reduces your appetite for other foods. Remember however, it contains no nutrients. Alcohol ingestion can become a particularly serious nutrient drain for women who are not eating sufficient calories. The depletion of B vitamins and Vitamin C can induce symptoms such as fatigue, uncomfortable menstruation, increased premenstrual syndrome, headaches, and dehydration.

As was mentioned earlier in this chapter, improper diet makes individuals who have a predisposition to alcoholism more susceptible to depen-

How Much Caffeine Do You Consume?

Beverages	Caffeine/ Serving (mg)
Brewed coffee, 6 oz.	83
Instant coffee, 6 oz.	60
Decaffeinated coffee, 6 oz.	3
Espresso coffee, 3 oz.	90
Leaf tea, 6 oz.	41
Jolt, 12 oz.	72
Mountain Dew, 12 oz.	54
TAB or Coca-Cola, 12 oz.	46
Shasta Cola (regular and cherry), 12 oz.	44
Sunkist Orange, 12 oz.	42
Pepsi or Dr. Pepper, 12 oz.	36
Root Beer, 12 oz.	0
Slice, 12 oz.	0

Drugs	
No Doz, 1 listed dosage	100
Vivarin, 1 listed dosage	200
Anacin , 1 listed dosage	32
Midol, 1 listed dosage	65
Excedrin, 1 listed dosage	32
Coryban-D capsules, 1 listed dosage	30
Triaminicin cold tablets, 1 listed dosage	30

Source: Coffee Information Institute, soft drink companies, and *Consumer's Union*

dency. To combat this tendency, researchers recommend a well-balanced diet low in refined sugar and high in complex carbohydrates.

Caffeine and Nutrition   Caffeine is everywhere in our culture. Over 200 billion doses of caffeine are consumed each year in the United States. It's in coffee, tea, chocolate, many kinds of soft drinks, even over-the-counter diet and pep pills. Soft drinks don't even have to have any color to contain caffeine—for instance, Mountain Dew has more caffeine than Coca-Cola. In fact, caffeine is actually a drug, a stimulant, to which millions of Americans are addicted. If you are addicted to coffee, you may be unable to get going each morning without your usual dose.

Studies have shown that one or two cups of coffee probably do not have any negative effects. In fact, a 1984 study revealed that aspirin or acetaminophen relieved pain more effectively when taken with coffee. However, excessive caffeine robs your body of nutrients, adds stress, and disturbs your normal sleep cycle. Because coffee and tea (both of which contain the stimulant caffeine) are diuretics, they cause your body to excrete not only more water but more water-soluble nutrients. Large amounts of tea and coffee at mealtime can rob your body of iron. Also, when you drink coffee and tea, the stomach may produce irritating excess gastric acid and enzymes.

Drinking decaffeinated coffee and tea—which, despite the term, still contain some caffeine—reduces the stress and sleep problems associated with caffeine, but may pose new health risks. First, these products do not help you avoid gastric irritation, because they stimulate acid secretions almost as much as their caffeinated equivalents. More important, many decaffeination processes use a solvent to extract the caffeine. The most common solvent used, methylene chloride, is a suspected carcinogen. An alternative solvent usually considered safer is ethylene acetate, a natural constituent of coffee and several other foods. Most coffees that have been decaffeinated using ethylene acetate are labelled as "natural" or "water processed." Many manufacturers are changing to this process to extract caffeine. Only if the label says "Swiss water processed" has the coffee been decaffeinated using charcoal filters but no solvent.

To minimize the nutritional and other physical costs of drinking caffeine, limit consumption. Two cups of coffee per day have far fewer side effects than four. Alternatives include: decaf coffee and tea, herbal teas, caffeine-free soft drinks, sparkling waters (some fruit-flavored, some with sugar, some without), as well as water, milk, and juice. Don't let your daily average consumption creep up.

Avoid caffeine within three hours of going to sleep. Caffeine reaches its highest level in the blood within 15 to 45 minutes of consumption. The halflife of caffeine (the time your body needs to eliminate half of the amount you drink) is three to four hours; if you go to sleep within that time period, the caffeine disturbs your sleep pattern even when you are asleep. If you're going to stay up late and want caffeine, drink it early in your study period. If you tire with one or two hours to go, take a brisk walk for ten minutes or climb up and down stairs a few times to increase the oxygen flow to the brain. Studies have shown that the ten-minute walk actually produces more alertness than a cup of coffee.

Stress and Nutrition   Good nutrition helps you minimize the effects of stress. Carbohydrates give you energy to persevere under stressful conditions, protein rebuilds cells damaged by stress, and vitamins and minerals keep your bodily systems in repair. On the other hand, poor nutrition can actually cause or exacerbate stress. Vitamin deficiencies, excessively low calorie diets, and other nutritional insufficiencies may make you more susceptible to illness, depression, fatigue, and other stressful conditions.

When you're under stress for any reason, you may be less likely to pay attention to eating well. You may ingest larger quantities of nutrient-depleting substances such as caffeine, alcohol, or sweets. Finally, you may also be shortchanging yourself on sleep, depleting your nutrient stores even further. Pay special attention to eating well during stressful periods. You'll feel the benefits almost right away. To learn more about how to manage stress effectively, see **Coping with Stress**.

Physical Fitness and Nutrition   A physically active lifestyle helps you nutritionally by keeping your digestive system working well and your circulatory system distributing nutrients to your body efficiently. Physical activity is also one of the most effective tools for weight loss and management.

On the flip side, good nutritional habits can support strenuous exercise. Most physical activities, from casual bike riding to most competitive sports, require nothing more special than overall good nutrition. If you're involved in an activity that favors a lean body mass (such as swimming, dancing, or running) you may be tempted to follow an extremely low calorie diet. However, overzealous runners and others in this category frequently experience bone breaks and develop osteoporosis, in part because their diets are calcium-deficient.

College Eating

At college you encounter more food choices and food abundance than at home. Your parents aren't around to provide balanced food choices for you. You probably eat most meals with friends, and it's natural to want to eat what you see others eating. Dining hall eating can be an ideal situation for overeating and other poor eating habits.

On the other hand, many students feel immense pressure to be in control and be slender; some, particularly women, fast or self-induce vomiting to attain this goal. Such behavior may signal not only a desire to control food and body shape but an overstressed life. For more information, see **Eating Disorders**.

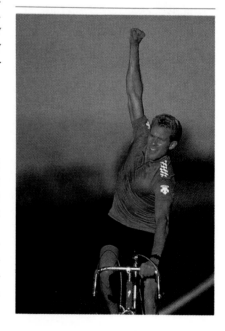

Influencing Residence Hall Food

Recently, food service personnel have become more sensitive to the dietary interests and needs of their student clientele. The growing concern with health issues and weight control among students has influenced many food service offerings. If your food service does not appear to be sufficiently enlightened about new nutritional information, tastes, or eating styles, you can help change that.

Form a student-oriented nutrition committee. Seek support from other students in your dining unit, then open a constructive dialogue with your food service manager. Some healthy changes will not cost the food service any extra money. Recommendations you might consider include: fresh, seasonal salad bars and vegetable selections; low-calorie and reduced-calorie dressings; sauces and butter served on the side; low-fat meats, cheeses and yogurts; reduced sugar and salt content; plenty of whole grains; vegetarian entrees without cheese or eggs.

By becoming more aware of the nutritional content of your food choices and then learning how to exercise that knowledge within the constraints of college eating situations, you can make choices that maximize your health and success at college. Here is healthy advice for the most common college eating situations: dining hall meals, snacking, parties, fast food restaurants, and cooking for yourself.

Dining Hall Eating

In the dining hall, not only what you eat but when you eat is somewhat out of your control. The food service offers each meal only during certain hours; you may feel you'd better eat dinner whether you're hungry or not, because the cafeteria won't open again for another ten hours, and you've paid for the meals in advance anyway. With those limitations in mind, here are some tips for taking control of what you eat in your campus dining hall:

- Think about what you want before you start through the food service line. Ask yourself—what will help me get done what I want to do today? What have I already eaten today? I'm tired and need some quick energy —I'll choose fruit instead of a sweet dessert. So, what would be best to have right now?
- Be creative. Make an entree of baked potato topped with broccoli and yogurt; a salad topped with tuna or cottage cheese; steam fresh vegetables from the salad bar in the microwave.
- Don't skip breakfast. If you're not hungry when you first get up, take with you for later a piece of fruit and a roll, or a low-fat yogurt. If you have something healthy with you, you're less likely to reach for doughnuts or other sweet but relatively useless snacks.
- Eat early in the meal service time period. If you eat later, the optimal choices may no longer be available.
- Sit facing away from the food service line. If you don't see the quantity of food waiting to be selected, you may be less tempted to go back for seconds unless your hunger prompts you.

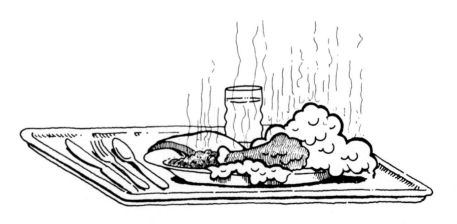

- Try not to compare what you eat with what your friends eat (at least not without considering how much exercise they get, how well they're doing academically, their basic metabolism, how much they snack between meals, and whether their parents are thin).
- If you eat less healthily when you're with certain friends, eat more carefully when you're not with them.
- Take control where you have it. Select nonfat milk, put sauces on the side, leave butter off the bread and go light on the salad dressing (lemon juice and olive oil are good).
- Work constructively to get the kind of residence hall food you want. The accompanying box, "Influencing Residence Hall Food," offers suggestions on what to request and how to get it.

Snacking

Ever noticed how study breaks turn into food breaks, particularly if a pizza arrives? Watch out for having a whole meal at ten or eleven o'clock at night, particularly if you've already eaten several full meals earlier. By that time of evening, your metabolism tends to have slowed down, so calories you ingest then are more likely to be stored as fat than burned.

If you do snack sometimes, keep good food available so you're not faced with the difficult choice of brownies or nothing. Try to select simple, whole foods as snacks. You might get a small refrigerator or share one with others. Some snack foods advertised as "health foods" actually have

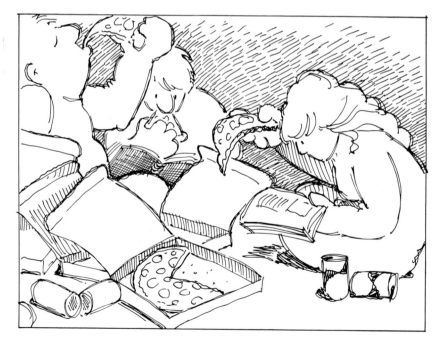

Nutrition Awareness

What are your favorite snack foods? (Multiple responses permitted.)

Fruit	52%
Pizza	41%
Cookies and brownies	37%
Potato chips and pretzels	37%
Ice cream	34%
Candy	27%
Popcorn	26%
French fries	25%
Hamburgers	23%
Yogurt	23%
Cheese and crackers	23%
Salad	29%

Source: *Newsweek On Campus*

high fat or sugar content. The accompanying chart lists truly healthy snacks as well as "health foods" to avoid if you're watching your weight or want to get the most benefit from foods you eat.

You may encounter snack opportunities almost anywhere on campus. Vending machines are everywhere, and many colleges have a campus store as well-stocked with food as any convenience store. If you frequently eat from vending machines, find the ones on campus that have the most healthful choices. Some offer raisins, crackers-and-cheese packages, chicken soup, pretzels, even fresh fruit (the crackers, soup, and pretzels may be high-salt choices). If you don't find good choices elsewhere, take snacks with you.

Parties

When your friends, family or dorm plan a party, get in on the process. Suggest that some of the food money go for whole-wheat pretzels or crackers, mineral waters, fruit, and/or fresh veggies. If you're watching your weight, try to get ingredients to make a dip based on cottage cheese rather than sour cream. You'll probably find that lots of people enjoy these alternatives.

Fast Foods without Fast Fat

Burgers, pizza, and other fast foods tend to provide many calories in a few bites. Here are a few tips on how to snack on fast food without consuming high levels of fat:

- Balance a fast-food lunch with a low-fat breakfast and dinner.
- Be selective about pizza toppings. You can make a healthy meal with toppings of bell peppers, mushrooms, onions, and tomatoes (and order a salad). Extra cheese, sausage, pepperoni, all meats, and olives are loaded with fat.
- When ordering burgers, get small ones without the "special sauces." Unlike mayonnaise, pickles and mustard are fat-free (though high in sodium). By leaving off the cheese, you'll save over 100 calories, most of which are fat.
- Skip most chicken and fish choices in fast-food restaurants; they are usually breaded and fried (which adds hundreds of calories of fat to otherwise healthy food). Some even contain ground-up chicken skin, which is pure fat.
- French fries are super-fatty. If you can't give them up totally, get just a small serving and split it with a friend.
- Salads and sandwiches (including those on pitas) can be great choices, if you limit the dressings and sauces. Stay away from croissants, which are loaded with shortening or butter.
- Drink nonfat or low-fat milk, mineral water with juice, or water instead of a milk shake.

Healthy Snacks

Don't trust that "health food" is truly healthy. Eat fresh foods as snacks. Read labels; look for minimal sugar and fat content.

Healthy Snack Foods	"Health Food" Snacks with High-Calorie Content
Fresh fruit	Granola and granola bars
Low-fat, low-salt corn chips	Dried fruit
Popcorn without butter	Trail mix
Low-fat crackers (such as Ry-Krisp, Ak-Maks, matzohs, rice cakes)	Nuts and seeds
Breadsticks	Cheese
Yogurt (non-fat or low-fat)	Fruit yogurts (whole-milk varieties)
Whole wheat pretzels	
Vegetable sticks (carrot, celery, bell pepper, cherry tomatoes)	
Sparkling water	
Herbal tea	

Cooking on Your Own

Living off campus can provide certain health advantages, for instance, it's great to have so much control over what and when you eat. Because meal preparation requires time, keep menu planning, shopping, and cooking simple. Try to post a shopping list in a handy place. If you can, spend ten minutes once a week jotting down what you'll need for the week, and make one big shopping trip a week. Shopping takes less time if you go to the same store every week, since you know where everything is. Plan your menus, use leftovers, and budget your resources.

Ask yourself: What do I eat for breakfast, for lunch, for dinner, for snacks? Select a variety of protein sources, vegetables, fruits, and carbohydrates, so you are satisfied with what you have available to fix. Try a few dinners a week based on rice, beans, tortillas, or other nonmeat sources of protein.

You can minimize food costs without sacrificing nutrition. For instance, if you like beef but are awed by its price, try mixing small amounts with rice or noodles, so you get the beef taste without the steak price. The best fruit and vegetable buys are those in season (they probably also taste best and have the most nutrients). Buy only as much milk and other perishable goods as you will use in a week or so. Refrigerate leftovers promptly so they won't grow harmful bacteria and spoil. Cook three times a week, and always prepare enough for two meals.

Allergies and Other Special Dietary Needs at College

You may have a special medical reason to be careful about what you eat. Perhaps you suspect or know you have food allergies. Other conditions affected by diet include diabetes, Candida, high blood pressure, and alcoholism.

If one of these situations fits you, get thorough dietary guidance from the health care provider who is treating your condition. You may want to consult a professional nutritionist as well. If you eat on campus, discuss your situation with your food service manager. Most food service operations are quite cooperative. If you don't get the results you need, ask the college health service to help you work with the food service.

Telling friends about your dietary limitations is usually a good idea. You are the only real supervisor of whether you stick to eating what you should, but friends are often quite helpful, and will stop tempting you if you stay within your guidelines fairly consistently. Emphasize what you can have, not just what is off limits. At parties, offer to bring foods prepared in a way that you can enjoy. Cookbooks are available for every type of dietary restriction. If you know you're going to indulge in "forbidden food" for some special occasion, compensate at other meals, if this is appropriate for your condition.

Attaining Good Nutrition

Now that you know intellectually what good nutrition entails, can you really eat that way? Can you eat more vegetables, reduce the sour cream on your potato, drink fewer sodas? You can successfully change your eating patterns only if you really believe that making such changes will help you achieve a goal you want. Eating appropriately may help you:

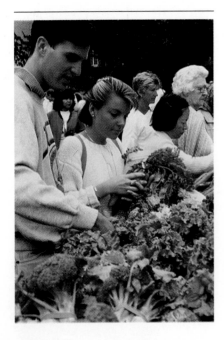

- Reduce tiredness and illness; maximize energy
- Attain and maintain an appropriate weight
- Maximize your appearance and energy
- Improve athletic performance
- Minimize diseases and other physical problems

Your Nutrition Plan

Practically speaking, actually achieving good nutrition will be much easier if you spend a few minutes preparing a personal nutrition plan. Review the suggestions earlier in this chapter; then list just one to two specific aspects of eating behavior you would like to change. You may decide to increase certain types of nutritionally valuable foods, reduce or eliminate your consumption of certain nutritionally undesirable foods, or eat differently in one particular setting (such as parties or studying).

Small manageable goals give you a chance to congratulate yourself more frequently, which builds a feeling of success. You'll find more suc-

A Healthy Diet—According to the National Research Council

Fat   Limit fat intake to 30 percent of your daily calories; keep saturated fat to less than 10 percent.

Cholesterol   Keep to less than 300 mg daily; eat low-fat dairy, lean meat, fish, and skinned poultry. Limit fried foods (fried in lard), egg yolks, and butter.

Complex Carbohydrates and Starches   At least 55 percent of your daily calories; six or more servings of whole grain breads, cereals, grains, legumes, pasta.

Fruits and Vegetables   Eat five or more half-cup servings every day, preferably citrus and green and yellow.

Protein   Eat no more than twice the recommended allowance (0.8 g per kg ideal body weight); two 3-ounce servings about the size of your palm.

Weight   Balance amount of food intake with physical activity to maintain appropriate weight.

Alcohol   Not recommended; if you do drink, do not exceed one ounce daily (two cans of beer, two glasses of wine, or two average cocktails). If you are pregnant, avoid alcohol completely.

Salt   Eat less than six grams daily (about one teaspoon). Avoid using table salt and eating salty foods to keep below this level.

Dietary supplements   You do not need more than the recommended daily allowance for vitamins and minerals.

Calcium   Keep intake up to Recommended Dietary Allowance (800 mg). If you are between the ages of 11 and 25, 1,200 mg is suggested. Drink low-fat milk or eat low-fat dairy products, and eat dark green vegetables.

Fluoride   Maintain optimal intake, especially during years of tooth formation.

---

cess with a specific target like "sauces on the side" than either a general goal like "eat balanced meals" or a radical and perhaps unattainable goal like "no snacking."

Pick the right time to start your nutrition plan. Changing your eating patterns takes some extra mental energy, so start when you are between exam periods and other commitments that already require special concentration. You'll have to maintain self-discipline and vigilance. Try not to consider yourself either on or off the bandwagon as far as your nutrition program is concerned. Think of this project as a transition to better eating habits.

Food Fears

In the early eighties fear of additives and preservatives led nutritionists to urge use of natural food products. By the late 1980s, the villains saturated fat and cholesterol sparked cholesterol-free everything and the removal of tropical oils from many foods. As we enter the nineties, national phobia of pesticides is sprouting an organic food revolution.

Many Americans harbor a grossly distorted view of the safety of foods, because we have been flooded with messages that pesticides in produce, additives in packaged foods, hormones in meats, Salmonella in chickens, and mercury in fish are killing us with cancer. The truth is, we have the safest food supply in the world.

There is no question that food safety warrants more attention from government agencies, food manufacturers, and yes, even you—consumers who need to sharpen their nutrition skills. But, as we wait it out or participate in this food cleanup, we should maintain a common sense perspective that not everything we eat is killing us.

Forbidden Fruit

1989 was the year of the forbidden fruit. An alarming report questioning the safety of apples for children set off a national chain reaction of produce phobia. A week later the federal government advised consumers to discard all fruit from Chile—the bulk of the fruit on the market—after two grapes were found to be injected with cyanide.

In the wake of dietary recommendations to eat less fat, sugar, and salt and more fruits, vegetables, and lean meats, it's no wonder Americans were left confused and questioning if

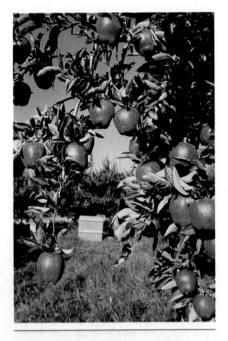

anything was fit to eat. Despite the fears generated by these two incidents, and the very real problem of pesticide residues, the benefits of eating fruits and vegetables still far outweigh the risks.

The best scientific estimates find 99.9 percent of carcinogens (cancer-causing agents) in the diet come from natural, not artificial, sources. Dr. Bruce Ames, chairman of the Biochemistry Department at the University of California at Berkeley, says plants make their own natural pesticides to protect themselves. Found in small amounts, these naturally occurring chemicals prove to be potent carcinogens in laboratory tests.

Man-made pesticides, subject to the approval of the Environmental Protection Agency (EPA) after proof of

safety, are applied to fruits and vegetables to kill the insects that would otherwise destroy the crops. Fungicides, the class of pesticides of greatest concern, are applied to extend shelf-life and make picture-perfect produce. The EPA also sets tolerance levels for pesticide residues, while the Food and Drug Administration enforces the residue-monitoring program.

Environmental activists such as the National Resource Defense Council (NRDC) and Americans for Safe Food (AFSF) charge that these government agencies are too lax in their approval process, regulations, and monitoring of pesticides. They claim that many of the pesticides in use have not been adequately tested for cancer risk and, in fact, many of those in use are not detectable by routine testing.

The controversy on the safety of pesticide residues has been accelerated by consumer concern. Pesticides have become our greatest food worry, despite mounting evidence linking dietary fat, not pesticides, to cancer risk from diet.

Still, it's time to clean up our produce. The best way to minimize pesticide residues is to reduce their widespread use in agriculture. Consumer power in the marketplace, outlined below, has the greatest influence on farmers, producers, and the government.

At the Store

- Buy organic. Either organically grown or home grown produce can come close to being pesticide-free.
- Buy domestically grown produce, especially from the western United

States, where they use fewer fungicides. Imported produce is not subject to U.S. regulations and generally contains more residues.

- Buy in season. Seasonal fruits are less likely to be treated with fungicides to preserve appearance during long-term storage.

In the Kitchen

- Wash all fresh produce (use water only).
- Peel or remove the outer layers of lettuce, cabbage, and other leafy vegetables, which usually contain the greatest concentration of pesticides. Peel produce with wax coatings, such as cucumbers, peppers, and some apples, that can prevent pesticides from being washed off.

In Your Living Center

- Encourage your dining hall manager to follow all the guidelines above.
- Eat a variety of the produce offered. Eating the same item over and over can increase exposure to the same pesticides.
- Keep a well-stocked organic fruit basket in your room.

At Home

- Grow your own fruit and vegetables. Tomatoes, lettuce, carrots, and many other vegetables do well in small containers suitable for apartments or small patios.
- Join an organic garden cooperative where everyone shares the land, work, and of course, the harvest of your efforts.

What's the Beef?

Among other consumer concerns, the safety of meat ranks high. More than half of American consumers rated antibiotics and hormones used in livestock to be "serious health hazards," in a survey for the American Marking Institute. Unlike pesticides, the case of antibiotics and hormones in meat may be "more hype than hazard."

Hormones used to enhance growth of muscle tissue have been deemed safe by numerous scientific bodies, including the World Health Organization and United Nations' Food and Agricultural Organization. The amount of hormones remaining in the meat you buy is negligible: 15,000 times less than the same amount of hormones produced daily in men and several million times less than that produced in women.

Antibiotics are used to prevent disease and promote faster weight gain. The residues of antibiotics are also minimal by the time the animal gets to market. But mounting evidence is linking cases of Salmonella infection in humans to the practice of feeding antibiotics to cattle, pigs, and poultry, specifically in people currently taking antibiotics who then eat Salmonella-tainted meat.

It is most often the result of mishandling that allows the Salmonella to multiply to produce Salmonella food poisoning. (See "Food Smarts" for more information on proper handling and prevention.)

As with produce, alternatives are available at the meat market. Meat that is free of antibiotics and hormones is sold in health food stores and by mail order. Your local market may stock these items if there is enough demand. Another option is to become a vegetarian and eliminate meat, poultry, and fish from your diet. You can still consume adequate protein by combining grains and vegetables.

If you continue to eat meat, your real health concerns should focus on reducing your intake of saturated fat by selecting lean red meat, chicken without skin, and fish and on handling these foods properly, as outlined below.

At the Store

- Select only lean cuts of meats (top round, flank steak, sirloin, pork tenderloin, center-cut chops).
- Select fresh meat and poultry with a nonslimy appearance.
- Buy chemical-free meat and poultry.

In the Kitchen

- Trim all visible fat from meat prior to cooking.
- Trim poultry of skin and external fat before cooking.
- Cook fish, pork, and poultry thoroughly.
- Rinse all meats with water before cooking.

In Your Living Center

- Eat a maximum of six ounces of all meats per day.
- Trim any visible fat from meat, remove skin from chicken.
- Eat only thoroughly cooked meats.
- Never take leftover meat or chicken back to your room.

Keep Informed

Consumers are more informed than ever regarding nutrition and food issues. The media has played a major role in shaping our views of these issues. Unfortunately, bad news makes better headlines than good news. Thus, the stories that get the biggest coverage are often the most frightening, not necessarily the most accurate.

To keep informed and maintain a common sense perspective, look for reliable sources that present both sides of an issue. Several excellent news-letters that you may want to subscribe to or read regularly at your campus library are included in the resource section of this chapter.

Environmental groups such as the NRDC and AFSF also distribute information that helps shape our views on food. These groups work to keep our food safe and are worthy of your support.

Most importantly, use your common sense. We have a very safe food supply that does, unfortunately, need some attention from growers, manufacturers, and the government. But our greatest fears should concern areas about which science has been able to provide evidence: the links between our high-fat, low-fiber diet and heart disease, stroke, cancer, and obesity.

If your reaction to daily news of mercury in fish, Salmonella in chicken, and Alar in apples is "Nothing's safe to eat, so I'll eat whatever I want," step back and put it all in perspective. Remember this recipe for a long and healthy life: A little of everything and a lot of moderation.

Food Smarts

Bacteria are naturally present in foods, but in minute quantities that can neither be tasted nor seen, nor generally cause us any harm. It is only when the organisms are given the proper environment to multiply and grow that the quantity of germs poses a threat.

Each year more than several million cases of food poisoning—typically a flu-like illness—develop as a result of contaminated food, most often undercooked meat, poultry, eggs, or fish. Of the one hundred or more species of microorganisms known to cause food poisoning, 85 percent of cases can be prevented by practicing the 3 C's: cooling, cooking, and cleaning.

Keep Food Cold

Microorganisms grow best at room temperature. Refrigerators should be kept at 40° F or below; freezers at 0° F.

- When storing leftovers, make sure you put them in the refrigerator immediately and in small batches to allow for quick cooling throughout the food.
- For picnics, pack coolers with plenty of ice or freezer packs.
- Thaw meats overnight in the refrigerator or microwave (just before cooking). Countertop thawing allows bacteria to multiply on the warmer exterior.

Cook Foods Thoroughly

- Never put cooked meat on the same dish that held the raw meat.
- Wash raw meats, poultry, and fish with water to remove surface microorganisms.

Clean Everything Thoroughly

- Wash hands with soap and water prior to and during food preparation.
- Clean all cooking utensils used on raw meat and poultry with *hot*, soapy water immediately after use.
- Never use the same cutting board for raw meats and chopping fresh produce. This encourages the transfer of contaminants from one food to another.

Fortunately, professional food handlers in the residence hall kitchens are required to participate in yearly training regarding food safety. If you live in a sorority, fraternity, co-op, or other living center, your local health department can provide some educational materials and training.

Trish Ratto, RD

Seeking Professional Help

You can probably make great strides toward nutritional health on your own. However, some circumstances require or benefit from the help of people with detailed knowledge of the relationship between eating and health.

Seek help if:

- You use fasting or self-induced vomiting after binging as weight control techniques.
- You find yourself eating compulsively.
- You have digestive upset or discomfort after eating that you have not been able to eliminate through adjusting what you eat.
- You suspect you have a food allergy or yeast problem.
- You have special dietary needs for medical reasons.
- You have gained or lost ten pounds or more without changing your eating patterns, as far as you can tell.
- You would like more specific guidance and support for your nutritional goals.

Types of Help Available

Physicians   Can diagnose if medical reasons exist for nutritional deficits, weight problems, digestive disorders, or other nutritionally related issues. May be able to tell if health problems have a nutritional cause, though some physicians are more attuned to this than others. Can advise regarding special dietary needs for any specific medical condition.

Nutritionist, Dietitian   Can help you analyze your current eating patterns and provide guidance in improving your nutrition.

Support and Maintenance

If you want support for your nutrition efforts, consult your health care provider, a nutritional counselor at the health center, or your coach. Your friends and family may be supportive, or undermine your efforts, or make you nervous about occasional slip-ups. You'll have to decide the extent to which they are helpful resources. Don't make changes just to please others; you're the one whose approval counts. So, in the long run, you are your best support system.

Vitamin and Mineral Keys to Good Health

Vitamin/Mineral	RDA Suggested Minimum	Maximum without Professional Supervision	Major Food Function in Body	Major Food Sources

Vitamin A	5000 IU*	4,000–5,000 IU; Beta-carotene: 25,000 IU	healthy skin
			eyesight
			hearing, smell, taste
			immune system
			healthy mucus
			    production
			teeth and bones
				dairy products fortified
				    with Vitamin A
				    (such as milk)
				liver
				egg
				dark green and dark
				yellow vegetables and
				    fruits, such as:
				    carrots
				    sweet potato
				    spinach
				    cantaloupe
				    broccoli
				    watermelon
				    leaf lettuce
				    apricots

Vitamin D	400 IU	8 mcg (400 IU)	builds and maintains
			    bones and teeth
				sunlight (not food source)
				foods fortified with
				    Vitamin D such as
				    milk)
				egg yolk
				fish: herring, salmon, tuna
				fish-liver oils

Vitamin E	30 IU	400–800 IU	protects cell membranes
			protects lungs
			red blood cell formation
			muscles
			protects Vitamin A and
			    others from
			    destruction
				vegetable oils (corn, olive,
				    peanut, safflower,
				    etc.)
				nuts, seeds
				green vegetables, espe-
				    cially leafy vegetables
				wheat germ; whole grain
				    products

Vitamin K	65–80 mcg	70–140 mcg**	protein formation
			blood clotting
			bone metabolism
				meats
				egg yolks
				liver
				vegetables, such as:
				    dark green, leafy
				    alfalfa
				    asparagus
				    broccoli
				tomatoes
				cauliflower
				peas

+ = includes vitamin and mineral intake from food sources
*IU = international units
**mcg = microgram

Vitamin and Mineral Keys to Good Health

Deficiency Symptoms	Overdose Symptoms	Comments

night blindness
rough, dry flakey skin
dry, brittle hair
mucous membranes dry or
    infected (including
    sinus problems,
    frequent respiratory
    infections or colds)
thin tooth enamel
	headaches
	blurred vision
	loss of appetite
	skin rashes
	insomnia
	menstrual irregularity
	irritability
	brittle fingernails
	hair loss
	very dry skin
		■ Beta-carotene, a food component that the body converts to Vitamin A, has few toxic effects, unlike preformed Vitamin A in liver and many supplements.
		■ Higher levels of beta-carotene correlate with lower rates of lung cancer and other cancers.
		■ Smoking inhibits Vitamin A absorption.
		■ Getting sufficient Vitamin A is difficult if your diet is predominantly fast foods and few vegetables.

bone softening poor teeth	fatigue kidney problems upset stomach nausea heart disease high blood pressure	■ Overdose may be dangerous. Excessive Vitamin D may cause calcification of soft tissue; damage is irreversible. ■ Excessive Vitamin D impedes body's ability to store magnesium. ■ The body makes Vitamin D from sunlight on the skin, but in winter the amount made is insufficient. ■ Insufficient Vitamin D intake is frequently associated with low levels of calcium and magnesium.

few (rare)	none definitely known;
	reports of headache,
	    blurred vision, fatigue,
	    muscle weakness
		■ If you live in area of high pollution, supplement of Vitamin E may prevent pollution-related health problems.
		■ If you have high blood pressure, consult with physician before taking supplemental Vitamin E.

slow blood clotting	relatively non-toxic	■ Increase Vitamin K if on prolonged antibiotic therapy. ■ Available only by prescription; consult with physician.

Vitamin and Mineral Keys to Good Health

Vitamin/ Mineral	RDA Suggested Minimum	Maximum without Professional Supervision	Major Food Function in Body	Major Food Sources
Vitamin B₁ (thiamin)	1.5 mg***	25 mg	promotes energy nervous system balance normal appetite, digestion	pork, beef, fish liver peanuts, seeds enriched/whole grains legumes oatmeal
Vitamin B₂ (riboflavin)	1.7 mg	25 mg	energy release from carbohydrates, protein, fats	dairy products eggs whole/enriched grains green, leafy vegetables meats, organ meats
Niacin (a B vitamin)	20 mg	50 mg	converts carbohydrates to energy skin tissue gastrointestinal system evens disposition	nuts lean meats, liver, fish, poultry eggs beans peas peanuts whole/enriched grains
Vitamin B₆ (pyroxidine)	2.2 mg	25–50 mg	facilitates use of proteins, fats, amino acids, carbohydrates red blood cells nervous system	whole grains (not en- riched) meats, organ meats, fish, poultry avocadoes spinach green beans bananas
Vitamin B₁₂	3 mcg	25 mcg	red blood cells builds genetic material nerve function energizer	lean meat, organ meats other animal products nutritional yeast fermented soy products (sometimes)

***mg = milligram

Deficiency Symptoms	Overdose Symptoms	Comments
nerve problems confusion, memory problems headaches weakness leg cramps constipation insomnia, fatigue hostility depression	deficiency of other B vitamins	■ Avoid coffee and tea (even decaf) within one hour of eating or taking B_1.
skin lesions cracked corners of mouth eyes unusually sensitive to light fatigue depression	none reported	
skin disorders diarrhea confusion irritability, anger and worry swollen or smooth tongue depression headaches insomnia	redness or tingling of face, neck, hands elevated blood sugar level	
nerve irritation muscle problems skin problems cracks at corners of mouth dizziness nausea anemia depression	neurological problems nerve damage with large doses symptoms reported with over 250 mg/day	■ Oral contraceptives may cause mild deficiency; take increased B_6 for oral contraceptives or PMS. ■ Usually take supplementary elevated level of B_6 only as part of B-complex supplement. ■ Zinc and magnesium help B_6 absorption. ■ Carpal tunnel syndrome (tingling, sharp pains in wrist and fingers) can often be cleared up by taking B_6. ■ Body levels decrease when under stress.
anemia pale skin numbness and tingling in fingers and toes psychiatric symptoms	none reported	■ Vegetarians who eat no animal products are often at risk for B_{12} deficiency.

Vitamin and Mineral Keys to Good Health

Vitamin/ Mineral	RDA Suggested Minimum	Maximum without Professional Supervision	Major Food Function in Body	Major Food Sources
Pantothenic acid	10 mg	10,000 mg	metabolizes foods hormone formation nervous system	plants and animals also formed in intestinal tract by microbes avocado nuts mushrooms broccoli poultry (dark meat) organ meats trout
Biotin	0.3 mg	no known oral toxicity	releases energy from carbohydrates formation of fatty acids	organ meats egg yolks dark green vegetables milk nuts legumes formed in intestinal tract by microorganisms
Vitamin C	60 mg	3000–5000 mg	forms intracellular material tissue bones and teeth blood vessels stimulates immune systems natural antihistamine	fruits and vegetables, including: citrus (oranges, grapefruit, lemons) strawberries tomatoes bell peppers cantaloupe broccoli greens
Folic acid	0.4 mg	800–2000 mcg	forms genetic material red blood cells	green, leafy vegetables eggs oranges nuts fish, beef, organ meats whole grain products legumes

Vitamin and Mineral Keys to Good Health

Deficiency Symptoms	Overdose Symptoms	Comments
fatigue may be sign	none reported	■ Lost in processed and heavily refined foods. ■ May be useful in frequent GI upsets. ■ May be useful in decreasing allergy symptoms.
eczema	none reported	■ Eating large quantities of raw egg white prevents absorption.
fatigue soft, bleeding gums easy bruising painful, swollen joints frequent infections	relatively non-toxic loose bowel movements kidney stones	■ Vitamin C can reduce effects of stress. ■ Alcohol inhibits absorption of Vitamin C. ■ May buffer reduced resistance caused by taking steroid medications. ■ Smokers require more Vitamin C.
anemia gastrointestinal problems diarrhea smooth tongue emotional lability (depression) low sex drive	none reported	■ Women on oral contraceptives may need increased folic acid. ■ Stress lowers body levels of folic acid.

Vitamin and Mineral Keys to Good Health

Vitamin/ Mineral	RDA Suggested Minimum	Maximum without Professional Supervision	Major Food Function in Body	Major Food Sources
Calcium	1200 mg	1600 mg	bones and teeth	dairy products dark green vegetables canned salmon, sardines dried beans tofu almonds
Iodine	.15 mg	150 mcg	metabolic regulation (thyroid)	marine fish and shellfish dairy products iodized salt most vegetables
Iron	18 mg	30 mg	helps form hemoglobin energy metabolism	lamb beans dark green vegetables prunes, apricots oysters, clams, shrimp peanuts, cashews whole grains
Magnesium	400 mg	200–400 mg	nervous system, nerves muscles converts food to energy protein synthesis	beans nuts avocadoes animal products green, leafy vegetables
Potassium	average intake is 2000–2500 mg	no known toxicity	fluid balance acid-base balance nervous sytem heart facilitates insulin secretion	oranges apples apricots avocado bananas broccoli carrots tomatoes potatoes chicken seeds fish; salmon instant coffee

Vitamin and Mineral Keys to Good Health

Deficiency Symptoms	Overdose Symptoms	Comments
osteoporosis stunted growth muscle cramps in legs memory impairment insomnia irritability	constipation	■ If increase calcium consumption, increase magnesium consumption. ■ Take calcium in the evening, because calcium can have a relaxing effect and is better retained then. ■ Calcium without sufficient Vitamin D cannot strengthen bone.
enlarged thyroid	depressed thyroid activity	■ Take only by prescription, because can cause toxic goiter. ■ Usually get enough from iodized salt.
anemia (weakness) fatigue pale skin irritability increased susceptibility to infection headaches	liver problems constipation or diarrhea	■ Coffee and tea (even decaf) inhibit absorption of iron if taken within one hour of taking iron. ■ If drink coffee or tea, may need more iron. ■ Extremely toxic to young children.
tremors nervousness muscle cramps mental apathy, anxiety poor appetite insomnia oversensitivity to loud noises PMS	high blood pressure	■ Magnesium may relieve nerves on edge or muscle tremors. ■ Heavy drinkers require more magnesium.
muscle weakness and aches poor reflexes	muscle weakness can be fatal due to heart arrhythmias	■ Only take supplement if advised by physician; may cause heart irregularities. ■ To maximize body's utilization of potassium in foods, keep sodium intake low.

Vitamin and Mineral Keys to Good Health

Vitamin/ Mineral	RDA Suggested Minimum	Maximum without Professional Supervision	Major Food Function in Body	Major Food Sources
Selenium	.2 mg	200 mcg	protects other vitamins and minerals stimulates immune system antioxidant	animal products most vegetables (depends on soil) whole/enriched grains
Zinc	15 mg	25–40 mg	absorption of vitamins growth digestion male sexual function (prostate) wound healing	beans seeds and nuts legumes milk wheat bran, wheat germ shellfish, especially oysters liver fish red meat

Deficiency Symptoms	Overdose Symptoms	Comments
rare, but anemia is possible	gastrointestinal problems	<ul><li>Considered an important anti-cancer agent.</li><li>Contributes to alertness in the elderly.</li><li>Works with Vitamin E.</li><li>Toxic—very dangerous.</li></ul>
loss of appetite, poor taste skin problems poor wound healing enlarged prostate poor night vision white spots on fingernails	fever diarrhea nausea vomiting	<ul><li>Dissolving zinc gluconate (not zinc sulfate) tablets in the mouth may decrease length of colds (look for good-tasting lozenges).</li><li>May cause iron or copper deficiency.</li></ul>

Beyond the Text

1. You have had your cholesterol tested at a shopping center testing site and the reading came back 240. Is it time to panic?

2. A cereal that contains hydrogenated coconut oil advertises itself as "healthy and cholesterol-free." Is there any reason to think otherwise?

3. Respond to the following statement: Alcohol calories don't count because there are no nutrients in alcohol.

4. Respond to the following statement: Osteoporosis is a disease of old women. I don't need to worry about that until I get there.

5. Every athlete needs large quantities of protein to build strong muscles. Do you believe this? Why or why not?

6. Respond to the following statement: A vitamin pill cancels out a poor diet.

7. Respond to the following statement: There is no more safe food left, so you might as well eat what you want.

Supplemental Readings

Diet for a New America by John Robbins. Walpole, NH: Stillpoint Publishing, 1987. Robbins, legacy of the Baskin-Robbins empire, offers us an extraordinary look at America's dependence on animals for food and how inhumane and unhealthy the conditions are for their growth. This book may change your eating habits forever.

Diet for a Small Planet by Frances Moore Lappe. New York: Ballantine, 1971. Now a classic, offers an excellent discussion on the nutrition, food combinations, and the economic and social aspects of food production.

Gluttons for Punishment by James Erlichman. Great Britain: Penguin Books, 1986. Discusses and documents the health hazards of the foods we buy and eat.

It's Not What You Eat But What Eats You by Jack Schwarz. Berkeley, CA: Celestial Arts, 1988. A world-renowned intuitive, Jack Schwarz presents a unique perspective on the mind-body connection between nutrition and vitality. Combining the subjects of health, diet, and nutrition, the author leads you to consider transformation on all levels.

Laurel's Kitchen by Laurel Robertson, Carol Flinders and Bronwen Godfrey. New York: Bantam, 1976. A homey and informative guide to nutrition and diet with emphasis on whole, fresh foods and vegetarianism. Contains comprehensive charts.

The Gradual Vegetarian by Lisa Tracy. New York: M. Evans and Company, 1985. An easy, gradual introduction to vegetarian lifestyle. A workable and forgiving plan to help you move toward healthier eating; includes delicious recipes.

The Whole Foods Encyclopedia: A Shopper's Guide by Rebecca Wood. Englewood Cliffs, NJ: Prentice-Hall Press, 1988. A gold mine of information about practically every food known to humanity, including an appendix on personal care products.

Key Terms Defined

additive substance added to another to improve its appearance, increase its nutritive value, and so forth

basal metabolic rate the number of calories required to maintain life-sustaining activities for a specified period of time

carbohydrate nutrient containing carbon, hydrogen, and oxygen; an efficient source of body energy

cholesterol steroid alcohol found in the human body (synthesized primarily in the liver) and in animal products; high levels of total serum cholesterol are associated with heart disease

complementary proteins incomplete proteins that, when combined, provide all the amino acids essential for protein synthesis

complete proteins proteins that contain all of the essential amino acids needed by the body for growth and maintenance, such as meat, milk, and fish

complex carbohydrates carbohydrates composed of long molecular chains containing many saccharide units (starch, glycogen, and cellulose)

fat lipids (oily substance) present in oils and food that have an exceptionally high energy content; saturated and unsaturated fats—all common unsaturated fatty acids are liquid at room temperature; through the process of hydrogenation (incorporating hydrogen into the fat), unsaturated fats are converted into solid fats

glucose simple sugar in foodstuffs and in normal blood; the chief source of energy for living organisms, glucose is the end product of carbohydrate digestion

high-density lipoproteins (HDL) compounds that bind with cholesterol and carry it to the liver for breakdown and excretion; considered "good" lipoprotein

insulin hormone secreted by the pancreas that regulates blood sugar; secreted into the blood in response to a rise in blood glucose and amino acids

low-density lipoproteins (LDL) compounds made up of a protein and a lipid that deposit cholesterol in the body cells; considered "bad" lipoprotein

nutrient nourishing substance, food, or component of food

nutrition includes all the processes by which the body uses food for energy, maintenance, and growth; particularly concerned with those properties of food that build sound bodies and promote health

protein one of the essential nutrients; any large organic compound made from one or more polypeptides, or amino acids

Weight Happiness

The vast majority of Americans believe they weigh too much. According to a *Newsweek* poll, almost one-third of college students see themselves as having a weight problem. In fact, many students (especially women) gain 10 to 20 pounds during their first semester at college. Some of this increase is a result of natural completion of the body's growth. However, college eating and drinking patterns contribute to weight gain—dining hall restrictions on when and what you eat, heavy late-night snacking, binge eating, and social activities centering on food and drink, including significant alcohol consumption.

Many individuals search for weight happiness—the secret diet or pill, or exercise through which they will finally achieve the same figure as a high-fashion model or a world-class athlete. The secret to weight happiness is not striving for perfection as measured by external standards, but recognizing, achieving, and maintaining the healthiest realistic weight for you. This chapter is designed to help you assess your attitude toward your weight and to develop a program that meets your unique needs.

Key Terms

Body mass index	Metabolism
Body image	Nutrition
Calorie	Obesity
Fasting	Plateau
Fats	Set point theory
Insulin	

Contents

Finding Your Desirable Weight

Why College Students Are Concerned About Weight

Surveys indicate that about one-third of women between 19 and 30 years old diet at least once a month. A recent Gallup Poll showed that 50 percent of teenage girls would like to lose weight. In contrast, 52 percent of teenage boys thought their own weight was appropriate, and 20 percent said they'd like to gain. Among young adults, weight control is a more important issue for women than men. As summarized by *American Health* magazine, thinness has great meaning for contemporary women. "Thinness has become symbolic of strength, independence and achievement, as well as attractiveness." In a survey of Wellesley college women, 80 percent wanted to lose weight.

Does the weight status of college students justify such concerns? Some individuals arrive overweight or gain unneeded weight at college; others have an inaccurate perception of themselves as overweight. Because weight has such psychological connotations in our culture, it's easy to confuse the reasons your weight status is important to you: physical health, pressure from parents, peer influence, or your own personal goals.

Being overweight (exceeding normal weight range guidelines) can have physical costs. It reduces your energy level, contributes to many diseases, and interferes with your physical agility. Being overweight is associated with higher rates of heart disease, cancer, joint problems, diabetes, and many other serious physical problems.

What drives most people to concern about their weight are social and emotional issues. Our culture associates certain body shapes with greater romantic, social, and even business and financial success. When these aspects of your life are not the way you want them to be, it's tempting, but often unrealistic, to think that if you lose (or gain) some weight, another problem would also improve. Sometimes our parents and friends also give us this message.

Should you conform to these norms or just think more positively about yourself and worry less about your body? How can you get your mind and your body to agree on the same ideal weight for you? How important is your weight? Worrying all the time about weight may get in the way of accomplishing other important goals. The correct balance is finding the right weight for you.

Self-Esteem and Weight

Self-esteem means how you feel about yourself—physically and emotionally. If you feel good about yourself, you can trust your physical and emotional impulses about what's right for you. Many of us have complicated attitudes about self-acceptance and food. For instance, you may sometimes eat to comfort yourself when another part of your life is stressful. On the other hand, you may feel people accept you only if you look or act

Weight Happiness

a certain way. When your self-esteem is high, you'll find it easier to discipline and regulate your eating according to internal rather than external signals.

College environments contain many persuasive external clues about when and what to eat—residence hall cafeteria, parties, study breaks, the campus coffee house, and off-campus eateries. It's natural to eat when you're in the company of others doing the same. When a friend or date offers food or drink, you don't want to be contrary. You don't want to draw attention to yourself or be different. In such settings, you may easily confuse emotional hunger with physical hunger and confuse your self-image with the image you want others to hold of you. Self-esteem can play a big role in what your weight is, whether you think your weight is a problem, and whether you choose to change your weight.

Determing Your Desirable Weight

Weight charts and tables give you a good external starting point for determining your ideal weight—the weight at which you'd have the greatest potential for health. But weight charts are incomplete—your ideal weight is the result of many individual factors for which no chart can fully compensate. Following the charts and techniques, you'll learn how to consider your own background, body, and lifestyle in determining your ideal weight.

Weight Tables   You've seen the standard weight table, developed by Metropolitan Life Insurance Company. Review this chart, but remember

Where Do My Calories Go?

Physical movement accounts for only about one-third of the calories spent in a day. For a normally active person, this might add up to 800 calories a day. About 1,400 calories are burned up by our metabolism, heart beating and lung exchange—all normal body processes.

Exercise can speed up your metabolic rate and, if you develop more muscles, you will spend more energy just to exist. Monitoring your calories and increasing your exercise is the healthiest way to lose or maintain your weight.

Source: *Hippocrates*, September/October, 1989

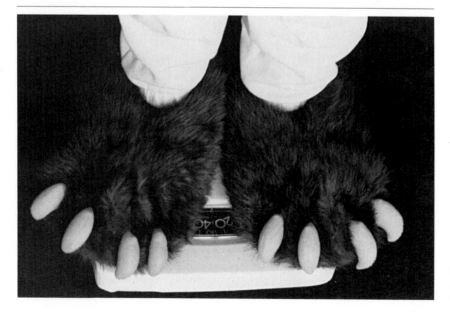

Weight Happiness

Weight Chart

This table was prepared in 1959 by the Metropolitan Life Insurance Company. Many nutritionists recommend using this version instead of the revised 1979 version, because the more recent table gives higher weight ranges, which may lead many individuals to greater complacency about their weight.

Desirable Weights in Pounds, According to Frame (in Indoor Clothing)

Height Men		Small Frame	Medium Frame	Large Frame
Feet	Inches			
5	2	112–120	118–129	126–141
5	3	115–123	121–133	129–144
5	4	118–126	124–136	132–148
5	5	121–129	127–139	135–152
5	6	124–133	130–143	138–156
5	7	128–137	134–147	142–161
5	8	132–141	138–152	147–166
5	9	136–145	142–156	151–170
5	10	140–150	146–160	155–174
5	11	144–154	150–165	159–179
6	0	148–158	154–170	164–184
6	1	152–162	158–175	168–189
6	2	156–167	162–180	173–194
6	3	160–171	167–185	178–199
6	4	164–175	172–190	182–204

Height Women		Small Frame	Medium Frame	Large Frame
Feet	Inches			
4	8	92– 98	96–107	104–119
4	9	94–101	98–110	106–122
4	10	96–104	101–113	109–125
4	11	99–107	104–116	112–128
5	0	102–110	107–119	115–131
5	1	105–113	110–122	118–134
5	2	108–116	113–126	121–138
5	3	111–119	116–130	125–142
5	4	114–123	120–135	129–146
5	5	118–127	124–139	133–150
5	6	122–131	128–143	137–154
5	7	126–135	132–147	141–158
5	8	130–140	136–151	145–163
5	9	134–144	140–155	149–168
5	10	138–148	144–159	153–173
5	11	142–152	148–163	157–177
6	0	146–156	152–167	161–181
6	1	150–160	156–171	165–185
6	2	154–164	160–175	169–189

Source: Metropolitan Life Insurance Company

Frame Size and Elbow Breadth

To measure your elbow breadth: Hold your arm horizontal, then bend your forearm up at a 90 degree angle. The inside of your wrist should face your body. Place the thumb and index finger of your other hand on the two prominent bones on either side of your elbow. Using a ruler or tape measure, have a friend measure the space between that thumb and index finger.

To determine your frame size: The following measurements are for men and women of medium frame. If your elbow breadth is below the range for your gender and height, you have a small frame. If yours is above the range for your gender and height, you have a large frame.

Height (in 1″ Heels)	Elbow Breadth for Medium Frame
Men	
5′2″ to 5′3″+	2½″ to 2⅞″
5′4″ to 5′7″+	2⅝″ to 2⅞″
5′8″ to 5′11″+	2¾″ to 3″
6′0″ to 6′3″+	2¾″ to 3⅛″
6′4″+	2⅞″ to 3¼″
Women	
4′10″ to 4′11″+	2¼″ to 2½″
5′0″ to 5′3″+	2¼″ to 2½″
5′4″ to 5′7″+	2⅜″ to 2⅝″
5′8″ to 5′11″+	2⅜″ to 2⅝″
6′0″+	2½″ to 2¾″

Source: Metropolitan Life Insurance Company

Calculate Your Body Mass Index

Body mass is obtained by dividing your weight in kilograms by the square of your height in meters.

To convert to kilograms, divide your weight in pounds (without clothes) by 2.2: _____

To convert to meters, divide your height in inches (without shoes) by 39.4, then square it: _____

Divide your weight by your height. Body mass = _____

Women Desirable body mass is 21 to 23. Obesity (20 percent above the desirable range) begins at 27.5. Serious obesity (40 percent above) begins at 31.5.

Men Desirable body mass is 22 to 24. Obesity begins at 28.5, and serious obesity begins at 33.

The National Institutes of Health urges those who weigh more than the desirable range to lose weight. The greater one's weight, the more urgent the recommendation becomes.

Source: *Medical Self-Care*

that these tables don't consider personal factors, such as genetics, health status, activity level, and how you feel.

To use this table effectively, you need to determine your frame size. One clue is how clothes fit through the shoulders and across the back. Again, looking at family members can help. Also, certain ethnic, cultural, and regional groups sometimes tend to have certain frame sizes. One objective and fairly reliable guide to frame size is elbow breadth. To measure your elbow breadth, follow the accompanying instructions and table.

Body Mass Index The National Institutes of Health regards the body mass index (BMI) as the most useful way to determine ideal weight because it compares weight with body fat. It doesn't tell you how much you should weigh or how much to lose; that's your decision.

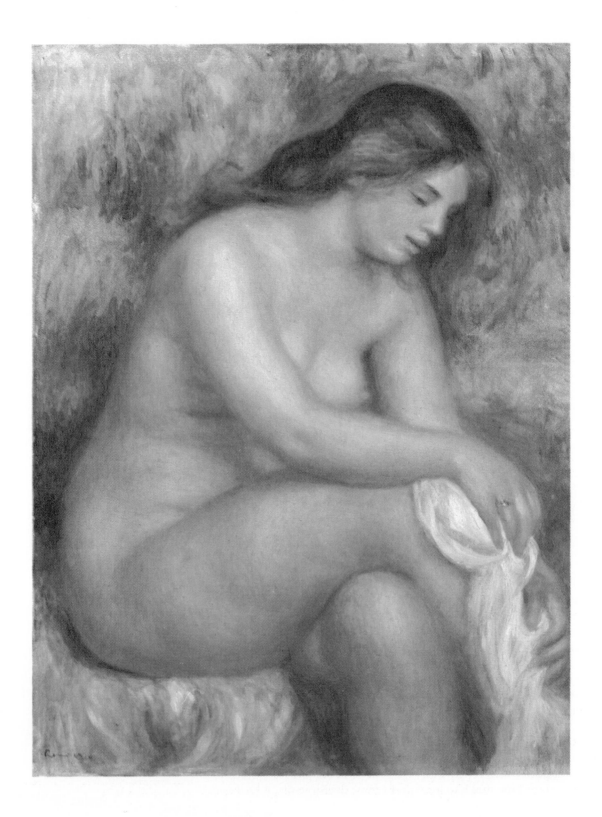

Personal Factors in Your Ideal Weight

Because your body and your lifestyle differ from everyone else's, personal factors influence whether you should set your ideal weight on the low or high side of the external ranges. Such factors include genetics, sex, health status, physical activity level, and self-image.

Genetics Physical characteristics of family members are often strong clues to your own size and shape. Bone size, metabolism, sensitivity to tastes—all these influences on our body shape have strong genetic components. For instance, a recent study of twins raised by adoptive parents showed that adult weight correlates much more strongly with the biological parents than with the family in which an individual grows up. If your family tends to be stocky, you'll probably do better giving up dreams of a dancer's body. If none of the men in your family is taller than 5'10", you probably won't be a basketball star. If you have to watch your weight more carefully than a friend who eats and eats but stays slender, don't blame yourself or resent your friend, who may just have genes that give her a faster metabolism.

Sex This plays an important role in weight and body composition. We know men tend to be taller; they also have a higher percentage of muscle mass. Women are biologically designed to carry a higher percentage of fat, because healthy childbearing requires fat stores. In fact, newborn girls have 10 to 15 percent more fat on their bodies than do newborn boys.

Personal and Family Health History Maintaining a relatively slender physique reduces your chances of contracting many serious illnesses—such as heart disease, diabetes, arthritis, high blood pressure, stroke, and several types of cancer. Many of these diseases have hereditary components, so if your family has a higher than normal incidence of such weight-related health problems, it is important that you adopt a relatively lean ideal weight.

Physical Activity Level Muscle weighs several times more than fat. If you lead an active life, you probably have a lower proportion of fat on your body than someone who weighs the same but is sedentary. So your healthy weight can be higher if you are active, because you'll have more muscle mass.

   In some athletic activities, you can expect to perform better if you have a low level of body fat. If you participate frequently in sports such as swimming, dancing, rowing, and running, you may want a relatively low ideal weight.

Self-Image Perhaps you weigh more than the charts indicate is an ideal range. Or perhaps you're on the low side of the range but would like to lose more. Is this necessarily a problem? If your weight exceeds or falls below the ranges by 15 pounds or more, consult your college health ser-

The Setpoint Theory

In recent years, some experts have proposed that the reason so many people lose weight, only to bounce back to their previous weight, is because their body weight is returning to its "setpoint." Your setpoint is the weight your body "wants" to be. A recent book by the University of California and *American Health* magazine comments, "There's an increasing consensus that fatness is regulated—that the body cares how much fat tissue it carries—and that some bodies are biologically suited to carry more fat than others."

Dr. William Bennett and Joel Gurin, in their book *The Dieter's Dilemma*, describe many studies that demonstrate that when you diet or lose weight, your metabolism slows down, conserving energy as a way to maintain or regain that weight level. If you exceed your setpoint, your weight loss efforts may succeed more easily, but only until you reach that setpoint again.

Does this mean you're trapped for life at only one possible stable weight? Though shifting one's setpoint may be difficult, a program by nutritionist Judith Stern and exercise physiologists Edward Bernauer and Paul Mole at the University of California at Davis showed that exercise could help keep metabolic rates high during dieting. In fact, exercise may help lower your setpoint. To accomplish this effect, you must reach and maintain your goal weight for quite a while—some say two years—by keeping your exercise high and your diet low in fat and high in complex carbohydrates.

vice to determine whether your weight (or losing more weight) puts you at medical risk. If it doesn't, you can choose; let the decision of whether or not to lose or gain weight depend on how you feel about your weight, on your external image, energy level, and amount of physical activity.

How to Achieve and Maintain Weight Loss Goals

Many traditional diets emphasize that if you want to lose weight, count calories. Ninety-five percent of those people who lose weight by counting calories regain their lost weight. Permanent weight loss is the result of selecting foods high in complex carbohydrates and low in fats, increasing and maintaining a vigorous exercise program, and making lifestyle and psychological changes.

Why Most Diets Don't Work

Many diets of college students are nutritionally unsound; most are ineffective for losing weight and keeping it off. Diets that emphasize counting calories often contribute to the perception that a calorie is a calorie is a calorie. If this were actually true, you might say, "Since one Snickers bar equals a tuna sandwich and an apple, I'll have the candy bar instead." However, because you burn more calories digesting complex carbohydrates than digesting fat, a high-fat snack (such as most candy bars, granola bars, and so forth) leaves more calories stored as fat.

College students often try fasting, low-calorie diets, and mono-food diets to lose weight. In an atmosphere filled with food options, eliminating most choices can seem like a simple answer, but such efforts often backfire. If you feed your body too few calories, your metabolic rate drops, which means your body starts conserving energy. Because your body then wants to extract every possible fraction of energy from your food, it burns less body fat, and you lose weight more slowly than you would on a diet higher in calories.

On rigid diets, the first several pounds of weight loss are often water, which you'll soon gain back as your body regulates itself. On quick-loss diets, your body tends to burn muscle rather than fat; you're not losing the undesirable flabby weight, just strength. Moreover, when you deprive yourself to such extremes, you're also more likely to binge later, setting yourself up not only for extra high-fat calories, but for disappointment and low self-esteem as well. No single or small group of foods can give your body the protein, carbohydrates, vitamins, and minerals you need for health. Not one of 11 popular weight-loss diets (including Atkins, Beverly Hills, Pritikin, Scarsdale, Stillman, and Richard Simmons) evaluated by Rutgers University provided sufficient essential vitamins and minerals. Fasting, low-calorie diets, and mono-food diets do not prepare you to eat sensibly (and maintain your weight) once you reach your goal weight. (To prevent nutritional deficiencies, women should usually eat between 1500 and 1800 calories, and men should consume between 1700 and 2000 calories.)

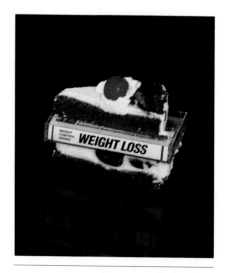

The Right Foods for Weight Loss

Unlike old weight-loss programs that emphasized weighing and measuring portions, more and more nutritionists now emphasize that the correct selections of foods make a greater contribution to achieving your objective than the amount of overall food consumed.

The guidelines for food selection for weight loss are similar to those for good nutrition in general—keep fat calories to a minimum; concentrate on complex carbohydrates, fruits, and vegetables. The single most important weight-reducing change you can make is to substitute high-carbohydrate foods for high-fat foods.

Americans spent more than $20 billion on diet foods and drinks in 1986.

Reduce Fat Consumption Fat contains more calories per gram than any other food source. Each tablespoon of fat contains 100 to 125 calories, all ready for your body to store as fat, with very little processing required. The average food use of fats by Americans has increased 15 percent in the past twenty years, and many of us are fatter as a consequence. Bestselling nutrition writer Jane Brody says, "Fat makes a far greater contribution to the weight problems of Americans than does sugar." So, limit fats to 25 percent of your total calories, just over half the American average.

Weight Happiness

Quick Nutrition Tips for Weight Watchers

Good nutrition tips for weight watchers (and anyone else):

- Eat a diet high in complex carbohydrates (whole grains, beans, noodles, rice, other starches).
- Limit fat consumption to no more than 25 percent of calories, especially by choosing low-fat protein sources.
- Limit or eliminate consumption of sugar (including soft drinks and juices).
- Limit or eliminate consumption of alcohol.
- Choose rich desserts infrequently; substitute fruit or sherbet.
- Eat a variety of fresh fruits and vegetables.
- Drink plenty of water; try for eight glasses a day.

Here are some quick ways to cut fat:

- Eat fewer nuts, including peanut butter (they're almost 100 percent fat).
- When you want a crunchy snack, choose unbuttered popcorn, fresh vegetables, fruit, and low-fat crackers (such as Ak-Mak, Ry-Krisp, rice crackers).
- Choose low-fat or reduced-calorie salad dressings.
- Eat foods without creamy sauces, gravies, butter, margarine, sour cream.
- Limit cheese consumption to only two to three ounces per week.
- Use non-fat dairy products instead of low-fat or whole milk. This is just as true for yogurt and cottage cheese as for milk itself.
- Avoid the skin of chicken (it's pure fat). When you do eat red meat, choose pieces with as little fat as possible, and cut off the fat you do find.
- Choose protein foods low in fat. (See **Nutrition** for a list of low-fat protein sources.)
- Limit frozen desserts and other treats to items containing no more than 3 grams of fat per serving.

Emphasize High-Carbohydrate, High-Fiber Foods   In spite of the myth that carbohydrates are the enemy of dieters, your true foe is not the baked potato but the sour cream, not the noodles but the alfredo sauce. Carbohydrates have low caloric density, so you can eat a lot, get full, and not have ingested many calories. For instance, University of Alabama researchers found that volunteers on high-carbohydrate foods felt full after eating 1,500 calories per day, but those eating foods high in fat and sugar needed 3,000 calories to feel full.

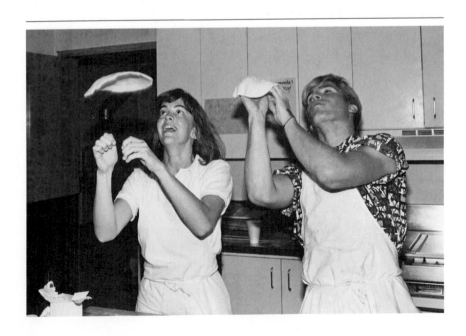

Many complex carbohydrates (such as whole grain cereals and breads) and raw fruits and vegetables are high in fiber, which also aids in weight management. High-fiber foods tend to have rather low caloric density, which means a large amount of that food has very few calories. For instance, a cup of apple juice has the same number of calories as three medium apples; yet eating the high-fiber apples requires more energy, time and calories to process. Your body begins to get the signal that it's full when you've eaten fewer calories, so you don't go on eating.

Reduce Sugar Consumption   Successful weight loss requires limiting the amount of sugar and sugar-containing foods (fruit yogurts, regular sodas, most jams, baked desserts, ice cream, and similar treats) you eat. When sugary foods contain more calories than you can use and process at one time, your body stores the excess calories as fat. Sugary foods often contain large amounts of fat. Ice cream, candy bars, cakes, cookies, pies, and most desserts are high in both sugar and fat. Moreover, a recent book by the University of California and *American Health* magazine states, "Refined sugars may be uniquely fattening because they increase hunger by raising insulin levels." A Yale psychologist working on this topic found that individuals who had a sugar drink with breakfast were hungrier and ate more at lunch than people who had eaten low-sugar foods and drinks for breakfast.

Substituting artificially sweetened foods for sugar-containing foods won't solve your weight problems. In a controversial report, American Cancer Society researcher Steven Stellman and his colleague Lawrence Garfinkel reported that after one year, women who used artificial sweeteners were more likely than nonusers to have gained weight. Results of several lab experiments also indicate aspartame may actually increase hunger, and none indicates that it reduces hunger.

In fact, some researchers believe that people often compensate for the "virtuousness" of using NutraSweet by rewarding themselves with something else—such as a piece of cake for dessert, or French fries—that turns out to be high in sugar, fat, or both.

Techniques for Parties, Snacks and Fast Foods   Even though you're trying to lose weight, you still want to have a good time when you get together with friends, and so many college social situations virtually focus on food and drink. Try to arrange to have foods and beverages you prefer available at parties, study sessions and other places you socialize. If they are not available, eat and drink lightly, or volunteer to bring what you'd like to have; if you bring extra, others may choose your fare as well.

Provide simple foods, such as plain popcorn, fresh fruit, crackers, raw vegetables; bring sparkling waters to substitute for alcohol and high-calorie soda. A small refrigerator in your room will help you keep your choice of food and beverages cold and convenient. (See **Nutrition** for more tips on parties, snacks, and fast foods.)

About Counting Calories

Many of us think of weight management as purely a calorie-management task. A "calorie" is actually the measure of how much energy food or drink contains. In scientific terms, a calorie is the amount of energy required to raise one gram of water one degree centigrade. Each dietary "calorie" is actually 1,000 calories, or one kilocalorie, but for simplicity, nutritionists refer not to kilocalories but calories.

Calories represent only part of your weight management picture. For instance, the amount of exercise you do influences how much energy your body conserves from the calories you consume. Your body also uses more energy processing calories from carbohydrates than those from fats; so concentrate on the nutritional content and fat content of what you eat rather than counting calories.

If you still want to know how many calories you are consuming, check one of the many paperback calorie books available. For instance, Barbara Kraus' *Calorie Guide to Brand Names and Basic Foods* includes most foods commonly eaten by college students. Remember, because fats are the most concentrated sources of calories, calorie count per serving often provides a fairly accurate guide to that food's fat composition.

At restaurants, choose pita bread sandwiches (not croissants, which are loaded with fat), baked potatoes (with vegetable toppings or cottage cheese), salads (with little or no cheese or fat-containing dressings), and low-fat or non-fat milk. If you crave a hamburger, get a small one and skip the sauce (mustard is fine).

Exercise Frequently

We all know that exercise helps with weight loss. Though any physical exertion expends calories, exercise that increases your body's oxygen consumption, called aerobic exercise, not only strengthens your heart, lungs, and circulatory system, but also burns more calories and increases your metabolism. Aerobic exercise ranges from brisk walking to high-paced dancing. In addition to the calories burned while exercising, aerobic activity enhances your metabolism for several hours post-exercise. During this entire period, your body keeps burning more calories than it otherwise would, and burned calories are not available to be stored as fat.

To achieve the desired results, you must exercise to increase your heart rate, then maintain vigorous activity for a specific period of time, generally about 20 to 25 minutes. Sports experts recommend aerobic exercise three or four times per week. Obviously, running and swimming burn more calories per minute than walking; but you can burn approximately the same number of calories by briskly walking three miles as by running three miles. The **Physical Fitness** chapter contains more information on aerobic exercise, how to identify and overcome your barriers to exercise, and how to integrate exercise as a permanent part of your college life.

Create a Healthier Eating Style

Your lifestyle has many components that influence your food choices, such as when you eat, with whom you eat, and what else you do while eating. To permanently improve your weight status, you'll have to change the aspects of your lifestyle that lead you to counterproductive eating behaviors. Small changes can have dramatically positive effects on your weight.

Improving inappropriate behavior patterns may be easier when you understand *why* you have those patterns. Did you learn them from your parents? Are you eating (or avoiding food) for security, comfort, power, reward, or as a call for help? Such issues are far too complex and controversial for this chapter to handle in the detail you may find helpful, so the Resources section includes several books on this subject. Counseling can often help receptive individuals sort out such issues.

To discover counterproductive behaviors, observe yourself as if you were a participant in a scientific experiment. For several days, pay attention to when, where, how, why, and with whom you eat. Keep a food diary if you can. Notice when you make food-related choices that hinder or contribute to achieving your weight goal. Here are some common eating-style problems and suggested solutions:

Lifestyle Habits

A lifestyle habit of regular exercise not only builds muscles, increases calorie needs permanently, and triggers the body to burn fat, but also protects you against heart disease and cancer.

Weight Happiness

Control Your Portions to Control Your Weight

How **much** you eat, particularly how much fat and sugar, plays a significant role in what happens to your weight. Because proteins often contain a significant amount of fat, if you want to lose weight, you need to pay special attention to the portion sizes of proteins (such as meat and cheese). Here are some visual memory aids to help you keep track.

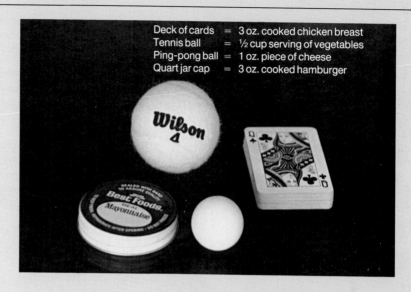

Deck of cards = 3 oz. cooked chicken breast
Tennis ball = ½ cup serving of vegetables
Ping-pong ball = 1 oz. piece of cheese
Quart jar cap = 3 oz. cooked hamburger

When You Eat

Problem: You skip breakfast, eat a small lunch or none, then binge at dinner or afterward.

Solution: Weight watchers should eat breakfast. Early in the day your body burns a higher percentage of its intake. Eat then and your body stays slimmer, with more energy for a busy day. If you skip breakfast, you'll more than make up for the calories later on, and at higher cost.

Alternatives to eggs (which are high in cholesterol) include oatmeal, cold cereal with fruit and milk, bagels, English muffins, yogurt, and cottage cheese. If you're not hungry when you first get up, take some breakfast with you; grab a bagel or English muffin and a piece of fruit. Eat them when you do get hungry.

Problem: At social events, you eat lots of high-fat party foods and drink alcohol.

Solution: Bring your own party food and drink. Organize or participate in social events that involve more physical or mental activity than eating and drinking. These could range from volleyball to dancing to campus projects. Achieving your

Weight Happiness

How to Lose Weight on Residence Hall Food

- *Salad bar*: Choose lots of vegetables and beans, less cheese, dressing, and bacon bits. Select cole slaw instead of potato salad if you crave a moist salad.
- *Vegetables*: Go for vegetables that are steamed rather than sautéed. Try to vary what you choose. Fresh, seasonal items are more appealing and more nutritious.
- *Entree*: Look for simple foods. Take a small amount of sauce or gravy on the side, or not at all. Eat meatless, cheeseless meals once or twice a week.
- *Beverage*: Non-fat milk (low-fat if you can't stand non-fat) or water is a good choice. So is herbal tea. Keep coffee and tea consumption moderate. Lemonade and other fruit juices are very high in sugar and, hence, calories.
- *Dessert*: Get only desserts you *really* want; don't select dessert just because it's there. Go back for it only if you're still hungry after dinner. If you want that *particular* dessert, but aren't hungry, save it for later. The lowest-fat desserts are fresh fruit, sherbet, frozen yogurt, and ice milk. Fruit crisps can sometimes be relatively low in fat, but pies, cakes and other pastries are filled with sugar and fat.

Problem: You eat while reading, watching TV, studying, talking with friends.

How You Eat

Problem: You eat too fast. Clues include: you swallow your food without chewing it well; while still chewing one bite, you're already putting the next bite on your fork; you try to finish your meal before your food gets cold.

Why You Eat

Problem: Whenever you see food, you want to eat.

Problem: You eat or drink whenever the people around you do.

weight goal while continuing to participate in social gatherings that revolve around food and drink requires significant self-discipline. The more you practice saying no, the easier resisting inappropriate choices becomes.

Solution: If you do something else while eating, you diminish the sensations you get from the food you eat, and so may wind up eating more than hunger or simple enjoyment would suggest. If you must have something to munch on during sedentary activities, try gum, fruit, non-calorie drinks, or plain popcorn. Here, too, you will probably have to develop self-discipline, but your new food habits will become easier as time goes on.

Solution: Concentrate on what your food tastes and feels like. Chew your food well. Put your fork down completely (actually let go of it) between bites. Take breaks from eating to involve yourself in conversations around you.

Solution: Discipline yourself to stay away from food situations unless you have already decided that it is an appropriate mealtime or snacktime. Minimize your visits to the kitchen, campus store, snack bars, vending machines, and your friends' refrigerators. At meals, sit facing away from the food service line or kitchen. Clear away your plate as soon as you finish eating. You may want to try taking only half of what you'll want at first; then you can feel the satisfaction of going back for seconds without overeating.

Solution: Learn appropriate choices for wherever you go with friends—an extra-big salad, lots of lightly flavored mineral waters. You probably notice more than anyone else notices when you skip the buttered popcorn at the movies, milkshake at the local hangout, or multiple beers at the party.

Recognize that true friends don't love you for what you eat or drink but for who you are. If your friends aren't supportive, remember that they may feel threatened when you're changing in other ways, or they may feel guilty about their own habits. Keep quiet about your dietary changes if they seem to bother your friends.

Problem: You eat to avoid or postpone unpleasant activity, such as studying.

Solution: Recognize that food will not solve your problems. The most effective technique is to face the conflict in a timely fashion. Alternatively, if you really need a little time, use a more constructive recreation, such as walking around the block or talking with a friend.

Problem: You eat when you're nervous or under stress.

Solution: Weighing more than you want and eating contrary to your weight management goals cause stress, too. Avoid these stressors by finding other ways of handling stress than eating inappropriately.

Develop effective techniques for dealing with stress more directly. See **Coping with Stress** to understand the stressors of college life, how to let go of unnecessary stressors, and how to use relaxation tech-

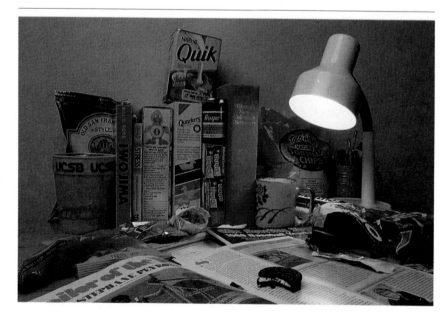

One College Student's Plan for Taking Off Pounds

Kimberley had gained 12 pounds since coming to college eight months ago. Here's what she decided to do about it:

What's my goal weight? Right now I weigh 137 pounds, but when I graduated from high school I weighed 125 pounds. Nobody in my family is really skinny, and I don't buy petite clothes, even though I'm 5'4", so I'm probably a medium frame. According to the charts and body mass index, my ideal weight range is 124 to 136 pounds. Even though I'm just above the top edge of that range now, I really felt better about how I looked and how my clothes fit when I weighed 125 pounds.

I'm going to set my goal weight at 125 pounds.

What will I do to lose that weight? I'll aim for three changes:

1. Lower-fat snacks: fresh fruit, plain popcorn, low-fat crackers, and sparkling water.
2. Take a jazz dance class that meets three times a week.
3. Don't eat while studying.

When will I start my weight program? Next week is finals week, so I won't try anything radical now. I'll start in two weeks, the first day of the upcoming quarter.

Weight Happiness

CHAPTER 8

niques to reduce the unwanted effects of stress on your body and mind.

Problem: You eat when you're lonesome, depressed, sad, or otherwise feeling down.

Solution: When you're feeling bad about yourself or your life, eating may appeal to you as comforting behavior, but it is really self-defeating. You feel good about the chocolate (or whatever) but later kick yourself for your fat-causing actions. And, of course, poor nutrition may make you feel worse. Instead, work on solutions for the negative feelings themselves, as discussed in the chapters on **Mental Fitness** and **Depression**.

How to Gain Weight

If you want to gain weight, you'll find far fewer resources to help you than to help people trying to lose weight. Some people may even think your goal amusing. If you think of yourself as weak and skinny, or believe that gaining weight would help you be a better athlete, have a better self-image, or be more attractive, here are some actions you can take to achieve your goal.

Warning: *Rapid, unexplained weight loss can be a sign of significant physical problems. If you've never had low weight and now find yourself chronically weighing less than you would like, and you are not aware of having changed your eating habits, consult your health care provider.*

Food Consumption

You don't have to eat all the time to gain weight. The secret to healthy weight gain is not simply to eat more but also to eat nutritionally valuable food. Following the nutritional principles discussed in the **Nutrition** chapter will contribute significantly to adding firm bulk to your body. Avoid consuming lots of empty calories in sugary foods, fatty foods and alcohol. Though you can certainly afford the calories in these foods, eating them fills you up and you run out of room for the nutritionally valuable foods you need for the body you want—protein for muscles, carbohydrates for energy, and vegetables and fruits for vitamins and minerals.

Pay attention to what you're eating—what do you skip as you serve yourself dinner? What do you leave on your plate? Look for ways to complete the nutritional components you may be avoiding. Because you can afford some of the more calorically dense foods that others may need to avoid, allow yourself the condiments that make food more palatable and attractive to you. If you'll eat a sandwich only if it has mayonnaise, or vegetables only with a sauce, fix your food the way you like, but then eat *both* the vegetables *and* the sauce.

To make sure you get sufficient food quantity, eat something from each food group at least three times a day—protein, complex carbohydrate, and fruit or vegetable. If quantity is a problem, you may want to consider "grazing"—eating small (healthy) meals frequently. An evening snack is often a good way to get in a bit more to eat—and your body retains more of the calories from food eaten late in the day. Fast snacks that include lots of compact nutrition include granolas, nuts, seeds, and dried fruit.

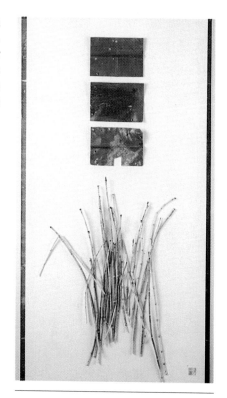

Physical Activity and Gaining Weight

Though physical activity burns calories, you don't have to become sedentary to gain weight. With such inactivity, you'd wind up with a heavier but fatter body (maybe even skinny everywhere but with a "beer belly" appearance). When you exercise regularly, your body converts the food you eat into muscle rather than fat. To develop muscle mass, concentrate on strengthening exercises (weights and calisthenics), discussed in **Physical Fitness**.

Positive Eating Situations

Many people who consider themselves underweight avoid eating with other people. You don't have to eat when everyone else does, but it is often a good idea. In the dining hall or kitchen you'll find nutritional food ready to eat, and friends to socialize with during the meal.

Observe yourself for a week or so to notice when you don't eat and others do. What are you doing and feeling at those times? Here are some common eating-style problems among people who want to gain weight, with suggested solutions:

Problem: You skip meals because you forget about eating.

Solution: Try to establish a routine of eating certain meals at your dining hall or home. Set up your schedule so you are at that place when it's time for a meal. The scent of the food and the activities of others may clue you to join in the meal. If you can only get meals at certain times of the day, you may want to set an alarm to remind you to eat.

Problem: You skip meals because you are too busy to eat.

Solution: College is full of deadlines and exciting activities, so you may have to consider meals as an element to work into your schedule. Resolve food-related time conflicts.

Combine a meal with something else, such as chatting with friends or reading. For busy mealtimes, some students use concentrated forms of nutrition, such as fortified cereals, blender smoothies, or all-in-one sandwiches.

Weight Happiness

Problem: You skip meals because you're uncomfortable with the social setting.

Solution: Avoiding people you live with by skipping meals just shifts your problems. You'll never work out social conflicts hanging out by yourself; getting proper food to enable you to improve your body and health may help you feel more self-assured in handling such situations.

Dining halls are some of the best places to meet and get to know other students. If the eating environment really isn't working, change the setting. Eat in a different dining hall, or change your living situation.

Problem: Eating makes you feel physically uncomfortable.

Solution: Investigate any physically unpleasant sensations associated with eating. If your teeth or mouth hurts, your stomach feels uncomfortable during or after meals, or you get headaches after eating, seek professional medical advice. Possible causes include physical problems, disease, food allergies, and stress. If your problem is stress-related (most common with stomach pains), you can improve your situation by adopting stress management techniques.

Making Your Weight Program Successful

Now that you have considered your own ideal weight and understand the roles of food, exercise, and eating behavior in weight management, you can establish your own program to meet your weight-related goals.

cathy®

by Cathy Guisewite

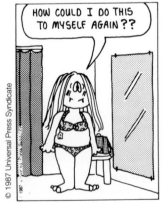

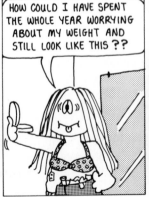

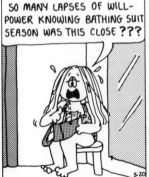

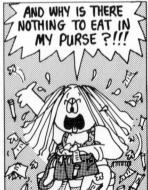

Set a Realistic Weight Goal

Few of us actually have the ideal body we often imagine society desires. In establishing your weight management goal, be realistic. In fact, you may not have the desire or energy to devote to attaining your ideal weight. Unless you are clearly obese, a more realistic target weight may be the weight you can reach and maintain without excessive dietary and lifestyle hardship. A realistic target includes consideration of your physical activity level, other stresses in your life, and how much energy you choose to devote to weight management at this time. If you've always weighed 125 pounds since reaching your adult height, chances are slim that you'll lead the rest of your life at 109 pounds. Focusing only on what you can change has a lot to do with successful weight management. Hanging on to an unrealistic ideal goal can jeopardize your physical, social, and psychological health.

You may want to lose weight even though the charts don't show you as overweight. That's OK, if you're just losing weight you've gained recently or since coming to college, or if you want to get to the lower rather than the higher end of the range given for your height and build. However, if you're already showing up in the charts as being underweight and you still want to lose weight, consult with a physician before trying to do so. You may be endangering your health or may have other issues related to weight and image that an outside perspective could help.

Anyone's normal weight fluctuates plus or minus two pounds. So give yourself not just a target weight goal, but a range. Make your weight goal incremental and as specific as possible. For instance, if you think you'd look great 10 pounds lighter, start with a 5-pound weight-loss goal. If you felt 10 pounds overweight before college and have gained another 15 since starting school, establish the 15 new pounds as your weight loss goal. If you'd like to gain sufficient bulk to increase your biceps two inches, start with one inch. You're more likely to succeed with smaller manageable goals, which give you a chance to congratulate yourself and evaluate how you feel at that intermediate weight.

Decide Specifically What You'll Change

You can successfully manage only a few focus points of deliberate change at a time. So set yourself up for success in weight management by not trying to change everything at once. Review the earlier sections of this chapter on food choices, exercise, and eating behaviors; identify two to three improvements you feel most motivated and able to accomplish. Be very specific about amounts and forms of food, frequency and duration of exercise. Write these down, and post them where you'll see them daily (such as on your calendar, bulletin board, or mirror). Every day, put a checkmark to show how well you're doing. When these behaviors become natural, review the chapter again and add a few new improvements.

No diet will remove all the fat from your body because the brain is entirely fat.

Without a brain you might look good, but all you could do is run for public office.

Covert Bailey

Weight Happiness

Seeking Professional Help

When To Seek Help

You don't have to be obese or skin-and-bones to seek help for weight-related problems. Seek help if:

- You experience sudden weight change (either gaining or losing 10 pounds or more) with no apparent cause. This could be the sign of a situation that needs medical attention.
- You'd like an informed opinion about whether you should lose (or gain) weight.
- You feel sad, hopeless or depressed about your weight, and can't seem to eat in a consistently healthy manner.
- You fast or purge (vomit) as weight-loss techniques.
- You want to lose (or gain) weight but can't seem to get started, keep going, or be successful.
- You want to better understand your personal issues related to weight—causes and solutions.

- You want support and encouragement for your weight management efforts.

Types of Help Available

- Medical diagnosis and treatment: For any health problems that may cause, contribute to, or relate to weight status. May include supervised development of exercise program for significant unfit or overweight individuals. Eating disorders are a growing medical specialty. (For more information, see the chapter on **Eating Disorders**.)
- Nutritional counseling: To analyze food consumption patterns and to establish a diet plan that contributes to attaining your weight goal.
- Psychological counseling: To examine personal issues relating to weight and eating patterns.

Start When You're Ready

Set a specific date to start your program. Pick the right time to start your weight plan, and give yourself a reasonable amount of time to accomplish your goals. For instance, weight losses of one to two pounds a week are usually the maximum your body can accommodate without burning muscle mass instead of fat. Trying to change your diet and eating patterns can be stressful. Avoid starting your program during times that are already high stress. During midterms and finals, just before holidays, and just before job interviews are often the worst times to start such changes. If you want to lose a bit more weight during those times, increase your exercise, but don't attempt to reform your eating habits.

Monitor Your Progress

The best place to keep track of activities related to weight management is the calendar you refer to every day. Here are some significant factors in weight fluctuation that you may want to record on your calendar:

- Exercise (and length of exercise period)
- When you skip meals
- Desserts or sweet snacks
- Fast foods
- Illness
- Travel, parties, academic deadlines, interviews, tests
- Other major deviations from your program

Mark your weight on your calendar periodically. Weigh yourself no more than once a week. Use the same scale every time, ideally one with weights like a doctor's scale (there may be one in the dressing room at the gym or in the health center). Weigh yourself about the same time of day, with the same amount of clothing.

You'll get a more accurate progress report with a tape measure than a scale. Because muscle weighs more than fat, you may actually have changed sizes without changing your weight that much. Measure your waist, chest, and thighs, and note your measurements on the calendar.

Support, Setbacks, Plateaus, and Maintenance

Getting support from others can be very helpful when you're involved in a program such as weight management. Truly supportive friends, who won't come down hard on you for minor failings, can be a great resource. Friends who continue to tempt you with "just one little bite" make your task more difficult. Your student health center may have nutritional counseling, peer support groups, or other services you might find helpful. Some campuses, and many off-campus communities, have support groups such as Weight Watchers, Overeaters Anonymous and Take Off Pounds Sensibly.

In the long run, you are your best support system. Learning to like yourself is the most supportive feeling you can experience in your search for the best body for yourself.

If you have setbacks or stop making progress, look on your calendar for a source, such as a change in exercise patterns, an increase in treats, more late nights of studying (with more snacks), poor weather (so less exercise), or becoming more casual about some element of your program.

If you want to keep losing weight and can't figure out and correct what's causing the plateau, exercise once or twice more per week. Look for additional alcohol or fat that may have crept into your diet. Have some patience, and remember that the weight will drop if you continue to exercise and watch your food and drink intake.

Once you've achieved your target weight, you probably won't just stay exactly at that level. Everyone's weight fluctuates a couple of pounds dur-

---

Counting Calories

Decide on your target weight. Multiply this weight by one of the following numbers:

- Sedentary—you walk sometimes, but never run or swim; no vigorous exercise. 10 for a woman; 13 for a man.
- Moderate activity—you exercise three times a week for at least 30 minutes. 13 for a woman; 15 for a man.
- Very active—exercise vigorously almost every day. 15 for a woman; 20 for a man.

After multiplying the weight you would like to be by this number, you will get an estimate of the calories you will need to maintain your ideal weight. For example, if you are a woman and wish to weigh 120 pounds and are moderately active, trim your calorie intake to 1550 (rounded off). Remember, you can also increase your exercise output to achieve the same goal. If you want to lose one pound a week, delete 500 calories a day and no matter what you weigh, you will lose weight. (Just one heavy-duty, chocolate-covered ice cream bar and you've done it.) Experts agree that cutting your daily intake to less than 1,100 calories requires professional supervision.

Source: *Hippocrates*, September/October, 1989

Weight Happiness

ing the week. Many women experience fluid and weight gain just before and during menstruation. If you go up by five pounds, put yourself back on a stricter regimen immediately, before that five pounds turn into ten. You'll have to maintain some vigilance, especially at first until your body gets used to the new you.

Beyond the Text

1. What would you say to someone who says, "Food is my only friend"?

2. You are struggling to stay on a diet. Your best friend, who doesn't need to diet, keeps tempting you. What would you do?

3. Your mother always nags you about your weight and your eating. What would you do?

4. Should colleges be required to provide special diets for students whose physicians recommend weight loss or weight gain for health reasons?

5. You eat almost the same foods in the same amounts as your roommate, but you gain weight when he/she does not. What factors could account for this difference? What should you do?

6. A friend has gained a lot of weight during the past few months but continues to indulge in high-calorie foods. What should you do?

Supplemental Readings

Food Habit Management by Jule Waltz. Seattle, WA: Northwest Learning Associates, 1986. An individualized workbook that teaches the reader how to manage eating behavior.

Getting Thin: All About Fat, How You Get It, How You Lose It, How to Keep It Off for Good by Gabe Mirkin, MD. Boston: Little, Brown and Company, 1983. One of the best general books on body fat control.

"Hunger is More Than an Empty Stomach" by Carol Ballantine. *FDA Consumer*, February, 1984. Explains the many physiological factors that affect the regulation of appetite.

Maximize Your Body Potential by Joyce D. Nash, PhD. Palo Alto, CA: Bull Publishing, 1986. A first-rate, comprehensive program for body fat control.

Slim Chance in a Fat World by Richard B. Stuart and Barbara Davis. Champaign, IL: Research Press, 1972. A thorough explanation of the factors leading to overweight and how those factors can be changed.

The Fit-or-Fat Target Diet by Covert Bailey. Boston: Houghton-Mifflin, 1984. A highly accessible—and enjoyable—guide for improving fitness and maintaining body weight.

Key Terms Defined

body mass index method of determining ideal weight by comparing weight with body fat

body image the total concept a person has about his or her body; may differ from another's concept of that individual's body

calorie amount of heat required to raise the temperature of 1 kilogram of water by 1 degree Celsius

fasting abstaining from intake of food

fats molecules composed of carbon, hydrogen, and oxygen with a particularly high energy content

insulin pancreatic hormone necessary for the metabolism of carbohydrates

metabolism process, physical and chemical, by which living substance is produced, maintained, and energized

nutrition process involved in ingesting and utilizing nutrients

obesity excessive accumulation of fat on the body; a condition of being 20 percent or more above ideal weight

plateau point at which weight levels off, neither increasing nor decreasing

set point theory theory that describes the weight range or point that the body strives to maintain by adjusting the metabolic rate

Physical Fitness

Physical fitness has emerged as one of the primary components of good health. Recent studies have proved conclusively that physical fitness reduces a person's chances of dying of heart disease, cancer, and other causes. In addition, being physically fit helps maintain desirable weight and helps people feel and look better. The other good news is that you don't have to exercise to the point of exhaustion or be a top-notch athlete to benefit from physical activity. Regular, moderate exercise is all you need to promote good health. The President's Council on Physical Fitness defines fitness as "the ability to carry out daily tasks with vigor and alertness, without undue fatigue, and with ample energy to enjoy leisure-time pursuits and to meet unforeseen emergencies." This chapter describes the major components of fitness, suggests how you can design your own fitness program, and offers tips on how you can avoid sports-related injuries.

Contents

Key Terms

Aerobic exercise

Anabolic steroids

Anaerobic exercises

Atrophy

Dehydration

Endorphin

Endurance

Exercise

Heat exhaustion

Heat stroke

Hypothermia

Metabolic rate

Physical fitness

RICE

Strength

Warm up

Physical Fitness: Why Me?

In *The American Way of Life Need Not Be Hazardous to Your Health*, author John W. Farquhar, MD, points out that for thousands of years, daily human existence and survival required physical exertion: hunting, farming, manual labor, and so forth. However, in today's high-tech environment, physical inactivity prevails. Driving replaces walking, elevators reduce stair climbing, and watching athletic events on television requires very little physical effort.

Medical research indicates that a physically unfit individual is more prone to experience health problems than a fit person. In a chronically inactive body, your heart and lungs have a lower capacity; muscles, joints and bones are weaker; your metabolic capacity is impaired. On the other hand, if you are active and physically fit, you will probably feel better, eat better, drink in moderation, sleep sounder, and have a generally positive disposition. Physical fitness increases your ability to overcome fatigue, cope more effectively with stress, and "fight off" pesky colds, the flu and other potentially unhealthy conditions. Heart disease, obesity and high blood pressure may not affect or concern you now, but during your college years you can lay the foundation for serious health problems in the future.

The college environment usually offers a wide selection of physical fitness opportunities. Many positive experiences are available, including organized exercise classes, intramural sports, club activities such as skiing or biking, and activities in the local community. Fitness programs offer social rewards and relief from academic stress. Peer pressure can reinforce physical fitness or divert you away from it. If your friends are physically active, you will be inclined to join them. If, however, they are sedentary couch potatoes or library dwellers, their example may not encourage you to maintain a healthy level of physical fitness. As with so many aspects of college life, the opportunities are numerous but the initiative and choices are up to you.

In the 1960s, heart disease gained first place on the American mortality charts. Among its causes was poor physical fitness. Experts launched serious efforts to reverse this alarming trend. Dr. Kenneth Cooper's *Aerobics*, first published in 1968, made an important contribution. The popularity of the widely televised 1972 and 1976 Summer Olympics fueled the running revolution of the 1970s. Today's interest in volleyball, tennis, cycling, aerobic dancing, health clubs, and so forth shows that quite a few Americans are involved in health and fitness. However, in spite of all the promotion surrounding the role of physical fitness in our health, only a small proportion of the population actually engages in vigorous physical exercise. The Department of Health and Human Services indicates that only 10 to 20 percent of U.S. adults (age 18 to 64) exercise enough to maintain healthy hearts. Many people participate in physically demanding recreational activities, but far fewer achieve physical fitness.

What is the difference between physical fitness and sports or athletics? As defined earlier in this chapter, physical fitness is a broader concept

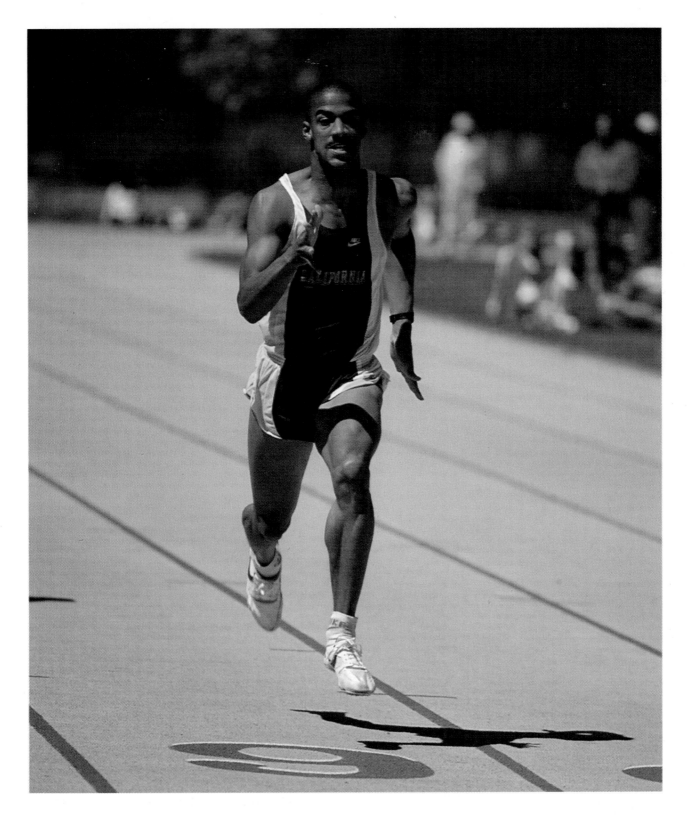

than sports performance or athletic endurance. Physical fitness will enhance your sports performance, especially activities requiring endurance, muscular strength or flexibility. In turn, certain sports contribute to physical fitness more than others. Cross-country skiing strengthens your cardiovascular system much more than downhill skiing does. Gymnastics classes help your posture and flexibility, but tennis doubles contribute little to your physical fitness.

How do you know if, in fact, you are physically fit? A general measure is whether you meet the criteria set by the President's Council on Physical Fitness. Fitness is a somewhat flexible concept, but there are minimal standards based on age, sex, weight, and other characteristics for each of the three main components: flexibility of muscles and joints, cardiovascular (aerobic) endurance, and muscular strength. To some extent, physical fitness is a relative condition. It is difficult to apply meaningful measurements to the average person's daily physical fitness status. Minimal standards for each physical fitness component provide a basis and a good starting point. Between minimal standards and world-class performance, there is a tremendous gap. And, your level of physical fitness changes according to how well you have kept up your exercise regimen. Achieving physical fitness can be fun, rewarding and healthy. A more complete list of fitness benefits for college students is presented in the accompanying table. What really counts is how you feel and how you feel about your appearance.

The material that follows defines and describes each fitness component, provides you with guidelines for assessing your present fitness status, and presents recommendations for designing your own fitness program.

Stretching for Flexibility

Flexibility is an important aspect of physical fitness. It increases your level of physical performance and decreases the chance of injury due to stress and strain on muscles and joints. Cats are excellent role models for flexibility; as we do, they achieve flexibility by stretching. The transition from an inactive state (such as sleeping or studying) to physical exertion places strain on your muscles. Stretching warms up muscles and gets you ready to move. A strong prestretched muscle resists physical stress more effectively than an unstretched muscle. In addition to providing this transition, stretching is an outlet for release of stress, especially neck and shoulder tension caused by long hours of high intensity study. Bob Anderson, author of the highly useful manual, *Stretching*, recommends that stretching become part of your daily activity because it relaxes the mind and tunes up the body. Stretching will:

1. Signal the muscles that they are about to be used. Strenuous physical activities such as aerobic dance, running, skiing, tennis, and cycling are easier when you are "warmed up."

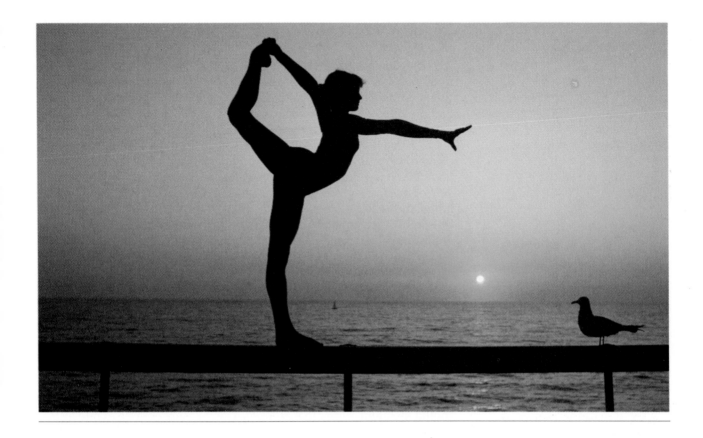

2. Help prevent injuries such as muscle strain, shin splints, sore elbows, stiff thighs, and so forth. Both warm-up and cool-down are instrumental in preventing injury.
3. Reduce muscle tension and make your body feel more relaxed. Since muscle tension results from long periods in uncomfortable positions (such as hunched over a desk) and stress, stretching can be a valuable stress management tool.

You can do stretching any time you feel like it: at your desk, in a car, waiting for a bus, walking down the street, or at the beach. Stretch before and after physical activity, but also stretch at various times of the day whenever you can. Here are some examples:

- In the morning before you start your day, even before you get out of bed
- At the library as a study break
- After sitting at a computer terminal for a long time
- When you feel stiff and sore from previous physical exercise
- To release nervous tension during examinations
- At odd times during the day, such as when watching TV, listening to music, reading, or sitting and talking

Physical Fitness

CHAPTER 9

203

Aerobics—The Heart of Your Program

Aerobic exercise, or "aerobics," is a relatively new fitness component. Experts have recognized the general benefits of vigorous exercise for centuries. However, Dr. Kenneth Cooper defined the benefits of aerobics and provided health and wellness enthusiasts with a comprehensive program in his 1968 landmark book, *Aerobics*.

Dr. Cooper defines aerobic exercises as "those activities that require oxygen for prolonged periods of time and place such demands on the body that it is required to improve its capacity to handle oxygen. As a result of aerobic exercise, there are beneficial changes that occur in the lungs, the heart, and the vascular system. More specifically, regular exercise of this type enhances the ability of the body to move air into and out of the lungs, the total blood volume increases, and the blood becomes better equipped to transport oxygen."

Aerobic conditioning can be achieved through walking, running, cycling, aerobic dancing, swimming, cross-country skiing, rowing, basketball, racketball, soccer, and many other vigorous activities. The goal of aerobic conditioning is to strengthen your cardiovascular system—heart, lungs and circulation network. A unique aspect of aerobics is that you, the participant, monitor and control the amount and duration of physical exertion. Your basic challenge is to complete 20- to 30-minute exercise sessions that tax your heart and lungs and result in an increased heart rate. Guidelines based on age and sex indicate how high a heart rate you should maintain during this exercise. You measure your heart rate by taking your own pulse.

Five Key Benefits of Aerobic Exercise

Aerobic exercise provides many benefits, including improved weight control, stronger and healthier bones, reduced risk of serious heart disease, improved management of the emotional stresses of daily life, and increased productivity.

Weight Control

The aerobic component of physical fitness plays an important role in the ability to control your weight. Combined with sensible eating, even moderate exercise can help you attain and maintain your ideal weight. As discussed in **Weight**, the body shape and weight most suitable for you is a function of heredity, sex, age, and other factors. Physical fitness and diet complement each other. Without dietary discipline, you cannot count on weight reduction or proper weight control based solely on physical exercise.

As you exercise aerobically, your metabolism speeds up. When you stop exercising, your metabolism continues to operate at that higher rate

---

Aerobic Potential

Activities providing the most effective aerobic exercise include:

- Cross-country skiing
- Swimming
- Jogging or running
- Aerobic dance
- Outdoor cycling
- Walking

Low-Impact Aerobics

Aerobics classes set to a disco beat are rewarding and fun. But, for too many enthusiasts, aerobic exercise has led to painful injury. The repetitive jarring movements of aerobic dance often cause injury to the shin, calf, lower back, feet, ankle, and knee. One research study showed that 76 percent of aerobic instructors and 43 percent of their students sustained injury from high-impact aerobics. The newer, less stressful format, called low-impact aerobics, substitutes sidesteps, marches, and simple dance/walk combinations for the jolting maneuvers of the earlier format. A popular variation, called hydro-aerobics, combines traditional aerobic movement with the buoyancy of a swimming pool. With the aid of a flotation device, you practice specific routines in deep water. This is especially helpful for individuals who are substantially overweight or recovering from a leg or knee injury.

for several hours. During this period, your body burns additional energy from the food you eat and from your fat stores. Because physical activity helps burn excess fat and build muscle, you look better and feel better.

Stronger and Healthier Bones

Like muscle, bone tends to get stronger and thicker with exercise, if dietary calcium is adequate. Stronger bones are less likely to break. This is very important for runners and dancers, who experience relatively high rates of stress fractures. New designs and construction of running shoes and a trend toward low-impact aerobic exercise have reduced these risks. However, bones tend to get thinner and weaker as you grow older.

Protection from Heart Disease

The build-up of fatty cholesterol deposits in the blood vessels, often described as "hardening of the arteries," is also known as atherosclerosis or arteriosclerosis. This can precipitate a stroke or massive heart attack. As a college student, you probably are not very concerned with how much cholesterol is surging through your system or how much plaque is building up on the walls of your arteries. However, studies show that college-age persons can and do show early signs of heart or blood pressure problems. Family history, obesity, smoking, and stress all conspire to promote heart-related problems. **Nutrition** contains a more detailed description of cholesterol and its sources. However, aerobic exercise can increase the level of your HDL cholesterol, a "good" type of cholesterol that helps clean the clogging ("bad") cholesterol from your body.

Couch Potatoes Arise!

The most significant study to date measuring fitness suggests that even modest amounts of exercise can substantially reduce a person's chances of dying of heart disease, cancer, or other causes. The study followed more than 13,000 men and women for an average of eight years to determine how physical fitness was related to death rates. The kind of exercise needed to move from the most sedentary level ("couch potato") to the next most fit entails only a brisk walk of 30 to 60 minutes per day. Because fewer than 10 percent of Americans over 18 years old exercise vigorously and regularly, these findings offer some incentive to those people who rarely, if ever, indulge in physical exercise.

Source: *Journal of American Medical Association*, November, 1989

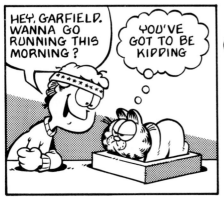
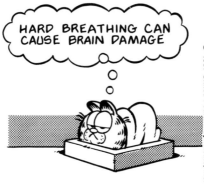
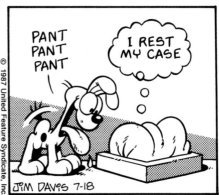

Are You a Runner or a Jogger?

If you usually run a mile in less than 9 minutes, you are described as a runner. Otherwise, you remain in the majority of enthusiasts as a jogger.

Control of Daily Life Stress

Since publication of Dr. Kenneth Cooper's *The Aerobics Program for Total Well-Being*, researchers have studied and documented the psychological impact resulting from aerobic exercise. Their results show that aerobic exercises facilitate the release of physical and mental tensions. Not only do subjects feel more relaxed directly following a workout, but this positive effect continues for a period of time thereafter. You can handle stressors of college life—academic schedules, performance objectives, social pressure, and so forth—more effectively when you maintain an aerobic exercise program.

Aerobic exercise affects the biochemistry of the brain. Most notable is the release of mood-elevating, painkilling brain chemicals called endorphins from the pituitary gland. Similar in biochemical makeup to morphine, endorphins enable the body to cope with the pain of prolonged physical exertion. Researchers suspect strongly that endorphins not only enable the body to endure the pain of a marathon but also produce the euphoria experienced by many long-distance runners.

Improved Intellectual Capacity Equals Increased Productivity

Research studies indicate that people who perform well on aerobic endurance tests show traits of greater creativity, increased duration of concentration, and quicker mental response time. In addition, such individuals can juggle more concepts simultaneously and show greater mental tenacity when working on complicated problems.

This correlation suggests that an effective exercise program can pay dividends in terms of your academic performance. College students who participate in aerobic classes report that they have more time for studies and social pursuits. Rather than losing time due to physical fitness sessions, they gain it. By clearing your mind and energizing your body, exercise contributes to increased productivity.

Muscular Strength and Endurance

The third major piece of a complete fitness program is developing muscular strength and endurance. Two effective methods of increasing muscular strength are weight training and calisthenics. When we think of muscular strength, many of us recall Olympic weight lifting, championship body building, and models featured in fitness equipment advertisements. However, many of your daily tasks and leisure time pursuits require muscle fitness but not gigantic biceps. Moving heavy furniture, carrying your bicycle to a third-floor apartment, or lifting a heavily loaded tray of dishes require muscular strength. To repeat certain efforts requires muscular endurance, for example, canoe paddling and snow shoveling.

Benefits of Weight Training or Calisthenics

Here are several reasons for including weight training and/or calisthenics in your workouts:

Reduced Risk of Injury   Muscular strength and balance make you less prone to injury when you engage in other sports or fitness activities. Sports such as soccer, softball and downhill skiing involve stress on your ankles, knees and legs. Strong muscles, ligaments and tendons can absorb such shock with less risk of injury. The danger for injury exists when, after a prolonged layoff, you take part in an active, stress-producing sport and attempt to match your earlier performance level. Your academic schedule may permit you to engage in some of your favorite recreational sports only occasionally. You may have limited opportunity to participate in seasonal sports such as downhill skiing. The occasional downhill skier is very prone to injury as muscle fatigue sets in late in the day. Statistics show overwhelmingly that most injuries on the ski slopes occur under conditions of fatigue or recklessness. When you strengthen your thigh muscles, you have more endurance and can ski in control for a longer time. Adequate warm-up helps prepare your muscles

Women need not worry about developing bulging muscles through exercise. Females do not have the same tendency to gain bulk as males.

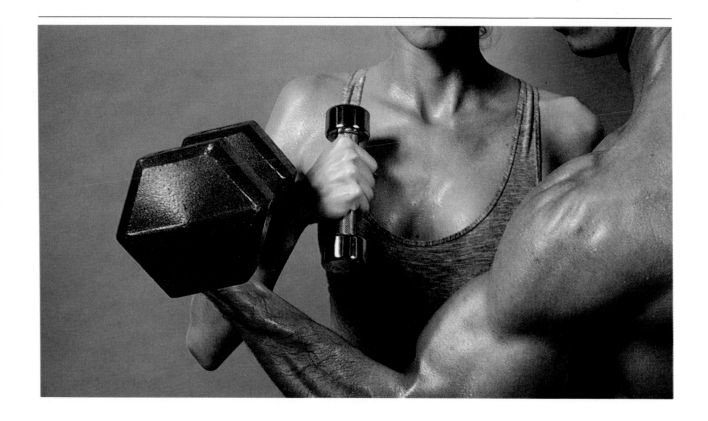

for the stress of exercise, but there is no substitute for muscular strength and endurance.

Relief from Lower Back Discomfort   People who suffer lower back pain usually gain some relief by strengthening their abdominal muscles. This is a specific illustration of muscle balance because the lower back muscles are usually stronger than the abdominals. Prolonged study sessions at a desk or table may result in back discomfort, especially when you hunch over your work. Stronger abdominal muscles help overall posture as well as reduce lower back discomfort.

More Attractive Appearance   Strength training helps you lose excess body fat as you build muscle. When you reduce fat content and build up your muscles, you may actually increase your weight. Muscles weigh more than fat but they are more compact. Thus, as a result of strength training, your body will take on a more firm and trim appearance. Not only will you look better but you'll feel better about yourself. You will depend less on diet alone for weight and figure control.

Enhanced Sports Performance   Sports trainers agree that strength training can enhance performance levels in competitive or recreational sports. The increasing number of serious athletes from all sports—not just football and wrestling—engaging in strength training demonstrates this fact. With stronger leg muscles you can perform better in soccer, lacrosse or field hockey; you can backpack and rock climb with greater assurance. Stronger upper body muscles will enable you to hit a tennis ball harder and a golf ball farther. Recreational sports become more enjoyable as you increase your proficiency. Building up your muscle strength and endurance may not set the stage for an Olympic tryout, but you'll perform better and safer.

Muscular Balance   The key concept in your muscle strength and endurance program is balance between major muscle groups. Dedicated athletes engaged in specific sports concentrate on the muscles emphasized in their specialty. However, fitness and sports enthusiasts seeking one or more of the previously described advantages need a program that exercises and strengthens all major muscle groups.

If your last experience with repetitive exercises, such as push-ups and jumping jacks, was during grammar school physical education, your interest in calisthenics may be negligible. Traditional calisthenics, as demonstrated in *Police Academy* and *An Officer and a Gentleman*, have given way to weight training, a more efficient and quicker way to strengthen your muscles. Even if you do not know the difference between a bench press and a reverse wrist curl, you don't have to be intimidated by weight training. Weight training comes in two main varieties: free weights and machines. Free weights include hand-held weights and the traditional bars with weights. Many fitness stores now promote wrist and ankle

Aerobic versus Anaerobic Conditioning

Physical exercise is of two types—aerobic and anaerobic—depending on how the body supplies energy to the muscles. The term *aerobic* means "in the presence of air." When you exercise, your muscles need energy. This energy is supplied by a fuel to be burned (glucose) and oxygen to support this combustion. The bloodstream carries glucose and oxygen to your muscles, where combustion takes place, releasing energy for muscle movement. The aerobic exercise system uses copious quantities of oxygen processed by the lungs and circulated by the heart and bloodstream to your muscles. Endurance activities—running, swimming and cycling—are common forms of aerobic exercise.

Anaerobic activity occurs "in the absence of air." In this mode, the body generates energy for your muscles in the absence of extra oxygen. The anaerobic system is energized by fuel stored in your muscles. For example, when you engage in exercise that requires short bursts of energy, such as a 50-yard dash or lifting weights, your muscles need energy more quickly than your lungs and heart can respond. Producing energy via the anaerobic system also generates lactic acid as a waste product. This substance causes muscle burning and fatigue; this is the pain referred to in the saying, "Go for the burn." Anaerobic exercise can be sustained for only short periods of time—usually less than two minutes—before your muscles become fatigued. This also reinforces the need for a slow deliberate warm-up prior to vigorous or strenuous exercise. Unless you shift efficiently from the "start-up" anaerobic system to the aerobic "endurance" system, you will experience much pain, little gain, and considerable fatigue.

weights for use during aerobic exercise. These assist with aerobic training but are not a substitute for weights used in strengthening major muscle groups; use them only after achieving a moderate strength base. Some physical fitness coaches believe the risk of injury does not justify the use of wrist or ankle weights during aerobic dancing or running. An alternative to lifting "free" weights is the use of specially designed fitness equipment, such as Nautilus, Taurus, Avita, and others. These machines provide exercise options ranging from abdominal crunch to shoulder press and vertical butterfly.

Your objective in either type of weight training is to stress the target muscle beyond its normal demands. By overloading the muscle, you cause it to react and adapt by adding more mass. But overdoing this process can result in muscle injury. Also, muscles that are exercised then need 48 hours of rest to allow muscle fibers to rebuild or regenerate. Your schedule of muscle strengthing sessions should allow for this recovery time.

Because there is a fine balance between sufficient and excessive overload, the inexperienced weight user should obtain professional advice regarding the weight (number of pounds or kilos) and number of repetitions to use for each exercise. Start with minimal weights or, if using fitness equipment, a low setting. It is easier to add the challenge of more weight than to endure the pain and inconvenience of injury. Furthermore, it is much more enjoyable to conduct weight training with another person. A friend makes the workout seem easier, gives you brief rest between reps, and provides a safety assist as needed.

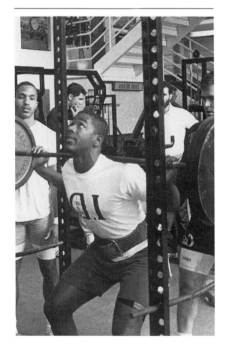

Developing Your Own Physical Fitness Program

The college environment offers varied and affordable opportunities for physical fitness. You can select from a variety of formal and informal programs and an array of athletic facilities to create an effective program. Perhaps you feel that lack of time and limited knowledge regarding how to set up your own program are obstacles. As described in **Time Management**, everyone has the same amount of time—24 hours per day. How you allocate your time reflects your priorities. If the benefits of physical fitness are of sufficiently high priority, you will find ways to make and keep a time commitment to fitness. Here are the key steps in developing your own program:

1. Assess your present state of physical fitness.
2. Select specific goals that seem both reasonable and attainable.
3. Determine the amount of time you are willing to commit to physical fitness or related activities.
4. Evaluate various physical fitness activities at your college that are convenient and potentially enjoyable for you.
5. Talk with other students about their experience and seek advice from athletic/fitness program coaches.
6. Determine how you'd like physical fitness to relate to other lifestyle aspects such as diet, use of alcohol and other drugs, coping with stress, and time management.

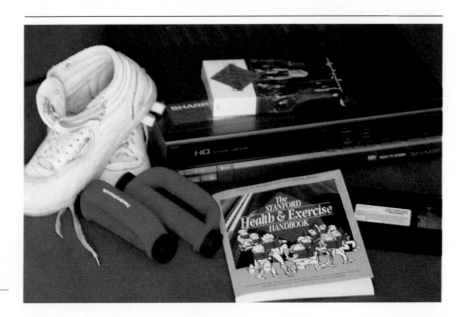

Self-Assessment

Most students arrive at college in good physical shape, thanks to active high school athletics and reasonably well-supervised diet and sleep habits at home. Of those who begin college in poor physical condition, most are overweight and underactive. Regardless of your condition at the beginning of your freshman year, it is highly probable that your fitness level will soon decline unless you pursue an effective fitness program. As the popular saying goes, "If you don't use it, you lose it." When completing your self-assessment, consider your family history and your own recent physical fitness status. Have your parents or grandparents suffered from chronic diseases? Were your parents in top physical shape when they were your age? If so, did they remain that way? Medical research indicates that during college years you can take positive steps to reduce the risks of suffering from heart disease, high blood pressure, obesity, tendonitis, arthritis, and other debilitating conditions in later life. Do these seem to be worthwhile goals or too distant to worry about?

- Consider your medical history. Physicians and physical fitness trainers recommend that you take precautions regarding potential medical problems. If you have a chronic condition (such as asthma) or prior injury (such as spinal fusion) that could be aggravated by vigorous exercise, consult with your family physician or with your college health center staff. If you are over 30 years old or not accustomed to regular physical activity, you should have a thorough medical examination, including a properly administered stress test.
- To determine your **flexibility fitness**, try the recommended stretching exercises in *Stretching* or other fitness books. Posters with stretching routines are available for purchase or perhaps on display at your college's physical education department. By starting with warm-up stretches and moving to ones that challenge your body, you will soon find your limits. When a stretch reaches the point of tightness, you are reaching your reasonable limit for that session.
- To determine your **aerobic fitness**, you can complete either of two tests: the 12-minute fitness test or 3-minute step test. The 12-minute fitness test is based on the distance that you can cover in 12 minutes. Guidelines for evaluating walking, running, swimming, and cycling results are contained in Kenneth Cooper's *The Aerobics Program for Total Well-Being*. The step test uses an 8-inch step and requires that you step up and down at a specific rate for 3 minutes. After resting for 30 seconds, take your pulse and check your level against a predetermined standard for your sex and age (these standards are included in most books on aerobics). This test indicates your heart's ability to recover from mild exertion. A quick recovery is considered to be a sign of fitness.
- You can assess **muscular strength** several ways. Two tests are commonly used: total number of push-ups and total number of sit-ups performed in sixty seconds. Push-ups are done by males with knees off the floor and by females with knees on the floor. Completing 24 or more

---

Your Training Heart Rate

To attain optimal training benefits, you should exercise within your training heart rate zone. The simplest method of computing this is to subtract your age from 220 to determine your maximum heart rate (MHR) and then multiply that figure by 60 percent and 80 percent. While you exercise, your heart rate per minute should fall between these two figures. For a 23 year old, the zone would be 118 to 158.

Some fitness enthusiasts prefer a more complicated formula that incorporates their resting heart rate (RHR). You can determine your RHR by taking your pulse when you are physically at rest, such as just before you get out of bed in the morning. Then calculate your maximum heart rate by subtracting your age from 220. Finally, use the following two formulas:

$0.6 (MHR-RHR) + RHR = $ Target Heart Rate (low)

$0.8 (MHR-RHR) + RHR = $ Target Heart Rate (high)

For a 23 year old with a resting heart rate of 68, the formulas work out as follows:

$0.6 (197-68) + 68 = 145$ (low)

$0.8 (197-68) + 68 = 171$ (high)

Training Heart Rate Zone = 145–171

Walk Into a Workout

Growing in popularity as an aerobic exercise and an alternative to jogging is walking. With a good pair of shoes as your only special equipment, you can firm up, burn calories, feel refreshed, reduce stress, and lose weight. Opportunities for a brisk walk across campus may coincide with your class or activity schedule. Fast-paced walking gives you more exercise than cycling. Naturally, walking takes more time than jogging or cycling. However, jogging a mile in 8.5 minutes burns only 26 more calories than walking a mile in 12 minutes. To get the most benefit from walking, you should use a long stride and involve your upper body by "swimming" with your arms. Many walkers add hand or ankle weights for extra benefit. Fitness experts recommend that you work up to brisk walks of 30–45 minutes at a pace that accelerates your heart to your target rate. As with other aerobic exercise, you should warm up and cool down. The chart on page 214 compares the calorie-burning effects of walking with those of several other physical activities.

push-ups in one minute gains you a rating of "good"; 40 earns an "excellent." Do sit-ups with your knees bent; cross your hands in front of your chest. 30 or more sit-ups in one minute earns a rating of "good"; 40 earns an "excellent."

Another muscular strength assessment method uses free weights or exercise equipment. Your present limits will become obvious quickly. Guidance from a qualified trainer is very helpful and can help you avoid injury. The chance of injury is quite high if you begin by lifting or moving weights that surpass your present strength level. Start with a light load and progressively work your way toward heavier ones. Nautilus and other equipment have variable weight loads or settings. Get advice from a qualified trainer and write down specific equipment settings that are appropriate for your initial workouts.

Setting Goals for Your Physical Fitness Program

Weight reduction or control is a very common physical fitness goal. This is only one of many incentives to working out. When considering the following list of fitness goals, remember that they are not mutually exclusive. Which ones are particularly attractive to you?

- Reducing or controlling weight
- Conditioning for sports or recreation activities
- Providing a diversion from academic schedules and deadlines
- Maintaining social contact with others who enjoy physical exercise
- Contributing to general level of health and wellness
- Increasing stamina to handle the pressures of academic work
- Obtaining more efficient sleep patterns (sounder sleep)
- Improving appearance through muscle toning
- Reducing stress
- Establishing good habits for later life
- Gaining skills for post-college recreational sports

Perhaps other factors motivate you to physical fitness: maybe you received a new cross-country bicycle for your birthday or your friends are more proficient than you in a recreational sport, such as wind surfing. Remember, to achieve weight reduction goals you need to relate physical exercise to your eating habits. Without diet discipline it is nearly impossible to lose a significant number of pounds. For more information, refer to **Weight**.

Time Commitment

Physical fitness is most effective when you work out on alternate rather than consecutive days. Schedule at least 30 to 40 minutes for each aerobic exercise session. Your program should include time for (1) warm-up, (2) aerobic exercise, (3) cool-down, and (4) muscle conditioning and strengthening exercises. Begin with a 5- to 10-minute warm-up, including stretching. Follow with an aerobic workout of at least 20 minutes. Allow 5 to 10 minutes for the third phase, cool-down.

The time required for developing muscular strength depends on your specific goals. If your objective is to balance your aerobic work, target three 10- to 15-minute sessions per week. When exercising major muscle groups, you can alternate upper body with lower body workouts. If you want to develop strength for a specific activity, such as windsurfing or rock climbing, consult one of many available fitness books or talk with a sports trainer at your school's physical education department.

In today's environment of rapid response and quick results, it is natural to seek signs that your fitness program is achieving immediate results. You should be able to sense some physical change after two weeks. The stiff muscles and soreness developed during the first week begin to recede by the end of the second week. You will notice almost immediately evidence of feeling and sleeping better. Most experts say that four to six weeks are required to see significant results.

An effective method of maintaining your program is to find a friend who will exercise along with you. This will increase your enjoyment and provide moral support as you move toward your fitness goals. Jogging alone may expose you to unnecessary personal risks, so a companion provides a measure of safety as well as good company.

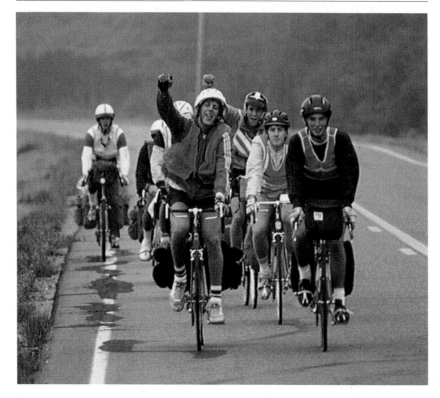

Physical Fitness

CHAPTER 9

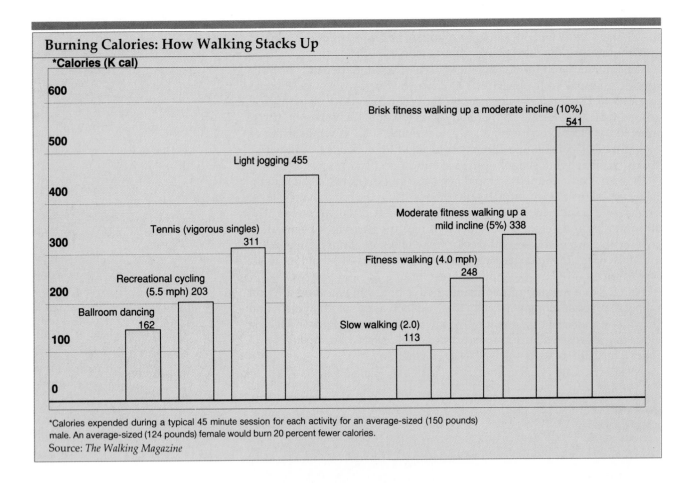

Burning Calories: How Walking Stacks Up

*Calories (K cal)

- Brisk fitness walking up a moderate incline (10%) 541
- Light jogging 455
- Moderate fitness walking up a mild incline (5%) 338
- Tennis (vigorous singles) 311
- Fitness walking (4.0 mph) 248
- Recreational cycling (5.5 mph) 203
- Ballroom dancing 162
- Slow walking (2.0) 113

*Calories expended during a typical 45 minute session for each activity for an average-sized (150 pounds) male. An average-sized (124 pounds) female would burn 20 percent fewer calories.
Source: *The Walking Magazine*

Your commitment to physical fitness may be more easily maintained by signing up for an aerobics class or participating in intramural sports. You will have to fit into prearranged schedules, but this can be an advantage. You know when the class or game will take place and you can plan other activities accordingly. Afternoon physical fitness programs give you a welcome change of pace between morning classes and evening study. As emphasized in **Time Management**, two techniques for using your time effectively are (1) establish specific goals and (2) write down your schedule commitments so you don't create conflicts or miss important events altogether. A word of caution: don't exercise within two hours of bedtime; it can disrupt sleep by energizing you at the same time you should be gradually shutting down your body.

Most campuses offer a wide range of physical fitness opportunities. Your college's course catalog or schedule of classes will list the sessions sponsored by your physical education or recreational sports department. Become familiar with your school's athletic facilities and when they are available for your use. For example, an indoor swimming pool may offer open time only between specific hours due to swim team or water polo practices. Tennis courts are usually in high demand, as are basketball

Physical Fitness

CHAPTER 9

Improving Fitness: Ratings for Popular Sports

Factors	Jogging	Bicycling	Swimming	Skating	Handball/Squash	Nordic Skiing	Alpine Skiing	Basketball	Tennis	Calisthenics	Walking	Golf	Softball	Bowling
Physical Fitness														
Cardiorespiratory endurance	21	19	21	18	19	19	16	19	16	10	13	8	6	5
Muscular endurance	20	18	20	17	18	19	18	17	16	13	14	8	8	5
Strength	17	16	14	15	15	15	15	15	14	16	11	9	7	5
Flexibility	9	9	15	13	16	14	14	13	14	19	7	8	9	7
Balance	17	18	12	20	17	16	21	16	16	15	8	8	7	6
General Well-Being														
Weight control	21	20	15	17	19	17	15	19	16	12	13	6	7	5
Muscle definition	14	15	14	14	11	12	14	13	13	18	11	6	5	5
Digestion	13	12	13	11	13	12	9	10	12	11	11	7	8	7
Sleep	16	15	16	15	12	15	12	12	11	12	14	6	7	6
Total	**148**	**142**	**140**	**140**	**140**	**139**	**134**	**134**	**128**	**126**	**102**	**66**	**64**	**51**

Using a scale of 0 to 3, seven experts rated each component of fitness with 0 indicating no benefit and 3 indicating maximum benefit.
Source: *Runner's World*

courts. By combining your interest with a scheduled PE course, you gain access to facilities and equipment on a regular basis. Your campus residence hall or fraternity/sorority may field numerous teams in sports ranging from Frisbee to volleyball and softball. Your college's health center may also sponsor certain classes such as aerobic exercise.

You will find information regarding student-organized skiing, hiking or cycling clubs in your campus newspaper. Or you may find a friend who can introduce you to a particular special interest group. Remember, all sports activities do not guarantee advancement in your physical fitness. You should continually compare their value to your fitness goals as well as their potential social rewards.

Physical Fitness and Your Lifestyle

The relationship between physical fitness and your overall lifestyle is rather astounding. Research studies continually document the positive impact fitness has on attitude and on eating and sleeping habits. Researchers are not exactly sure why, but subjects consistently report that they eat fewer rather than more calorie-loaded foods as a result of moderate exercise. People who endure the discipline and effort of achieving physical fitness become more in tune with their bodies and develop a sensitivity regarding what's good and what's bad for them. Physically fit people are much more likely to be nonsmokers and to drink alcohol in moderation.

A Winning Diet

The fitness boom of the 1970s and 1980s stimulated new interest in the relationship between diet and athletic performance. Recent research has dispelled many long-standing myths. Nutrition experts now say:

- High protein (such as steak and eggs) is not the recommended "pregame" meal. Complex carbohydrates (such as pasta) are more efficient. When muscles require energy, the body will utilize its store of carbohydrates before fat (much of which is found in protein).
- Eating a candy bar or other high-sugar snack immediately before exercising will not give you a sustaining burst of energy. Your body's fuel comes from foods eaten hours, even days earlier, not from what you consume just before exercise.
- Fluids during exercise will not cause stomach cramps. During periods of prolonged, intense activity, drink small quantities of water (3 to 7 ounces) every 10 to 20 minutes.
- Salt tablets are not necessary to replace sodium lost in sweat. Sodium and potassium are lost in small quantities that can be easily replaced by normal diet. For example, foods containing significant amounts of sodium include yogurt, crackers, cheese, soup, and pizza. Salt tablets should be taken only when prescribed by a physician.

As summarized by the *University of California, Berkeley Wellness Letter*, "The dietary needs of athletes and other active individuals are, with a few small adjustments, not very different from those recommended for all healthy people." Most sports nutritionists advise against diet manipulations such as carbohydrate loading or taking mega-doses of vitamins or supplements. The *Wellness Letter* concludes that "the best advice for all recreational exercisers is to stick to the balanced, high-carbohydrate diet they should be eating on a daily basis."

Nutrient	Importance for Exercise
Carbohydrates	The most efficient fuel for the body. Emphasize complex carbohydrates (starches not sugars).
Protein	Needed to build, maintain and repair tissue. Used as an energy source only when carbohydrates and fats aren't available.
Fats	The most concentrated and abundant form of energy in the body, fat stores serve as the primary fuel during prolonged aerobic exercise.

| Vitamins | Needed for the metabolism of carbohydrates, protein and fats to produce energy. |
| Minerals | Needed for the metabolism of carbohydrates, protein and fats to produce energy. Iron is vital for oxygen transport. Sodium and potassium help maintain the body's water balance. |

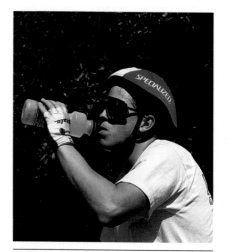

For more information on these nutrients and how to get them from the foods you eat, see **Nutrition**.

Fluid Replacement—A Critical Part of Your Exercise

Sweating away just 2 percent of your body weight without compensating for it can hurt your performance by causing lethargy, nausea and circulatory problems. And greater losses can lead to cramps, heat exhaustion or heat stroke as the body's ability to cool itself fails. Unfortunately, thirst isn't always a good indicator of the body's need for fluids. Because of the strain and excitement of physical activity, it's possible to lose four pints of water before you notice your fluid loss. You should make a deliberate effort to drink enough fluids—and the right ones—when exercising.

- Plain water is the ideal fluid replacement. Cool water (40 to 50° F) is more quickly absorbed than warmer liquid and won't cause cramps.
- If you drink a sugar-loaded liquid just prior to exercising, you may decrease your exercise endurance by as much as 25 percent. Following a hefty dose of sugar, the body triggers an insulin response that lowers the blood sugar level. Continued low level of blood sugar may result in depletion of glycogen stores and premature fatigue.
- Soft drinks containing caffeine are diuretics, so they may increase dehydration. They can also cause the jitters.
- Alcohol, also a diuretic, can promote dehydration. Beer, wine and hard liquor are poor sources of energy and have a depressing effect on the heart and nervous system. They also hamper coordination and impair performance.

How to Avoid Sports Injuries

Tendonitis, runner's knees, swimmer's ear, tennis elbow, shin splints, sprained ankles, eye infection, stress fracture, blisters . . . the litany of sports-and-exercise-related injuries is endless. Whether you are a seasoned athlete, a fitness buff, or an intrigued novice, the risk of injury is a constant specter. Whether you have a gymnastics class tomorrow or are looking forward to biking in the hills with your friends, an injury stops you cold and may leave you feeling frustrated and depressed. But injury

Physical Fitness

need not happen—common sense and good preparation are the only deterrents you need.

Most injuries are not the result of thrill-seeking (you saw the cliff and you had to climb it), competitors who ruthlessly sabotage their opponents (a player kicked you with her cleats when the referee's back was turned), or an extraordinary accident (lightning struck a tree and a limb fell on your bike). The majority of injuries make dreary (if not downright embarrassing) stories because they are the result of common inattentiveness to the proper conditioning, technique or equipment required for maximum safety and performance. Fortunately, most sports-and-fitness-related injuries are preventable.

Lack of Knowledge Can Be Detrimental to Your Health

Numerous myths about exercise prevail and contribute directly or indirectly to injury. Below are examples of some of the more harmful.

Faulty Comparisons   Through television, newspapers and magazines we have become spectators of an incredibly wide range of athletic events and sports conducted on a world-wide basis. Many amateur athletes make their sports look so easy that we begin believing that we also can perform in similar fashion. Then, every fourth year we are treated to Olympic competition covered by the media in microscopic detail. This inspires us to equal these performances when we finally get into the athletic arena. For any high-level amateur contest, the competitors have trained for weeks or months. A lifetime of training and conditioning goes into one Olympic performance. Everyone can become fit, but not everyone can be a star.

When working on your physical fitness program or participating in recreational sports, forget the competition, the broken records, and your roommate who runs ten miles a day, takes an aerobics class, lifts weights, and doesn't sweat. Recognizing the differences between yourself and others, and knowing your individual physical strengths and limitations, are crucial in preventing injuries.

No Pain, No Gain   Nothing has done more to skew our perception of healthy exercise than the prevailing notion that pain is vital to physical fitness progress. Its corollary—that the best treatment for pain is to ignore or "work through" it—is equally bad. Pain is a warning signal that means "Stop!" Closely related to the pain theory is the "go for the burn" myth. Learn to differentiate between healthy muscle soreness and an unremitting burning sensation. Some discomfort may follow more intensive conditioning, but a powerful "burn" causes extreme muscle stress with accompanying fatigue. This sets the stage for injury.

If You Don't Have a Perfect Body, You're Not There Yet   Health and fitness magazines picture recreational sports enthusiasts as slim, trim, toned, and tanned—hardly a population in need of advice on diet and exercise. A combination of designer leotards, expensive athletic shoes, and high-tech equipment does not necessarily result in achieving physical fitness. Being fit means having enough energy to meet your daily needs with vigor and alertness, responding to unexpected challenges without stress, and feeling good about yourself. Setting attainable goals and committing to a modest program will yield positive results and rewarding experiences.

Avoiding Injuries During Fitness Training

The chance of minor injury is a constant companion. You can sprain an ankle by stumbling on a stair or stepping on a half-empty beer can. However, your exposure to potential injury increases as your physical activity becomes more vigorous. Athletes who participate in intercollegiate sports have special training regimens and a retinue of coaches, physical therapists, and sports medicine clinicians to monitor their practices and performances. Students have the resources of the PE department, but they lack supervised training and attentive coaching that may help avoid or treat injuries properly. Injuries interrupt your fitness progress, cause you to lose your conditioning level, and disrupt your active lifestyle. The pain, discomfort, inconvenience, and expense caused by injuries are undesirable as well.

Today's sports injuries are concentrated in the highly popular activities of running and aerobic exercise. These two involve more injuries than most other exercise because they are *weight bearing*. The repeated pounding and accompanying stress are transmitted through joints and ligaments—up to three or four times body weight with each footfall. This soon translates into knee, hip or foot problems. Swimming and cycling, although extremely popular, have lower injury rates because they are not weight bearing.

The Fitness and Health Handbook, published by the University of California at Berkeley, identifies the key ingredients to minimizing the risk of injury from physical fitness or sports activities: physical capabilities, technique, equipment, conditioning, pain and fatigue awareness, and progressive training.

Physical Capabilities   When undertaking vigorous exercise, you should review your physical capabilities. If you are generally physically active and in reasonably good condition, you don't have to be overly concerned. However, if you are a physical fitness novice, be cautious. Don't try to accomplish too much too soon. If you have a potentially serious medical condition (high blood pressure) or a previous sports injury (runner's knee), you should obtain qualified medical advice regarding your fitness program. A substantial weight gain or loss can also affect your physical capabilities. A fitness test and some helpful advice from your college health center will assist you to evaluate your capabilities. Attempting to perform beyond your capabilities too early in your program is very risky.

Most Common Injuries to Runners

1. Runner's knee
2. Heel spurs
3. Tibial stress syndrome (shin splints)
4. Achilles tendonitis

Physical Fitness

Choosing Safe Sports

You may seek the personal challenge and thrill of participating in relatively high-risk sports. If so, you probably know what you're getting in for when you launch yourself down a hill on skis or a skateboard. If you are uncomfortable with a new sport, be cautious and do not try to imitate the proficient athlete. Popular sports are grouped below in terms of risk of injury:

Sports Ranking in Terms of Injury Risk

High Risk	Medium Risk	Lower Risk
Football	Ice hockey	Swimming
Rock climbing	Soccer	Hiking
Skateboarding	Basketball	Bicycling
Downhill skiing	Wrestling	Tennis
Hang gliding	Field hockey	Softball

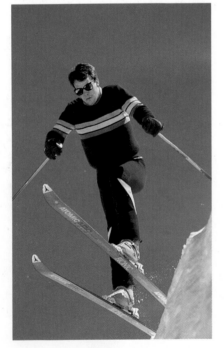

Technique   Proper technique is a very important part of preventing athletic injuries in any sport. Improper tennis-serving technique can result in arm soreness or tendonitis of the elbow. You can severely injure an ankle or knee sliding into base during a softball game. Seek proper instruction when you begin any new sport or exercise. This approach will enhance your performance, increase your rewards, and reduce both self-consciousness and injury risk.

Equipment   Proper equipment, especially footwear, makes a big difference. For aerobic dancing and all running sports (basketball, soccer, jogging, and so forth), athletic shoes are essential. More advice on shoes is presented later in this chapter. Boots for hiking or skiing must fit properly, not only to protect you from wear and tear, but also to minimize the risk of injury from a bad fall. When you become involved in a new sport you may need specialized equipment. When renting or purchasing equipment, make certain you are properly fitted. Check that rented or borrowed gear is in good shape. Gloves, goggles, knee or shin guards, and other accessories are important as well. If participants usually wear them, there must be a valid reason, and so should you.

Selecting sports equipment can be very confusing because of the great variations in designs and prices. Your options often range from barely adequate to high-tech or designer. You'll find such choices in every item, from leotards and shoes to bicycles and tennis rackets. Observe what others are using and ask experienced participants. If in doubt, rent at first and buy later.

Athletic Shoes: Getting In Step

Selecting athletic shoes involves more than choosing a color or deciding between low-cuts and high-tops. If you wear athletic shoes every day, you may assume these shoes are so versatile you can use them for almost any athletic activity. Not so! Athletic shoes have become very specialized. Running shoes have different features than tennis shoes or aerobic exercise shoes. The April 1988 *Runner's World* survey actually reviewed 36 different shoes designed just for runners. At least eighteen major companies compete in the multimillion-dollar-per-year athletic shoe market. As a prospective buyer, you can select among several hundred models.

You may wonder, "Isn't all this just hype to sell more shoes?" The answer is no. Extensive research has given shoe designers more data on the physiology of the foot. Comfortable, well-supported feet are essential to sports performance and contribute greatly to minimizing the risk of injury. The correct shoes help your feet stay free of blisters, cool in warm weather, and warm in cold weather. If you are a first-time exercise enthusiast, the wrong shoe choice can nullify a potentially rewarding experience before you have a chance to get into step. So how should the average person shop for shoes? First, consider your feet and your intended physical activity; second, talk to people who participate in that activity; and third, shop at a reputable store that offers a wide selection of athletic shoes.

Before heading for your local shoe outlet, here's what to consider:

Your prior experience with athletic shoes Do you own one or more pairs now and how comfortable have they been? If this is your initial serious purchase, you need to know something about your foot construction.

Your foot type There are three foot types: normal, rigid and flat. If your feet are normal, you'll have the widest choice of shoes. The rigid, or high-arched, foot requires special consideration because this type of foot does not absorb shock well. Such feet need shoes with extra cushioning to absorb the shock of running or other exercise. Flat-footed individuals experience excessive flopping or flattening of the foot in mid-stride. This tendency is a prime cause of foot, ankle and knee problems. If you have flat feet, shop for a shoe that provides extra stability.

Your intended use Shoe design has become specialized, because each sport—running, basketball, aerobic dance, tennis, racketball, and so forth—puts different stress on your feet and legs. For example, the running shoe is unique to that sport and does not adapt well to basketball or other court games. After convincing sports enthusiasts that three or four different shoes were needed for full protection, manufacturers recently introduced multisport shoes. The marketing manager for one major shoe company was quoted as stating, "We've been telling people for ten years that they need a different shoe for each sport. Now, promoting one shoe that fits several sports may confuse the potential buyer." The truly serious one-sport athlete will stick with specialization, while the recreational sports enthusiast will be attracted to the multisport model. Footwear experts agree that you should purchase shoes designed for your intended sports activity. To be properly outfitted, a versatile athlete owns several pairs of sport shoes.

The surface on which you will play or practice Concrete, asphalt, wood flooring, grass, cinder, and dirt all have their unique features. If most of your exercise time will be spent on concrete or asphalt, purchase shoes that provide maximum cushioning.

Use a shoe outlet that carries a wide selection of athletic shoes, preferably a store that caters to students. Explain your special needs to the sales clerk. Bring along socks that you would normally wear for exercise. Since your feet swell during the day, shop in the afternoon or evening. Most people have one foot slightly longer or wider than the other. Get a good fit on the larger foot. Try on several pairs and inspect them carefully for minor flaws or misaligned parts. Jog around the store, play aerobics music over your Walkman, and generally make a fool out of yourself. For $30 to $60, you can purchase very adequate shoes. You can also get custom-made beauties, created to your own specifications, for about $150. They make good conversation pieces as well.

Steroids: Illegal and Dangerous

A practice potentially dangerous to your health is the use of anabolic steroids. Evidence suggests fairly widespread use of black market (illegal) steroids among both male and female athletes trying to increase muscle mass and strength. Most steroid use is illegal, so it is difficult to run open, objective tests on athletes who conceal their steroid practices. Thus, researchers cannot conclusively prove the effect of steroids on muscle mass and strength. What scientists do know about is the alarming and dangerous side effects of steroids, including feminization in men (such as atrophy of the testicles), masculinization and temporary infertility in women, liver damage, and clogged arteries. Common features of the female athlete using steroids are leathery skin, bulging muscles, and a five o'clock shadow. Recent research conducted by McLean Hospital in Belmont, Massachusetts on steroid-using body builders has linked psychotic episodes (paranoia, hallucinations, violent tendencies) to the use of steroids.

Conditioning   You've arrived late and the exercise class or basketball game is already underway. You are inclined to jump right into the activity. Putting such great stress on muscles, ligaments and joints without proper warm-up can result in injury. Going from a dead stop to full running without any warm-up puts extra stress on your cardiovascular system. Preparing your body for action ("conditioning") includes stretching, warming up and cooling down. Procedures vary for each activity, but the process remains the same. Bob Anderson's *Stretching* provides helpful instruction for many common physical activities. Search out special-interest magazines that include helpful conditioning tips and instructional material for beginning as well as experienced enthusiasts.

Pain and Fatigue Awareness   Pain is a clear indication of trouble; you should pay attention. Persistent pain in bones, muscles or joints is a signal to stop exercising and seek medical help. When exercising with gusto to burn off calories or achieve a certain distance on your bike in less time, you can easily reach the point of fatigue. When you are fatigued, your muscle control weakens and you are highly vulnerable to injury. Nearly 80 percent of ski injuries occur near the end of the day; most of these are related to fatigue. When one portion of your body tires during exercise, shift to another exercise that gives a good workout to another part of your body. For example, stationary cycling gives your lower body a good workout; your upper body is exercised when lifting weights.

Progressive Training   Trying to achieve ambitious performance goals too quickly involves a high risk of injury. You may be eager to step up your pace and reach higher levels. Achieving physical fitness and performing well on the playing field require pacing and patience. Fitness experts continually advise that you start any new physical activity slowly and then gradually build more frequency, intensity and duration into your program.

Treating Sports Injuries

Fitness experts, sports trainers and orthopedic surgeons all agree that the best common-sense approach to injury prevention is to listen to your body. When it yells "pain," stop what you are doing immediately. Muscle soreness is natural, especially when you begin a new sport or routine that calls upon muscles that you've not used recently. If soreness persists for more than a day or two, you should analyze the problem. Exercising or continuing to play a sport while in pain aggravates injuries and may lead to a chronic condition.

Initial Self-Care   For many common athletic injuries—even those that need clinical attention—there is a simple treatment formula: RICE. This acronym provides helpful guidelines.

Rest	Immobilize the injured part of your body.
Ice	Apply ice to dull the pain and reduce blood flow to the injured area. This also helps control swelling. A plastic bag with crushed ice is best, but a cold can or bottle will work temporarily.
Compression	Wrap a towel or elastic bandage around the injury to apply pressure, then place the ice over the towel or bandage; use the remainder of the wrap to secure the ice pack. Immerse an injured foot or hand in ice water for a maximum of 15 minutes at a time. This may seem impossible at first, but once you have left it there for a few minutes, the pain of cold goes away.
Elevation	For the first day or two after an injury, keep the injured area above the level of your head as much as possible. This facilitates drainage of excess blood and fluid. If necessary, remain prone and ask your roommate or a friend to serve you meals and snacks while you recuperate.

Application of ice is both important and helpful. During the first two days you should apply ice for 10 to 20 minutes every hour or two during waking hours. Symptoms indicating that your injury should be treated with RICE include:

- localized pain
- joint stiffness
- swelling
- muscle tear or pull
- unexplained redness of skin or black and blue marks

When To Seek Medical Help A few signs indicate something serious has occurred. You should seek professional medical help when:

- Your experience or intuition tells you that you are injured. Especially dangerous are blows to the head that cause you dizziness.
- Your injury causes you severe pain, disability or numbness.
- You have injured a joint.
- You have loss of movement of a finger, toe or limb.
- Injury bleeds substantially, or scrapes or cuts have dirt or foreign substances imbedded in them.
- What appeared to be a minor injury does not respond to a few days of RICE.
- You have infection, pus, red streaks, swollen lymph nodes, or fever.
- You experience continued nausea or breathing difficulty following an injury.

Running Safely

Attacks on joggers occur both on-campus and off-campus, in darkness and during daylight hours. After a brutal attack on a jogger in Central Park, the New York City police provided the following guidelines:

- When possible, run with a partner.
- Avoid isolated areas. Run where others run.
- Inform other people concerning when you are running, where you plan to run, and when you expect to return home.
- Avoid using personal stereos. They are targets for theft, and wearing a headset can make you less aware of your immediate surroundings.
- Run with confidence and determination.
- Avoid wearing jewelry or other valuables when running.
- At night, wear reflective or light-colored clothing.

Source: *New York Times*, July 31, 1989

Physical Fitness

Weather conditions can pose hazards for the physical fitness enthusiast. The effects of temperature and wind on your body range from causing mild discomfort to total collapse. People experiencing the effects of heat and cold often do not realize how quickly their condition is deteriorating, so they do not respond to the threat. Surrounding air temperature is only one variable to consider. Others include intensity and duration of your exercise, velocity of the wind, and your level of conditioning. People suffering from heat stroke or hypothermia (cold) require immediate emergency treatment because either condition can have fatal results.

Exercise in the Heat

During exercise, your body generates substantial heat; more than 70 percent of the energy used to power your muscles is lost as heat. To keep the body's heat-regulating mechanism functioning, water lost via perspiration must be replenished. Insufficient water replenishment can result in several types of sudden heat illness. The relatively minor forms are **heat cramps** and **fainting**. A more serious condition is **heat exhaustion**, the inability to continue exercise due to dehydration or excessive salt depletion. The most serious, **heat stroke** is a true medical emergency because the body's heat-regulating mechanism can no longer function. Football practice, long-distance running, and endurance cycling in conditions of high temperature and humidity can and do result in heat exhaustion and heat stroke. Heat stroke is second only to head and spinal injuries as a cause of death among young athletes in the United States. Warning signals for heat injury are important to know.

Warning Signals of Heat Injury

Heat Exhaustion	Heat Stroke
Headache	Headache
Fatigue	Bizarre behavior or convulsion
Weak, slow pulse	Full, rapid pulse
Tingling sensations on arms	No tingling sensations
Pale, moist, cool skin	Dry skin
Profuse sweating	Little sweating
Chills or shivering	Very high temperature

Adequate training, respecting your limits, and proper fluid replacement are your best deterrents against heat problems. The following will help you prevent heat exhaustion and other heat-related illness:

1. Get in shape for hot-weather exercise before hot weather arrives. Then take it easy on the first few hot days to allow your body to acclimate.

Seeking Professional Help

When To Seek Help

The two most important occasions when it is appropriate for you to seek professional help are (1) when you are starting a new physical fitness program and (2) when you suffer an injury. As stressed earlier in the chapter, you should receive clearance from a physician prior to starting a fitness program if you suffer from a physical disability, chronic illness, or sensitive condition (pregnancy, recovering from an illness). You should receive professional guidance when undergoing the various fitness tests or upon commencing an aerobics program. The sections on sports injuries and on exercising in heat and cold provide guidelines for seeking professional help when injuries occur under those conditions.

Types of Help Available

The best help for physical fitness evaluation, training and guidance usually comes from coaches and other instructors in your school's PE department. If you are injured, the student health center or school nurse can direct you, as appropriate, to physician, physical therapist, orthopedic specialist. For the serious athlete, some physicians now specialize in sports medicine.

2. Follow the fluid replenishment guidelines in the fitness diet section earlier in this chapter. Don't let thirst be your guide. Continue to drink proper fluids at appropriate intervals.
3. If you feel weak and tired during exercise, stop and drink several ounces of water.
4. Do not take salt tablets unless prescribed for you by a physician.

The primary treatment for heat illnesses is to cool the body: fluids, water from a hose, rubbing ice on the body, pouring cold drinks on the body, and so forth. The victim should rest out of the sun. Summon emergency assistance. For more information, see **First Aid**.

Exercise in the Cold

When exercising in the cold, you must take into account the combined effect of the temperature and wind, called the wind-chill factor. For example, if the outside temperature is 30° F, a 15 mph wind will give the effect of a temperature of 10° F. As you exercise and give off heat, your body temperature can drop to a dangerously low level.

The most common cold illnesses are **frostbite** (frozen tissue) and **hypothermia** (drop in body temperature). The areas most sensitive to cold are fingers, ears and toes. By protecting these with mittens, hat, wool socks, and so forth, you reduce the discomfort of cold temperatures.

Guard against wearing wet clothes, especially non-wool garments like cotton jeans, because they give you little protection. Individuals who get caught in unseasonably cool rains while hiking in the summer frequently experience hypothermia. When temperatures reach extremely cold levels, your toes, fingers, cheeks, and other exposed areas are likely candidates for frostbite. Do not rub snow on frostbitten areas; doctors recommend treating frostbite with warm water (102–104° F). Some people believe that breathing very cold air will freeze the lungs. This is not true.

Warning Signs of Hypothermia

1. Shivering and slurred speech
2. Loss of control over fingers
3. Difficulty walking
4. Inability to think clearly

Treatment for cold victims is warmth. Warm fluids, warm bodies, and other warming agents are the recommended effective remedies. For more information, see **First Aid**.

The Fitness Movement in America

American History Is Sprinkled with Populist Movements That Strove to Reshape the Country

Erich Segal, author of *Love Story* and other bestsellers, taught Frank Shorter in one of his classics classes at Yale. Segal tells stories about Frank's negative attitude toward marathoners and marathons. Shorter felt marathons were a waste of time and a pointless diversion. On overcast days in late winter when Segal was flogging himself at the track in preparation for his annual trek to the Boston Marathon (where he consistently ran under three hours), Shorter would come out, do a casual track workout, make a good-natured snide remark to Segal about his mentality—or lack of it—and jog off, while Segal continued his incessant circling of the track.

Ironically, Segal was serving as commentator for ABC-TV a few years later in 1972 when Shorter stunned everyone at Munich by breaking away from the world's best marathoners early in the race and winning the event as though it were an exhibition run. Shorter was the first American to win the Olympic Marathon since Johnny Hayes did it back in 1908.

Many observers cite Shorter's achievement as the beginning of the running revolution that swept America. His influence upon his contemporaries was certainly profound. Hundreds of thousands of post-graduate Americans who were beginning to notice a slight paunch took up jogging and running and revolutionized America's concept of how adults are "supposed" to act. The 1970s saw an inordinate number of people in their 20s running around in public in their underwear.

Frank Shorter's contribution to his generation was not unique. In the very early 1960s, Americans who had disdained formal physical education classes because they were boring, militaristic (with their reliance on platoon-like calisthenic drills), and *required* were inspired by the example of the youthful, energetic President John F. Kennedy. When he challenged America to take up walking—even walking as much as 50 miles at a time—Americans of all ages responded with thousands of blisters, a million sore muscles, and a feeling that they'd done something significant.

In 1968, with the publication of *Aerobics*, Dr. Kenneth Cooper became an inspiration to sedentary Americans, many of whom were successful business people who became convinced that a healthy body would contribute to better and more creative business. Cooper's modest, quantified, easy-to-follow program of regular aerobic exercising became as integral as ledgerbooks. Dr. Cooper, at his Dallas Aerobics Institute, continues to host a series of races each year among the upper echelons of American business leaders, while he continues to guide their aerobic futures.

Frank Shorter's inspiring marathon win in the Olympics in 1972, and his silver medal in the Montreal Olympics in 1976, served as the catalyst that put fitness on the front page of every newspaper in the country. Shorter's contemporaries had been the post-World War II baby boom generation, the largest segment of population to ever move through the demographics of America. They were the generation that had revolted against a series of what they perceived as unconscionable moves by certain government officials in the mid- and late-1960s and early 1970s. They had also been indoctrinated by the feeling of power their accomplishments had produced into believing that anything was possible. After graduation from college and assimilation into the job market, they began to notice signs that perhaps not all things were possible. Chief among these suddenly impossible things was the extension of their youth. Sedentary jobs for which they'd been trained in college offered no physical outlet. The college graduates from the late 1960s and early 1970s began to lose muscle tone, gain body fat, and notice a lessening of their vital energies. Generations before them had placidly accepted this slow physical deterioration as part and parcel of the process of aging.

A generation fascinated by the powers that youth had bestowed, and raised on the supposition that anything is possible, decided to revolt against one more injustice.

Literally millions of Americans in their 20s and early 30s took to the roads in the late 1970s, shedding body fat, building cardiovascular capacity, pumping endurance into muscles that had been on the downslide. In 1977 there were 3000 entries in the Boston Marathon; two years later there were 7866. In 1977 there were 40,000 marathoners in the United States; in 1982 there were 112,000. Demographic research indicated that the overwhelming majority of people who were getting into running and entering marathons were college-educated, white-collar professionals with substantial earning power.

Suddenly the three-martini lunch gave way to the three-mile lunch run. Business was conducted on the run, new contacts were made, previously unphysical people became incredibly fit, and with that fitness came an increased sense of self-esteem that carried over into their jobs and personal lives.

The concept of mandatory physical education became outmoded in a matter of years. The reality of voluntary physical fitness had arrived. And just in time. Cutbacks in funding for certain school programs severely undermined many physical education programs, and voluntary involvement in a personal physical fitness program was suddenly all that stood between thousands of Americans and the severe consequences of being unfit.

Scientific studies conducted in the wake of the running revolution and the later, wider-reaching fitness movement unanimously point up the benefits of a regular, aerobic fitness program. The famous, far-reaching Framingham Study and the ongoing study of Harvard alumni point out that a moderate amount of exercise coupled with good nutrition add both quality and quantity to a person's life. A fit lifestyle decreases the chance of disease, prevents premature death from heart disease, provides additional energy stores, increases productivity, and even stimulates creativity by increasing the amounts of oxygen and nutrients that are delivered to the brain.

Unfortunately, despite all the publicity and favorable scientific studies, physical fitness of this type is enjoyed by a surprisingly small proportion of the American population. Although not quite as exclusively the reserve of the highly educated as it was during the days of the running revolution, physical fitness has not percolated throughout all segments of society. Indeed, a large segment of the population harbors a deep-seated resistance to physical activity unless it's related to their work.

Fortunately, for more people than ever before, a voluntary commitment to achieve and maintain fitness is emerging as part of the modern lifestyle. Knowledgeable Americans who want to reap the most from life realize that the likelihood of achieving their goals increases if they are fit and healthy. The race doesn't go to the sluggish. It goes to the sleek and the fit.

What does the future portend for fitness? We've already seen the beginning of a shift in the medical community. Many hospitals (especially HMOs) now place an emphasis on fitness as a positive preventative alternative to the traditional stance of waiting to get sick to go to the hospital. It is much more cost-effective to teach and encourage fitness instead of treating catastrophic illness. And on a personal level, the alternative of a healthy, active lifestyle as opposed to a constant, downward health spiral isn't even a contest. The scenario of a hard-working business person reaching the pinnacle of success only to become incapacitated and out of the business arena due to heart disease or death has become outmoded.

The exciting prospect for the future of fitness is that the fitness pioneers have refined the science of becoming and staying fit to the point where most major diseases that killed or debilitated Americans are now optional. Today's college graduate is in the enviable position of being able to pretty much choose how healthy and physically happy he or she wishes to be 10, 25 or 50 years from now. And that's patently revolutionary.

Richard Benyo

Richard Benyo, former editor of Runner's World *magazine, is the author and co-author of numerous fitness books, including* Dynastrid! A Complete Walking Program for Fitness After 50. *Mr. Benyo, who resides in St. Helena, California is also a fitness columnist for the* San Francisco Chronicle.

Beyond the Text

1. Respond to the following statement: If you don't look good in Spandex shorts, you aren't fit yet.

2. Respond to the following statement: Exercise doesn't do any good unless you do at least an hour of demanding exercise every day.

3. A member of your soccer team is on the ground clutching her ankle. What would you do?

4. You have been hiking in a light, drizzling rain and the sun is beginning to set. Your companion's speech is a little slurred and he seems slightly disoriented. What would you do?

5. What is the relationship between physical exercise, nutrition, and weight control?

6. Comment on the following: Two valid excuses for avoiding physical fitness are (1) I'm not a very good athlete, and (2) I can always exercise when I have more time.

Supplemental Readings

Getting Stronger: Weight Training for Men and Women by Bill Pearl and Gary Moran, PhD. Bolinas, CA: Shelter Publications, 1986. An illustrated resource guide that gives a wide variety of exercise options for every part of the body.

Health and Fitness Excellence. The Scientific Action Plan by Robert K. Cooper, PhD. Boston: Houghton-Mifflin, 1989. Features a comprehensive seven-step approach to developing your optimal health and performance. Topics range from stress and nutrition to exercise and positive attitude.

Stretching by Bob Anderson. Bolinas, CA: Shelter Publications, 1980. Offers a safe, comprehensive guide to stretching for everyone from novice to the very limber. Illustrations enable the reader to easily master the appropriate stretching exercises.

The Aerobics Program for Total Well-Being by Kenneth Cooper, MD. New York: Bantam, 1982. Follows his 1977 classic, *The Aerobics Way* and includes guidelines for dozens of exercises as well as information on nutrition, emotional balance, and the importance of monitoring your body through periodical medical examinations.

The Complete Sports Medicine Book for Women by Mona Shanghold and Gabe Mirkin. New York: Simon and Schuster, 1985. Provides practical advise on a wide range of women's health and fitness topics, including safe training, proper diet, preventing injuries, and keeping fit during pregnancy.

The Sports Performance Factors by James Rippe, MD, and William Southmayd, MD. New York: Putnam Publishing, 1988. Describes the links between health, fitness, and daily performance; includes mental strategies, aerobics, nutrition, strength, and lifetime training.

Key Terms Defined

aerobic exercise form of physical exertion for an extended period of time, usually at least 20 minutes, without disturbing the balance between intake and use of oxygen

anabolic steroids any group of synthetic derivatives of testosterone

anaerobic exercises activities that require sudden bursts of energy, such as sprinting, when energy is drawn from stored fuel rather than conversion of oxygen

atrophy to waste away from disuse

dehydration loss of fluids from body tissues

endorphin group of brain substances that bind to opiate receptors in various areas of the brain and thereby raise the pain threshold

endurance ability to withstand the stress of physical exertion

exercise performance of physical exertion for improvement of health or correction of physical deformity

heat exhaustion (or heat prostration) disorder resulting from overexposure to heat or to the sun

heat stroke severe, life-threatening condition caused by failure of the body's heat-regulating mechanism due to prolonged exposure to heat

hypothermia generalized cooling of the body core resulting from exposure to cold temperatures or immersion in cold water

metabolic rate rate or intensity at which the body produces energy

physical fitness state of well-being in which a person has enough energy to meet daily needs and unexpected challenges

RICE acronym for Rest, Ice, Elevation, Compression

strength physical power; the maximum weight one can lift, push, or press in one effort

warm up mental and physical preparation for exercise

Your Personal Image

Your personal image is a reflection of how you feel about yourself and your health. A healthy individual projects energy and confidence. Your exterior—skin, hair, eyes, teeth—provide important clues regarding your overall wellness. Poor complexion, peeling nails, bloodshot eyes, straggly hair, and cavity-riddled teeth are clues to neglect or possible illness. Poor dietary habits, sleep deprivation, and neglected personal hygiene may show up initially as a deteriorating personal image but later result in an illness. For example, neglecting proper tooth and gum care may lead to gingivitis, a painful and potentially serious condition. Equating a dark suntan with sex appeal can put you at risk for skin cancer if you experience overexposure to the sun's dangerous ultraviolet rays.

This chapter discusses how your skin and hair function, and why they need your continued care. Your teeth and eyes do, too. Frequent headaches may signal eye strain or weakened eyesight. Perhaps you need eye glasses or a new prescription if you use them now. The importance of continued dental care is discussed, and a comprehensive chart identifies common oral/dental problems and their treatment. Taking care of yourself and your health includes paying attention to all these important elements.

Key Terms

Acne	Exfoliation	Sebaceous gland
Blackhead	Hangnail	Self-image
Cellulite	Myopia	Sunburn
Cosmetic	pH	Toxin
Dandruff	Plaque	Ultraviolet radiation
Dermis	SAD	
Epidermis	Sebum	

Contents

Skin—Beautiful or Not

Perhaps beauty is more than skin deep—but how your skin looks is important to you. Your skin, all seventeen square feet of it, is the largest organ of the body and a very important one. Together with the kidneys, lungs and intestinal tract, it aids your body in the elimination of toxins and wastes. Your skin is composed of millions of cells and thousands of blood vessels, nerve endings and sweat glands. Though seemingly simple, skin is actually a very complex organ that requires care. Your skin needs more than a daily bath and an expensive moisturizer to look good; to give your skin what it needs, you should understand how the skin works.

The Inside and Outside of Skin

Your skin is made up of three layers: the epidermis, the part you show to the world; the dermis, made up of connective tissue, nerves, blood vessels, sweat glands, and oil glands (which cause so many problems during adolescence); and the subcutaneous, or fatty layer.

At the base of the epidermis is a layer of cells that constantly reproduce to form new cells. These new cells push outward and upward toward the surface of the skin. As they arrive on the surface, they dry out and are sloughed off and replaced by new cells from below. You've probably heard that your skin is completely replaced every seven years—this process goes on continually so that at any given moment cells are dying and being replaced. When layers of dead cells lie flat against each other, they appear smooth. When they are uneven and turned up at the edges, the skin appears dry, lifeless and dull.

The millions of cells on the surface of your skin exist in a bath of liquid similar in content to seawater. The water from sweat glands and the oil

What Your Skin Does for You

- Protects your body from invasion by bacteria, viruses and fungus
- Helps eliminate waste products
- Helps guard the inside of your body from destructive ultra-violet rays
- Relays certain messages from the outside world to the brain
- Records sensations of pleasure and pain, a way of letting you be aware of what is a pleasant or a dangerous stimulus

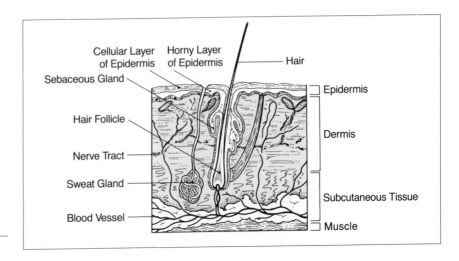

Cellular Layer of Epidermis — Horny Layer of Epidermis — Hair — Epidermis — Sebaceous Gland — Hair Follicle — Nerve Tract — Sweat Gland — Blood Vessel — Dermis — Subcutaneous Tissue — Muscle

Your Personal Image

CHAPTER 10

from sebaceous glands also form an oil-in-water film that acts as a natural moisturizer and protects your skin by maintaining an acid balance. On the pH scale, which ranges from 0 to 14, your skin is slightly acid, between 4.5 and 5.5. (A pH below 7 indicates that a solution is acidic, and a pH above 7 indicates that a solution is alkaline.) This acid coat helps protect against invasion of any kind, so it is important to maintain the right pH. Any number of substances can disturb the skin's pH: soaps, most of which are alkaline; cosmetics and moisturizers, most of which are not acid-base balanced.

The outer layer of your skin is not only affected by its pH balance but also by exposure to the elements. Sun, wind, pollution, and general wear and tear all take their toll. But it is the dermis, or underlayer, that ultimately determines the beauty of your skin. Though outside elements affect this layer, "inside" health is really the most important. Such things as the food you eat and the stress you experience will influence the health and quality of your skin.

Diet and Your Skin

Without proper nourishment your skin simply cannot look healthy. Dull, lifeless or uneven skin signifies internal neglect. Your skin needs a well-balanced diet, with proper vitamins, minerals, proteins, essential fatty acids, trace elements, and complex carbohydrates. Take a minute and look in the mirror. What do you see? If you observe poor skin quality and you don't know whether or not you are deficient in any of the above, read the **Nutrition** chapter and learn about healthy eating. Make sure your diet includes lots of fresh fruits and vegetables, especially green leafy ones, eight glasses of water daily, and vitamin and mineral supplements. Also, cut down on foods containing high proportions of fat, sugar or refined (white) flour. Try this regimen for a few weeks, then take a second look in the mirror.

For your skin to do its job of eliminating wastes, other organs must also be efficiently ridding your body of internal pollution. When you are constipated, your colon is blocked; this allows more toxins to assimilate into the body. In turn, this leads to both poor cell nutrition and added stress on the toxic-cleansing functions of the skin. Even if you are having a bowel movement every day, your bowel may not be emptying completely, or material may be passing through the bowel so slowly that toxins are reabsorbed. Refined and heavily processed foods can take up to three or four days to pass through the system; a diet of raw or unrefined foods can transit in a few hours.

One of the most effective methods to improve waste elimination is the addition of fiber to your diet. By correcting intestinal stasis, adequate fiber enables every organ in your body to function more efficiently, and your skin will appreciate the difference.

To increase the fiber in your diet from the average 15–20 percent to the ideal 30 percent, include lots of whole grains, such as brown rice, oats,

Vitamins and Minerals for Healthy Skin

- Each day of your life, 10 percent of the cells in the skin's basal layer (the layer that creates the outer skin) reproduce themselves. Vitamins and minerals help supply the energy needed for this process.
- Vitamin C protects the collagen fibers in the dermis and the capillaries so that they can bring necessary nutrients to the cells.
- Vitamin A is important for the growth of new skin cells.
- Zinc is vital to the production of collagen. Twenty-five percent of the body's zinc is stored in the skin.
- Magnesium is essential for the storage and release of energy in your skin at the cellular level.
- Selenium, an essential micronutrient, helps preserve the elasticity of the skin by preventing oxidation of fatty acids.
- Vitamin E, another antioxident having antiaging properties, works closely with selenium. Vitamin E also helps heal rough, dry skin.
- Silicon, found in apples and avocados, helps to prevent loose, flabby skin.

The skin is a major organ of elimination, helping rid the body of toxins and wastes. In fact, the composition of perspiration is very close to that of diluted urine. The skin eliminates about two pounds of material daily.

Recipes for Beautiful Skin

If you have oily skin: Put fresh mint, ice cubes and cold water in a blender. Blend for several seconds, strain through gauze or a clean nylon, and use this mixture to clean your face.

If you have dry skin: Use mineral water or NaPCA from an atomizer before applying moisturizer or makeup.

millet, rye, and wheat, as well as vegetables (preferably raw) and fruits. Since meat, fish, eggs, dairy products, and highly processed or refined foods are practically devoid of fiber, limit your intake of such foods.

TLC for Your Skin

Your skin, just like the rest of you, deserves consistent, tender, loving care. Daily external care keeps the pores from clogging up and maintains a healthy, clean surface. Whether you choose to use soap and water or lotion and water, the actual procedure of cleansing is important.

Washing with Soap or Cream   Soap is an excellent cleanser, but it can penetrate the outer surface of the face and leach away the lipid film, making your skin dry. Also, if your skin tends to be oily, soap may stimulate the already overactive sebaceous glands to produce even more oil; therefore, the more you wash with soap, the more oil your glands produce, creating a vicious cycle. If you are committed to washing with soap, choose a pH-balanced soap, not an alkaline one. Remember, you want to preserve the natural acidity of your skin.

Another alternative is to cleanse with oil or cream. These substances cut grime and makeup efficiently, but many women feel oil and cream do not leave their skin feeling clean. If you use this method, you may want to complete the cleansing routine with a tonic or freshener. If you live in a large city known for its air pollution, you may want to employ both methods. First, use the oil cleanser to remove makeup and oil-soluble dirt. (If you are short on funds, simply use a pure vegetable oil, such as safflower, sunflower or corn oil.) Remove oil with a damp cotton ball followed by washing with pH-balanced soap and water to remove the oil and any remaining surface dirt; then rinse thoroughly in warm water, and complete your facial routine with a cold splash. Try to follow this regimen twice daily—if this takes too much time, at least do it before bedtime. Your skin needs time to recover from the daily hassles.

Your Skin at Night   During the night a number of changes and repair processes take place in your skin. Cell metabolism increases; glycolysis (the breakdown of sugars for energy and the assimilation of amino acids) takes place; and the body synthesizes collagen and elastin. Going to bed with clean skin helps preserve its integrity. Better yet, apply a light night moisturizer. You are not too young—even at twenty—to begin to prevent dry skin. A night cream is not useful if you have a bad case of acne. In this case, consult your dermatologist.

Why Exfoliate?   Notice how many men have a healthy, rosy skin glow. How do they do it? It is very simple when you consider that every day a man shaves and removes a layer of dead cells. Rather than shaving, some women use a procedure called epidermabrasion. This process resurfaces the outer layer of skin by using a brush, polyester mitt, or cream formula that contains abrasive particles. Any of these methods, called exfoliation, can benefit nearly every type of condition—from acne to dull and lifeless skin.

When you use exfoliation regularly—at least two times a week and, if needed, every day—you will notice your skin becomes clearer and more translucent. It no longer looks dull and gray, but refracts light and attains a healthy, rosy glow. Exfoliation has been found to have a positive effect on acne. In a study of 285 people with acne, exfoliation with a polyester web, together with regular acne treatment, showed significant skin improvement. (If you are using Accutane™, a prescription drug for acne, consult with your doctor before using this technique.)

Skin Brushing   To give the skin on your whole body a treat and improve your energy level, try an all-over form of exfoliation, a bizarre-sounding technique called skin brushing. With just a hemp-bristle brush, you can give yourself a simple, safe, amazing treatment that will probably do more to improve the vitality and beauty of your skin than anything else.

Before your shower, while your skin is still dry, begin to brush from the top down. Always brush toward your heart. Imagine that you are soaping your body and brush, using a variety of motions, your neck, shoulders, trunk, arms, and so forth. As you reach your waist, stop brushing down and begin to brush from the feet up, covering every square inch. The entire procedure should only take three to five minutes. Be a little gentle at first, since your skin may be quite sensitive. After you have completed the skin brushing, take your shower.

What does this technique accomplish? Skin brushing removes the top layer of dead skin cells. At the same time it stimulates the oil-secreting glands to moisturize your skin. In fact, this process will clear up a dry skin in a few days. If you don't believe this works, take a damp cloth and go over your skin after the brushing. Within a few days, the smell on this cloth will convince you to adopt the skin-brushing technique.

Continue with this for two months; then evaluate your energy level. The waste material removed by skin brushing is normally carried by your blood through the bowel or kidneys for removal. Remember, well-functioning skin assists the other organs of elimination to do their job.

Once you have removed the dead skin cells and your skin is clear and clean, it is very receptive to a moisturizer. If your skin is dry, you might want to choose a fairly rich cream or lotion, because you will get excellent absorption. If you have acne, apply your acne treatment after exfoliation.

Protect Your Asset with Moisturizers   You have probably heard that once over thirty, your skin will need special care that includes everything from expensive cosmetics and moisturizers to facials. Current thought is that age twenty might be the time to start paying attention to your skin. Prevention now can retard aging skin, wrinkles and loss of elasticity.

Your skin is always losing moisture, both through sweat glands and through evaporation. This evaporation occurs constantly, even when you

How to Care for Large Pores

First, cleanse your skin thoroughly to keep the surface of the pores clean. Use only fine-grained exfoliating agents; large granules bruise the surface. If you use these agents gently, without grinding them into your skin, they will leave your skin glowing. As a natural remedy for large pores, apply chamomile tea (that you have previously brewed and chilled in the refrigerator) several times a day as a skin freshener.

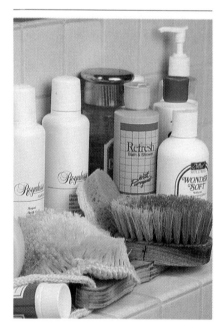

233

Always clean your skin before applying a moisturizer; otherwise, your pores will become clogged and your skin will be in worse shape.

aren't perspiring in warm weather. The lower the humidity, the more rapid the fluid loss. Humidity in a centrally-heated room is comparable to humidity in the Sahara Desert—almost nil.

The body's own moisturizing agent is sebum, a substance that coats the outer cells and prevents rapid evaporation of water. Sebum seals—water lubricates. You can protect your skin against moisture loss. First, minimize evaporation by controlling your indoor environment. If you live in a building that uses central heating, use a humidifier or at least put a pan of water on the radiator to evaporate in the room during the months the heating system is operating. An air moisture level between 75 and 90 percent will preserve the skin's water balance. Humidifiers also help protect you against colds and flu.

Second, consider some form of surface protection against dry skin. Just to complicate matters, researchers have now discovered that a different moisturizer is better for winter weather than for summer. This awareness is based on the work of a Japanese scientist who discovered that skin temperature is higher in the summer and lower in the winter; that skin pH is lower in the summer than during any other season; and that loss of water through evaporation during the summer is twice the amount as in winter.

This means that we need two different types of moisturizers. In the winter, choose a formula higher in fatty acids (this does not mean baby oil); this is a formula with a high level of lipids and is effective at low temperatures and low humidity. In the summer, choose a moisturizer high in glucose and one that will assist in retaining water. You may want to do some research on your own or ask for literature from cosmetic companies. If drug and department store products are too expensive, visit your health food store and purchase an inexpensive cream composed of collagen, elastin or both. For under ten dollars you can buy all the protection you need. If you use a product on your skin that causes a slight red, itchy rash, probably you are allergic to that product. Switch brands to a hypo-allergenic variety. These solutions to dry skin don't just apply to women —men also have dry skin and can benefit from using light moisturizers.

Acne—A Devastating Condition

From little eruptions to large elevations, how your skin looks makes a difference—mostly to you. Everyone is self-conscious of how they appear to others. Seeing yourself as unattractive in any way affects the whole of your "I": your self-image, your self-confidence with others, your social relationships, and your self-esteem. What if you do have zits or acne? Whether skin blemishes are a little or big problem to you, you probably would like to see them disappear. There are several alternatives to dealing with acne. Some are traditional methods, medications and professional dermatological care, and others are natural or nontraditional treatments.

Causes of Acne   The exact cause of acne continues to evade researchers. We do know that the sebaceous glands secrete an oil that changes to a

Helping Dry Skin

If you ski, cycle, swim, sail, or participate in almost any other outdoor sport, your skin may suffer from dryness. Snow, cold, wind, as well as indoor heating, are all tough on your skin. It may itch, flake and feel very dry. What actually seems like a lack of oil is really lack of moisture or dehydration. Thus, the best cure is moisture. How do you achieve this?

- Drink lots of water, at least 8 glasses a day, so you have enough moisture in your system.
- Humidify the air. Use a humidifier in your home or room; put a pan of water on the radiator to evaporate into the air; or keep several green plants in the room.
- Apply moisturizers to your face and body. These creams cut down on water loss and protect the skin from the elements. (The most effective products contain humectants, which help hold water.) If you are acne-prone, do not use oil-based moisturizers.
- You can increase blood flow through the capillaries that feed the skin via a five-minute facial massage—include it in your daily routine and notice the rosy afterglow.
- When you come inside from the cold, splash your face with cool water to facilitate the transition from cold to warm; then apply a moisturizer.
- Use a moist lipstick or substance like Vaseline to protect your lips.
- Bathe your body, not your face, less frequently; surface oils, which help to keep moisture in, will not be leached from your skin. Add a small amount of apple cider vinegar to your bath water to maintain acid mantle.
- Spray your skin every day with an atomizer of mineral water or, better yet, NaPCA, a natural, liquid moisturizer found in your local health food store.
- Use a moisturizing mask once a week. Mix one teaspoon of mayonnaise with one egg yolk, and if you have an aloe vera plant handy, add a teaspoon of the pulp. Mix all this together and spread on your face. Leave on for 15–20 minutes, then remove with warm water.
- A recent study at the University of Pennsylvania found that Vaseline, applied for 14 days on the legs, eliminated dryness, cracks and scales. Lanolin worked second best.
- Skin brush your body at least once a week to remove the dead skin cells and open up the pores.
- Try nutrient supplements like cod liver oil, one capsule a day (terrific for dry skin), or evening primrose oil from Great Britain (available at most health food stores).
- Instead of using oil (which may only mat down the scales), try a plain yogurt massage and switch to an acid-based cleanser.
- Panthenol, a derivative of Vitamin B_5, helps fortify the skin's defenses against the drying effects of central heating.

solid white substance called sebum. This travels to the opening of a hair follicle and erupts on the skin's surface. This process may be due to an infection of these glands or to excessive amounts of male hormones called androgens.

Blackheads appear when sebum mixes with skin pigments in plugged pores. Whole blackheads look like dirt. They are actually a mixture of sebum and skin scales that have closed off a hair follicle. When this condition is severe, the clogged hair follicle cannot contain the build-up of sebum mixture. When it closes off, a white pimple (whitehead) appears at the skin's surface, which may leak into the surrounding tissue. The blackhead now becomes a boil-like eruption that may contain bacteria. If these lesions are not treated, they may leave permanent scars. Since the exact source of acne is not known, it is often difficult to determine a treatment

Your Personal Image

How to Clean Your Skin

- Complete the following cleansing process twice daily, morning and night.

  Normal skin: Use pH-balanced soap (not alkaline) or oil-based or cream-based cleanser.

  Oily skin: Use cream-based cleanser; may use pH-balanced soap and water.

  Dry skin: Use oil-based cleanser.

  If you live in an area of high pollution: Use oil-based or cream-based cleanser. Follow with pH-balanced soap and water.

- Rinse thoroughly with warm water.
- Splash with cold water.
- Apply freshener to restore pH balance.
- Moisturize.

Flaky, Dry Skin   A frequent side effect of acne is flaky, dry skin, with or without dandruff. When the pores are plugged, dead skin falls off in clumps, and the skin looks dry. This condition may be caused by poor diet, stress, active hormones, lack of exercise, poor cleansing habits, or generally ill health.

If the follicles are completely plugged, oil cannot reach the surface, so the skin will be dry. This may be caused by too much oil, either from diet or hormones, from failing to keep the skin clean and free of buildup, or from greasy cosmetics.

Insufficient oil may be as troublesome as too much. If your diet is deficient in oil, there may not be enough oil in your skin to seal in the moisture. If you live in a dry climate, the water in your skin evaporates quite quickly. Soaps and shampoos can also contribute to dry skin. Check the ingredients listed on your soap or ask for a natural product in a health store.

Diet and Acne   Many physicians and nutritionists believe that diet does affect acne. Examine your patterns of elimination. Try more roughage, salads, bran, and at least eight glasses of water every day to get things moving so that your skin does not have to be burdened by wastes the alimentary tract cannot handle. A diet high in fat and sugar contributes to acne. Chocolate probably does not directly result in zits, but if your diet is high in fat and sugar, your skin is not receiving the nutrients it requires for health. Limit fat intake to 15 to 20 percent of your diet, eliminate sugar, and increase complex carbohydrates to 50 to 60 percent, leaving protein at 20 percent. Allergies may also play a role. You might try eliminating milk, dairy products, wheat, and food preservatives. Ask your physician to do a complete allergy test, and eliminate foods suggested by the results.

Diet Supplements   Vitamin and mineral supplements have helped many acne sufferers. Vitamin A helps restore balance and maintain a clear skin, Vitamin B complex helps reduce excess sebum, and Vitamin C can help reduce infection. Vitamin E will help reduce scarring on the skin. Zinc is the most useful mineral and one that by itself may make a considerable difference in the quality of your skin. Studies have shown that zinc has helped cure acne in 50 percent of the cases for which it was prescribed. Essential fatty acids (linoleic acid, linolenic acid) are necessary for healthy skin.

External Treatment   Clean your skin by washing it with warm water twice a day. As we have already discussed, use a gentle, pH-balanced soap that does not contain sulfur, bactericidals or other chemicals or perfumes. Remove all dirt and excess oil without damaging the skin. In addition, you might want to steam your face a couple of times a week to open the pores and allow waste material to escape. Mild exfoliation will clear away the dead skin. To avoid transmitting bacteria to open sores, touch your face only with clean hands. Wash your hands frequently, and particularly avoid touching your nasal area and then your skin.

Over-the-counter creams containing benzoyl peroxide may control mild to moderate acne. For difficult problems, you may choose to consult a dermatologist, who can prescribe medications effective for treatment of acne.

Internal Treatment   If your acne seems totally uncontrollable through diet, herbs, cleansing, external medications, and stress management, consult a dermatologist and together work out a program of treatment. You don't have to live with acne—one of these methods or several in combination will help.

Tetracycline, an antibiotic, has been found to be useful in clearing the skin of most acne sufferers. It is usually given in doses of 250 milligrams two to four times per day for several weeks. Occasionally, this medication will work for the first few weeks then cease to make a difference. It is successful in only 70 to 75 percent of the cases. This drug should be taken on an empty stomach at least one hour before the next meal. If you are taking tetracycline, discuss the proper protocol with your doctor. According to *Modern Medicine*, the failure of tetracycline to work effectively may be because it is taken at mealtimes. Foods such as milk or other dairy products interfere with its absorption. Be aware that if you take tetracycline or other antibiotics short-term, they will upset the bacterial balance in your gastrointestinal tract. Read more about inner ecology and yeast in the **Nutrition** chapter.

Accutane® has proven to be almost a miracle drug to many young people with severe acne. Accutane (13-cis retinoic acid), a derivative of Vitamin A, is often given for several months; following this course, the skin is usually clear. However, this process is not easy. First, during the course of taking this drug, facial skin is tender, peeling and dry. Your lips will be dry, maybe even cracked, and you may suffer from frequent nosebleeds because of dry nasal membranes. More important, Accutane can have severe potential side effects which must be monitored. Your physician will insist that you have blood tests every few weeks, because this drug can damage your liver or raise fat levels in the blood. Pregnant women should not take this drug, because it can cause birth defects. If you complete the course of Accutane successfully, your skin should remain clear. Acne scars will also improve tremendously. If you have tried other methods and nothing helps, discuss Accutane with your doctor.

Retin-A™ (tretinoin) is a second prescription medication that has improved the appearance of many individuals with acne-scarred faces. Retin-A is a topical cream derivative of Vitamin A. This substance increases your skin's sensitivity to sunburn. Users are cautioned to protect treated areas from exposure to the sun, wind or extreme cold. Other skin medications should be used at the same time only on your physician's advice. For example, use a mild, nonmedicated soap when also applying

---

Accutane®—Wonder Drug or Hazard?

When introduced in 1982, Accutane® was heralded as a revolutionary treatment for cystic acne; a miracle treatment for young and older adults who suffer from this disfiguring form of acne. But there is a problem: pregnant women using Accutane are vulnerable to birth defects in their babies. The active ingredient in Accutane is isisotretinoin, one of 1,500 retinoids, and a relative to Vitamin A. This component is known to pose a risk to a developing fetus because it affects cell division. Mothers who take Accutane have a one-in-four chance of having a malformed baby. The FDA has not banned this drug, but the agency instigated preventative steps: a one-page signed consent form verifying that the woman knows the risks; a pregnancy test no more than two weeks before starting the drug; and the woman cannot begin treatment until she has started her menstrual period. Even with these safeguards, some critics believe only dermatologists should give the prescription.

Cellulite, aptly named by the French, *peau d'orange*, spoils even the most svelte figure. As a woman ages, she tends to accumulate unsightly cellulite bumps on her hips, thighs, buttocks, and even upper arms. Over 90 percent of women experience this condition in varying degrees. There is no definitive cure, but women can take steps to begin to reverse the problem. One of the most important factors is diet. Avoid the primary culprits: refined carbohydrates and sugars, additives, saturated fats, salt, and alcohol. Smoking is also discouraged. Dry skin brushing, external rubbing, and buffing all contribute to increased blood flow. Certain foods will aid in the removal of toxins: lemon juice in a large glass of water every morning to help eliminate the impurities, garlic to purify and cleanse the blood, and lots of onion to improve lymphatic drainage. Common herbs such as rosemary, tarragon, parsley, and fennel all are good diuretics and help flush toxins and excess fluids out of the body. Perhaps women don't have to live with these unsightly bumps after all.

Retin-A. While treatment may initially cause some discomfort or peeling, these effects usually subside within two to four weeks. It may take six to twelve weeks for you to notice a major improvement. And, once your acne is under control, you may need to continue regular application of this cream until your physician instructs otherwise.

Conjugated Estrogens are still another treatment for young women that they may take just before menstruation. Birth control pills can accomplish this, particularly those with a higher estrogen balance. However, this treatment has potential complications; for example, delay of menstruation and imbalance of the endocrine system. Consult your physician about this alternative.

Cosmetics

For most women, whether or not to use cosmetics is not a question. If you feel comfortable without cosmetics, you don't need them to maintain healthy skin. But if you do use cosmetics, also know that you can use them in an effective fashion so that you will feel better about your outward appearance. Since cosmetics generally enhance natural attributes, they can provide an important adjunct to your self-image.

More relevant to total skin care is buying cosmetics that fit with you, do not cause allergic reactions, or make you look like a high-priced model (this is the nice way of putting it). The essence of using cosmetics well is allowing them to enhance your natural beauty. Try variations of different cosmetic applications. Ask your friends (prefacing the question by telling them you really want an honest answer) how they like your use of cosmetics, and use your own good judgment.

Natural or Synthetic Cosmetics? Unfortunately, the label of "natural" is misleading. Even cosmetics called "natural" may contain chemicals that are not derived from plant, herb or other natural substances. In fact, at least 100 ingredients used in cosmetics are suspected of being cancer-causing agents. Even though cosmetics are regulated by the FDA, many name brand products contain these ingredients. If it is important to you that your cosmetics contain only natural ingredients, shop around for these products. Most natural cosmetics contain no petroleum-based substances. Their formulas include no chemical additives or preservatives, artificial dyes, or animal products. Instead, the manufacturers use herbs and other plant ingredients.

The truth about cosmetics is that most commercial lines differ only in label, not ingredients. In fact, there are about five ranges of quality, and all major cosmetic firms use the same manufacturing formulas and similar combinations of ingredients. One important consideration when you are buying cosmetics is whether you are allergic to the ingredients. To test your sensitivity, apply a small amount to the inside surface of your arm and leave it for several hours. If your skin remains clear, you are probably not allergic to this substance. If in any doubt, purchase hypo-allergenic cosmetics.

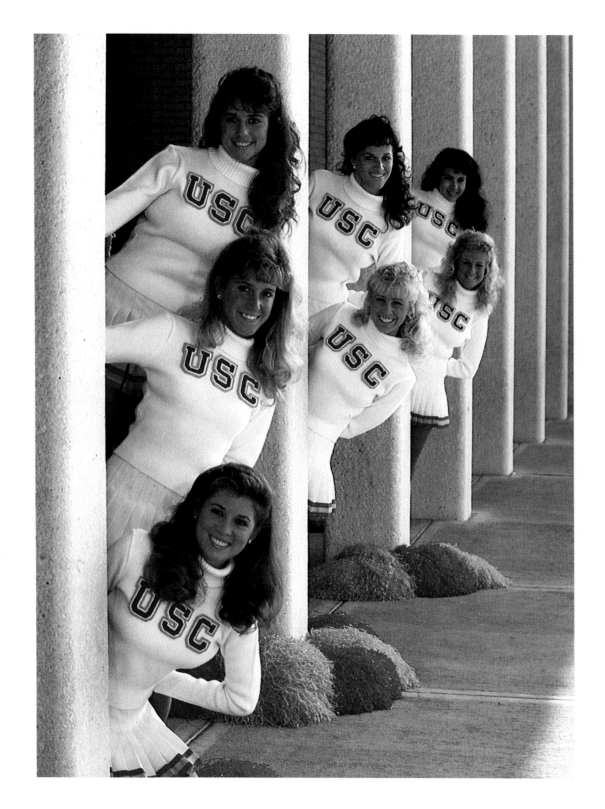

Even if you are not dramatically allergic, you may find mascara irritating to your eyes. If this occurs, stop using it for a few days to avoid an eye infection. Replace mascara tubes frequently, because mascara brushes may provide a supportive breeding ground for bacteria.

Makeup should be thoroughly removed every night before going to bed. Be very gentle when cleansing the delicate skin around the eyes. Follow the cleansing and moisturizing rituals outlined earlier in this chapter.

The Elements and Your Skin

Sun and Your Health　Wherever you see the sun shining, you see people of all ages basking in its warmth. Today many are still in search of the "Great American Tan." Often these sun worshippers are college students who identify with the images associated with a dark tan. Through advertising and the extensive use of bronzed, beautiful models, we have come to relate a good tan with health, wealth, glamour, and social status—a tanned person epitomizes an active, successful man or woman.

Although a tan might project these outward qualities to some people, in reality sunning has its dark side. Premature aging and skin cancer are two facets of the tanning craze to which college students should pay attention. Recently, experts are seeing an epidemic of skin cancer, and people in their twenties are among the fastest growing number of cases. But you can tan safely. By using common sense and appropriate sunscreen products, you can have an attractive, healthy tan while minimizing the risks of unhealthy side effects.

The Healing Power of Sun　It's definitely important to be well-informed about the harmful consequences of the sun. But luckily, in moderation, tanning also has some beneficial effects. A moderate amount of sun helps mild cases of acne. When the top layer of skin peels off, it carries away blackheads and potential breakouts. (Note: Be careful. The sun has adverse effects on serious acne. As with anything else, pay attention to your body; then you can decide what's best for your personal health care.)

Natural sunlight helps the body utilize Vitamin D, which in turn aids in the absorption of calcium that keeps bones strong and healthy. Sunlight can help to lower your blood pressure and promote high energy and endurance. It also maintains biological rhythms and the secretion of hormones and now is even believed to affect emotional stability.

SAD　One of the most enlightening discoveries has been that sunlight can improve your mood; or, conversely, insufficient sunlight can throw you into a mild depression. In 1980, Alfred Lewy and his research team found that bright light decreases pineal gland function and darkness accelerates it. The pineal gland is a small organ located deep in the brain. This gland secretes the hormone melatonin, which, scientists have learned, times the onset of puberty, stimulates sleep, and influences mood levels. Lewy's team speculated that melatonin levels change as the season changes—all according to the amount of sunlight available.

Biometeorologists (scientists who research how the weather affects our moods) continue to study the effect of the seasons and variations of weather on moods. These results may explain why we feel good or up on a sunny day and down or depressed on a dreary day. They also provide an explanation to the disorder known as seasonal affective depression, or SAD. With awareness of this disorder—directly connected to the amount of sunlight a person receives—comes even stronger affirmation of the importance of sunlight in your life.

People with SAD notice changes in their moods depending on the weather. Usually, people feel better, more relaxed, happier and content during summer, when days are longer. Researchers believe that exposure to sunlight is responsible. Now, when you come back from a day at the beach in a great mood, you'll know why! There is a caveat, however. Too much sunlight can be damaging.

The Hidden Harm of Sunlight   Ironically, while a tan might project a young, healthy image, it actually accelerates the aging process. The drying effect of the sun on skin, especially on faces, causes the skin to wrinkle. Most college students don't worry about premature aging, but the term "premature" implies that you should at least start thinking about it.

Even more frightening is the prospect of getting skin cancer. Doctors used to think only older people who had spent many years in the sun could develop skin cancer caused by overexposure. Recently, though, younger people have fallen victim to the dangerous, and sometimes deadly, disease.

How can sunlight be so potentially dangerous, especially when we feel so terrific after a day in the sun? The sun produces ultraviolet rays (UVR's), which are believed to stimulate the production of free radicals in the skin. These free radicals can damage DNA molecules (the blueprint for all life activity). Usually, when these molecules are damaged, the body recognizes the problem and repairs it. If this does not occur, mutations develop and cancer may result. Any substance that produces free radicals in the body can be said to be potentially cancer producing.

Another theory regarding the effect of UVR's suggests that these rays depress the immune system. The immune system protects you by fighting foreign invaders or removing errant damaged cells. Regardless of exactly how sunlight is connected to an increase in skin cancer, scientists believe there is a definite link; and brief, high-intensity exposures to strong sunlight are the greatest threat.

Skin Cancer   Each year over 300,000 new cases of skin cancer are reported. The Skin Cancer Foundation believes that overexposure to ultraviolet rays from the sun is the primary cause in 90 percent of the cases. There are three major types of skin cancer. The first two, basal cell and

Does Sun Help Acne?

If you think you've found an acne cure because your face looks better after a few rays, beware. According to dermatologists, the sun may temporarily improve acne by peeling off the top layer. The pimples drain and look better for a while. Then the pimples may return even more severely; now, you not only don't have your tan (that disappeared in a few days) but you have a worse case of acne. If your acne is severe, stay out of the sun.

Your Personal Image

squamous cell carcinoma, are the most common and usually occur on the areas most exposed to the sun—face, ears, neck, chest, and hands. Melanoma, the third type of skin cancer, is less common but much more dangerous. The relationship between this cancer and sunlight is not as definitive, but ultraviolet overexposure appears to be a contributing factor. More frequently, these cancers develop from pre-existing moles. If you notice that a mole has grown or changed color or that the pigment has become uneven, see a physician right away. Skin cancer has the highest cure rate of any cancer. Melanomas that are diagnosed early can be curable. If untreated, skin melanomas can be deadly.

All this talk about the harmful consequences of the sun may tempt you to want to hide inside and seek a golden tan on a tanning bed. A word of advice—don't. The modern tanning bed has ultraviolet x-rays which tan the skin at a very slow pace. Because you need to spend a longer period of time under a tanning bed than in the sunlight in order to tan, the prolonged exposure can lead to wrinkling and even decrease your skin's ability to fight off cancer.

The Heart and Sol of Tanning   Safe tanning is a three-step process: 1) know your skin type and your body's ability to handle sun exposure; 2) use the appropriate tanning and sun screen products; and 3) use your best judgment—be careful not to burn.

First, it's important to understand what a sunburn really is. When exposed to the sun, your skin activates a protection system. Cells in the top layer of skin produce a pigment known as melanin—this is what gives you the tan color. But if you're fair, or stay out too long, your skin can't produce melanin fast enough. The redness caused by a burn is related to dilated blood vessels in the second layer of skin; this condition allows

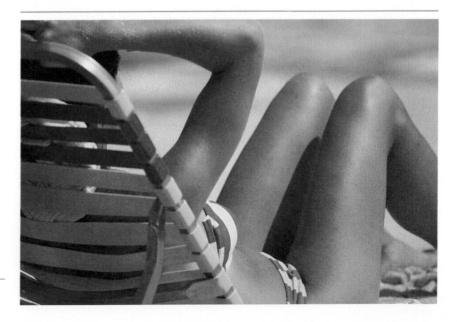

Burn or Tan—What's Your SPF?

Eye Color	Hair Color	Complexion	You Are	SPF Range
Blue Green Gray Hazel	Blond Lt. brown Red	Very fair	Likely to burn	15 to 29
Dark blue Gray Hazel	Brown	Fair	May burn	8 to 15
Brown	Dark brown Black	Olive skin Black skin	Likely to tan	4 to 15

When Your Risk of Sunburn Is Greatest

- In the direct sun from 11 AM to 2 PM
- If you are taking certain drugs such as antibiotics, sulfonamides, antipsychotics, diuretics, oral contraceptives, or Accutane
- At high altitude—above 5,000 feet
- In the snow—white reflects sunlight
- Near water or sand—both reflect sunlight

more blood to flow to the burned area, turning the skin red and swollen. When plasma forms under the damaged skin, blisters occur. In a few days, the dead skin peels off. A sunburn not only looks bad and feels bad, but does some pretty harsh damage to the skin; foremost, it's a preface to cancer.

SPF To prevent burning, wear appropriate sun protection products. Lotions sold today are identified by a sun protection factor (SPF) number. The accompanying chart will help you identify your skin type and its corresponding ability to take the sun. If the chart indicates that you're prone to tan or burn, you should always wear a strong sunscreen with at least a SPF 15 when you first hit the beach or other tanning hot-spot. If you have medium-toned skin, start with at least a SPF 8. For black and olive skin tones that never seem to burn, start with a number 4, and always protect sensitive spots such as your nose, under your eyes, your shoulders, chest, and so forth. To figure out which SPF to use, calculate the hours it would take you to burn if you weren't wearing any protection. Multiply this number by the product's SPF. For example, if you would burn in two hours, you would burn in four hours if you wore a lotion with a SPF of 2. Neutrogena makes a Paba-free SPF 15, and Presun makes a SPF 29 for individuals extremely sensitive to the sun. Make sure to always watch dangerous areas: lips, eyelids and nose. Bullfrog works great for these spots—and it's waterproof for several hours.

Don't be fooled into thinking that you can't burn after you have a base tan. Keep using a sunscreen; slightly decrease the strength if you find you aren't burning and want to gradually darken your tan. Remember to reapply sunscreen after swimming, exercising or a few hours of sweating— it can't protect you if it has washed off! Aloe-up and several other products provide a variety of waterproof sunscreens.

Your Personal Image

Protecting the Rest of You From the Sun   Skin care is imperative, but protecting your eyes, hair and lips from harsh extremes is also important. Your eyes can burn just like your skin, so wear good sunglasses that block out at least 95 percent of both the ultraviolet and infrared rays. When skiing, be extra careful because the snow can reflect up to 85 percent of ultraviolet light. Snow blindness occurs when the cornea is burned by these harmful rays, and may lead to cataracts. Also, the area around the eyes is extremely sensitive and prone to wrinkles if overexposed to the sun.

Your hair's health needs are an important consideration. The sun, wind, salt, air, and chlorine all take their toll. Be sure to wash your hair frequently—especially after swimming in a chlorinated pool—and use a conditioner to avoid dryness. You can also purchase hair gels and conditioners that have sun screen in them to seal in moisture and protect against the sun.

One part of the body people don't often think about protecting is the lips. Lips lack the protective melanin layer your skin has, so they often burn. Regular lipstick can't protect them, so be sure to use a high SPF emollient. Bullfrog works and Bain de Soleil and Clinique make special protective lip balms. Zinc oxide also works well to block the UVRs. Whatever product you choose, wear one because damaged lips are especially prone to skin cancer.

For Great Skin Twenty Years from Now

If you start taking care of your skin right now, you will be slowing down the aging process, preventing wrinkles, while at the same time enjoying a healthy, radiant skin. To accomplish this, remember the three cardinal rules of external skin care

- Regular, thorough cleansing—a minimum of once per day.
- Protection from loss of moisture.
- Protection from the ultraviolet rays of the sun.

You also may want to incorporate healthy internal skin care: a healthy elimination system maintained by adequate fiber and fluids; vitamins and minerals to supplement deficiencies; stress-coping techniques; and the avoidance of substances that destroy skin such as smoking, alcohol and caffeine. Work this plan into your life, and twenty years from now when you return for your college reunion, your friends will be asking how you stay so young.

Hair Care

Most women and more than a few men want beautiful hair, and most are not totally thrilled with what Mother Nature gave them. If your hair is naturally curly, maybe you prefer straight; if it is brunette, you might wonder if blondes have more fun. Whether your hair is thin, thick, straight, curly, or grows fast or slow depends on inheritance. The condition of your hair depends on you. For hair to be beautiful, the hair follicle must be healthy; for the cuticle and cortex of the hair shaft to be healthy, it must be fed from inside. You can influence the condition of your hair by diet, your overall health care, and good care of the hair itself. This section will discuss care of your hair—from the inside out.

A Closer Look at Your Hair

Hair is primarily protein; in fact, it is 97 percent protein. The remaining component is moisture. Hair, like your nails, is lifeless. Why then would something that we eat make a difference if hair is already dead? This is a mystery not yet solved. We do know that the follicle beneath the scalp depends on adequate blood and oxygen for nourishment to produce healthy hair. You are born with approximately 90,000 hair follicles. Though the number does not change with time or health, they may shut down or not work properly.

Each strand of hair has three layers: the cuticle, or outside; the medulla, or center; and the cortex, the part in between, which is made up of amino-acid chains. The cuticle is the part that protects the underlayer and preserves moisture. If this part is damaged, your hair will look dull and lifeless. The cuticle is composed of a keratin coat that is also layered. When these layers lie flat, they shine and reflect the light. When they are damaged or peeling, your hair becomes dull. The cortex is the part of the strand that gives your hair its color. If the amino-acid chains that make up this cortex break as a result of poor treatment (hair dryers, hot rollers, alkaline shampoos, or over-processing with permanents), you will have broken strands and split-ends. The third layer, the medulla, is the component that transports nutrients to the other layers.

Your hair grows in cycles that last from two to seven years. Each strand has its own seven-year cycle until it is finally shed as a normal part of brushing or washing. The shedding of one strand triggers the follicle to produce another strand, and so the process continues. Your hair tends to shed more rapidly in autumn and grow more rapidly in the spring and summer.

You can expect to lose between 100 and 200 strands of hair each day. However, if your hair is coming out by the handfuls, something is definitely wrong. This may not be anything to worry about if you can identify the cause, such as a recent illness, alteration in hormonal balance (as in childbirth), or an emotional crisis that has passed. If this is not the case, however, and your hair continues to fall out at an alarming rate, contact a physician for a complete medical workup. Such hair problems can indicate more serious bodily malfunctions. They can definitely be related to stress, so do not forget to consider your emotional health. If you are under stress and your hair is falling out, consider seeking professional help for reducing the stress in your life. For moderate hair loss improve your diet by adding more complete protein and vitamin-mineral supplements.

Dramatic Hair Loss

If you're losing lots of hair, consult a physician for a complete workup. This could be an indication that your overall health may be in jeopardy. For moderate hair loss (not by the handfuls), improve your diet, adding more complete protein and consider adding supplements: zinc (30 to 40 mg/day), Vitamin B-complex, Vitamin C (2,000 to 3,000 mg/day), sulfur, and iron. Wheat germ is an excellent natural supplement for hair loss. Some nutritionists also recommend Vitamin E (200 to 400 units/day), cysteine, and manganese.

Vitamins and Minerals for Healthy Hair

Just like any other part of your body, the hair follicle benefits from good nutrition. Perhaps the worst thing you can do to your hair is go on crash diets. A diet of inadequate nutrients does not allow the cuticle to receive the oxygen and nourishment it requires. Research has documented that hair begins to deteriorate as early as the second or third day of a strict diet; this is how closely your hair condition is tied to internal health.

What nutrients does your hair require? The most important mineral for healthy hair is iron. Studies reveal that a majority of American women are at least mildly iron deficient. If you are deficient in iron, your hair will reflect this deficiency by appearing brittle, dull and hard to manage. If this describes your hair, ask your physician to test the iron content in your blood. If you decide to take an iron supplement, remember to take it with Vitamin C, as this enhances iron absorption. Calcium must also be present in your body in the appropriate levels for iron to be efficiently absorbed. As always, vitamins and minerals work synergistically—one affects the other.

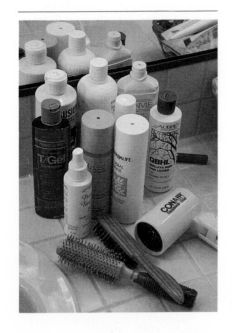

Another mineral important for healthy hair is sulfur, which keeps your hair smooth and silky (remember the cuticle layers that are supposed to lie flat). Sulfur is found in amino acids. The best sources are eggs, fish, beans, nuts, and meat. If your diet is inadequate in protein, the amino-acid chains are deficient and your hair will suffer.

Zinc is also an important mineral, and a deficiency will probably show up as excessive hair loss, lack of sheen, and difficulty with control. If you are taking contraceptive pills with estrogen, which depletes zinc levels, you might consider a zinc gluconate supplement. At the same time, remember that zinc is necessary for healthy skin and in many instances will clear up pimples. So if neither your hair nor your skin seem in good condition, think about taking zinc.

Vitamin C and B complex are important for healthy hair. A lack of any B vitamin will cause problems. Deficient B_{12} will result in dandruff, scaling and hair loss. However, because the B vitamins work together, if you are deficient in one, you probably also will be deficient in others—thus the B-complex model.

Megadoses of vitamins and minerals are not necessary for healthy hair. In fact, it would be preferable to eat a well-balanced diet and not have to take supplements. The truth is, however, if you are living on campus, dining in a residence hall or eating many fast-food meals, you are probably not ingesting all the nutrients you need to remain healthy and this will be reflected in your skin, hair, energy level—every part of your life. Also, be aware that if you are taking medications, such as birth control pills, thyroid medication, cortisone, diet pills, or aspirin, your hair may appear dull and brittle and you'll have some hair loss. If you do choose to supplement your diet with vitamins and minerals, make sure you take safe dosages. Review the tables in the **Nutrition** chapter for appropriate dosage.

Washing Your Hair

Many of us simply buy a shampoo that is attractively packaged or that we've seen advertised. Choosing the right shampoo is important for the health of your hair. An alkaline shampoo, in general, is not good because hair, like your skin, is mildly acidic. Choose a shampoo that is pH-balanced or slightly acidic.

Most shampoos today are detergent based. This is preferable to soap-based products because soap leaves a film on your hair. Choose a shampoo with a conditioner. This substance coats the hair shaft and makes it look thicker. Finally, most of the numerous formulas ranging from herbs and plants to protein provide the basis for most shampoos. These shampoos are good for your hair, providing they are pH-balanced. The accompanying box gives a few hints on buying the right shampoo for your hair.

How frequently you wash your hair is entirely up to you and the condition of your hair. If you have dry hair, you might limit washings to a couple of times per week; if you have oily hair, you may choose to wash every day. If you do wash your hair daily, use a pH-balanced shampoo and only wash once; more than that removes too much of the natural oil.

Treatment for Hair Problems

At various times during your busy, hectic life you may need a little extra help to keep your hair in good condition. If your hair or scalp needs a boost or special treatment, try one of the following recipes.

Oily Hair   Lemon shampoo or a lemon-and-water rinse helps control the oil in your hair. You might choose two or three lemon-based shampoos and alternate them so they maintain their effectiveness. Another option is to add spearmint leaves (about four teaspoons) to one quart of natural water and heat the mixture until it boils, then cool and use as an after-shampoo rinse.

Dry Hair   If your hair is naturally dry, an oil treatment will help. An efficient, inexpensive way to give yourself an oil treatment is to massage olive oil into your hair and scalp, then cover your hair with plastic wrap or aluminum foil. Cover this with two wet towels that you have heated in a microwave oven for two minutes. Keep towels on for twenty minutes, then remove oil with two washings.

If you have dry hair, remember to use a hair dryer only on medium and cool settings, stay out of the direct sun, and limit the use of heated rollers (which are very drying). Also, supplement your diet with B-complex vitamins. If your hair is dry from over-processing (strong permanents left on too long) or over-coloring, an oil pack will not work. Purchase a protein pack and apply; in this case, the more, the better.

Guidelines for Selecting Shampoo

- For damaged or fine hair, use protein shampoo labeled substantive protein. With exceptionally fine or dry hair, your shampoo should be more than slightly acidic. The other option is to rinse your hair following shampoo with white vinegar and water or lemon and water. This acid rinse will help to restore a smooth cuticle and the shine to your hair.
- For healthy hair, regular protein shampoos are fine. If you are a blonde, you might try chamomile, which has mild bleaching properties.
- For oily hair, use a lemon-based shampoo.
- For fine hair with little body, try a balsam-based shampoo.
- For all types of hair jojoba-based shampoo is good. Jojoba is successful in treating scalp conditions as well as dissolving sebum build-up. It leaves your hair squeaky clean and shining.

Your Personal Image

Dandruff   When your dandruff is caused by a dry, flaky scalp condition, brush frequently to remove the flakes, massage your scalp to improve circulation, and avoid using alkaline-based shampoos. Try a pure jojoba oil-based shampoo and use it regularly.

You may also apply an over-the-counter dandruff shampoo once a week to keep this problem under control. Buy one that contains zinc pyrithione or selenium sulfide to remove scales. Coal-tar formulas are also very effective. Do not over-use these shampoos—more is not better. In some rare cases, a selenium-based shampoo can cause more dandruff, so be watchful! Another effective age-old remedy is to use a final rinse of one cup of warm water mixed with two to three tablespoons of white vinegar. This also brings out the highlights in your hair and makes it shiny.

Still another dandruff remedy is to massage table salt into your dry scalp before shampooing with an acid-based shampoo. And don't forget those C and B-complex vitamins.

Split Ends   Everyone has some split ends that occur naturally. But, when your entire head is covered with split ends and your hair does not shine or glow, it is time to do something. Start by cutting off the ends to prevent further splitting. Take better care of your hair—blow dry on medium or cool only, stay out of the sun, change shampoos to acid-based, and do not brush with a short-bristled or nylon brush. Trim the ends frequently and protect the hair shaft with hot-oil treatments. Also, avoid permanents for several months.

Difficult-to-Manage Hair   Build-up of residue from shampoo may coat the hair shaft, making it dull, lifeless and hard to manage. The best solution is to rotate shampoos or use Neutrogena shampoo one week out of every month. This natural shampoo will remove the buildup and restore the shine to your hair.

Building Body and Shine   Try a do-it-yourself massage. Take a tablespoon of vegetable oil—jojoba oil is best because it closely resembles natural scalp oil—warm it and rub into your scalp when hair is dry. Massage scalp with firm strokes for 5 minutes, wrap with a warm, damp towel and leave for 10 minutes. Notice the difference in body and shine.

Care of Hands and Nails

Your hands and nails give others many cues about you—your health, your age and your personality (and even your wealth, if you tend to wear it on your hands). Any good palm reader will tell you that she or he can read your life, health and even innermost thoughts by simply looking at the shape of your fingers, lines on your palms, and your fingernails. Yet, both women and men often neglect these parts of their bodies.

Most of us admire clean, reasonably long, beautifully shaped, manicured nails on a woman. How can you create beautiful nails? There are two major areas to consider—a healthy diet and protection from environmental damage.

Protection for Nails and Hands   Your nails, like hair, need complete protein. They also require Vitamins A, C and B complex; minerals, especially zinc, iron, calcium, iodine, and sulfur; and trace elements. Vitamin A is important to prevent splitting nails; Vitamin C to prevent peeling and hangnails; B complex to prevent ridges and fragile nails, as well as fungus infections; and iron to prevent weak, dry, thin nails. Calcium is a must for healthy nails. A well-balanced diet with all of the nutrients is necessary for healthy nails. If your diet is inadequate, consider vitamin and mineral supplements.

Both nails and hands suffer from exposure to harmful liquids and harsh weather. Putting your hands in water with detergents, disinfectants, soaps, or chemicals damages both skin and nails. The best cure is prevention—wear gloves when you can. Heavy-duty creams will also both protect and repair damage to your hands and nails. Cold, inclement weather, wind, and low humidity are all hard on your hands and nails. If you live in a section of the country where winter weather is extreme, wear a protective cream daily, put polish on your nails, and wear gloves.

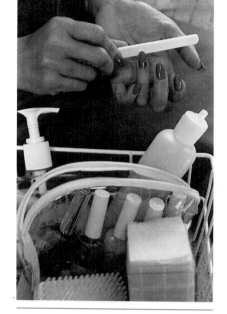

Solving Nail Problems

In addition to a balanced diet, you can take other steps to prevent and improve troublesome nail conditions.

Hangnails   Every day, in addition to taking adequate doses of Vitamin C, rub Vitamin E around your nail-bed and use a light pumice stone to remove loose skin.

Brittle Nails   This nail condition, often manifesting as dry, brittle nails that constantly break, can be related to several causes. Diet is one of the most important. For a well-balanced, healthy diet, refer to **Nutrition Awareness**. Nail polish remover is very drying to nails and cuticles, and should be used sparingly. Nail product ingredients, such as enamels, are drying as well as protective. Do not cover the cuticle but keep it moist with healthy oils. Try a combination of oils (evening primrose oil or Vitamin E). Also, look for a natural or hypoallergenic enamel, one without the formaldehyde resin. Nail hardeners containing formaldehyde make brittle nails more brittle. You might try white iodine, found in health food or drug stores. This substance, applied three times per week, will strengthen your nails. Don't worry if your nails become yellow. Their quality will improve and the yellow will go away. Beware of artificial nails, nail wraps, or sculptured nails. These products are composed of acrylics and peroxide that may damage your natural nails.

Peeling Nails   Make sure your diet is well balanced and includes many fresh fruits and vegetables. Keep your nails out of water by using rubber

White spots on nails: may relate to zinc or Vitamin B_6 deficiency. Deep ridges on nails: may relate to B complex deficiency or high stress.

gloves. Wear a polish that does not contain formaldehyde for protection, and, if you are desperate, you might try a nail hardener temporarily.

Broken Nails   Keep a nail-mending kit on hand so that when a nail snags you can fix it immediately, before it totally breaks. Use glue to mend a broken tip, then apply polish.

Tips for Pretty Hands

Rough, Red Hands   Use the same exfoliator that you use on your face to rid the skin of dead cells. Or you might use sugar mixed with mineral oil—apply and rub all over, then rinse off. Follow with a rich cream.

Dry Hands   After rinsing your hands in warm water to open the pores, apply a rich cream, put on white cotton gloves, and get a good night's sleep (preferably alone, unless you want to be considered weird). An age-old cure for dry hands is glycerine. Buy it in the drug store and apply it every night; you will notice a significant difference in just a few days.

Future Protection   Put sun-block on the backs of your hands whenever you're going outdoors for long periods of time. One easy way to tell the age of women over about 33 is to look at the backs of their hands. Those unsightly brown splotches (also known as aging spots) do not get there overnight. What you do as a 20 year old will affect your appearance for the rest of your life.

Eye Care

Eyesight is a capability you probably take for granted—until you experience a vision problem. Nearly 120 million Americans wear glasses or contact lenses. As a student, you depend heavily on your eyes for reading and writing. Though most people who wear glasses are past usual college age, more and more students are experiencing vision problems which require corrective lenses. This section will identify the more common vision impairments, describe the warning signs of eye problems, and discuss the conventional treatments for these conditions.

Vision Exams and Corrective Options

Under normal conditions, have your eyes checked annually. If you experience one or more of the warning signs listed in the accompanying chart, have them examined immediately. Eye exams are given by optometrists and ophthalmologists; the latter is a medical doctor. Using the familiar big "E" chart, the examiner will determine if you can see clearly. A rating of 20/20 is normal. A visual acuity of 20/30 means that what a normal person can see at 30 feet, you can see only at 20 feet. The most common vision defects are nearsightedness, farsightedness and astigmatism.

Warning Signs for Eye Problems

- Difficulty focusing or seeing close or distant objects
- Blurred or double vision, spots, or ghost-like images
- Vertical lines looking wavy or distorted
- Difficulty adjusting to darkened rooms
- Halos (colored rings around lights)
- Dark spot at vision center
- Black spots or flashes of light
- Excessively watery eyes
- Dry, itchy or burning eyes

Nearsightedness (myopia) means that you can see near objects clearly but far objects appear fuzzy. A farsighted (hyperopic) person has sharp distance vision but poor near vision. With astigmatism, vision is blurred at all distances. Other potential eye deficiencies include problems with eye coordination and muscle balance, focusing, and eye diseases, such as glaucoma.

Opticians make and adjust eyeglasses according to prescriptions from eye examiners. Refractive problems, such as farsightedness, nearsightedness and astigmatism, are treated with either eyeglasses or contact lenses. Some types of vision problems respond best to contact lenses. Depending on your vision deficiency, you may need to decide between glasses and contact lenses.

Only about 15 percent of people requiring vision correction use contact lenses consistently; many try contacts but give them up within the first year. Contact lenses come in several varieties: hard, soft, gas-permeable, and extended-wear. Each has advantages and disadvantages in terms of comfort, convenience, durability, and price. Ask your optometrist or ophthalmologist to explain these advantages and disadvantages as they apply to your specific needs. Regardless of whether you choose glasses (with glass or plastic lenses) or contact lenses, their effectiveness depends on getting a good fit. Not only must the lenses effectively aid your eyesight, but they must also be comfortable.

Hints for Contact Care

If your vision correction requires contacts or if you find contact lenses comfortable, convenient and attractive, here are some hints for contact care.

- Give your eyes a chance to adjust to being awake before inserting your contacts.
- Wash your hands before touching contact lenses so you don't introduce bacteria into your eyes.
- Don't wear contacts to bed unless you have extended-wear lenses; they will cause irritated corneas and interfere with fluid circulation in your eyes.
- Be meticulous about cleaning your lenses, especially soft contacts. Sloppy cleaning techniques can lead to eye infection or even permanent damage.
- If you find your contacts aren't working or your eyes are continually irritated or painful, get retested by a professional. Your eye acuity may have changed.
- If you are a woman, insert your lenses before you put on mascara or makeup and be careful about using hair spray near your eyes.
- If your eyesight is poor without contact correction, always carry a pair of glasses with you in case you lose a contact lens (so you can still function).

Contact Lenses and Cosmetics

Women who wear contact lenses should avoid eye cosmetics that are "waterproof." Small amounts will find their way into the eye, and a particle could become trapped under the lens. This can be extremely painful. If you use oil to remove the mascara and any gets in your eyes, it will cause cloudiness of the lens. Even when you take out the lens before removing makeup, a trace of oil remains in the eyes and is enough to cloud the lenses when they are inserted the next day. This clouding can last up to 24 hours and is perhaps the most common complaint of those who wear contacts. "Frosted" eye shadow products contain minute flakes of mica, and mascara contains small particles of nylon, neither of which breaks down in the tear fluid that naturally lubricates the eyes. These particles can also cause extreme pain by getting under contacts and scratching the surface of the cornea. Use only water soluble makeup and insert your contacts each day before it is applied. This reduces the risk of carrying makeup into the eye with a lens, a slip that, with soft contacts, could necessitate purchase of a new pair.

Source: Adapted from *Healthwise*

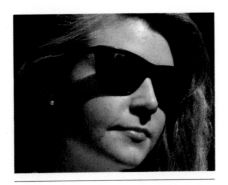

Sunglasses—More Than a Fashion Statement

The well-equipped student is never without a pair of trusty sunglasses. Not only do proper sunglasses make you look cool, they also reduce eye exposure to potentially damaging ultraviolet rays and reduce eyestrain and accompanying headaches. When selecting a brand name (Varnet, Ray-Ban) or design (aviator, wraparound) you should consider more than just style. New evidence points to the potential dangers of very dark glasses that cause pupils to dilate, allowing potentially harmful ultraviolet rays to penetrate deeper into the eyes than they would without sunglasses or with lighter lenses. Green and darker grey tints are recommended over yellow or rose. Bright yellow and orange lenses may also distort color perception and cause you to fail to recognize traffic lights. To guard against excessive exposure to sunlight, lenses should absorb at least 95 percent of ultraviolet and infrared radiation. Before purchasing sunglasses, inspect the label on the glasses or ask the sales clerk whether the glasses meet this standard. However, if you always venture outside with your shades on or worse, wear them inside, you may also be initiating negative long-term effects. Never allowing your eyes to accommodate to bright light lessens their capability to do so. Eye exercise is important, so give your eyes a chance to accommodate to light changes. Wear sunglasses when in the full sun or when there are glare conditions; otherwise, squint a little. If you plan to wear sunglasses while cycling or participating in recreational activities, make certain that the lenses are made from a high-impact plastic rather than glass. The frame should be as impact resistant as the lenses.

Your Eyes and Video Display Terminals

Eye care specialists have become aware of several eyesight problems related to extensive use of video display terminals (VDTs). If you are farsighted, you may experience blurred vision and discomfort while using a VDT. Nearsightedness is usually not much of a problem because you can see close objects, such as the video screen, more clearly than distant ones. If you suffer from astigmatism, working at a VDT will cause you discomfort. Any eyesight problem causes your eyes to try to adapt and serve your needs. In the process, such efforts may cause discomfort such as soreness, headache and fatigue. This reduces your efficiency and compounds the stress with which you are already dealing.

The following steps will minimize eye fatigue while using a VDT: use indirect room lighting, block excessive sunlight with shades or drapes, and maintain a high contrast between the characters and the screen background. Finally, both your body and eyes need relief. A 15-minute break to stretch your body and rest your eyes is recommended every two hours. Other tips for minimizing stress are to use an adjustable chair for body comfort, a work station that allows you to place the keyboard in a comfortable position, and an adjustable copyholder so that you can place the reference copy close to the screen. This reduces the strain of making head and eye movements from copy to screen, and so forth.

Dental Care

When you were a kid, someone else was responsible for your dental health. Not wanting to go to the dentist was the standard attitude. Now that you're in charge of your dental health, you should know the good news. Tooth decay and gum infections—the two major disease processes that take place in the mouth—are nearly 100 percent preventable. The bad news is that you are the one responsible if you let things go to pot.

To understand why certain techniques are important in keeping your teeth and gums healthy, you need to know what causes problems in these areas.

Tooth Decay

Two things must be present in order for the decay process to take place, bacteria and sugars. When bacteria and sugars come together on the surface of the teeth, the bacteria metabolizes the sugar to form acids. These acids then dissolve the tooth structure. You can interfere with the decay process by (1) reducing the number of bacteria in the mouth through brushing and flossing and (2) controlling the frequency and duration that sugars are in the mouth.

Gum Tissue Infections

The plaque that forms on teeth, whether you eat or not, becomes the matrix and the medium for bacteria to grow and multiply to high concentrations. The soft tissue of the mouth, especially the gums, react like any other tissue when subjected to concentrations of bacteria. They become inflamed, swollen and likely to bleed. Effective flossing and brushing removes the plaque and bacteria from the teeth. This leaves no place for the residual bacteria to multiply and prevents most gum tissue infections.

Preventive Dental Care

As you may have noticed, whether these problems develop in your mouth or not depends on your actions. If you avoid thinking about your teeth because of the pain you associate with dentists, you'll probably wind up in need of serious dental work—with accompanying discomfort. The best way to avoid long, uncomfortable (and expensive) hours in the dentist's chair is to take good care of your teeth and gums now. Here are the activities and materials that can help you achieve and maintain a healthy mouth.

- Some individuals now use a special plaque rinse. This product, which you swish in your mouth for 30 seconds before brushing, is specially formulated to loosen newly forming plaque from your teeth, plaque that brushing and flossing then carries out of the mouth. Though such rinses are not necessary, they can help reduce plaque.

Be true to your teeth or your teeth will be false to you.

Your Personal Image

If a tooth is knocked out, a dentist or oral surgeon can sometimes successfully reinsert it in place, if you:

- Do not wash the tooth or the mouth.
- Place the tooth back in the tooth socket in the mouth if possible. Otherwise, place the tooth in milk for transport to the dentist.
- Go to the dentist's office immediately.

- Brush at least once a day, preferably as many times as possible following eating. Fluoride has been proven to be a great preventive against cavities and we certainly recommend using a toothpaste with fluoride. Avoid hard-bristle brushes, which may encourage receding gums. If you have a small mouth, use a toothbrush with a narrow or small head, so you can brush your back teeth thoroughly. Brush the gums as well as the teeth. To really clean your mouth, brush your tongue as well (this will also help clean your breath).

- If you experience problems with tooth decay or accumulated plaque, ask your dentist to review your brushing technique. Obtaining the right toothbrush and using the right technique, especially if you brush after every meal, will contribute to effective prevention. Other methods of dealing with these problems include using special devices such as the Water Pik® or the Interplak.® Recent studies reveal that one of the best deterrents to gum disease (which ultimately affects nine out of ten Americans) is the frequent removal of plaque. If plaque is not removed daily, the accumulated bacterial film may lead to gum disease and tooth decay.

- Floss at least once a day. If you're new to flossing, have the hygienist show you how to floss properly. You may want to try various thicknesses (and flavors) of dental floss until you find the best one for you. Floss in front of a mirror so you can see that you get the floss down the sides of each tooth. Rub the front, back and sides of every tooth until it squeaks, even if there's not a tooth next to it and even if the gums are tender and bleed. Within a few days of flossing daily, you will notice that your gums do not bleed any more. This technique is perhaps the best way to prevent receding gums.

- Visit your dentist and/or dental hygienist twice a year, even if you feel no discomfort. Trained dental care personnel can often spot problems before they become painful. Early treatment of dental problems is usually less painful, traumatic, and expensive. These semi-annual visits usually include a thorough cleaning, an optional fluoride treatment, or x-rays, and a visual inspection by a dentist.

- Avoid causing your teeth unnecessary trauma. Don't tempt fate by ripping open plastic snack bags or other items with your teeth; that's what scissors are for. Wear protective head and mouth gear when playing football, riding motorcycles, serving as hockey goalie, or engaging in other activities involving high risk to teeth.

- Don't use tobacco. Nicotine stains teeth, and tobacco users suffer much higher rates of gum and mouth cancers.

For More Beautiful Teeth

Now, at college, may be the time to consider correcting imperfections in your teeth that you used to think you were stuck with for life. If your teeth are misaligned, or poorly spaced, orthodontics can straighten them. Clear braces are now available, though they are more expensive than traditional metal arrangements. Certain dental procedures can correct teeth discoloration. Bonding is a recent development in which a composite material is applied to the teeth which can alter the surface, shape and contour of the teeth. This technique can make a dramatic difference in how your teeth look—and perhaps in your total self-image.

Dental Problems and Treatments

When dealing with dental problems that occur in the mouth, it is helpful to first identify the type of symptom: pain, bleeding or swelling. Then consider the specific discomfort. The following material describes common dental discomforts, then suggests possible causes and treatments. The causes and treatments are listed by number and can be found in the list at the end of the section.

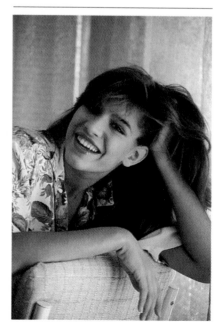

Dental Problems and Treatments

Symptoms	Possible Causes	Treatment
Pain		
A. An individual tooth hurts and		
The tooth has a hole, dark stains or an old filling that may be broken or loose.	3,4,5	1
A front tooth is darker than the other teeth.	3,4,5	1,2
The tooth surface along the root next to the gum is sensitive to touch, hot/cold or sweet and sour foods.	15	3
The tooth is the upper first molar (the furthest forward big tooth on the top), and this tooth aches, throbs or is sensitive to pressure.	11	7
B. Several or many teeth hurt and		
The teeth that hurt are the upper back teeth.	11	7
You feel a general aching, mostly in response to pressure, of all or most of the teeth.	12	8
C. You feel a dull ache, throbbing or sensitivity to pressure behind the last teeth in back corners of the mouth.	6	4,5,6
D. You feel pain, sensitivity, clicking, popping, or a sensation of slight distortion in the temporomandibular joint (TMJ), which is just in front of the ear.	12,17	8,9
E. The bump of tissue on the roof of the mouth just behind the two front teeth is painful to touch or sensitive to spicy or acidic foods.	1	4,10
F. The gum tissue is sore or painful in a specific area such as between two teeth.	2,6,7	4,6,10
G. The gums are generally sore and sensitive in most of the mouth.	7,8,9,10	4,6,10
H. You have small painful sores on the lips, cheeks or floor of the mouth.	16	4,10
Bleeding		
A. You have bleeding from the gum tissue behind the last teeth in the back corners of the mouth.	8	4,5,6,10
B. You have bleeding of the gums from a specific area of the mouth such as between two teeth.	2	4,6,10
C. You have generalized bleeding of the gums upon touching, brushing or flossing.	2,7,8,9,10	4,6,10
Swelling		
A. You have swelling of the gum tissue behind the last teeth in the back corners of the mouth.	8	4,5,6,10
B. You have swelling of the gum tissue in a specific area such as between two teeth.	2,7,8	4,6
C. You have generalized swelling of most of the gum tissues of the mouth.	2,7,8,9,10	4,6,10
D. You have a small swelling on the inner side of the lips or cheeks that looks like a water blister. The swelling may disappear and then reappear later.	13	11
E. You have a swelling in the floor of the mouth under the tongue. The swelling may come and go.	14	12

Possible Causes	Treatment
1. Trauma, caused by hot foods, rough foods, excessive brushing	1. This can be serious. It could lead to an abscessed tooth and need for a root canal. You should consult a dentist for a temporary sedative filling or a permanent restoration.
2. Food packing between teeth or under the gums	2. This can be serious. There is a possibility of an abscess around the root of the tooth. You should consult a dentist to determine if a root canal is necessary.
3. Decay—new decay or secondary decay under an old filling	3. This may not be serious. Try using a toothpaste formulated for sensitive teeth. You can purchase this at a drugstore. If the symptoms do not subside after about one week, you should consult a dentist.
4. Broken or cracked filling	4. Rinse vigorously with hot salt water (one teaspoon salt to one cup of water) for two minutes, three times a day.
5. Abscessed tooth	5. If you can see a flap of gum tissue in the back of your mouth behind the teeth, get a small rubber baby syringe and use it to irrigate with hot salt water (one teaspoon salt to one cup water) under the flap of tissue.
6. Impacted wisdom tooth or teeth	6. Use dental floss once or twice a day. Follow guidelines described earlier in this chapter.
7. Lack of flossing and/or brushing	7. If the upper teeth are hurting, your sinuses may be the cause, so take a decongestant for a day or so. If the symptoms go away, this may not be a dental problem.
8. Infection in the gum or around an impacted tooth	8. This is a difficult condition to treat. Try to determine when you grind or clench your teeth and what you're doing at these times. Consciously make an effort to instruct yourself not to grind or clench during these periods. Since this often occurs during the night, tell yourself to relax as much as possible and not grind or clench while asleep. Program your subconscious. If this problem is not resolved, see your dentist about a mouth piece to wear at night.
9. Stress due to factors such as heavy schedules, personal relationships, academic requirements and so forth	9. Traumatic biting produced by behaviors such as grinding, clenching, bad occlusions, excessive chewing, a bump to the jaw, or even an extra big yawn can irritate TMJ. When this happens, try to give the joints a rest. Avoid chewing gum, change to a softer diet (avoid food like a tough steak), reduce the use of the jaw (even by less talking), and don't keep testing it by opening wide to see if it's getting better. The symptoms should subside in a few days.
10. Lowered resistance due to lack of sleep, poor diet or ill health	10. Take aspirin as necessary for minor discomfort.
11. Congested sinuses, due to colds, flu, hay fever, or other allergies	11. This is a mucous gland that fills with fluid and occasionally drains. This condition is not serious and does not need treatment unless the gland becomes so enlarged that it is a nuisance. In extreme cases, it may need to be surgically removed.
12. Habitual grinding or clenching of the teeth	12. This is a plugged salivary duct. If it doesn't become unplugged on its own within a few days, you should consult a dentist.
13. Blocked mucous gland	
14. Plugged saliva duct	
15. Some portion of the root is exposed due to the recession of the gums. This part of the tooth can become sensitive but it isn't serious	
16. Possible cold sores or canker sores	
17. Trauma to the temporomandibular joint (TMJ)	

Beyond the Text

1. What warning would you give your roommate who borrowed some Accutane from a friend to see if it worked?

2. Respond to the following statement: Skin cancer is a threat only to elderly people who live in Sun Belt retirement communities.

3. Respond to the following statement: All shampoos are about the same. The ad agencies just try to confuse you.

4. If I look good outside, I feel better about myself inside. Do you agree or disagree with this statement? Explain.

5. Respond to the following statement: A dental checkup twice per year really is an unncessary expense for anyone between the age of 18 and 28 who has not experienced any dental problems before.

6. A roommate says, "If your friends are really true friends, they won't care how you look." How would you respond?

Supplemental Readings

Color Me Beautiful Make Up Book by Carole Jackson. New York: Ballantine Books, 1987. A practical, helpful guide for analyzing your color essentials. Includes skin, hair, nails and make up lessons, and helps you put it all together.

Skin Secrets by Joseph F. Bark, MD. New York: McGraw Hill, 1988. An informative guide to maintaining healthy skin and treating various skin conditions. Directed at the whole family.

The AMA Book of Skin and Hair Care edited by Linda Allen Schoen. Philadelphia: J. B. Lippincott, 1976. Detailed information about skin and hair-care problems and products. Helpful advice on how to deal with common problems.

The Consumer's Common Sense Guide to Better Dental Care by Jerry F. Taintor, DDS. New York: Ballantine Books, 1989. A comprehensive consumer guide designed to help the reader obtain quality dental care at a reasonable cost.

Your Skin by Fredric Haberman, MD. New York: Berkley Books, 1983. A dermatologist's guide to dealing with acne, avoiding sun damage, skin cleansing, and many other helpful topics.

Your Skin, From Acne to Zits by Jerome Z. Litt, MD. New York: Dembner Books, 1989. Helpful advice on keeping your skin healthy. Explains causes of skin ailments and suggests effective over-the-counter remedies.

Key Terms Defined

acne   disorder of the skin with eruptions of papules or pustules; *acne vulgaris* an increased production of sebum in the form of blackheads and whiteheads that plug the pores; usually occurs in adolescents and young adults

blackhead   plug of keratin and sebum within the dilated orifice of a hair follicle

cellulite   rough, uneven, fatty deposits under the skin that accumulate on the hips and thighs of women in their middle years

cosmetic   beautifying substance or preparation

dandruff   scaly material shed from the scalp; the condition may spread unless checked, and in rare cases may spread to the eyebrows

dermis   the second, connective tissue layer of the skin

epidermis   the outer, protective, neurovascular layer of the skin

exfoliation   falling off in scales or layers

hangnail   shred of skin at one side of a nail that can cause infection; prevented by gently pushing back the cuticle instead of cutting it

myopia   nearsightedness; seeing near objects clearly, but far objects fuzzy

pH   a measure of acidity or alkalinity numerically equal to 7 for neutral

plaque   soft, thin film of food debris, mucin, and dead cells deposited on the teeth that provides a medium for the growth of various bacteria; plays an important role in the development of dental caries

SAD   seasonal affective disorder; changes in mood and feelings of depression in winter due to decrease in sunlight

sebum   oily secretion that can change to a solid, white substance; secreted from the sebaceous glands

sebaceous gland   glands in the skin that secrete an oily substance

self-image   picture one holds of himself that encompasses his beliefs, attitudes, and convictions about himself

sunburn   actual burn of the skin caused by exposure to ultraviolet rays of the sun

toxin   harmful, poisonous material

ultraviolet radiation   light rays of a specific wave length emitted by the sun

Committed Relationships

Regardless of your age, sex, economic status, or family situation, close relationships with other people are crucial—not just for your personal happiness, but for your health. People involved in close, stable, loving relationships tend to have fewer illnesses and live longer than individuals who are single, divorced, separated, or widowed. The days of the lonesome cowboy are over in our modern, high-speed, pressure-cooker society. Our environment is filled with so many psychological stressors that finding true health and contentment through isolation is nearly impossible.

This chapter describes the nature of some of your most important adult relationships—friendship, romance, intimacy, and marriage. Alternatives to marriage are discussed as well. The emotional trauma of ending relationships cannot be overlooked, because most people experience relationship failures during their lives. This chapter is designed to help you recognize how forming and ending relationships may affect your health and wellness.

Contents

Key Terms

Bonding
Cohabitation
Commitment
Conflict
Developmental task
Divorce
Friendship

Homosexual relationship
Intimacy
Marriage
Monogamy
Passionate love
Personality development
Platonic

Relationship
Romance
Self-esteem
Traditional marriage
Trust
Values

Relationships

From the time we are born, we seek to connect ourselves with others, to form relationships. One of the most critical connections that occurs in life is an infant's bonding to a parent. Through our relationships, we develop our sense of self and our humanity. Regardless of our status, sexual orientation, or career path, close relationships with other people are crucial—not just for personal happiness, but for health. People in close, stable, loving relationships are known to live longer and have fewer illnesses than people who are single, divorced, widowed, or separated. In fact, the lack of social relationships per se heightens people's susceptibility to illness. Studies of recent widows and widowers show they are highly vulnerable to disease and death. Sadly, many die shortly after their partners. Some say these people virtually die of a broken heart, that they lose the will to live after losing a beloved partner. Researchers now recognize that loneliness and isolation weaken the immune system, which can lead to premature illness and death.

Relationships and Our Personal Development

Abraham Maslow, identifying a hierarchy of human needs, studied healthy, fulfilled individuals. He proposes a theory that each of us has a set of basic needs divided into two classes—deficiency needs and being needs. Deficiency needs are necessary for life and are the focus after our essential physical needs (for food, shelter, sleep, exercise, and so forth) are met. A critical deficiency need, placed immediately after safety, is the necessity for belonging and love. Failure to meet deficiency needs may result in immature and guarded behavior and lack of adaptability, and also it negates fulfillment of such higher needs as respect, self-esteem, and self-actualization. In any sense, love is critical to life and growth. An example of this phenomenon is illustrated by an infant who suffers "failure to thrive." This syndrome is characterized by an infant's failure to grow and develop. Without intervention the infant may die—not from lack of nutrients, but from lack of love. One of the primary causes of this condition is the nature of the mother–child relationship—the mother is unable to provide a warm, loving, nurturing environment for the infant.

Erik Erikson, one of the foremost theoreticians on personality development, presents a structure for healthy growth and development. Erikson theorizes that we move through eight distinct stages of development from birth to death. At each stage we may encounter a crisis, at which time it is essential to master the developmental task of that stage. For the purpose of understanding how relationships work, Erikson suggests that mastery at one stage increases our power to adapt and move successfully to the next stage. Thus, an infant must develop a sense of trust versus mistrust with the significant person in his or her life. This stage, which occurs during the first year of life, establishes the foundation for healthy growth. A child matures and moves through the stages of autonomy, in-

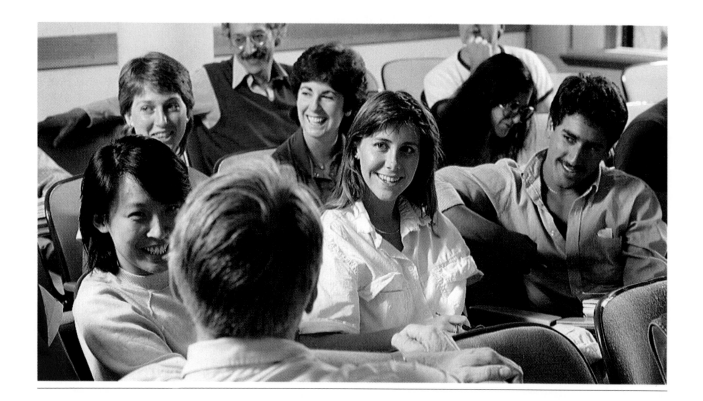

itiative, industry, and self-identity to the stage of intimacy. An adult must master the task of intimacy and solidarity versus isolation in order to form lasting relationships with others. Erikson and Maslow are only two of the many researchers and therapists who have suggested that a healthy, self-actualized adult is one who can develop intimate, long-term relationships with others.

Relationships take many forms, spanning a wide spectrum from short-term friendships and romantic liaisons to lifelong relationships between close friends, parents and children, husband and wife, or committed partners. Despite their many variations, long-term relationships all share several common features: interpersonal interaction, intimacy, commitment, collaboration, rewards, and frustration. This chapter explores the chain of human ties that gets lumped together into the catchall word, *relationships*.

Friendship

Aristotle described friendship as "a single soul dwelling in two bodies." Any time two people are attached to each other by affection, esteem, and good will, there is friendship. Friends provide needed companionship,

Committed Relationships

CHAPTER 11

succor, emotional support, and help during life transitions and emotional difficulties. They also enhance our self-esteem because friends like us, care about us, and think we are okay. Because friends are usually outside the family, they help foster independence and deepen our sense of self. In addition, best friends are good medicine. Research indicates that people who are isolated from families and friends double their chances of sickness and death.

Judith Viorst, in *Necessary Losses*, talks about the different kinds of friends we have as we progress through life. She describes several categories.

- *Convenience friends*: not too close but close enough to provide convenient reciprocation and meet various needs.
- *Special-interest friends*: sharing an interest both partners enjoy but never getting really close.
- *Historical and crossroads friends*: high school, college, special-period relationships that are maintained by intermittent communications and may be resurrected at various points in life, such as our twenty-fifth college reunion.
- *Close friends*: people with whom we relate emotionally by sharing feelings and mutual trust, and by knowing these friends will be there when times are tough.

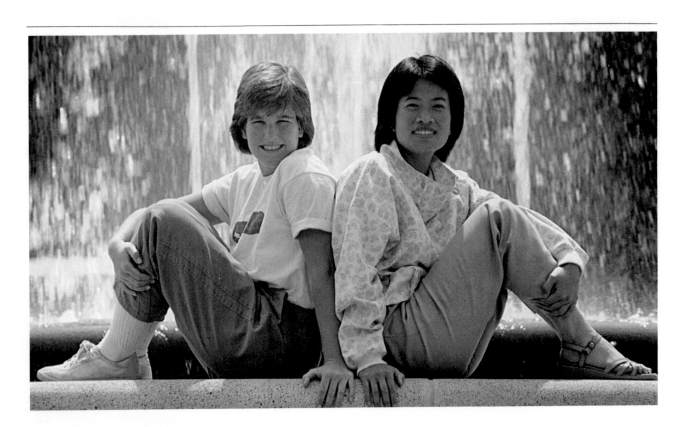

Making Friends: Do's and Don'ts

- Join a club or group on campus in which you will share an interest with others.
- Sit beside and introduce yourself to an unknown person in one of your classes. Call that person and ask for clarification about a class assignment.
- Practice starting conversations with someone when you are waiting in line at the dining hall, movies or other queue.
- Ask a person you don't know well for advice on a decision. People like being asked for their opinion or advice, and this may begin an interesting exchange.
- Feel and look friendly. Smile when you are walking around campus. Look up and at people, not down. Act like you will be a fun person to meet.
- Ask to join someone sitting alone in a dining hall, coffee house or campus hang-out and introduce yourself.
- Pay a person a compliment—

make it honest. Positive feedback is very reinforcing for beginning a relationship.
- Don't monopolize a conversation. Give the other person a chance to contribute and then respond.
- Don't focus all conversation on yourself, your needs, problems and interests. In fact, the more you focus on the other person, ask them about themselves, what they think, and so forth, the more they feel open to your friendship.
- Don't come on too strong in your opinions or comments. You may frighten away a potential friend.
- Don't always project yourself as being glum and down. Others are not attracted to "doom and gloom" personalities, as your vibrations will affect their own mood. Try to portray an up, happy person—one with a sense of humor.

A person without a few close friends may feel lonely and isolated from others, and even depressed. Love relationships may disintegrate, but if you have even one close friend with whom you share your innermost feelings, you have an important coping resource to sustain your emotional balance and to keep you from feeling isolated. An extensive study of friendship conducted by *Psychology Today* found the following factors to be the most important in sustaining friendships.

- Friends confide in each other and share intimate aspects of their feelings and personal lives.
- Friends can share bad news as well as good.
- Friendship involves the right to ask for help and the obligation to reciprocate when asked.
- The qualities most valued in a friend are loyalty and the ability to keep confidences.

The ability to form close, intimate friendships is not inherent in every person. While some people seem to do it with ease, others struggle and

> **Lovers come and go but best friends last forever.**
>
> Sol Gordon, PhD

Committed Relationships

feel inadequate and uncomfortable. Perhaps this latter group never mastered Erikson's milestones of trust and intimacy. Like all forms of relationships, however, friendships require work—they involve give-and-take interactions that enhance our lives.

Friends just do not drop through a keyhole as a gift. Often, we must develop the skill of making friends before we have to work at maintaining the friendship. If you are feeling lonely and wish to broaden your relationships, try a few of the suggestions on how to make friends, "The Do's and Don'ts."

Romance

Movies, literature, fantasy, and dreams—what do they have in common? The image of romance. Swept away by visions of moonlight and roses, gondolas and Chianti, we bring to many of our relationships a vision of romantic expectations. Our ideas about love, marriage, and happiness

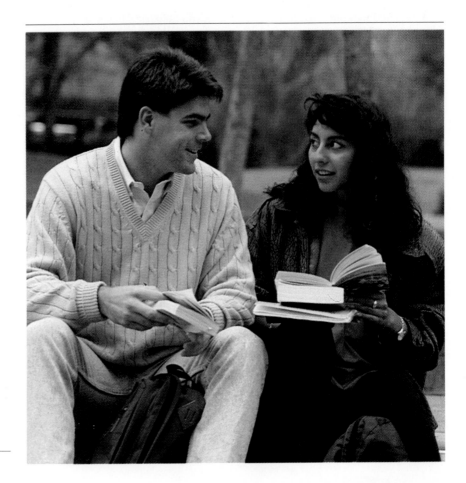

are often colored by our beliefs about romance. The dictionary defines romance as "a strong, enthusiastic attachment or involvement with another person." The nature of this attachment often becomes idealized and unrealistic as our enthusiasm clouds our judgment.

Fictional romances and dreams are not practical standards for real-life, enduring relationships. This doesn't necessarily mean there won't be any moonlight and roses in your life; it is just more likely that there will be moonlight and mortgages, and roses and toilet paper rolls. Romance, for all its heady, thrilling power, is not the total substance of love. Romantic love may fade, but it can fade into the next stage—the deeper, more mature, more enduring stage of love.

Love

What is love? No one has ever so completely defined love that it is accepted by everyone. Perhaps because of its mysterious, unpredictable nature it is almost impossible to define. Dr. Scott Peck, in *The Road Less Traveled*, suggests a definition with which most people will agree: "The will to extend one's self for the purpose of nurturing one's own or another's spiritual growth." One of the difficulties in defining love is that what may seem to be love is not really love at all, but actions that are totally self-serving. An example is a mother who keeps a child totally dependent on her, even into the teenage years. And, while love must encompass self-love ultimately, it must also include love directed toward another person.

Falling in love, being "madly" in love, or "crazy" in love are labels we apply to the erotic feelings—usually having to do with sex—that we experience in relation to another person. The illusion that this feeling will last forever and that destiny has finally delivered our soulmate is perpetuated by fairy tales, the media, and romantic novels. Many a psychiatrist's couch has been occupied by those who attempt, against all odds, to perpetuate the myth of a perfect, everlasting relationship. The ancient Greeks had three words for different types of love: *philia*, *agape*, and *eros*. We moderns, on the other hand, have only one: *love*. It is a profound human wish to be loved. More than anything else in life, people want to love and be loved.

Despite our succinct vocabulary, our way of thinking incorporates love's diversity without question. Love, our most transforming and expansive emotion, is simultaneously subtle and varied, complex and simple, well known and elusive—and easier to feel than define. As human beings, we can experience many kinds of love. Erich Fromm, in his classic book, *The Art of Loving*, discusses different levels of love, the final manifestation of which is mature love. Mature love follows the principles, "I am loved because I love" and "I need you because I love you," (not the reverse). Fromm goes on to describe four criteria that define a mature love relationship: caring, respect, assuming responsibility for each other, and developing joint understanding.

> **Sophia returned my kiss and the earth went under my feet; my soul was no longer in my body; I touched the stars; I knew the happiness of angels!**
>
> From an old German novel

As the Greeks Would Say

Philia is love for or benevolence toward friends or humanity in the aggregate.

Agape is love of God, nature, or any affection freely given without concern for reciprocation.

Eros is any grand passion, including sexual love.

265

> **Earth's the right place for love: I don't know where it's likely to go better.**
>
> **Robert Frost**

Most people long for a deep emotional attachment to one person: someone to love and be loved by in return, someone they can reveal themselves to as they truly are, and someone who will reciprocally embrace them in their acceptance. The route to this kind of enriching, enduring, exclusive love is intimacy.

Intimacy

Perhaps the word intimacy is so much a part of our everyday vocabulary that its precise meaning has become diffuse. Intimacy is the quality of a relationship between two people—a shared experience of trust in their personal lives. The ability to be intimate with another person depends on many factors. Perhaps going back to the development of basic trust (Erikson's trust versus mistrust) in infancy, the capacity for intimacy also rests on parental relationships, past experience with others, and one's ability to love. Intimacy is a feeling, not an act. Intimate relationships tend to grow deeper and richer over a period of time. Intimacy does not just happen: it is hard work. Becoming intimate means taking risks: you must be willing to reveal your feelings and thoughts, openly and honestly. In order to establish genuine trust and caring, partners need to share significant experiences. This means you must be willing to place your trust in the other person.

Intimacy is based on trust: trusting your partner to love you for yourself, trusting yourself to let go enough to let your partner in. When you trust, you are able to share your feelings openly, without fear that your

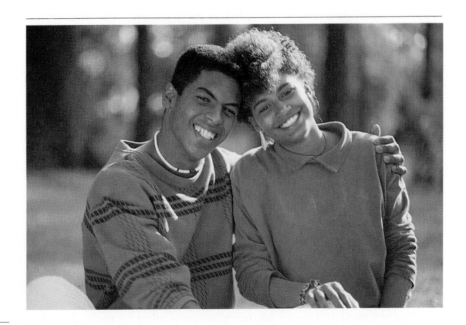

partner will misunderstand or betray you. When you trust, you can be yourself without having to deny your feelings or values to please the other person. According to a study by Julian Rotter, a professor of psychology at the University of Connecticut, the way to build trust is to be trusting. The more trusting a person is, the more likely he or she is to be trusted in return.

According to Herbert Zerof, author of *Finding Intimacy: The Art of Happiness in Living Together*, the following universal transitions determine the direction of intimacy for a couple. To be on your way to true intimacy, you must move beyond

- Romantic love to liking and knowing a mate.
- Disappointment with a partner to acceptance of differences in each other.
- Frustration with a mate to fairness between partners.
- Boredom to self-direction within a relationship.
- Isolation to intimate ties.

Sometimes sex is mistaken for intimacy. This happens because love and affection are feelings associated with both sex and intimacy. However, emotional intimacy, although it may include sexual intimacy, goes far beyond sex. You can be sexually intimate with your partner, yet at the same time feel emotionally alienated or separate from him or her. Some people become sexually indiscriminate as they search for intimacy or approval. Paradoxically, indiscriminate sex does not promote intimacy; it prevents it. One study of college students found that they are apt to use addictions and dependencies—including sexual addictions and relationships—to cope with their stress-filled lives. The unhealthy addictions become the means by which they hope to achieve affection, approval, a sense of connection, and emotional fulfillment. For more effective ways to manage stress, refer to the chapter on **Coping with Stress**.

Sex can be emotionally fulfilling or stressful, depending upon the values and expectations of each partner. This aspect of a dating or romantic relationship calls for an assessment of the goals and commitments that each partner has toward the other. Especially difficult are situations in which one partner expects a physically intimate relationship to accompany romance while the other partner resists this kind of intimacy.

Loving someone means being able to see the other person as she or he is, unadorned by hoped-for or fanciful attributes. Be scrupulously honest when evaluating your partner's strengths and weaknesses—because that is what there is to love.

Some people are concerned that if they let their true selves show, no one would love them. They may act helpful or conciliatory when they are actually hurt, or they may acquiesce instead of speaking out about their wishes. This kind of emotional dissembling eventually catches up to the person; long-term resentments and self-sacrifice eat away at self-esteem and create hard-to-break, destructive cycles in relationships.

Satisfied with Your Love Life?

A 1989 Gallup survey of 800 adults showed that 72 percent of married people are "very satisfied with their love lives," whereas only 44 percent of singles feel this way.

Source: *American Health Magazine*, 1989

Committed Relationships

Intimacy

The word "intimacy" derives from the Greek "intima," meaning essential, private, close to the blood.

When we consider intimacy we often think only of sexual intimacy. This is a limiting view, for your life has many more opportunities for intimacy than physical closeness. Intimacy really means to feel emotionally connected to another person.

It is a condition that many struggle with throughout a lifetime and is an adult developmental task some never complete. Few of you know how to care for your relationship well-being at the level that you now care for your bodies. Individuals repeatedly identify intimate relationships as a major stressor in their lives. You can probably benefit from looking at your current relationships in terms of intimacy—and decide if you are happy with the degree of intimacy you can sustain or if you need to learn new skills to enhance your functioning in this area.

Intimacy has four major components

- Physical—touching, playing, allowing private time, caressing, proximity, shared physical activity, and sexual interaction
- Intellectual—the ability to discuss honestly and respect political, social, economic, religious, and moral views, including exchanging core ideas, thoughts and dreams
- Emotional—the use of "feeling" versus "thinking" vocabulary, (for example, "I feel upset that you are neglecting me" versus "I think you are spending too much time studying and playing basketball"); using a here-and-now orientation when discussing your relationship; honestly and openly commenting on the dynamics between the two of you and how each of you feels about those dynamics
- Spiritual—co-creative activity combining individual talents to create something together, for instance, as parent, as lover, as worker, as artist; sharing a vision that reaches beyond the two of you and transcends individual desires

Intimacy is not a static state but open to change and adaptation as your life circumstances or desires require. It is not dependent upon one person to be complete and you can experience several intimacy states at one time.

What types of intimacy are you experiencing and with whom? Family, friends and work colleagues can all be a part of your total intimacy configurations; it is important to realize that no one person can complete the intimacy quotient, no matter how much you might like them to do so or believe they "should"!

What balance would you like among these forms of intimacy? How does that contrast with what you are currently experiencing? If you are in a committed relationship with another person at this time, how do you imagine he or she would view your current intimacy status? Do you think that he or she desires similar patterns of intimacy?

Although no match is perfect, there are compatibility considerations. If your primary partner would like 75 percent of your intimate relations to be in the physical arena and you are more likely to desire a 25 percent portion to go to each of the intimacy components, it could cause problems. This type of pairing would demand compromise and a rich circle of friends to supplement the areas where neither of you is getting your desires met. Again, there is no value judgment placed on how these areas are divided. Only an acknowledgement that people's desires can vary vastly and that each member of a dyad needs to share or work out compatible desires.

If you are experiencing loneliness, shallow relationships or feelings of emptiness, you may want to review your current intimacy status. Achieving and maintaining a desired degree of intimacy is not an easy task. However, if you are willing to work at it and take the prerequisite risks, the rewards will be exciting.

Here are some of the many possible actions you can take to enhance your current intimacy status.

Physical Intimacy

- Try new behaviors and learn new activity skills.
- Take advantage of the myriad physical activity options available on the college campus or in the surrounding community.
- If you are particularly interested in exploring your sexuality individually or as a couple, growth-oriented groups or individual counseling related to sexuality is often available through the college counseling center.

Intellectual Intimacy

- A desire for intellectual expansion is relatively easy to accommodate on the college campus via lecture series, philosophy classes, debate competitions, political activities, and public forums dealing with a plethora of relevant topics.
- Learn to understand and acknowledge others' views even though they may be different from your own.
- Master these skills through activities such as assertiveness training groups, and practice with understanding friends!
- Another way to enhance your intellectual intimacy is to risk sharing important dreams for your future with someone you trust.

Emotional Intimacy

- This component depends most heavily on clear and honest communication. It is important to be able to recognize what you are feeling "in the moment" and to acknowledge it, not to defend, explain, deny, or rationalize.
- Invest in an on-going relationship; be willing to risk vulnerability and "being wrong."
- Initiate candid discussion about the two of you, how you feel about one another, and the relationship you are experiencing. This process can be both painful and pleasurable.
- This is often a skills-deficit area but you can seek assistance in the form of communication classes, groups, couples or individual therapy in order to augment your repertoire.

Spiritual Intimacy

- The least tangible of the intimacy components, this co-creative functioning is often spontaneous and impossible to "manufacture." Having a mutual dedication to a cause arises from our emotions and values as often as from our intellect.
- Truly believe and dedicate yourself to a vision of how things can and should be; this is not jumping on the bandwagon because someone you care for is involved. It is imperative that you learn the things that are truly important to you and that they fit with your values and belief systems. Seek out others who share this vision.
- Another tactic to enhance the spiritual arena is to allow yourself and others to share in quiet time together; a sunset viewed, a symphony heard, a poem read, may be the spiritual connection you desire.

Barbara Thomas, PhD

Love and Conflict

Many couples who love each other expect to live happily ever after. Even if the partners love each other deeply, conflict is inevitable in relationships. Maggie Scarf, in *Intimate Partners*, suggests that the qualities that first attracted partners to each other are often the same attributes later identified as major sources of conflict. The woman who was initially attracted to a stable, calm, reliable man may, in subsequent years, complain that he is dull, boring, and predictable. Conflict can produce reactions such as anger, sadness, fear, insecurity, pain, disappointment, and irritation. Sources of conflict arise from incompatible goals and expectations. For example, one partner may feel burdened by the time it takes to sustain a relationship. In another situation, one partner may focus on the relationship to the exclusion of everything else, causing the other partner to feel resentful. Or, one partner may become complacent or take the relationship for granted after the groundwork has been laid. Any time one partner is frustrated or unhappy, the resulting tensions and anxieties produce strain in the relationship.

Unrealistic expectations can also cause conflict. All relationships begin with expectations about how things *should* and *ought* to be. For the most part, these expectations come from each individual's desires and needs. People often believe that their partner will satisfy their every need, regardless of whether the need is emotional, intellectual, spiritual, or financial. When expectations are not met, partners may become frustrated and disappointed.

Relationships improve when people let go of their expectations. Relationships flourish when the partners are free from preconceived ideas about themselves and their relationship. This freedom from unrealistic expectations allows intimacy to grow in its own natural way. Accepting your partner as he or she really is—without the burden of unrealistic expectations—is an essential component of a successful relationship.

> **Kissing is a means of getting two people so close together that they can't see anything wrong with each other.**
>
> **Rene Yasenek**

cathy®   by Cathy Guisewite

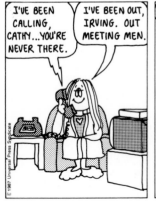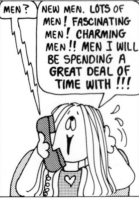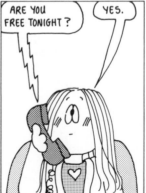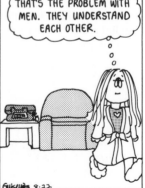

How conflicts are resolved determines whether intimacy is fostered or eroded. Psychologist Carl Rogers believes that learning to be good partners should be part of our education. "An individual can get a college degree today without ever having learned anything about how to communicate, how to resolve conflict, or what to do with anger and other negative feelings," says Dr. Rogers.

Often, when you are upset with your partner, your first response is to defend or protect yourself. There are many ways to do this: you may deny your feelings and automatically comply with the other person's wishes. Or, you may attempt to control the other person through nagging or guilt. You may even withdraw and pretend to become indifferent. When you try to protect yourself, you reduce the probability of finding a solution to the problem. Resolving conflicts means using your feelings to learn about yourself, so that, together with your partner, you can overcome the conflict and help the relationship grow.

Sometimes problems go so deep they cannot be solved without outside assistance. Warning signs can be long-term, unresolved resentment or hostility, the feeling that communication is at an impasse, depression and suicide threats, or even violence. One study of college students showed that 45 percent have experienced violence in dating relationships, including hair pulling, slapping, throwing objects, and sexual aggression. More than half the incidents caused injury, but not the end of the relationship. If you are in such a relationship, you may wish to seek some counseling. Referrals for local psychiatrists and licensed marriage and family counselors are available through your college health service or by contacting the American Association of Marriage and Family Therapists (AAMFT).

> Love, the magician, knows this little trick whereby two people walk in different directions yet always remain side by side.
>
> Notes on Love and Courage
> by Hugh Prather

Commitment

A commitment is a mutually agreed upon bond with explicit and implicit expectations. When you make a commitment to one person, you are making a choice—and with that choice comes obligation and responsibility. Partners who have made a commitment to each other have placed their trust in each other; an agreement that they willingly devote time, understanding, trust, and affection to each other. An implicit expectation of making a commitment is that you are willing to stay with your partner during periods of difficulty or hardship. It may also mean you will be sexually exclusive or that you intend to stay together for a long time. A commitment is more binding than a simple promise. Promising to "love forever" is not the same as being willing to commit yourself to the ups and downs of a partnership for as long as "you both shall live." According to Dr. Scott Peck, whether commitment is shallow or not, it is the most important foundation for any genuine relationship.

For long-term relationships to be successful, strong feelings of commitment and dedication are required. According to psychologist Carl Rogers, dedication in a partnership means that the partners commit themselves to

Features of a Mature Relationship

- Intimacy
- Sense of humor
- Honest communication
- Common sense of purpose
- Equality
- Sense of adventure
- Shared experience
- Respect for each other's feelings and wishes
- Passion
- Sharing in domestic duties

Source: *Why Love Is Not Enough*, by Sol Gordon, PhD

working together on the changing process of the relationship, because the relationship is enriching their love and their lives together, and they want the relationship to grow. Couples also continually need to reaffirm their commitment to each other: "A partnership is a continuing process, not a contract," Rogers says. "The dream of a marriage 'made in heaven' is totally unrealistic. Every relationship must be worked at, built, rebuilt, and continually refreshed by mutual growth."

Marriage

Despite people who point to high divorce rates (one out of two marriages in the United States ends in divorce) as evidence that marriage "doesn't work," marriage remains the most popular institution in the world. The possibility of intimacy, love, security, family life, companionship, commitment, and a steady sexual partner is appealing to people of all types and all ages. In addition to the emotional feelings of intimacy and love, marriage also offers financial, social, moral, familial, and political benefits.

Today, nine tenths of young adults say family is the most important focus in their lives. They believe marriage is the optimal way of life, and they want to have children. The young are not the only group who embrace the idea of marriage—the sentiment is universal. By age 45 to 54, 90 percent of American women and 95 percent of American men have been married. Another noteworthy trend is the increasing average age of people getting married for the first time. Many delay marriage until they have completed their educations or have established their careers.

People like marriage so much they keep trying it again, even if it did not work the first or second time. About 40 percent of the marriages in the 1980s have been remarriages. Dr. Samuel Johnson referred to the tendency to remarry as "the triumph of hope over experience." In the United States, the odds are 87 in 100 for men and 75 in 100 for women that they will remarry.

The myth of romantic love is a major lie that has a great effect on marriage, says Dr. Scott Peck. He relates how this myth has caused untold millions to suffer as they try to make the reality of their lives conform to the unreality of what they believed would be an ideal union. Many experts say that marriage really begins after romance fades. You are no longer answerable only to yourself; when you are married, another person's welfare and happiness become your concerns. As a couple, you will face many decisions regarding where you live, how you pursue mutual interests, and many other lifestyle choices. All these need to be worked out or negotiated within the context of the relationship. Married women who work or go to school may find themselves juggling multiple responsibilities that include being a spouse, wage earner, student, parent, and housekeeper all at the same time. Men are increasingly sharing these roles, too.

The best way to approach marriage is with a clear-eyed view of what it is: a day-to-day committed partnership that will see good and bad times, happiness and sorrow, love and anger, and much change over time. Marriages do not succeed for many reasons. In the last few years numerous studies have revealed that unrealistic expectations upon entering marriage are often at the root of major problems. Once the myth is discounted that true love is all you need for a successful marriage, a couple can begin to seriously work at the relationship. The unrealistic expectations must

A World Record

Mr. Glynn de Moss "Scotty" Wolfe holds the world record for greatest number of marriages accumulated in the monogamous world: 26.

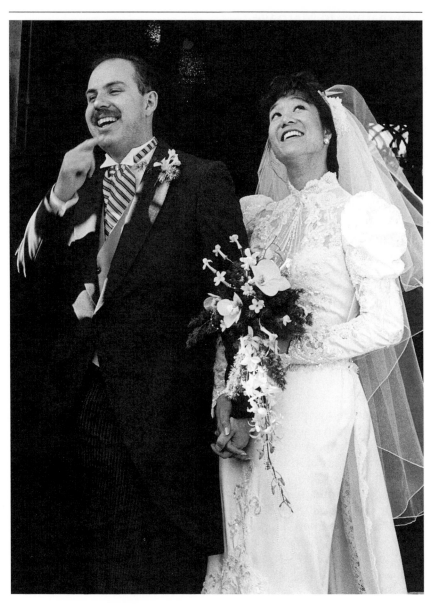

Committed Relationships

CHAPTER 11

accommodate to the realities of living with another person. Couples who are able to adjust and continue a loving, committed relationship while maintaining a sense of humor and a sense of self are the most likely to remain in a satisfying relationship. They are also able to withstand the stress of change that is inevitable in a marriage. So, for anyone contemplating a permanent union, it is worthwhile to not only focus on love and intimacy, but also to make the effort to explore the degree of commitment each partner is bringing to the relationship.

Alternatives to Marriage

Many people choose not to marry. Others who are disenchanted with traditional forms of marriage (or marriage as an institution) seek alternatives to marriage. The institution of marriage has been repeatedly taken to task by idealists, as well as by those who object to monogamy. Other, more feminist arguments suggest that marriage, as traditionally structured, demands that women give up their identities, career options, and opportunities for self-growth in order to raise children and provide emotional support to their husbands. Most modern women disagree with these assumptions, but they do provide a rationale for alternative lifestyles.

Although many women work as many hours as their husbands and contribute equally to household expenses, studies show that men do not share the responsibility of housework and childrearing equally with women. For all these reasons and more, many people seek alternatives to marriage, such as cohabitation, gay relationships, and remaining single.

Remember, personal happiness is not determined by marriage alone, but by the quality, effort, and sincerity we bring to our work, our friends, our interests—and ourselves. You can lead a rich, happy life enjoying the affection, comfort, and companionship of friends—as well as sensual pleasures—even if you never meet the "right" person.

Being Single

Being single has lost much of its social stigma. As recently as twenty years ago, a 30-year-old single man or woman was looked upon with suspicion by family, neighbors, and community members. A woman who hadn't married by the age of 30 was written off as a spinster. But the trend toward living alone, away from nuclear families, groups, or marriage has risen dramatically within the last 20 years. Thirty-one percent of persons age 25–44 now live alone—twice as many as in 1970. Those who choose to be single cite career interests, not having met the right partner, wanting to experience life on their own, easy availability of sexual partners, and personal freedom among their reasons for choosing to be single. Overall, studies show single people have high self-esteem and tend to be happy with their lives.

Despite social and numerical gains, single people still do not enjoy the same benefits as married people, either socially, legally, or financially. Tax laws, government programs, health insurance providers, and employers continue to favor married people. And, despite the more relaxed sexual climate brought about by the sexual revolution in the 1960s, sex outside of marriage is still not universally accepted.

Although many people choose to be single, the majority of women become single as a result of separation, divorce, abandonment, or death of a spouse. The number of women either married with their husband absent, single (never married), widowed, or divorced is eight times higher than the number of women married with husbands present. For these women, being single is financially and emotionally difficult, particularly if there are children. Many, particularly those with limited educations, must take low-paying, unskilled jobs to provide subsistence-level living for their families.

Many single people do not want to remain single indefinitely; they view being single as a time to actively search for a partner. Sexually active single people need to be more concerned about pregnancy and sexually transmitted diseases than married people who know their partner's background, sexual history, and beliefs about monogamy.

Even if you do not intend to remain single indefinitely, it is important to maintain friendships and social support networks. As stated previously, close relationships with other people enhance both personal happiness and health. Studies show that loneliness and isolation affect men particularly severely. Isolated men are two to three times more likely to die than men with close social ties. The risk for isolated women was only one and one-half times as great as for women with close ties.

Cohabitation

The more informal term for cohabitation is "living together," which actually means "living together as partners and lovers without marrying." For many people, cohabitation is a trial marriage or a prelude to marriage, a time to experiment and see how the partners function as a couple. For others, it is a personal or political statement about their lack of faith in marriage as an institution, or their belief that ceremonial or government approval is unnecessary to sanction a relationship that is as valid as marriage in every way except that it lacks a piece of paper to prove it.

Other cohabiting couples see their union as temporary, feeling that they will stay together only as long as the relationship is rewarding. These couples enjoy the relative ease with which they can dissolve the relationship, unencumbered by the legal requirements of divorce. Although cohabiting couples may experience the same emotional trauma when they separate as divorcing couples, they are not permanently labeled "divorced."

Like single people, couples who live together do not enjoy the same social, legal, and economic benefits as married people. Couples may feel

---

What Are the Odds?

- A man enters a singles bar. What are the odds that he really is single? 45–50 in 100
- A woman in the USA receives a proposal of marriage. What are the odds she will accept? 1 in 3
  The average woman refuses two proposals before accepting.
- An adult runs away from his or her spouse (and possibly children). What is the probability that this person is a woman? 1 in 2
  Before 1960, the odds were 1 in 300.
- A girl marries in her teen years. What is the probability she will still be married five years later? 1 in 4
- Pick one baby at random born in the USA. What are the chances that the child's parents were not married to each other when the child was conceived? 1 in 3

Source: *The Odds Almanac* by James Fix and David Daughton

Committed Relationships

CHAPTER 11

this acutely if one partner is hospitalized and the other partner is restricted from being at the bedside because the hospital allows only family members to visit the patient. Cohabitation can be socially awkward if the couple wishes to have children together. Unmarried couples cannot share health insurance or tax benefits.

Homosexual Relationships

Many gay people have warm, loving relationships and would like to marry, but our legal code prohibits them from doing so. Approximately 6 percent of men are predominantly gay and 4 percent of women are lesbian. Many homosexual couples have long-term relationships, and some of them marry, seeking out ministers, priests, and rabbis who are willing to bless their unions. Nevertheless, these marriages are not legally recognized or socially sanctioned. For these reasons, many gay couples do the next best thing: cohabitate.

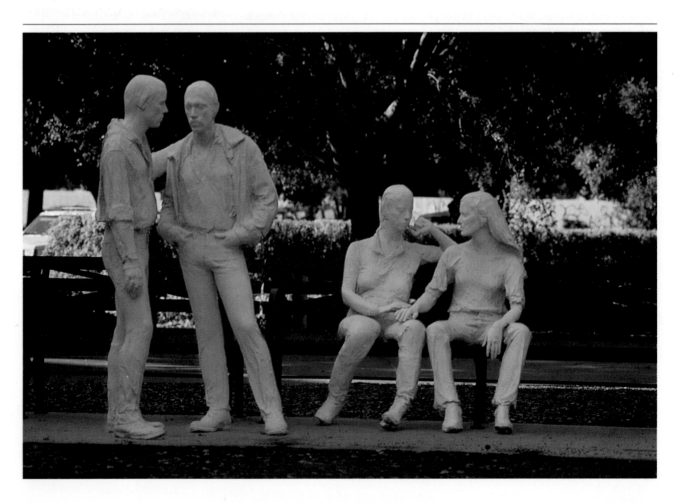

Gay couples face the same legal, financial, and social restrictions in their relationships that unmarried heterosexual couples do—only more so. They cannot share health insurance, are not counted as family members in hospital emergencies, and cannot receive joint tax benefits. Homophobia, confusion about homosexuality, and intolerance often make daily life difficult, sometimes even dangerous, for a gay couple. Restrictions tighten further if the couple wishes to adopt children. To date, gay couples have not been able to adopt a child as a couple; only one partner in the couple can be the adoptive parent. A recent court case in Washington state granted adoption rights to both partners of a lesbian couple, but so far this is a major exception. Despite social obstacles to their unions, gay couples of both sexes continue to form committed, loving relationships: 28 percent of gay women and 10 percent of gay men are in long-term, committed relationships.

Divorce Statistics

The Census Bureau estimates that of all women who have been married, 24 percent have had at least one divorce; for men, the figure is much higher.

When Relationships End

No one likes to think a relationship will end. When you begin a new relationship, or when your relationship is going well, breaking up may seem unlikely, even impossible. However, relationships do end, and it is wise to occasionally ask yourself what you would do if your relationship were to end. For some people, the end of a relationship brings relief, whereas for others it brings grief and depression.

Romance

Students who become severely depressed frequently cite romantic problems or relationship breakups as the main cause of their emotional distress. When you become immersed in a romantic liaison to the point of neglecting other relationships, you make yourself vulnerable to isolation. During the course of your relationship, make an effort to maintain personal friendships and outside interests so that, if the relationship should end, you have supporting emotional ties.

> There is no enterprise which is started with such tremendous hopes and expectations and which fails so regularly as romantic love.
>
> Erich Fromm

Divorce

Reno and Las Vegas were known as the divorce capitals of the United States. Nowadays, as the divorce rate climbs, this notorious claim to fame is fading. Circa 1900, the divorce rate was a mere .7 of a percent. Since then it has risen sharply: the rate for white women is 45 percent; for black women it is even higher. On the average, one out of two marriages ends in divorce.

According to the Holmes and Rahe Stress Scale, only death of a spouse causes more stress than divorce. People going through divorce develop myriad health problems: depression, insomnia and sleep loss, loneliness, memory problems, and a sense of failure. In addition, people may turn to destructive behaviors such as overmedication, alcohol and drug abuse,

Committed Relationships

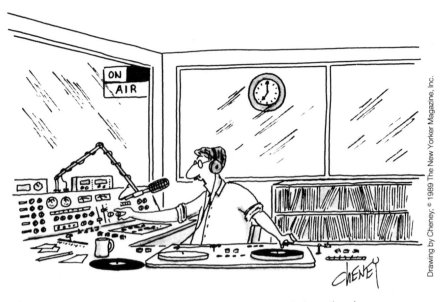

"This next one goes out to all those who have ever been in love, then become engaged, gotten married, participated in the tragic deterioration of a relationship, suffered the pains and agonies of a bitter divorce, subjected themselves to the fruitless search for a new partner, and ultimately resigned themselves to remaining single in a world full of irresponsible jerks, noncommittal weirdos, and neurotic misfits."

recklessness, and increased smoking, that may have been previously held in check by family obligations.

Although much less so than in the past, divorce still carries a stigma. Married couples often do not know how to incorporate a divorced friend; the result may be a new, awkward social isolation. If there are children, custody arrangements as well as property settlement can be lengthy and emotionally draining.

Divorce has a financial, as well as an emotional, toll. In community property states, men who have worked hard to accumulate security for retirement may suddenly find their assets halved and the future not so secure. Of course, women also experience diminished economic security, especially if they have only limited job skills. Statistics indicate that only a small percentage of women actually receive full support payments or a large settlement from ex-spouses. Women who have remained at home to raise a family or help put their husbands through school often find themselves without money or job skills. Many have to take low-paying, unskilled jobs to make ends meet. If the woman has custody of the children, the financial picture worsens.

The effects of divorce affect the children as well. A recent study showed that the effects of divorce on children can linger for years, even decades, afterwards. The findings include the following:

- Three out of five youngsters felt rejected by at least one parent.
- Half grew up in settings where the parents continued to fight with each other.
- Two thirds of the girls had difficulty making lasting commitments later in life.
- Many boys failed to develop a sense of independence, confidence, or purpose.

The study pointed out, however, that how well children cope depends on the parents' attitude toward each other and the children's ability to resolve crises.

Seeking Professional Help

You can resolve most relationship problems with honest, caring discussion between yourself and the other person. Sometimes a relationship does not work, so you face the loss and let it go. With some situations you may need help. Here are some circumstances that would benefit from talking with a counselor.

- If your low self-esteem leads you to depression or thoughts of suicide.
- If your sense of failure in a relationship influences other aspects of your life so that you begin to see yourself as a failure in everything.
- If your degree of shyness prevents you from making friends and you feel isolated from virtually everyone else.
- If you experience one failed relationship after another and are ready to examine new patterns of relating to others.
- If your feelings of possession,

jealously or insecurity are beginning to damage the quality of a relationship.
- If your romantic relationships are OK but your friendships cannot be sustained (or vice versa), you may want to examine your behaviors in both types of relationships.
- If you have tried but simply cannot relate to certain people (professors, peers, member of same or opposite sex), you may want to develop new skills in relating.

For help with an issue involving your self-esteem or personal relationships, contact your student health center or dean's office to ask for an appointment with a counselor. Most colleges have excellent and qualified counselors ready to talk with students about personal problems. Don't feel shy—they are there to help you.

Beyond the Text

1. Respond to the following statement: It is less painful to end a relationship suddenly than to waste time and energy trying to resolve conflicts.

2. You figure if it doesn't work, you can always get a divorce. What does this show about commitment?

3. Your definition of an intimate relationship is "intellectual closeness" but your partner's is "physical closeness." What problems would you anticipate and how would you resolve them?

4. You have experienced a romantic relationship with a person who says, "I just want to be friends." What is the difference and what would you do?

5. Respond to the following statement: You can learn enough about each other by living together to know if a subsequent marriage would be successful.

Supplemental Readings

Becoming Partners by Carl Rogers. New York: Delacorte Press, 1972. A classic book by a renowned psychologist that discusses partnerships and love, and offers suggestions on how to build successful relationships.

Intimate Partners by Maggie Scarf. New York: Random House, 1987. The author addresses the problems that often develop in today's stressed and "overworked" intimate relationships. Methods of recognizing problems and resolving them are also offered.

Loving Each Other by Leo F. Buscaglia, PhD. New York: Random House, 1984. Author of several other books on interpersonal relations, Dr. Buscaglia discusses how relationships work, what they mean, and how we can enhance them.

The Road Less Traveled by M. Scott Peck, MD. New York: Simon and Schuster, 1978. This book has remained a best seller for ten years because it is written for all of us. Dr. Peck presents us with a guide to loving relationships and a formula for solving our problems on the way to developing a more spiritual self.

Why Love Is Not Enough by Sol Gordon, PhD. Boston: Bob Adams, Inc., 1988. Nationally-known psychologist discusses the essential factors for a successful relationship or marriage, how to identify the right person for you, and when to walk away from certain people and relationships.

Key Terms Defined

bonding important, initial feeling of intimacy established between a newborn and its adult caregivers

cohabitation living together as lovers and sexual partners without marriage

commitment willingness to act over time in a way that perpetuates the well-being of a relationship

conflict a state of disagreement and disharmony between two or more people in a relationship

developmental task term identified by Erik Erikson to denote personality tasks we all must master at various stages of development

divorce the legal dissolution of a marriage

friendship close relationship between two people involving feelings of mutual trust and support

homosexual relationship partnership that includes sexual intimacy with another of the same sex

intimacy a shared experience of trust and a feeling of mutual closeness in a relationship

marriage legal union of man and woman as husband and wife

monogamy sexual exclusiveness with one partner

passionate love powerful, ardent, adoring, sexual emotion for another

personality development stages of growth resulting in one's unique emotional, physical, social, and behavioral relationships

platonic companionship between two people that does not include a sexual relationship

relationship the condition of being related; may be close, intimate, sexual or friendly collaboration

romance love affair or loving involvement, often short-lived

self-esteem sense of self-worth; valuing oneself as an individual

traditional marriage marriage in which the couple assumes the roles prescribed by society; excludes cohabitation, gay marriages or relationships, and communal marriages

trust degree of confidence felt in a partner or in a relationship, related to ability, integrity, and character

values criteria by which you evaluate yourself, others, and the events in your life

Sexual Health

College is an excellent time to develop sound knowledge and values regarding sexuality. You are in an environment in which you can develop relationships that have the potential of being life-long. These are years of great personal growth. So learn and experiment at your pace, not someone else's. You learn about sexual issues from many people—friends, health care providers, family members, and, of course, sexual partners. The most effective way to maximize this learning is to share what you know and feel; hear what others have to say.

This chapter discusses women's and men's sexual health, identifies major sexually transmitted diseases (including symptoms, treatment, and prevention), and describes the common methods of contraception. Common methods of abortion are described and the current legal and moral issues are explored. A special section focuses on acquaintance rape, a topic of serious concern on college campuses throughout the United States.

Key Terms

Abortion	Homosexuality	PMS
AIDS	Hormones	Prostate gland
Amenorrhea	Impotence	Rape
Contraception	Mammogram	Sexually transmitted diseases
Epididymis	Menstruation	(STDs)
Genitalia	Pap Smear	Sterilization

Contents

Learning About Sexuality

Learning about sexuality has several stages. You won't go through these stages neatly, or perhaps even in order, but you do need to go through them to approach sexual health. In the first stage you become aware that you are a sexual being and accept that fact. If you deny that sexuality is a part of you, you will have difficulty accepting responsibility for your sexual actions; you will simply react to or withdraw from your environment, or experience consequences like unwanted pregnancy or sexually transmitted diseases.

In the second stage, you seek to learn about your sexual self. People experiment with their bodies and emotions. They search for answers in books and from friends. A respected educator of our time has said that we can't learn to play with other people until we learn to play with ourselves. This means that you need to know yourself before you can share yourself with a partner. This second stage is very important; yet people receive very little guidance in this area. We have little training in identifying and expressing emotions. We all have intimacy needs, but we often confuse them with physical expression of sexuality. On college campuses, most sexuality education focuses on this stage.

The third stage involves sharing yourself with a partner. As you do, all sorts of new and strong emotions become evident. In this stage "book" knowledge about sexuality is not as important as the ability to openly communicate feelings, needs and desires with a partner. You don't usually get this right the first time. "Dating" involves "practicing" sexual communication. This happens no matter what age dating starts. One college professor would ask her class to identify the largest sex organ in human beings. The correct response she was looking for, but the response seldom given, was the brain. So much of our sexuality and our ability to communicate with others is centered in the brain, and yet we tend to focus on the genitals. Communication is the most important part of sexuality with other people.

Even though intoxicants, especially alcohol, are fused with media images of sexuality, they seldom enhance sexual learning when used in large amounts. Sexuality is too important to learn about with anything more than minimal amounts of intoxicants. Intoxicants lower inhibitions, sometimes to the point where judgment is impaired. One seldom fully remembers—or learns from—behaviors engaged in during intense intoxication. This is why so many people who have chemical dependency problems also have problems with sexuality and relationships.

This chapter will focus on the second stage of this process—learning about our sexual selves. Most college students are experiencing the second stage and making significant inroads into the third. If you are already well into the third stage, use this chapter as a review of everything from anatomy to contraception. See how much of the basics you have already learned correctly; fill in any gaps you may have missed. You may find this chapter includes some new helpful specific skills.

Sexual Health

CHAPTER 12

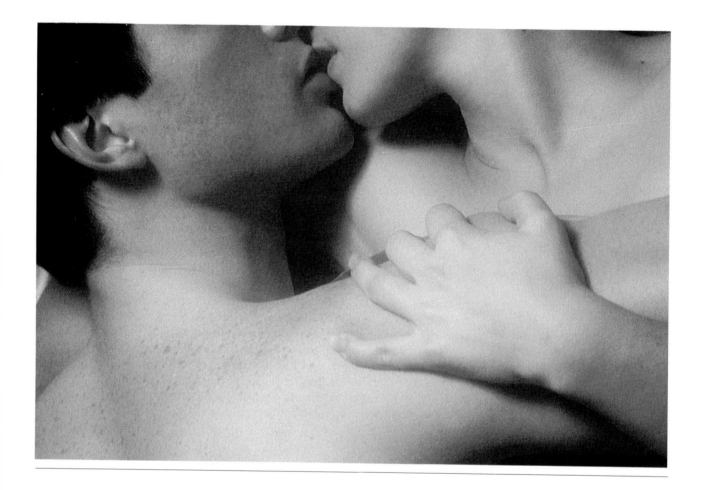

Men should read the section on Women's Sexual Health, just as women should read the section on Men's Sexual Health. Because many of our sexual relationships are with people of the opposite gender, it helps to know about our partners.

In all that follows, keep two points in mind. First, how does this relate to me and my knowledge of myself? Second, how would I communicate about this topic with other people—whether they are a partner or a health professional.

Women's Sexual Health

An important part of the women's movement in the United States over the last twenty years has been women learning about, understanding, and taking responsibility for their own sexual functioning. All three steps mentioned above are important: recognizing that we are sexual beings,

Sexual Health

learning about ourselves, and communicating with other people. A frequent description found in a physician's office twenty years ago was "Doctor, I have a pain down there." Many women were unaware of basic anatomy or physiological functioning. Women's growing awareness about themselves has led to improved health status as well as better communication with other people, including partners.

Female Anatomy

One of the reasons that neither women nor men are very knowledgeable about female anatomy is that only the vulva is visible on the outside. The vagina, cervix, uterus, fallopian tubes, and ovaries are inside the pelvic region and not easily observable.

The **mons pubis** is the soft mound of tissue covering the pubic bone. The vulva is external genitals—what you see when you look at the perineum. The vulva has several parts: right below the mons pubis is the **clitoris**, which leads to orgasm when appropriately stimulated; the **labia majora** and **labia minora**, the outer and inner lips surrounding the vaginal opening; and the **urethra**, the pathway for urine to leave the body. As with other bodily features, the external genitals vary greatly in size and shape from person to person, as does the amount of pubic hair. The vulva plays an important role in sexual arousal and often becomes the focus of foreplay before intercourse and during masturbation.

The **vagina** is an extremely flexible canal connecting the vaginal opening to the uterus. It stretches to accommodate a penis during intercourse

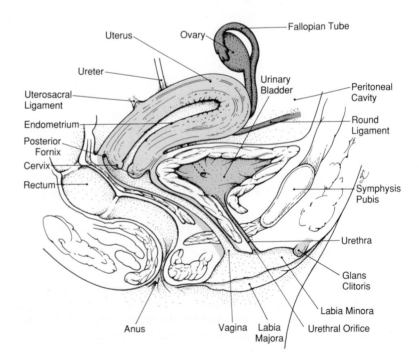

or a baby during birth. The vagina is distinguished from the urinary opening, or urethra, by its larger size. A thin layer of perforated skin (the hymen) covers the vaginal opening in some women who have not had intercourse. This membrane is often stretched before intercourse and its presence is not an indication of virginity. Virginity means that a woman has not had sexual intercourse.

The **cervix** is the entrance to the uterus at the back of the vagina and is a doughnut-shaped structure about the size of a half dollar. In the center of the cervix is the cervical os; this is a tiny tunnel that serves as the pathway for semen to travel into the uterus. Hence, it is a point of application for barrier forms of birth control such as the sponge and the diaphragm.

The ovaries, fallopian tubes and uterus are involved in the release, fertilization, and implantation of an egg which, if fertilized by a male sperm, can lead to the development of a fetus.

Menstruation

Reaching puberty and beginning to menstruate, which occurs somewhere between 10 and 17 years of age, indicates that the female reproductive organs are mature and capable of conception. The menstrual cycle becomes an important indicator of health status until menopause, or the end of ovulation. Few functions of the human organism are as misunderstood or surrounded by myths as menstruation.

Very simply, **menstruation** is a three-part feedback cycle that prepares the body for implantation and nurturing of a fertilized egg. To understand why women menstruate, and what regulates this process, requires a clear understanding of female hormonal changes. The average cycle takes about 28 days, although it may vary from 20 to 36 days or more.

The first phase is the menstrual period, or flow, and the first day of menstrual bleeding is day 1 in the cycle. This bleeding signals the release of uterine material accumulated in preparation for the fertilized egg. When an egg is not fertilized, the uterine lining is sloughed off. The second phase involves the release of a mature egg, or ovum, from the ovary and a thickening of the uterine lining. This is triggered by a release of follicle-stimulating hormone (FSH) and luteinizing hormone (LH) from the pituitary gland.

About 14 days before menstruation begins (day 14 from the first day of bleeding in a 28-day cycle), an increase in LH occurs, which causes a follicle in the ovary to rupture, releasing an ovum into the fallopian tube. The sperm usually fertilizes the egg in the first third of the fallopian tube. Once fertilized, the egg and sperm become an ovum. The ovum then journeys down the fallopian tube and implants on the thickened uterine lining. This takes about 24 hours. However, since sperm can live in the uterus for at least 48 hours, fertilization can take place during a two- to four-day range of time surrounding ovulation. So you can get pregnant on Monday from sperm deposited during intercourse on Saturday. Since young women's menstrual cycles are often irregular and ovulation can occur more than once a cycle, predicting periods of fertility accurately is very difficult.

The third phase involves the further thickening of the lining of the uterus, or endometrium, so that it can nourish a fertilized egg. If fertilization does not take place, progesterone and estrogen levels decrease, causing the endometrium to be shed as menstrual flow through the cervix and vagina. This menstrual flow lasts from three to eight days and generally consists of about two ounces of blood, mucus, endometrial tissue, and the unfertilized egg. The falling estrogen levels stimulate the pituitary gland to begin secreting FSH, and then another cycle begins.

Women should keep track of when periods start and when they expect their next period; this not only helps determine pregnancy, but also helps women and their health care providers evaluate other reproductive health conditions. A number of symptoms surrounding menstruation can cause a great deal of worry. Most fall within the "normal" range of symptoms, but a woman needs to pay attention to all symptoms to determine what is "normal" for her. If you are uncertain, seek the advice of a health professional. Here are some common menstrual problems and suggestions for assessing and alleviating them.

Amenorrhea is an absence or abnormal stoppage of menstruation. In college women this can be associated with stress, severe dieting including eating disorders, increased levels of exercise, and illness. Or, it could indicate a pregnancy. In any case, if you have kept track of your cycles and know what is normal for you, you can help a health professional evaluate the missed period.

Dysmenorrhea is painful menstruation. It is normal to experience some pain and cramping as part of the menstrual cycle. If menstrual pain interferes with your normal activities, ask your health care professional for advice. While keeping track of your cycles, you might also want to develop a personal index that measures how uncomfortable you are throughout your cycle. If pain increases over "normal" for you it would be helpful for the health professional to be able to assess both the length of the cycle, number of days of flow, and intensity of the pain.

Premenstrual Syndrome (PMS) refers to a combination of symptoms experienced by many women during the menstrual cycle, usually just before menstrual bleeding begins. The intensity and range of symptoms vary widely. Symptoms may include temporary (water) weight gain or a bloated feeling, headaches, cramps, tender breasts, tension, skin outbreaks, and depression. All of these may occur to some degree when hormonal balances change. Women are encouraged to keep track of their cycles and symptoms to document for themselves their own pattern. Diet (low sodium/salt, increased fluids, high fiber, high complex carbohydrate, low fat, and low sugar), exercise, massage, relaxation techniques, and prescription medications may be of help in alleviating symptoms. Researchers are investigating the relationship of PMS to certain vitamins and minerals. Check with your health care provider about the advisability of taking extra nutrients to relieve PMS.

Toxic Shock Syndrome is a rare bacterial-caused illness occurring mostly in young women during their menstrual periods, especially in women who are using high absorbency tampons. Symptoms include the sudden onset of a fever over 102° F, vomiting, diarrhea, and a rash on the hands or feet. These symptoms can rapidly lead to loss of blood pressure and shock. If these symptoms occur, consult a physician or go to an emergency room immediately.

Other Female Reproductive Health Problems

Some vaginal discharges are normal; some are not. Normal amounts of estrogen produce vaginal discharge much in the same way as tears or ear wax are usually part of normal functioning. Cervical mucus and secretions from glands in the walls of the vagina and vulva produce a healthy, moist environment. Normal sexual stimulation also increases secretions as a lubricant which minimizes abrasion and pain during intercourse. Women should know what is "normal" for them so they can be aware if their discharge becomes heavy or changes appearance or odor. Douching, or using fluid to flush the vagina, changes the environment and can lead to irritation or infections. It is not an effective means of birth control and should be done only on the advice of a health professional.

Vaginitis is a general term used to describe an inflammation or infection of the vagina. A number of organisms can be the underlying cause including bacteria, protozoa, fungi (yeast), parasites, and allergens. Some of these may be sexually transmitted, but most are not. Some women may have symptoms such as an unusual discharge, itching or odor, but many have no symptoms and the infection is first diagnosed in the partner. A woman with vaginitis who has kept careful track of signs and symptoms surrounding menstruation and vaginal function can help the health professional diagnose and treat the underlying cause. Recurrent vaginitis may result from stress, multiple sex partners, restricted diets, poor nutrition (including eating disorders), fatigue, tight clothing, synthetic underpants, routine use of antibiotics, or sensitivity to spermicides in cream, jelly, foam, sponges, suppositories, or spermicidal condoms. If you take antibiotics, discuss with your doctor the advisability of taking acidophilus to increase normal, "good" bacterial flora. Also, wear cotton underwear and avoid tight pants and pantyhose.

Cystitis, urethritis, bladder infections, and other urinary tract infections are infections, usually bacterial, of the urinary tract that cause painful urination, frequent urination, lower abdominal pain, or pain during intercourse. Some are sexually transmitted, but most are not. They are usually treated with sulfa drugs or antibiotics. Simple hygiene rules minimize the risk of these infections including wiping from front to back after defecation, keeping the urethra, vaginal and anal areas clean, urinating when the urge is felt rather than postponing for a long time, and drinking plenty of fluids, such as water or fruit juices (especially cran-

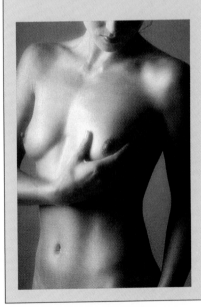

berry or cherry juice), to keep the urine in the bladder diluted and the urinary tract "flushed out." If you use a spermicide, switch brands.

Pelvic inflammatory disease (PID) is a general term for an infection anywhere in the female pelvic organs including the lower abdomen. Having multiple partners may increase a woman's risk of contracting PID. The condition usually starts as an infection of the cervix and spreads upward to involve the uterus, Fallopian tubes, ovaries, and into the abdominal cavity. Two common sexually transmitted diseases (STDs), chlamydia and gonorrhea, are responsible for a large share of PID among college students. Therefore, since most women do not have immediate symptoms of these STDs, tracing through male partners becomes a high priority to prevent PID in women. The symptoms may be minor, such as a slight fever and aching in the lower abdomen, to a sudden high fever up to 104° F and severe pelvic pain that resembles appendicitis. It is important to see a health care provider immediately, for two reasons: the infection and its complications may be life-threatening, and PID is now the leading cause of infertility problems in young women due to scarring and blockage of fallopian tubes as a result of the infection. Regular annual pelvic exams can include tests for PID. Condoms help women avoid PID (and other STDs).

DES daughters are women born to mothers who took a nonsteroidal estrogen, called diethylstilbestrol (DES), to prevent miscarriage from the late 1940s to the late 1960s. DES daughters are at risk for several female reproductive tract cancers and abnormalities. Relatively rare cancers of the vagina and cervix are more common among these daughters. DES daughters and women who have had PID may have higher risk pregnancies. Research indicates that women who took these drugs during pregnancy may have a higher rate of breast cancer. All women born during this period should find out if their mothers took DES. If the mothers were on these drugs, then the daughters should determine with a specialist the advisability of routine, yearly pelvic examinations whether or not they are sexually active.

Breast Self-Examination

Though the breasts are not part of the female pelvic organs, they are an important part of a sexual health inventory. Breast sizes vary from woman to woman, as do individual breasts on any given woman.

Why is breast self-examination important for young women? One in five women in America dies of breast cancer. Some develop breast cancer in their late teens or early twenties. Many young women don't feel at risk, but no one needs to take unnecessary risks for cancer. Early detection of breast cancer can mean the difference between survival and premature, painful death.

You should do your exam on the same day of your menstrual cycle each month so that you are not finding natural changes due to differing hormonal levels. The size and texture changes during the menstrual cycle

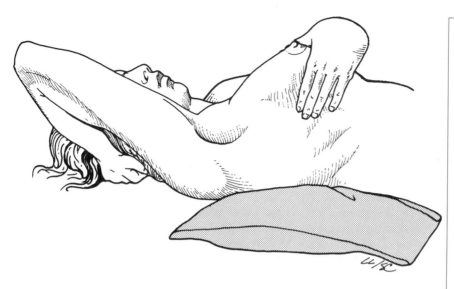

How to Do a Breast Self-Examination

- Choose the same day every month—two or three days after your period ends.
- Start the exam in front of the mirror where you can visually inspect your nipples for any changes or discharge. Look at size and shape.
- Stand with your hands at your sides, then move your hands behind your head. In both positions, look for any changes in size, symmetry or contour of both breasts.
- Stand with the first arm raised or lie on your back with one arm above your head and a pillow under the same breast you will be examining.
- Use three fingers and, in a circular motion, press against your breast tissue. Feel for any lumps or nodules. Start at the outer edge and work toward the nipple.
- If you note any changes or you are concerned, seek the help of a health professional.

and during pregnancy. The best time is immediately after your flow has stopped each month. Once again, you are determining what is "normal" for you and reporting changes to a health professional. You should ask a health professional or a certified representative of the American Cancer Society to teach you to examine your breasts since a "hands on" approach to teaching is far more effective than diagrams or even films. Once you reach age 35 to 40 you should have a baseline mammogram and a yearly breast examination by a clinician in addition to your monthly self-examinations. Women are more at risk of developing breast cancer after age forty and if they have a family history of breast cancer. All women should examine their breasts on a monthly basis throughout their life. Most of you will discover small normal lumps in breast tissue. Some of these are fibrocystic breast disease, which is usually considered noncancerous. Most breast cancer lumps are discovered by women themselves rather than by their doctors. A good time to learn and practice is when you are young and healthy. Early detection is critical to a positive outcome of the second largest killer of adult women in the United States. (What's first?—Lung cancer just passed breast cancer one-and-a-half years ago, due to an increase in women smokers.)

Men's Sexual Health

For years most people have assumed that men are very knowledgeable about their sexual functioning, in part because most of the male sex organs are easily visible, accessible, and men often play with them. The truth is many males have less knowledge about their sex organs than their female counterparts have about theirs. Most young boys learn about their anatomical functioning from their mothers, and mothers often do not know enough themselves. Men have also been encouraged to act as if they are sexually knowledgeable, so few take the opportunity to inquire and learn. Both men and women should be familiar with the following material.

Male Anatomy

The **penis** is made up of three parallel tubes which become engorged with blood, and thus erect, during sexual excitement. This erection makes penetration of the vagina possible during intercourse, but can also be a source of embarrassment to young men when erections are sometimes frequent and visible.

The head, or **glans**, of the penis is normally covered by a retractable foreskin. In a surgical procedure called circumcision, the foreskin is often removed at birth for social, religious, or hygienic reasons. This procedure is rapidly becoming less common in the United States except for religious purposes. Males can easily be taught to retract the foreskin and wash away a normal secretion called smegma to retain cleanliness.

The **scrotum** is a pouch that hangs below the penis and surrounds two **testicles**. The testicles produce sperm and the hormone testosterone. In addition to protecting the testicles, the scrotum is very sensitive to heat, cold and emotion as it attempts to maintain a constant temperature slightly below that of the body. This lower temperature is so essential for sperm production that men experiencing fertility problems are often told to change from jockey shorts to boxers and to stay out of hot tubs. (By the

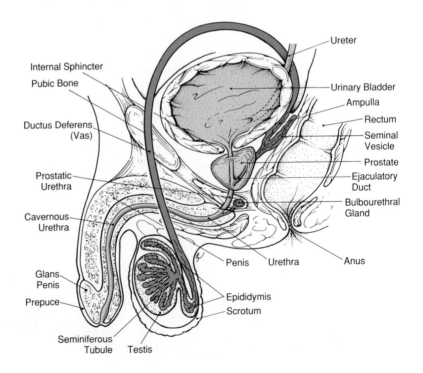

way, jockey shorts and hot tubs are not an effective form of birth control.) The left testicle usually hangs a little lower than the right because of its blood supply. This allows men to comfortably cross their legs.

The testicles develop inside the abdomen and descend into the scrotum shortly before or after birth. If one testicle doesn't descend, a condition called an undescended testicle, it is brought down surgically. Because the blood vessels and nerves for the testicles originate in the abdomen, a blow to the testicles may be felt much higher in the abdomen. After the testicles descend, the weak spot left in the muscle layer at the bottom of the abdomen is a potential site for a hernia, a bulging of intestine through the muscle layer. When health professionals feel above the testicle and ask you to turn your head and cough during a physical, they are looking for a beginning hernia. (By the way, you only turn your head so that you don't cough on the doctor; it is not important to the exam.)

Sperm collects at the back of the testicle in a structure called the **epididymis** and then follows a spermatic cord from each testicle up into the **prostate** where these cords join the urethra. The prostate provides the fluid that is the primary component of semen. During ejaculation, a small valve closes to allow semen to be discharged through the urethra, which runs the length of the penis. Most of the time this same tube is the pathway of urine.

A small gland near the prostate secretes a clear fluid during erection which neutralizes urine in the urethra and provides lubricant for intercourse. This fluid usually contains many sperm and therefore any contact with the female vulva or penetration of the vagina during sexual excitement can deposit sperm which can lead to a pregnancy.

Male Reproductive Health Problems

Urethritis—an infection of the urethra, the pathway for urine and semen—is one of the more common infections in men. This infection is marked by pain or a burning sensation during urination or erection and a discharge from the urethral opening on the tip of the penis. Although there are several possible causes, sexually transmitted diseases such as chlamydia and gonorrhea are very real possibilities for those who are sexually active. (See section on STDs.) Most cases of urethritis can be treated with antibiotics, but one should refrain from sexual intercourse until all signs of infection are cleared up so you do not transmit the infection to a partner.

Prostatitis is an inflammation or infection of the prostate, the organ between the bladder and the penis through which the urethra passes, and the source of fluid found in semen. Prostatitis may result from several types of bacterial infection, and even a physician may not be able to distinguish between prostatitis and urethritis. In prostatitis, in addition to a burning sensation and a discharge, beginning a stream of urine may also be difficult and painful because the prostate swells, causing the urethra to narrow and constrict. Though prostatitis is caused by STDs less often than is urethritis, both are treated with antibiotics.

In a medical examination for a swollen prostate, a clinician inserts a gloved finger into the rectum to feel the prostate through the wall of the bowel. This examination becomes part of a routine physical for men over age 40 to detect signs of prostatic cancer—a cancer that almost never affects young men but is frequently seen in older men. This usually slow-growing and most-often-treatable cancer is so common that it has been theorized that if all men lived to 100 years of age, all men would develop prostatic cancer.

Testicular Self-Examination

Just as women should perform monthly breast self-examination (BSE), so should men perform testicular self-examination (TSE) on a monthly basis. The idea is to become very familiar with your own sex organs and note any changes. TSE, like BSE, is performed to identify a number of conditions, primarily cancer. Testicular cancer is a relatively rare form of cancer with only about 5,000 cases in the United States each year. However, unlike breast cancer, which usually occurs after age 40, testicular cancer often occurs between 15 and 25 years of age and is the third highest cause of cancer deaths in this age group. If detected early, testicular cancer is second only to skin cancer in terms of a successful cure rate. However, since TSE is not widely known or practiced, many deaths occur that could be easily prevented. Your health professional should make certain that you know how to perform TSE at the time you have a routine physical. If this is not included as part of the physical exam, speak up and ask!

The best time to examine yourself is during a warm shower when the heat of the water can relax the scrotum and the soap reduces friction as you feel the scrotal contents. First, identify each testicle and the epididymis on the back of the testicle. Rotate each testicle between thumb and forefinger, feeling for a round, firm surface. If you discover a small, painless lump on the surface of the testicle that does not appear to be the epididymis, consult a health professional immediately. Testicular cancer is almost always painless, so do not wait for the lump to grow or pain to develop. Second, examine the rest of the contents of the scrotum. Any one of the following conditions may be found.

Epididymitis is a painful condition that occurs when the tubular structure on the back of a testicle becomes infected. Often there is a fever and a discharge from the penis. This infection should be treated by a health professional and usually requires antibiotics and bedrest.

Varicocele is an enlargement of veins above the left testicle, an enlargement that may disappear when you lie down. Varicocele is very common (about 40 percent of men have it). Men may discover varicocele during self-examination. It is often described as feeling like a "bag of worms." It does not need treatment unless there is pain associated with it. If you have problems with low sperm count in an attempt to produce a pregnancy, your physician might want to surgically correct a varicocele since it is sometimes associated with fertility problems. (Note: fertility refers to sperm count and not to potency, which is the ability to have an erection and ejaculate. Low sperm counts are definitely not an effective form of birth control!)

Hydrocele and **spermatocele** are small lumps separate from the testicle that are filled with fluid or sperm. These usually are not treated unless they become large enough to be painful or interfere with functioning. A health professional can reassure you if you are uncertain. It is important to note that these are always separate from the surface of the testicle. Any lump that appears to be part of the testicle, and is not the epididymis on the back of the testicle, should be evaluated by a health professional immediately.

Torsion of the testicle is a condition in which one of the testicles twists, cutting off its own blood supply. The result is extremely painful and, like any severe pain, should be evaluated by a health professional immediately. Surgery, often needed to save the testicle, is usually successful if done promptly.

Male Problems with Sexual Functioning

Because men are often expected to be all-knowledgeable about sexual functioning, and since admitting to questions or problems might be viewed as a sign of being less than masculine, men seldom honestly compare notes in terms of sexual functioning problems. The "stories" tend to exaggerate size and potency; in reality, most men spend a great deal of time worrying about performance—in most cases without cause.

Potency refers to the ability to achieve and maintain an erection and to ejaculate semen. The opposite of potency is impotence. Fertility refers to the number of functioning sperm in semen and is seldom related to potency. Most infertile, or sterile, men can have an erection and most men who are impotent are not sterile. Potency and fertility have nothing to do with the size of one's penis or testicles—nor does size have anything to do with sexual performance. Though penis size varies greatly in the non-erect, flaccid state, the variation is much less among erect organs. The small tend to get much larger and the large tend to get only somewhat larger. If men had opportunities in average life situations to compare themselves with other men, they would find that they are not so different.

Men sometimes experience situations in which they expect to have an erection but don't. This temporary form of **impotence** is usually associated with fatigue, nervousness, or large amounts of alcohol or other drugs. In young men the problem becomes one of performance anxiety; if you worry too much that you won't have an erection, you won't. Because of the distress this often produces, males need to learn how to communicate their concerns with either a partner or a compassionate listener. Worrying about this condition and thinking you are the only one experiencing it only makes it worse. During an average night's sleep, men have several erections and will often awake with an erection that is as-

Erections are the great "equalizer" among men.

Sexual Health

sociated with a need to urinate. These erections are usually an indication that there is not a physical cause for impotence with a partner. As males age, several health problems such as diabetes, heart disease, and smoking (which causes blood vessel damage in all organs, including the penis) can cause physical impotence.

Unintended ejaculation is a term that is much more descriptive than another phrase frequently used, premature ejaculation. It simply refers to experiencing an ejaculation before you want one to happen. Probably no other situation causes so much misunderstanding between heterosexual partners—in part because neither partner is able to communicate about this "problem" with the other. Men become sexually excited and can reach orgasm—ejaculation—faster than women. Often, and especially with new partners, a man may ejaculate "too soon," often before the woman has had an opportunity to begin to reach her own orgasm. If the man is embarrassed, or inconsiderate, sexual activity stops there. Perhaps the most understanding phrase people can say is "that's all right, it will be better the next time." This opens communication and implies a commitment to continue sexual activity until the needs of both partners are met. If unintended ejaculation continues, partners can easily be taught techniques to improve ejaculatory control.

Prolonged sexual excitement without ejaculation can sometimes cause painful cramping feelings in the testicles and/or urinary tract, also known as "**blue balls**." One of the oldest excuses men have used with women after heavy foreplay or petting suggests that since the woman has caused this "excitement," it is "important" that intercourse proceed or the man will be "hurt." Nothing is further from the truth, and today's male should expect a reply along the lines of "I'm sure you can find some other solution." Masturbation is successful in relieving these cramps and is certainly preferable to unwanted, pressured, or even forced intercourse.

Sexually Transmitted Diseases

Sexually transmitted diseases are an important public concern because of the severe health consequences associated with many of them. Unfortunately, concern over medical issues often becomes confused with moral issues because society is still not comfortable with sexual topics—even though we have supposedly undergone a "sexual revolution."

Just a few years ago the term "venereal disease" was changed to "sexually transmitted disease" (STD) in an attempt to recognize a wider range of conditions that can be sexually transmitted and to lessen the moral stigma associated with venereal disease. Many of these diseases, such as syphilis and gonorrhea are "diseases as old as the Dark Ages, still acquired in the dark, and when acquired, kept in the dark." Unlike in the Dark Ages, scientists now know that these diseases are caused by specific bacteria, viruses, or other organisms. These organisms do not know or care about sexual preference, religion, political ideology, what grades you

Sexual Health

Doonesbury

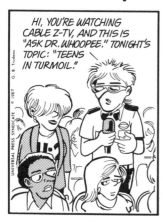
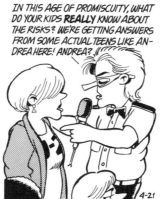
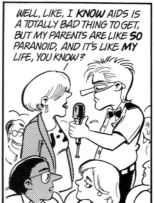
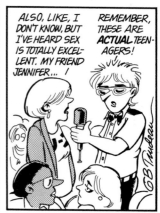

get in school, or anything else, other than the fact that you are an accommodating host.

Most STDs can be treated, many can be cured, but some may go undetected for years, though causing serious damage. One STD in particular, acquired immune deficiency syndrome (AIDS), is fatal. With all STDs, prevention is much, much, more important than treatment. In general, prevention of STDs begins with communication with your partner. Why talk to your partner? Because you can't always tell from looking at your partner or his or her sexual organs or functioning whether he or she has an STD. You must talk to find out, and if you don't trust the answers, ask yourself . . . do I want to have intercourse with this person? After all, though most STDs can be cured, at least one, chlamydia, has no symptoms for most people but can cause infertility; AIDS has no cure and it kills. STD prevention involves knowing yourself well enough to determine that the appropriate time for you to be clear about STDs is *before* intercourse. Be open enough to discuss previous sexual histories honestly *before* intercourse. Be able to look and examine your partner's sex organs *before* intercourse. Talk about your choice of birth control *before* intercourse; some forms (such as birth control pills) provide little protection against STDs, while other forms (such as condoms) provide a great deal, but not total protection. Prevention involves limiting the number of sexual partners. If all of this leads you to think that intercourse is far too important to let happen spontaneously, with no preparation, just like in the movies . . . you are right!

Chlamydia (Chlamydia trachomatis)

With an estimated five million cases per year, chlamydia is the most common sexually transmitted disease in the United States today. One reason that the term "chlamydia" is relatively unknown is that for many years

Sexual Health

C H A P T E R 12

the organism causing chlamydia was difficult to identify. The medical community referred to it simply as non-gonococcal urethritis (NGU) or non-specific urethritis (NSU in males, NSV in females) because the symptoms were similar to gonorrhea. Now that tests for chlamydia are available, clinicians are recognizing how common it is.

Chlamydia is spread primarily through sexual activity where infected mucous membranes come in contact with other mucous membranes. It is more common in heterosexual couples than homosexual, and both chlamydia and gonorrhea may occur at the same time. Though almost all males show symptoms if they are infected, almost all females *do not*. This is very serious because untreated chlamydia in women is now thought to be the leading cause of pelvic inflammatory disease (PID). Not only does PID cause many women chronic pain, but every year 60,000 women in the United States become infertile because of PID and 25–30,000 have ectopic pregnancies. Therefore, it is vitally important for all men infected with chlamydia to identify all of their partners to a medical practitioner and for sexually active women to have yearly pelvic examinations that include tests for chlamydia. Both partners should abstain from sexual activity until both are tested and free of infection to avoid re-infecting each other.

Symptoms

Incubation is 7 to 28 days.

In women (Note: Most women will have no symptoms)

- Itching and burning in the genitals
- Unusual vaginal discharge
- Urinary frequency
- Mild pain with urination
- Bleeding between periods
- Inflammation of the cervix
- Symptoms of PID:
    pelvic pain
    fever
    abnormal vaginal discharge
    ⚹painful intercourse
- No symptoms

In men

- Mucus or pus-like discharge from penis one to three weeks after exposure
- Painful, frequent urination
- Symptoms may be so mild as not to be noticed

Diagnosis

- Laboratory tests on urogenital secretions

Treatment

- Full course of oral antibiotics (tetracycline or doxycycline)
- Follow-up cultures taken 2 to 3 weeks after treatment
- All partners referred for evaluation and treatment
- Avoid sexual activity until cure confirmed

Prevention

- Reduced number of sex partners
- Consistent use of barrier contraceptives: condoms and spermicides

Gonorrhea

Gonorrhea, like chlamydia, is caused by a bacterial infection. With an estimated one-and-a-half million cases per year in the United States, gonorrhea is the most prevalent reportable disease. Long experience with gonorrhea, as well as its easy treatment with antibiotics, have led many to believe that this disease is not serious. However, its complications can cause serious infections, sterility, arthritis, and blindness. Even more important, there are now several strains of gonorrhea that are resistant to penicillin. This is why most health professionals will ask you to have a follow-up examination one to two weeks after initial treatment. As with chlamydia, most men have symptoms and most women do not. Therefore, it is important to identify, evaluate, and treat all partners. Since gonorrhea is so common and can cause blindness in babies delivered through the birth canal of an infected mother, all newborns are treated with protective eyedrops or antibiotic ointment at birth.

Symptoms

Incubation is 2 to 10 days.

In women (Note: Less than half of the women will not develop symptoms)

- Vaginal discharge
- Urinary frequency and pain
- Complications—PID, can lead to sterility
  Abdominal pain
  Fever
  Nausea and vomiting

In men

- Profuse, yellowish discharge from penis (within 2 to 5 days of initial infection)
- Pelvic pain
- Fever

- Inflammation of posterior region of testes—pain, tenderness, and swelling
- Complications—post-gonococcal urethritis and spread of infection to urethra, prostate, and seminal vesicles; systemic gonorrheal infection

Treatment

- Amoxicillin, oral 3 gm or ampicillin 3.5 gm. With concurrent chlamydial infection, add tetracycline or doxycycline
- Most clients will respond to treatment in 12 hours with resolution of symptoms within three days
- Inform client you are required to report all cases to public health officials
- Avoid sex while completing treatment and have follow-up cultures taken one week after finishing medication

Prevention

- Reduced number of sex partners
- Use condoms to avoid future infection
- Women need to have frequent screening if sexually active (because they may not have any symptoms of the infection)

Syphilis

Fortunately, syphilis is now relatively rare in the United States (approximately 34,000 cases in 1989 compared with 5,000,000 cases of chlamydia). Some experts anticipate that rising incidence in heterosexuals may return caseload to 60,000 level of the early 1980s, before AIDS brought about changes in gay sexual activity. Caused by the treponema pallidum bacteria, this disease is characterized by four well-defined stages. Aggressively identifying and treating cases is important because the late stages of syphilis can mimic almost all serious chronic diseases including severe mental illness.

Symptoms

Primary (21–90 days after exposure)

- A painless, red-rimmed, indented, sore (chancre) on the penis, anus, rectum, vagina, cervix, or mouth. The chancre disappears two to six weeks later with or without treatment.

Secondary (6 weeks to one year after healing of chancre)

- Rash on palms of hands and soles of feet, fever, sore throat, headaches, lack of appetite, nausea, and/or inflamed eyes. These symptoms may be severe or mild and usually disappear after 2 to 6 weeks.

Latent (1 to 30 years after secondary symptoms)

- No symptoms at all but blood tests remain positive.

Tertiary or late stage

- At least 25 percent of people with untreated syphilis will experience one or more of the following: central nervous system deterioration including paralysis and senility, heart disease, blindness, and death.

Diagnosis

- Examination of fluid from chancre
- Blood test

Treatment

- Primary, secondary or early latent—single IM injection of Bicillin, 2.4 million units. Later latent stage—full course of penicillin. With treatment, syphilis is curable at any stage.
- No intercourse until cured
- Blood tests for one year

Herpes Simplex Type I and II

In the 1970s and 1980s, until AIDS came along, the media often portrayed herpes as the most frightening STD. Because "herpes is forever," which simply means that once infected the virus stays in the body, our cure-oriented society reacted with more panic than common sense. It is important to put all herpes viruses into context.

The herpes family contains many familiar viruses including the Epstein–Barr virus, which causes mononucleosis, chicken pox (in which the virus retreats into nerves and can "reactivate" many years later as shingles), and the common "cold sore," or herpes simplex type I. Over 85 percent of children have antibodies against herpes simplex type I, which simply means that many have at one time or another been infected with a cold sore. A cold sore, sometimes called a fever blister, is a small, painful blister that ruptures to form an open sore that soon heals. Herpes simplex type II is simply a "cold sore" that occurs in the genital region. However, because of oral-genital contact, and the similarity of type I and type II, one can have type II "above the waist" and type I "below the waist." In fact, most health professionals do not bother to culture out secretions to determine whether a lesion is type I or type II.

Half the people who are infected with herpes simplex type I will have a lesion, develop antibodies, and never have another outbreak. The other half experiences an average of one or two outbreaks a year. No one needs to panic. Simply take an outbreak in stride. Avoid kissing people if you have a cold sore because herpes in this stage is very contagious. Herpes simplex type II should be approached in a similar manner. Half of the people infected have only one outbreak and the other half will experience an average of one or two outbreaks per year. To avoid spreading the virus, avoid sexual contact during an outbreak. However, though you

> **As illnesses go, herpes is a minor health problem. Twenty million Americans now have it, and despite the media's sensationalized view, traumatic reactions are the exception, not the rule.**
>
> **Sam Know, Program Director**
> **Herpes Resource Center, Palo Alto, California**

may see a cold sore on our partner's lip and refrain from kissing, you seldom look for "cold sores" on your partner's sex organs and then refrain from sexual contact. This virus can be spread even though no lesions are visible.

Though herpes cannot be "cured," the prescription drug acyclovir is being used with some success in minimizing outbreaks of simplex and shingles. The one very serious complication of herpes simplex type II is that it can cause great damage to a newborn if the baby passes through the birth canal of a mother who has an active herpes lesion. It is very important that health professionals caring for a pregnant woman know of previous herpes simplex infections. Women should be cultured for herpes during the ninth month of pregnancy. If the culture is positive, or there is a lesion, the woman will deliver by planned Caesarean to avoid having her baby acquire herpes as it passes through the vagina.

Symptoms

Incubation is 7 to 10 days.

- One or several groups of small painful blisters on the sexual organs. In women, the labia are most often affected, but the clitoris, the outer part of the vagina, the anal area, and the cervix can also be involved. In men, the head (glans) and the shaft of the penis are most often affected. Men or women who have anal intercourse may get blisters in or around the anus.
- Blisters rupture to form soft, painful, itching, open sores. The sores may be covered by a yellow-grey secretion or pus if infected with bacteria.
- Enlarged lymph nodes, fever, and flu-like symptoms may be present.
- Painful urination or intercourse.
- Sores may reappear once or many times. The virus is most likely to be re-activated during times of stress, fever, cold, exposure to sun and wind, or fatigue.
- The most common complication is spread of the lesions to other sites—usually mouth, eyes or cuticles.

Diagnosis

- Physical examination of sores
- Laboratory culture of secretions for herpes virus

Treatment

- No known medical cure. Clients receive oral acyclovir capsules (Zovirax) 200 mg 5×/day for 10 days. Acyclovir oral dosage is given for first and subsequent outbreaks, as well as for routine prevention between. Acyclovir cream spread on lesions can minimize symptoms of an outbreak in many people. The 5 percent topical ointment is useful only during the first outbreak. Active stage resolves itself in ten to twenty days. The skin is gradually replaced, starting from the edges of each sore.

- Keep infected area clean and dry, and wear loose clothing.
- Refrain from sexual contact, including intercourse, during outbreak, but virus may spread between outbreaks as well.
- A woman infected with herpes simplex type II should have a pap smear annually.
- If you become pregnant, discuss your herpes history with your obstetrical clinician.
- Obtain counseling to assist you to live with this condition.

Prevention

- Condoms offer some but not total protection, due to breaking or incorrect application. For best results, use latex condoms, and use them every time.
- Wash hands after using bathroom to avoid spreading infection.
- Maintain overall health and avoid stress.

Genital Warts

Every year an estimated 400,000 to 600,000 Americans develop genital warts, a disease caused by the human papilloma virus (HPV). The virus infects the cervix, urethra, and anus in women, and the penis, scrotum, and anus in men. It may go undetected because it usually has no symptoms other than lesions. One to two months after exposure, warts may appear. They are transmitted either by skin-to-skin contact during intercourse or by oral-genital contact. The major concern is that clients with a history of genital warts are at increased risk for certain types of cancer, primarily cervical. (The human papilloma virus is associated with up to 90 percent of cervical malignancies and may play a role in other cancers of the genital organs.)

Symptoms

- Small to large wart-like growths on the genitals. The warm, moist environment of the genital area seems to favor the wart growth. The warts may be very small or larger with a red, indented, cauliflower-like appearance.
- Outbreaks exacerbate during pregnancy or with a defective immune system.

Diagnosis

- Examination of growths in genital area; very small warts must be identified with a colposcopic exam of the cervix or vagina.
- Pap smear.

HPV—A Frightening Development

Genital warts, caused by the little known human papilloma virus, are increasing. Experts estimate there may be one million new cases a year in the not too distant future. Some forms of the virus have been linked to cervical cancer. Presently, there is no cure.

Treatment

- There is no cure for genital warts, and treatment may be uncomfortable.
- Cyrotherapy with liquid nitrogen and a weak acid (podophyllin) are commonly used.
- Electrocautery, excision, and laser surgery are also used, but they are painful and have the risk of scarring.
- Podofilox, 0.5% applied twice daily to external genital warts for three consecutive days has recently been shown to be less expensive, safe, and effective. (Lancet, April, 1989)

Prevention

- Similar to any other STD—limit sexual contacts and use condoms.
- Those with HPV should have a Pap test every year (due to the cancer risk).

Hepatitis B

Hepatitis B (HBV) is a viral inflammation of the liver contracted by exposure to blood or body fluids of an infected person. Sharing of contaminated needles or sexual contact are the primary means of transmission. In addition to being a serious disease in itself, hepatitis B is associated with later development of liver cancer.

This STD is increasing at an alarming rate—from 200,000 new infections in 1978 to a current 300,000 cases per year. Approximately 10 percent become chronic carriers, most of which have a high risk of developing cirrhosis of the liver or liver cancer. This disease is more infectious than HIV because household members can become infected (unlike the risk of AIDS). Those in identified high-risk groups should be counseled as well as immunized to prevent the spread of this disease, which is both a killer and a costly public health burden. In the next 20 years, the total cost of caring for chronically ill HBV-infected persons is expected to exceed that for AIDS.

Concern with the problem is prompting discussions at the Centers for Disease Control (CDC) on developing a comprehensive immunization program for the future. Fortunately, effective vaccines are available. In 1982, a plasma-derived vaccine was introduced, and in 1986, a vaccine manufactured from yeast cells became available. The latter vaccine is entirely safe and effective (if somewhat expensive), and it does not carry the fear of HIV transmission through the plasma. The preventative costs of immunization far outweigh the long-term costs of caring for the chronically ill and dying.

Symptoms

- Early stage may include skin eruptions and joint pain.
- Acute phase may include gradual onset of fatigue, loss of appetite, nausea, diarrhea, headache, fever, joint pain, muscle ache, and abdom-

inal pain. These symptoms are common to many viral diseases including mononucleosis and require a blood test to isolate the causative agent.

- Within two weeks dark urine and grey stools are produced, and a yellow coloring of eyes and skin called jaundice appears. The liver becomes tender and enlarged.

Diagnosis

- Presence of above symptoms confirmed by laboratory blood test

Treatment

- Symptom management, since there is no cure
- Limitation of activity
- Alcohol and other drugs metabolized by the liver must be avoided to minimize liver damage

Prevention

- Education of health care workers to be immunized and to counsel immunization for high risk persons
- Immunization of high risk groups:
    Students and workers in the health professions
    Heterosexual, sexually active persons
    Homosexual, sexually active persons
    IV drug users
    Persons who are natives of Alaska, Pacific Islands, Asia, or Africa, or persons who travel for extended periods of time in the above geographical areas
    Persons who are sexual or household partners of identified carriers

Pubic Lice/Crabs and Scabies

Pubic lice, sometimes called crabs, are a common form of body lice, and scabies are small mites. Both are very common and are transmitted by close contact with an infected person or close contact with the clothes, towels, and sometimes hairbrushes of an infected person. Both lice and scabies are difficult to see but cause itching that may lead to local infections. It is a shock to have been with someone you care about and find yourself infected with "crabs" the next day. Did you get them from him? Who has he been with? Will he think he got them from you? If you are in a relationship and pubic lice become apparent, it is time to talk openly with your partner. Though they may not necessarily have come from your partner (bedding, camping, etc.), avoiding placing blame may be difficult. This situation may be a terrific opportunity to really open up your sexual communication.

Symptoms

- Itching
- Infected "bites"
- Nits look like cotton on hairs and crabs look like pepper
- Rash in spread of fingers

Diagnosis

- Examination of pubic hair for lice or eggs
- Examination of skin for tracks of bites—red streaks

Treatment

- Apply pediculocide shampoo, lotion or cream (Kwell or Eurax), usually obtained by prescription for scabies; over-the-counter products will kill lice and nits.
- Avoid scratching infected areas.
- Boil, treat or dry clean infested clothes, bed linens and other sources of re-infestation including cloth-covered chairs and carpets.
- Treat all partners and members of the household.

AIDS (Acquired Immune Deficiency Syndrome)

Probably no other disease in the last twenty-five years has aroused as much fear and concern as has AIDS. Many college students recognize that AIDS is a growing threat on campus. Because AIDS has such unremitting consequences, and because students often have inadequate information about AIDS, this book devotes a chapter specifically to this disease—its prevention, transmission, symptoms, and prognosis. Turn to the chapter on the **AIDS Crisis** for information that will help you make wise, safe and informed choices—choices that can affect your future and your life.

The Pap Smear Test

The Pap smear is a screening and testing procedure used to detect cervical cancer. This procedure has greatly contributed to a dramatic decline in cervical cancer deaths since it was introduced in 1943. The test is conducted as follows: vaginal and posterior fornix secretions are swabbed and smeared on a glass slide for examination under a microscope.

The traditional method of categorizing the cells is according to specific pathological classifications.

- Class I   No abnormal or atypical cells detected
- Class II   Atypical or abnormal cells present, but no malignancy found—a repeat pap smear is advised
- Class III   Cytology, suggests malignancy
- Class IV   Cytology, strongly suggests malignancy
- Class V   Cytology, concludes malignancy

The Delicate Art of Talking About Sexual Histories

Healthy sexual discussions begin by finding out about your partner's health and sexual history and discussing your own. While you may feel that talking—especially about STDs and previous sexual partners—inhibits spontaneity and passion, being open and honest with each other can "take the worry out of being close." Since talking isn't always easy, here are some ideas. . . .

How to Talk Be direct. Be prepared to talk about your past experience. Persist even if the other person wants to brush your concerns aside. Be prepared to postpone or not have sexual relations if the other person isn't responsive to your concerns or is not taking you seriously.

When to Talk Admittedly, discussing these issues is difficult because it may seem that you are assuming intimacy and your partner is not. It is important that you view talking together as a process and not a one-time event.

- Talk with your partner before you are physically intimate. The best time to discuss your sexual history and the kind of sexual intimacy you are comfortable with is *before* the passion becomes the moment.
- Talk with your partner while you are being physically intimate. You can tell your partner what you are/are not comfortable with or you can stop at any point. While this may seem awkward, you will be protecting your health and your peace of mind.
- Talk with your partner after you have been physically intimate. It's never too late—talking after the fact is better than not talking at all. You can learn that:
    there was nothing to worry about;

you may have been exposed to a STD and need to see a physician;
    you want to use condom protected sex or sexual practices that do not include an exchange of body fluids;
    you don't want to have sex again with this person.

What to Say

- Acknowledge that you are feeling awkward or uncomfortable talking about these issues.
- Let your partner know that you care for him/her.
- Volunteer information about your health and sexual history.
- Ask for information about your partner's health and sexual history.
- Decide together what you both feel comfortable doing sexually.

Source: Cowell Student Health Center and the Office of Residential Education, Stanford University

---

Today, many physicians prefer to use the Richart classification system that is based on three grades of intraepithelial neoplasia (CIN).

- Grade I Mild dysplasia (cell changes)
- Grade II Moderate dysplasia
- Grade III Carcinoma in situ

The Richart system is based on the concept of a continuum from dysplasia to invasive cancer. If the woman's test indicates cytology with atypical or abnormal cells, or CIN, a repeat test with a follow-up colposcopic evaluation is normally recommended.

Cases of cervical cancer, as evidenced by increased numbers of abnormal pap smears, has been on the rise since the early 1980s. This alarming trend is considered to be related to the increased presence of the human papilloma virus (HPV).

Sexual Health

> **Last night I discovered a new form of oral contraceptive. I asked a girl to go to bed with me and she said no.**
> **Woody Allen**

Contraception

Sexual urges and activity are normal. Heterosexual contact in which semen is deposited in or near the vagina can result in pregnancy. Therefore, a man and a woman engaging in sex should expect pregnancy to occur if they do nothing to avoid conception. Unfortunately, although that is the rational way of thinking, human beings are anything but rational when it comes to sex.

People who choose not to take precautions against pregnancy do so for a number of reasons. They may be uncomfortable talking about sex with partners. They may believe the popular image that discussing sex beforehand is less romantic. They may not want such discussions to lead their partner to decide not to have sex. Few role models in the media teach us that contraception is a part of sexual activity. The percentage of pregnancies that result from sex in the media is far, far fewer than in real life. Many people don't feel that they are at risk—it won't happen to them. Wrong. *Over 20 percent of college women become pregnant.* Some college men and women just don't think about contraceptive options; some don't know or are afraid to ask. The average couple requesting contraception information from Planned Parenthood clinics has been sexually active for nine months. Others mix intoxication with sexual activity; this minimizes the chance that they will take reasonable precautions. Several religions limit contraceptive options. However, these same religions usually restrict sexual activity to marriage.

Sex is too important to be left to chance. Pregnancy is too serious to think that it won't happen to you. If you are ready to put your hands on someone else's sex organs, and theirs on yours, there is nothing in the world that you can't talk about, and one of the things you should be talking about is contraception. An unwanted pregnancy takes a sizeable toll in both emotional and physical health. It can be very expensive, interrupt education and life goals, and put a tremendous strain on relationships. Those who are philosophically or religiously opposed to abortions should be especially careful not to become involved in an unintended pregnancy, since most college-age pregnancies outside of marriage end in abortion. A few minutes of discussion before sexual activity and a little advanced planning can prevent a lot of pain.

Contraception is a shared responsibility. Some methods are more oriented towards a woman and others towards a man, but both partners have a responsibility to be informed and openly discuss what will work best for them. Women are becoming more involved in traditionally male-oriented contraception. For example, a high percentage of condoms are now bought by women. What methods leave you and your partner most comfortable ? You may experiment with several types of contraception before finding one that works best for you. Some important questions to be considered in making your decisions are:

- Are you aware of medical reasons that would make a certain form of contraception unsafe? For example, women who smoke cigarettes should not use birth control pills.

- Are you afraid of any methods?
- Have you had difficulties with any methods in the past?
- How often are you having intercourse? Are you having intercourse? It is probably not advisable to be on birth control pills for long periods of time "in case" you might have intercourse (because of potential side effects, which will be discussed later in this chapter). Condoms and foam may be a more appropriate alternative.
- How do you and your partner feel about an unplanned pregnancy? If pregnancy would be especially disruptive, consider a combination of two methods or abstain.
- How many partners do you have? Having multiple partners increases your chance of contracting STDs, including AIDS; in such cases, condoms would be a preferred choice (or condoms plus another method).
- How much cooperation can you expect from your partner?
- How do you feel about touching yourself or your partner?
- How well can you openly discuss personal things with your partner? If you can't talk about contraception, perhaps you are not ready to enter into a sexual relationship.

Not all means of contraception are equal. Each has its own rate of effectiveness, convenience level, and potential side effects. Here is some material about contraceptive methods college students use most often. For more information about these choices, or for professional input in making such choices, consult either your college health center or a family planning group, such as Planned Parenthood.

Hope

Hope is the most common method of birth control among college students. It can "work" for some for a while. Hope is a form of "Russian roulette"; if it works by chance one time—you avoid your fertile time one month—you may be tempted to use it the next month. Over 80 percent of couples who use this "method" become pregnant within one year.

Abstinence

An important, but sometimes overlooked, form of contraception is simply not to have intercourse with another person. This is an effective way of preventing not only pregnancy but also STDs. Many couples form close relationships but decide to postpone sex until they are ready or until marriage.

Sexual Activity Short of Intercourse

Many couples include kissing, massage, and mutual masturbation as part of their sexual intimacy but do not have intercourse. As long as semen, including pre-seminal fluid, is not deposited in or near the vagina, there is little risk of pregnancy.

> **More than 40 percent of condoms are now bought by women.**

Sexual Health

Contraceptives: A Buying Guide

Type	Estimated Effectiveness	Advantages	Disadvantages	Comments
Birth-control pill (oral contraceptive)	98% (combination) 97% (mini)	Most effective reversible contraceptive. Results in lighter, more regular periods. Protects against cancer of the ovaries and uterine lining. Decreases risk of pelvic inflammatory disease, fibrocystic breast disease, and benign ovarian cysts.	Minor side effects similar to early pregnancy (nausea, breast tenderness, fluid retention) during first three months of use. Major complications (blood clots, hypertension) may occur in smokers and those over 35. Must be taken on a regular daily schedule.	Combination types contain both synthetic estrogen and progesterone (female hormones). Mini-pill contains only progesterone and may produce irregular bleeding. Available by prescription only.
Intrauterine device (IUD)	95%	Once inserted, usually stays in place. Remains effective for a year.	May cause bleeding and cramping. Increased risk of pelvic inflammatory disease. If pregnancy occurs, increased risk that it may be ectopic.	Only two types currently available in the U.S. Must check for placement after each period. Requires annual replacement. Available by prescription only.
Condom (rubber, prophylactic, sheath) Condom with foam	90% 95%	Protects against STDs, including AIDS and herpes. May protect against cervical cancer.	Must be applied immediately before intercourse. Rare cases of allergy to rubber. May break. Blunting of sensation.	More effective when the woman uses a spermicide.
Vaginal spermicide	70–80% (used alone)	Available over the counter as jellies, foam, creams, and suppositories.	Messiness. Must be applied no more than one hour before intercourse.	Best results occur when used with a barrier method (condom or diaphragm).
Diaphragm	90–95% (with spermicide)	No side effects. Can be inserted up to six hours before—rather than during—intercourse.	Increased risk of urinary tract infection. Must be replaced every few years or refitted after pregnancy.	Must be used with spermicide. Proper fit is essential. Available by prescription only.
Cervical cap	95%	Half the size of a diaphragm and can be held in place longer (48 vs. 24 hours).	More difficult to position and woman's cervix must be physically adaptable.	Does not require additional spermicide for repeated intercourse, unlike the diaphragm.
Vaginal sponge	76–83%	Easy to use because spermicide is self-contained. May be inserted as much as (but no more than) 24 hours prior to intercourse.	May be hard to remove; may fragment. May irritate vaginal lining. Cannot be used during menses.	Must be left in for 6 hours after intercourse, but not longer than 24 hours due to danger of toxic shock syndrome.

Source: *University of California, Berkeley Wellness Letter*

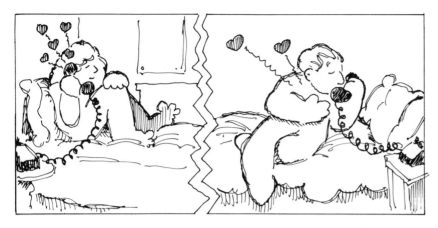

Safe sex

Women's Choices

Percentage of U.S. women (aged 18–44) using the following contraceptive methods:

Methods	Married	Unmarried
All methods	97%	87%
No method	3	13
Sterilization, female	28	12
Sterilization, male	24	1
Pill	22	48
Condom	15	16
IUD	3	3
Diaphragm	4	4
Foam	3	1
Sponge	1	4
Periodic abstinence	5	3
Withdrawal	5	6

Source: *Family Planning Perspectives*, Ortho Pharmaceutical Corp

Withdrawal

Some couples think that as long as the man does not ejaculate into the vagina, there is no risk of pregnancy. This is not an effective form of contraception, for two reasons. Pre-seminal fluid that lubricates the penis during sexual excitement contains sperm. Recognizing impending ejaculation in order to "pull out" in time is difficult, especially if you have been using alcohol or other drugs.

Natural Family Planning

Natural family planning, also called the rhythm method, or fertility awareness, is a form of contraception based on detailed knowledge of female reproductive cycles. Women, or couples, keep track of body temperature, vaginal discharge, and menstrual cycles to help identify the few days when a woman can become pregnant. Since many younger college women may not have regular menstrual cycles and since sperm can live in the female reproductive system for several days, this may not be an effective method for many college students. It is especially risky for women with irregular or infrequent menses. A clinician or family planning counselor should be consulted for training in this method, and back-up methods should be available. This method is more popular among couples in long-term relationships in which concern about STDs is minimal, since there is no protection from infection.

Birth Control Pills

Birth control pills contain one or both of the female hormones estrogen and progestin. "The pill" suppresses ovulation by making cervical mucus inhospitable to sperm and by altering the uterine lining so eggs won't implant. When used consistently and correctly, birth control pills provide

Sexual Health

C H A P T E R   12

the most effective contraception protection aside from sterilization and abstinence. However, birth control pills are hormones, and they should always be used under a health care provider's supervision. Users should be familiar with possible side effects. Although dangers are slight, and pill use is less of a risk than pregnancy, women who are not sexually active on a regular basis might want to choose a different form of contraception. Furthermore, it cannot be stressed enough that birth control pills do not offer protection against STDs.

Morning-After Pill

Some women who have intercourse without contraception, or who know or fear that their contraceptive method has failed, may hear that they can take a morning-after pill to prevent pregnancy. Certain prescription synthetic female hormone drugs can prevent survival of a fertilized egg, if taken within 72 hours of intercourse. But the morning-after pill isn't a casual, easy way out of an uncomfortable situation. None of these drugs has been approved by the U.S. Food and Drug Administration for use as a morning-after pill. Side effects of the most common morning-after pill include nausea and vomiting. (A woman who vomits within one hour of taking the drug may need to repeat that dosage.) Side effects of DES, which is used very occasionally as a morning-after pill, can include not only nausea and vomiting, but also breast tenderness, headaches, dizziness, and changes in menstrual cycles. DES can cause dangerous reactions in women who cannot take estrogen. A woman who takes DES and experiences severe headaches, leg cramps, or deterioration of vision or respiration requires immediate medical attention. Morning-after drugs should not be used regularly as contraceptives—only in an emergency.

Intrauterine Device (IUD)

Until a few years ago, IUDs were a popular form of contraception for women who had already had children and for whom STDs were a remote possibility. They are copper or plastic loops or coils which are placed in the uterus. The presence of a foreign material is thought to interfere with the implantation of a fertilized egg (ovum). All IUDs must be inserted by a clinician. Because of the risk of infection which may cause fertility problems later, IUDs are generally not recommended for college women. At least two types of IUDs have recently been approved for the U.S. market. If you are interested in more information about this product, check with your health care provider.

Diaphragm

The diaphragm is a dome-shaped latex cup with a firm, flexible rim. When coated with a spermicidal cream and fitted inside the vagina to cover the cervix, it prevents sperm from entering the uterus if left in place during intercourse and for six to eight hours afterwards. A clinician must size and fit a diaphragm as well as instruct a woman on its proper use. Because the vagina stretches with regular sexual activity and childbirth, users should have the fit of a diaphragm professionally checked on a regular basis. The diaphragm is attractive because it is a barrier method that has few physical risks and no chemical or hormonal risks. It may present some side effects, such as bladder infections and sensitivity to spermicides.

Cervical Cap

The cervical cap is similar to the diaphragm but smaller. It is a thimble-shaped cup that is held in place on the cervix by suction; it is used with spermicidal cream or jelly. Like the diaphragm, the cervical cap must be fitted by a clinician. The cervical cap is being tested by the Food and Drug Administration and is not yet widely available. Your local clinic or family planning agency can direct you to a clinic that provides the cap.

Contraceptive Sponges

The contraceptive sponge is a spermicide-containing polyurethane sponge that is inserted into the vagina against the cervix. It is effective when left in place during each act of intercourse and for 24 hours afterward. Because of a slight risk of toxic shock syndrome, the sponge should never be left in for more than twenty-four hours. The sponge is easily available in drug stores without a prescription and is becoming a very popular form of birth control. However, be certain to read all of the instructions carefully and then read them again! As is true for any method, use with a condom helps prevent STDs (including AIDS) and provides double contraceptive prevention.

Vaginal Spermicides

Spermicides are special jellies, creams, foams, and vaginal suppositories that contain agents to kill the sperm. To be effective, a spermicide is inserted into the vagina before intercourse. Nonoxyl-9, the commonest spermicidal ingredient, is currently being tested for its effectiveness in killing the AIDS virus. They are available without a prescription in drug stores. Even though some couples may find them "messy," they do provide lubrication, which makes intercourse more comfortable. Use vaginal spermicides as a backup with a condom for double protection and STD prevention!

Condoms

The condom was the major form of birth control and protection against sexually transmitted diseases for many years before the advent of the

Sterilization

Almost 20 million U.S. men and women have chosen to be sterilized—tubal ligation for women and vasectomy for men. These procedures are 99.6 percent successful, and clearly are the most effective form of birth control. While sterilization is meant to be permanent, it is estimated that 25 percent later regret the decision, and at least 10 percent have the procedure reversed. Reversals are about 60 percent successful for women and 65 percent for men.

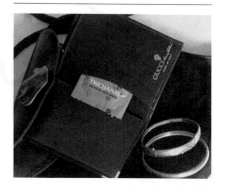

Using Condoms Effectively

Condoms are the only form of contraception that does not come with extensive usage instructions either from a clinician or in printed form. Anyone considering using them should keep these points in mind:

- Condoms are made of thin latex rubber and should not be exposed to prolonged heat or pressure. Glove compartments of cars and wallets are not good places to store condoms. Condoms have expiration dates, so it is important to note these dates.
- Use only latex condoms; the virus responsible for AIDS may penetrate natural lambskin condoms.
- Condoms should not be used with petroleum–based lubricants, such as Vaseline, which weaken the latex. They can be used safely with saliva, spermicidal foams, creams, jellies, suppositories, and KY Jelly.
- Condoms come in many shapes, textures, colors, flavors, lubricated and non-lubricated, but condoms come in only one size. They can be blown up to almost three feet before breaking, so no human male can use the excuse that they are not large enough for him!
- Leave room at the tip, especially in the condoms without the reservoir end, for the ejaculate.
- Put the condom on the erect penis *before* the penis comes into contact with the vagina. After ejaculation, hold the rim of the condom on the penis as the penis is withdrawn from the vagina so as not to spill any semen.
- When used with lubricants, condoms rarely break. If one does, apply an extra dose of spermicidal foam.
- Use a condom only once and then throw it away.

birth control pill. Today, with the rise of STDs and especially AIDS, many couples use the condom because it is a fairly effective preventive measure for both pregnancy and infections. Condoms are inexpensive, easy to obtain, and quite safe. Some males feel that they may slightly decrease sensation. However, this should be viewed as a positive advantage, since some young men have trouble with unintended ejaculation, and condoms help lengthen the duration of the erection. Latex condoms used in conjunction with a spermicide or a sponge provide almost 100 percent protection, as well as sufficient lubricant for comfortable intercourse. As the **AIDS** chapter explains in more detail, latex condoms provide more effective AIDS protection than do natural lambskin condoms.

Pregnancy

You miss a period, and if you have been sexually active in the last month, you wonder if you are pregnant. Suddenly your life might be changed. Your first step should be to find out if you really are pregnant. Many things other than pregnancy cause women to miss a period, especially young women who are not yet regular in their cycles. You can purchase a pregnancy testing kit without a prescription in a drug store. If the results from the kit indicate that you are pregnant, confirm these results with a health professional. You will need to line up support to help you consider a wide range of options before making a decision. Your partner, your parents, your friends, clergy, and counselors and clinicians are all possible sources of support, but you will want to communicate with them that you need and require support. Just as communication is essential when entering into a responsible sexual relationship, communication and support are essential to feel good about your decision. Your attitude helps to ensure a healthy outcome.

If you are pregnant, you will need to protect your own health by following your health care provider's advice regarding prenatal care, even if you do not intend to carry the fetus to term. If you intend to have the baby, early prenatal care will benefit the health of both you and your baby. Initial guidelines are presented in the chapter on pregnancy. The most important reason you need to move quickly is to have the healthiest baby possible or the safest abortion possible. Early evaluation and decision making is critical for both.

Abortion

The subject of abortion is highly charged. It was one of the most controversial issues of the 1980s, and people for or against it will continue to have heated confrontations during the 1990s. Even the terms that label the opposing sides are argumentative: "Prolife" for the antiabortion group and "Prochoice" for those in favor of allowing unrestricted legal abortions.

Historical Perspective

Until the mid-1800s, abortions were legal in the United States. Based on English common law, abortion was not a legal matter until quickening, the moment when the fetus could be felt moving in the womb. Although abortions were legal, they were not safe. The first laws concerning abortions were aimed at abortionists, whose dangerous practices harmed or killed women they purported to treat. By 1871, the American Medical Association (AMA) had begun to criticize abortion on moral grounds. Its committee on Criminal Abortion wrote that a woman who sought an abortion is "unmindful of the course marked out for her by Providence."

Home Pregnancy Tests

Product Names: Factplus, Answer Plus, Advance, e.p.t., First Response, QTest, Daisy 2

What They Do: Measure the amount of a hormone called human chorionic gonadotropin (HCG) in urine. This hormone is produced by the developing placenta and excreted in the urine.

Procedure: A urine sample is taken and mixed with chemicals in a test tube. With one-step tests, the solution will change color if the result is positive.

Time for Results: 10 to 30 minutes.

Cost: About $8 to $12 for a single test, or $10 to $17 for a double test kit.

Comments: The first morning sample of urine contains the highest concentration of HCG, and therefore should give the most reliable result. Any traces of soap in the container can produce a false result. Home pregnancy tests are particularly useful for women who must wait several weeks to get a doctor's appointment. Some manufacturers report that their tests will pick up a positive result the same day as a missed period.

Furthermore, the AMA maintained that women were "shirking their responsibilities of maternity." By 1900, every state in the nation had made abortion a crime, but these laws were rarely enforced. When pressure mounted to make abortions illegal, the discussions turned more to moral issues than health or medical professionalism.

Until after World War II, the situation drifted along and illegal abortions were generally accepted, but not publicly approved. During the 1950s, the national mood turned conservative, and women who chose abortion were described as "bad girls" who became "pregnant out of wedlock." Then, in the 1960s, the pendulum swung back toward a more liberal position and, with the insistence of the National Organization for Women, abortion again became a public issue. Several state legislatures passed laws allowing abortions to be performed under specific criteria, such as when pregnancy threatened the mother's life or when it resulted from rape. State laws prohibiting abortion were challenged on the basis of an inherent constitutional right of privacy.

Abortion Medical Procedures

Abortions are most commonly performed by widening the cervix and removing the contents of the uterus with a suction device. A curette is used to remove any remaining tissue. Later in pregnancy, forceps may be used and occasionally labor is induced so that the uterine contents are expelled.

Abortions typically cost about $200 at a clinic and the majority of them (about 90 percent) are performed in the first trimester. Later abortions may have to be performed in a hospital at much higher cost.

The majority of abortions take only ten minutes, but a woman having an abortion must plan to spend at least two or three hours at the clinic. During this time she can receive counseling, give her medical history, and prepare for surgery. Most first-trimester abortions are performed under local anesthesia and are not painful to the woman; a second-trimester abortion may require a pain-killing drug. There may be cramping during the procedure and bleeding afterward. As with any procedure, there are risks, particularly infection and hemorrhage; and, the later the abortion is performed, the more risky it becomes. However, studies show that abortion is safer than childbirth for women of all ages, especially for teens and older women, both prone to delivery complications. Planned Parenthood says that up to 25 weeks, abortion remains safer than childbirth.

Having an abortion does not affect a woman's chances for having a successful pregnancy later. A recent report from the Surgeon General's office indicates that infertility, miscarriage, and premature births are no more common among women who have had abortions than those who have not. Studies do show, however, that there is an increased risk if a woman has had several abortions and experienced at least one infection.

According to reputable physicians, such as Dr. David Grimes at the University of Southern California School of Medicine, the fetus does not feel pain because the brain and nervous system are not developed to the stage where the sensation of pain can be felt. Right-to-Life proponents disagree with this conclusion, citing the fact that a fetus reacts to touch as early as eight weeks, as evidence of the pain sensation being present.

Abortion Techniques and Risks

Abortions should be performed before the twelfth week, if possible, because the complications and risks are less during this time. First trimester abortions are performed by two methods.

Vacuum Aspiration Developed in China in the late 1950s, this method has become the preferred technique because it lessens the chance of uterine perforation, reduces blood loss, and reduces the time of the procedure. A hose-linked curette, a metal, spoon-like instrument, is inserted into the dilated cervix. The hose is attached to suction, and the uterine contents are emptied in 20 to 30 seconds. A little cramping may occur during the procedure. So that no fragments of tissue are left, the physician scrapes the uterine lining with the curette. After two or three hours in the recovery room, the woman is usually feeling well enough to be discharged. She is instructed not to douche, use tampons, or have intercourse for at least one week following the abortion. A follow-up visit is important to determine that the abortion was complete and that no infection is present.

Dilatation and Curettage (D & C) The cervical canal is dilated with a series of instruments, increasingly graduated in diameter size. After the cervix is dilated, the tissue is removed with forceps and the lining of the uterus is scraped with the curette to assure that all products of conception are removed. The procedure takes fifteen to twenty minutes and is usually done under local anesthesia. Recovery time is a little longer than vacuum aspirations due to a greater blood loss.

Hysterotomy A second-trimester abortion technique, this method is a major surgical procedure. It is performed between the fourteenth and sixteenth week of pregnancy. An incision is made through the abdominal wall into the uterus and the products of conception are removed with forceps; the uterine cavity is then curetted to remove remaining tissue. The client requires general or spinal anesthesia and several days of hospitalization.

Intraamniotic Injection or Prostaglandins Abortion These methods, also performed between the fourteenth to sixteenth week of pregnancy, have largely replaced the hysterotomy. The procedure is to replace a certain amount of amniotic fluid with hypertonic saline. The increased osmotic pressure of the amniotic fluid causes the death of the fetus. Uterine contractions usually begin in about twelve hours and the products of con-

"Abortion Pill" in the News

RU 486, an "abortion pill" currently available in France and China, has sparked controversy in the United States. Used experimentally by 12,000 French women, experts say it works 80 to 95 percent of the time. Used alone, it is most effective within five weeks of a missed period. The only side effect reported is bleeding which has been reported in .01 percent of the cases.

One side of the controversy, Prochoice, believes that this drug could make ending an unwanted pregnancy safer, cheaper (it costs about $100), and more private than abortions are today. They believe RU 486 will be available in the United States within five years, legally or illegally.

The opposing view is that this drug can cause birth defects, bleeding, and infertility. At present, Right-to-Life groups are keeping this drug out of the United States, believing the drug to be dangerous and, in fact, opposing all methods of abortion.

No one knows which side is correct, and currently there is no testing in progress. It could take two to five years of testing to actually find the answer. No U.S. pharmaceutical firm has applied for a license to begin testing, partly due to concern over boycotts and possibility of liability lawsuits.

Sexual Health

ception are expelled in 24 to 30 hours. Drugs to stimulate contractions may be given if they do not begin naturally. Recovery period is slightly longer than for the suction method.

Prostaglandins, hormone-like acids, cause abortion by stimulating the uterus to contract. They may be administered IV into the amniotic sac or inserted through the cervical canal into the uterus. The IV method is less effective and has more possible side effects than the cervical method.

Abortion Complications

The incidence of complications following abortion is greatly reduced if, in addition to it being performed early in the pregnancy, there is the use of the suction procedure rather than a major surgical one. Local anesthesia is safer than general, and good client care is essential. When the abortion is performed by a well-trained clinician and the client is counseled about follow-up care and a return visit, complications are significantly reduced.

Bleeding during or following the procedure is unlikely with the vacuum method. Hemorrhage can occur with medical procedures, but vigilant monitoring will help prevent a serious outcome.

Infection is another complication which can be reduced by preabortion testing and counseling to determine the presence of a sexually transmitted disease. Also, the use of antibiotics given routinely for abortion has reduced the incidence of infection. Again, counseling and a postabortion examination reduce the chances of serious complications.

Uterine perforation, while uncommon, can occur. Using a well-trained clinician who understands the importance of early abortion (or the methods appropriate to later abortion), as well as the necessity for careful and slow dilation of the cervix in order not to create trauma, is important to reduce the risks.

Risk of Death

Legal abortions have greatly reduced the risk of death. Statistics show that only 1 in 400,000 deaths occur when abortion is performed on pregnancies of less than nine weeks duration, and 1 in 100,000 between 13 and 16 weeks; after 16 weeks, the death risk is 1 in 10,000. These figures, when compared to the risk of death by continuing the pregnancy (1 in 10,000) or by having an illegal abortion (1 in 3,000), are quite dramatic. In fact, the most fearsome possibility, according to Prochoice leaders, is the return to murderous, illegal abortions. In the years prior to *Roe*, abortions performed in filthy conditions using bleach, coat hangers, and knitting needles left some women dead—11 in 1972—and others unable to have children.

Abortion Issues

The issues surrounding abortion are complex and thought-provoking. Each separate argument for and against abortion has relevant points of view. A major study done on abortion in 1984 by Luker (*Abortion and the Politics of Motherhood*), identified four major positions on the issue.

- *The moral status of the embryo.* The status of the embryo has long been ambiguous. One philosophical position is that only beings with a capacity for conscious self-reflective intelligence are considered living beings. Arguments centering on the legal status of the fetus, the timing of abortions, and the value of children are central to this position.
- *When life actually begins.* Even though the heartbeat of a developing fetus can be observed by the end of the first month, no one agrees on what this fact means. Does the presence of a heartbeat prove that life exists; if so, what does the ability to breathe mean? If life requires both functions, when does life for a fetus begin? Since it is still nearly impossible to save an infant before the 23rd week because the lungs are not sufficiently developed, this issue is difficult to resolve.
- *Is the embryo a person?* One valid argument centers around the issue of when a fetus becomes a person who is able to assume the inalienable rights to due process associated with a living human being. A corollary issue is the allocation of scarce resources, which also impacts on the belief of worth and value of every person. A final question that relates to the issue of personhood: if an embryo can be destroyed, what is to stop our society from deciding that another segment of our society should not receive care?
- *The woman's role in our society.* The woman's rights as an individual and her role in society is the final controversial issue. A woman's right to determine what happens to her body, as well as her right to exercise control over her reproductive system, is one side of the argument. Opponents to this view fear that the role of motherhood may be threatened and devalued if legal abortion is allowed to exist.

Paths to the Abortion Clinic

Why do women make the choice to have an abortion? Their reasons for ending a pregnancy are complex and varied and seem to be based on their own individual situations. The circumstances most frequently cited by the 1.6 million women who receive abortions every year fall into six major areas. According to studies by the Alan Guttmacher Institute, an independent research center, women cite the following reasons for choosing an abortion. Here are the stories of six women—all of whom chose an abortion.

- *An unmarried woman whose partner is afraid of fatherhood:* "I would have this baby in a second if my boyfriend weren't so set against it." The man is either unwilling to marry or not ready to father a child, so the woman chooses not to go it alone.
- *A teenager is not ready to bear the burden of an adult:* "I'm not ready for the responsibility of a baby, even if my boyfriend were willing to marry me." Teenagers feel overwhelmed and unprepared to accept the emotional and financial responsibility of a baby.

Abortion Statistics and Religion in College Students

A Gallup survey was done to determine how religion affects sexual attitudes and practices of college students. Five hundred thirty-nine undergraduates were randomly selected from 100 institutions, including two and four year colleges and universities. Protestants, Catholics, and "Born-Again" Christians were the predominant religions represented. Forty-two percent said religion was very important in their lives.

- One in ten women now attending college has had an abortion at some time in her life.
- Nine percent of the women surveyed said they had had at least one abortion, fifteen percent of the men said at least one of their sexual partners had had an abortion.
- Four percent of the students said they had been treated at some time for a sexually transmitted disease.

These findings, while startling to some, are consistent with the number of estimated abortions in the country every year. Of 6 million pregnancies in 1982, 46 percent were unintended. Based on 1982 figures, 14 percent of women between ages 15 and 19, and 27 percent of women between ages 20 and 24, have had abortions at some time in their lives.

Sexual Health

- *A drug abuser cannot cope with her own life and cannot even contemplate accepting responsibility of a baby*: "I've had four abortions and, for most of them, I've been on so many drugs it seemed like the right decision." This woman went on to say, "Birth control, as easy as it seems, is not easy when you're out rockin' and rollin'."
- *No room in the home for another child*: Many families who are not financially secure feel that another child will place an undue emotional or financial burden on them. "My baby is too young for me to have another one"; or more commonly, "We have low-paying jobs and can barely make ends meet. Another baby would really increase the financial pressure."
- *Bad luck, bad timing*: A moment of indiscretion and lack of planning resulted in an unplanned pregnancy. "I'm the kind of girl who doesn't sleep around, but this time it was just a spur of the moment thing; I don't even really know the guy, and I certainly don't love him."
- *A career woman sees her life goals falling apart*: An unplanned pregnancy at this point would put her career on hold. "I want to work, make money, and achieve things in life—a baby just won't fit into these plans."

The abortion issue is so laden with emotional responses that a rational, scholarly debate seems impossible. It remains for each person to consider this issue, not only from a personal point of view, but also from a philosophical, moral, ethical, and even health perspective. None of these aspects, however, will be relevant if, ultimately, the courts choose to decide the issue.

Abortion and the Courts

When does life begin? At the time of conception when sperm and egg meet, or when a baby can survive on its own outside the mother's womb? Is it a woman's right to choose abortion for herself, or the government's right to choose it for her? If women are required by law to have children, should the lawmakers be forced to pay for their support? Whose life is more important, the fetus's or the mother's? Should the government pay for abortions? Does a woman's right to an abortion mean she does not have to inform the father—or her parents—if she chooses to have one? What are the rights of the prospective father? Is abortion a sin? Is it a crime?

These are only a few of the questions haunting the issue of abortion in the United States today. Political and judicial lines have been drawn between people who believe in a woman's right to choose and those who champion absolute right to life. The controversy continues to rage in abortion clinics, on the streets, in state legislatures, and in the courts. Once again the U.S. Supreme Court has been asked to rule on abortion, and its decisions will shape the legal answers to the nation's many questions concerning abortion—questions that involve personal freedom, morality, religion, politics, money, and the meaning of life and death itself.

A landmark Supreme Court decision in 1973 confirmed the privacy issue by ruling 7 to 2 that abortions were legal during the first trimester. The *Roe vs. Wade* decision marked the beginning of acknowledging that our nation's constitution gives a woman the right to an abortion on demand. States could not restrict abortions during the first trimester of pregnancy, but they were allowed to maintain certain controls over conditions

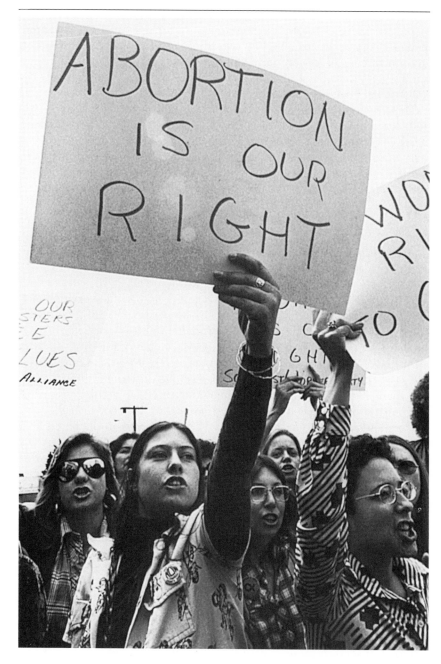

for abortions during the second and last trimester. Questions such as whether states or the Federal government could withhold funds for abortion were not addressed in *Roe vs. Wade*, and the controversy surrounding these issues has continued in the courts since 1973.

Abortions in the United States increased after the *Roe* decision and leveled off at around 1.6 million per year. About 30 percent of all pregnancies, excluding stillbirths and miscarriages, are terminated by abortion. One-fifth of American women above the age of 15 have had an abortion; 81 percent were unmarried at the time, and more than 25 percent were teenagers. The reasons given by two-thirds of those having an abortion were that they could not afford the child or were not ready for motherhood. The Gallup Organization announced in early 1989 that 9 percent of college women surveyed admitted to having at least one abortion.

The emotional battle over abortion has continued to rage between the right-to-life advocates and those who are committed to keeping abortion legal. Abortion cases continued to be heard by the Supreme Court. One case, *Webster vs. Reproductive Health Services*, centers around a 1986 Missouri law that states life begins at conception. Because of the law, any doctor, clinic, or hospital in Missouri receiving state monies is prohibited from performing abortions except to save the life of the mother. On July 3, 1989, the Supreme Court decided to uphold the Missouri statute. Although this ruling does not take away a woman's right to abortion, the Court's decision signals a possible shift. Broad Federal policy may now begin to give way to state-by-state abortion rulings.

If the U.S. Supreme Court ultimately turns the abortion issue back to the individual states, the controversy is certain to become very political. Individual states may enact laws to obstruct abortion by prohibiting government funding, increasing the cost (now about $200 to $250), adding paperwork burdens for doctors and hospitals, and discouraging abortion counseling. With the abortion issue in the states' political arena, impact from the opposing sides may throw legislative and gubernatorial races into chaos. Each state could become a battleground with antiabortion and Prochoice candidates vying for support from their constituencies.

Ten states continue to have pre-1973 abortion laws on the books, but whether they will be implemented is not known. Legislatures in six states have already said they will ban abortion. On the other side are states with a long tradition of favoring abortion rights—California, New York, Oregon, Washington, and Hawaii among them. These states are among the 16 that permitted abortion before the *Roe* decision. Several states protect privacy in their state constitutions which is a powerful tool for Prochoice advocates; these states include Hawaii, California, Illinois, Montana, and New Jersey.

Another option for each state is to put the issue on the ballot. Recent elections in Virginia and New York were strongly influenced by the abortion issue. Prochoice candidates narrowly won over Prolife candidates, and while their success cannot specifically be attributed to the abortion issue, political analysts believe that it had a critical impact.

While the Prolife and Prochoice groups capture headlines with massive demonstrations, what are the views and thoughts of millions of others in America? Interestingly, the National Opinion Research Center shows that the country's stance on abortion has changed little since the first opinion poll in 1965. The center's polls show that the majority of the United States citizens support legalized abortion when the pregnancy results from rape or when the baby is likely to have a serious birth defect. Other reasons for abortion (the woman is unmarried, poor, or does not want another child) are not as acceptable to the general population; less than half think that a legal abortion should be available. Specific percentages from a 1988 Gallup poll indicate that 57 percent believe abortion should be legal under certain circumstances; 24 percent, legal under many circumstances; 17 percent, under all circumstances; and 2 percent have no opinion. However, as the opposing sides become more polarized and more visible, there may be shifts in public opinion. These philosophical viewpoints may manifest as political victories or losses in state elections.

The controversy over abortion is far from concluded. If anything, it seems destined to be a main issue for the 1990s in state politics as well as the courts. If each state decides the issue independently, it may never be resolved on a national level.

Sexual Orientation

A frequent concern of college students is whether they are straight or gay. This is probably more of a concern today because of a new openness toward homosexuality and the proliferation of a number of different role models. It can also lead to a great deal of confusion.

Unfortunately, there is no simple test and no easy answer. Are you straight or gay? The answer is a definite yes, maybe, both, and sometimes.

Most people experience close attachments to members of the same sex and some form a sexual relationship. The sex researcher Kinsey used to claim that on a scale of one to seven, with one being exclusively heterosexual and seven being exclusively homosexual, most of us would fall on a bell shape curve with an average of about four. Societal pressures keep people from admitting this, even to themselves.

Most people who begin to worry about their sexual orientation first try to find answers in books. This is usually not helpful since there are books that will support almost any point of view. The trick is to find out what you want to be and then find the books and other resources, including support groups, to help you and reinforce that choice.

Most helpful is to find an understanding counselor or friend who will talk the whole subject out with you over a period of time, but who will not enter into a sexual relationship with you. Discovering who you are is not a process that can be done in a couple of hours. You have to experiment.

Sexual Health

You have to try on new ideas. Above all, you have to be honest with yourself. Experience alone is often not enough for college-aged students. All of these things have to come together with the realization that you are always changing. No matter what you decide, you will feel more comfortable if you reach out to other people with similar lifestyles. Join support groups. Remember, almost everyone goes through similar questioning and, therefore, no matter what your questions, you are not alone. No matter what you decide your sexual orientation is, be aware of open communication and methods to prevent sexually transmitted diseases.

Why Are Some People Homosexual?

As more and more research is done, there is a move away from the idea that homosexuality is pathological and that whatever causes it is pathological (like domineering mothers, distant fathers, or child abusers). The idea that homosexuality is not an illness is becoming more and more accepted. In fact, according to James Krajeski, chairman of the American Psychiatric Association's committee on gay, lesbian, and bisexual issues, many are now suggesting that early influences may be biological. Gay activists generally endorse such theories, proposing that sexual preference is really not a matter of choice—the child is born this way and that it is a normal state for a segment of the population. Of course, there are numerous dissenters to these theories; many believe that the idea that people are born into one type of sexual preference is foolish—homosexuality is a behavior, not a condition. This controversy will not be resolved until hard scientific data are available to validate one side or the other.

Rape and Sexual Assault

No one has the right to touch you sexually if you do not want to be touched. If you firmly believe this, you can be clear in your messages and set firm limits. Exceeding those limits against your will is sexual assault or rape and is clearly against the law in all states. You have a right, and perhaps a duty, to file complaints with appropriate authorities when sexual assault takes place. When community standards are clear that sexual assault will not be tolerated, then less sexual assault will occur.

Most people think that forcible sexual penetration of a woman by a male stranger is the most common form of rape or sexual assault. However, in reality, that is the least common. Sexual assault does not have to involve penetration. Moreover, most sexual assault takes place between people who know each other. If the people involved are related, then it is called incest. Males have been sexually assaulted by men and women, and are less likely than women to report it.

College students can easily get into situations called date rape or acquaintance rape. The psychological trauma can be just as great as assault by a stranger. In date-rape situations, one or both members of the couple have usually been drinking and therefore inhibitions and controls are

The key to rape prevention is to increase women's independence, confidence, assertiveness and self-esteem.

Leslie Simon
Coordinator, Anti-Rape Workshop
University of California
at San Francisco

A Definition of Terms

Masturbation   Excitation of one's genital organs by manual contact or a means other than intercourse. Masturbation is a common sexual outlet for many people and contrary to myths, it does not cause sterility or blindness. For those who are incarcerated or require long-term care, this may be the only means for gratifying sexual needs. Very frequent or inappropriate masturbation, however, may be harmful to one's health. Also, this form of gratification is not a substitute for maintaining a loving, intimate relationship with another human being—it is meeting a physical-sexual need for gratification, not a human need for interpersonal contact.

Transvestite   This term refers to one who enjoys wearing clothes of the opposite sex—the person may or may not be homosexual and often is not. It is simply an individual who wishes to wear clothing, either undergarments or outer, that is usually worn by the opposite sex.

Transsexual   A person who has an overwhelming desire to be the other sex and who chooses sexual reassignment. This is a very complex procedure and involves surgical intervention as well as psychological and social counseling as a part of the process of assuming the gender identity, sex, role, sexual object choice, and sexual behavior of the opposite sex.

Homosexual   A person who prefers and establishes patterns of intimacy and sexual behavior with a member of one's own sex. This sexual object choice has a strong influence on the person's lifestyle—for example, the choices of whether or not to be a parent, where to live, and even what career path to follow.

Self-Help Hotlines

National Gay Task Force; Crisisline: (800) 221-7044; (212) 807-6016 in NY, AK and HI.

National Abortion Federation: (800) 772-9100; (202) 546-9060 in Washington, DC area.

Bethany Lifeline: (800) 238-4269. Referrals to professional counseling, adoption services.

National Pregnancy Hotline: (800) 233-6058; (800) 831-5881 in CA.

PMS Access: (800) 222-4767; (608) 833-4767 in WI.

VD Hotline: (800) 227-8922; (800) 982-5883 in CA.

lessened. Messages about what each partner wants are often unclear because of miscommunication and unclear signals. Respect your partners. Believe that no means no. Limit alcohol consumption in situations where sexual activity might take place. Openly state your limits in clear, unambiguous language, and avoid situations in which you might feel at risk.

If you are sexually assaulted, you will most likely feel ashamed and dirty. The terrible thing about sexual assault is that the victim suffers more than the assailant. Remember that you are not alone. Others have experienced this and are willing to support you. Contact your campus women's center, college health service, or local sexual assault counseling center. They can help you with the immediate crisis of feeling helpless as well as provide medical and legal advice. Seriously consider filing charges; that means do not destroy evidence by bathing or changing clothes. Sexual assault is a community-wide problem that we all have a responsibility to prevent.

Sexual Health

Acquaintance Rape—A Serious Campus Problem

Beginning college is an exciting, enriching experience for most students, but for some, this period of transition from adolescence to adulthood is marred by sexual violence in the form of acquaintance rape. Betrayal in this fashion by a friend or lover is an alarmingly common experience for many college women.

What is Acquaintance Rape?

Rape is an act of violence. In most states, it is legally defined as vaginal, oral, or anal penetration with a penis or other object, committed against the wishes of the victim by the use of force or threat of harm.

Even though the legal definition does not address the social factors involved in the situation, a lot of confusion surrounds acquaintance rape simply because of the relationship between victim and offender. For example, factors such as prior sexual contact between the two, whether she allowed him to buy her an expensive dinner, or if she went alone with him to his room are legally irrelevant when determining whether a rape has occurred. However, some people consider that these social factors minimize the forced nature of the act and justify the intercourse that follows. As a result, many people avoid calling it rape. But sexual penetration is rape whenever the act takes place against the will of the victim, no matter how well people know each other. And the fact is that more women are raped by boyfriends, dates, or people they know than by strangers.

Acquaintance rape, then, is forced intercourse by someone the victim knows. It may be her boyfriend, her roommate's brother, or someone she hardly knows, such as a classmate or member of a study group. The term "date rape" is often used interchangeably with "acquaintance rape" to indicate that the rape has occurred in a social situation.

How Serious is the Problem?

Most women deny the reality of rape because it is such a threatening prospect. However, research indicates the problem is widespread and that this denial is dangerous. Over 50 percent of college women report having been the victim of some form of sexual assault or offense, and 25 percent say they have experienced an attempted or completed rape. More than 10 percent of college men report having forced a woman to have intercourse against her will at least once, while 35 percent report they would rape if they could be assured of no detection or penalty.

Acquaintance rape occurs most frequently between the senior year of high school and the end of freshman year of college. During this transitional period both male and female students risk involvement in sexual coercion. The statistics are too high to ignore. Although the overwhelming number of victims are female, males are also victims of sexual aggression. In most of these cases the offender is another male. Once again, the key element of a sexual assault is the victim's lack of consent.

The Date Who Rapes

It is a myth that rape is sex. Rape, in fact, is an invasive, violent act which uses sex as the weapon. It is intentional, interpersonal harm of the most intimate nature.

Contrary to popular belief, men who rape do not have overwhelming sexual desires that need immediate gratification. They are neither sex starved, nor have they become aroused to the point when they are no longer responsible for their actions. Men who rape do so to satisfy unmet psychological needs to feel adequate and powerful or to express their anger and hostility. The rapist is aroused by the struggle of the victim rather than by the sexual activity itself. Nonrapists respond very differently to the resistance of a sex partner. They interrupt lovemaking at the first sign of their partner's distress or resistance. They are excited by passion and pleasure, not power and pain.

Research informs us that men who rape tend to be extremely traditional in their attitudes toward women, and they are often described as "macho." Dating is a contest in which there are winners and losers. The sexually aggressive male believes he is justified to force sex under certain conditions. For example, if he spends a lot of money on a date, he thinks he is entitled to sexual compensation. He may also believe that if he and his partner have had sex before, or if she agrees to have sex and then changes her mind, then he is entitled to force intercourse. Frequently, this sexually aggressive male believes a woman would never admit to wanting sex, and he sees his role as conquering her resistance. He hears her say no but is convinced she means yes. Because he is sexually aggressive, he won't take no for an answer.

Men who rape don't view women as friends or equals, but rather as sex objects. Their major motivation is to "get some," "grab a piece," or "get laid." The wishes or welfare of their women are of no concern. Women are viewed as interchangeable objects serving only one purpose—to gratify the man's need to be powerful and in control.

The Date Who is Raped

Little is known about acquaintance rape victims because so few share their experience with anyone. In a major study of 35 college campuses, only five percent of the women students who said they had been raped reported the event to anyone in authority. Many carry the traumatic feelings and consequences associated with rape long after the event.

The most disturbing factor in these statistics is that the common denominator of acquaintance rape seems to be dating. Simply stated, women who date are at a higher risk than those who do not because they are accessible to more sexually aggressive behavior. It is an unfortunate fact that the act of socializing presents risk for all women. The fact is that

the risk of victimization can be reduced, and the most important element of prevention is education.

Students who are especially vulnerable are those who are unaware that acquaintance rape exists. The belief, "It will never happen to me," is illusory, and it does not prepare the individual to cope with coercive sexual situations as part of the dating scene. Studies show that women who escape rape recognize danger early in the interaction and get out of the situation. These "early avoiders" act immediately. Therefore, the more women learn about sexually coercive situations and offenders, the more they will be prepared to deal with the scenarios that can arise.

Another vulnerable group of students are those who have not developed their own sexual value system, including an awareness of their personal sexual limits. Recognizing your sexual limits immediately alerts you when someone is violating your personal sexual boundaries or value system. The situation can thus be handled before it escalates into a dangerous confrontation.

Many experts believe that sex role socialization predisposes women toward greater vulnerability. Women who are socialized in the traditional feminine role of passivity and submission may have an increased risk of rape. Early socialization of females often teaches them to be agreeable and to provide only positive responses to male requests. These women may have difficulty communicating sexual limits for

fear of rejecting a date and hurting his feelings. Unclear communication patterns create double messages. This allows the sexually aggressive male to select the message of his choice. The man who is overly aggressive sexually counts on a woman's reluctance to offend or assert herself even at the expense of her own well-being.

Contributing Factors

Certain factors exacerbate the occurrence of acquaintance rape. Dating expectations between males and females often differ. In general, women are more interested than men in forming close relationships involving love and commitment. Many men, on the other hand, are more interested in casual sex without the complications of a serious relationship. Unless clear communication is practiced by both parties, these different goals and expectations of the relationship may create misperceptions and misunderstandings. Sexual violence is sometimes a result.

Peer pressure is another prominent factor in sexual aggression. Very often men rape as a way of gaining status with other men, not for sexual gratification. Sexually aggressive men, therefore, reinforce sexual violence in others as a measure of masculinity. Unfortunately, this view presents a very narrow picture of masculinity, since being a man is much more than achieving sexual conquest. In this context, women are not considered friends, but a means by which men can display dominance and masculinity. It is interesting that sexually aggressive men almost never identify their behavior as rape.

The use of alcohol and drugs cannot be ignored as contributing factors in acquaintance rape. Alcohol is often used to impair a victim's judgment so that she is unable to recognize coercive clues to which she would ordinarily respond. Alcohol also reduces the aggressor's inhibitions about using force, and provides him with an excuse for inexcusable behaviors—under the guise that he did not know what he was doing. Drinking is, in fact, reported by 75 percent of offending males and 50 percent of female victims.

What Women Can Do

Unfortunately, there is no guaranteed way to avoid acquaintance rape. The best protection is your awareness that the possibility exists. You may find yourself in a situation in which you have to defend yourself. It is vital that you remain aware of your surroundings and stay tuned in to your feelings. At the first sign of uneasiness, act! Think back to those times when you had a feeling that something was wrong. Did you act on it? Learn to listen to that voice now, and use your sixth sense to protect yourself.

You may want to consider incorporating these 3 R's into your repertoire of responses:

Reduce the possibility of assault by

- Learning all you can about acquaintance rape in advance.
- Avoiding places that isolate you from support assistance.
- Eliminating the use of drugs or alcohol around people you do not know well.

Resist his efforts

- To wear down your resolve. Ignoring his partner's protests is the most common strategy used by sexually aggressive males. Do not do anything you do not want to do. This includes drinking more than you can handle or doing things sexually for which you are not ready.
- To make you feel guilty. You do not owe him anything. It is your right to say no, just as it is your responsibility to firmly communicate your sexual limits.

Remember, if you become a victim

- It is not your fault. No one asks to be raped.
- You do not deserve it. No matter what the circumstances, rape is never acceptable as a punishment or power play. It is always a crime, and the criminal is the rapist.
- Tell someone you trust. It helps to talk. This is the first step to your recovery.
- There are some circumstances in which rape is totally unavoidable no matter how much you know or how well you are prepared.

What Men Can Do

Our culture puts a tremendous amount of pressure on males to perform and conform. Often your individual needs are ignored as you try to meet everyone's expectations. This is especially true of sexual performance as a measure of masculinity. This pressure can create tensions with you that are sometimes expressed as sexual aggression against dates and friends. Using someone else in order to gain status within a group is never acceptable. Males who are comfortable with their own sexuality do not have to rape to feel like real men. Remember real men take *no* for an answer.

To avoid serious consequences for yourself, consider the following suggestions:

Stop

- Believing the myths about rape, the victims, and victimizers. Learn the facts about the acts and actors involved in rape.
- Confusing rape with sex. Learn the difference between seduction and rape. Recognize that struggle and sex do not go together. Sex and caring do.

Look

- At the facts. The FBI predicts that one out of three women will be a victim of sexual assault. Someone you know and care about will be a statistic.
- For ways to reduce the occurrence of sexual victimization, learn all you can about rape.

Become part of the solution, not part of the problem.

Listen

- To what your partner says. Assume "no" means "no," not "maybe." The question of consent is crucial. A "yes" can never be assumed, and a "no" should not be ignored. Be sure you hear verbal consent before you proceed sexually. Without it you risk a rape charge.
- To someone who tells you about her rape experience. Your understanding and concern will impact strongly on how she recovers. Learn how you can help her on the road to recovery.
- Do not listen to rape jokes. They present rape as funny and acceptable.

A Last Word

Rape is rape. You cannot disguise it to make it look good, acceptable, or not harmful. It always involves coercion, and one person always suffers as a result. One communicates personal values, feelings of self-worth, and feelings about a partner through sexual activity. Indeed, it is the most intimate form of communication. When we make love, it is an act of human bonding. It is anticipating responding, giving pleasure to another. Rape, on the other hand, is an exploitative activity in which one person uses another in an effort to feel more adequate or powerful.

Claire P. Walsh, PhD

Seeking Professional Help

When to Seek Help

Health care professionals can help you take care of your sexual health in many ways, whether you are suffering from discomfort, are evaluating contraceptive options, are worried that you might be pregnant, or just have a couple of questions about sexual issues. Definitely seek professional help if:

- You are sexually active (or are considering being sexually active) and are not consistently using effective methods of contraception and STD prevention.
- You want to be able to discuss sexual issues more clearly with your partner but are unsure what to say.
- You suspect (or know) that you or a sexual partner has been exposed to an STD.
- You experience any of the symptoms of STDs listed earlier in the chapter (including, but not limited to, itching, rash, sores) and have been sexually active.
- You experience pain, difficulty, or burning while urinating.
- You discover any lumps or other unexplained changes in your sexual organs.

If you are a woman, see a health care provider if:

- Your period is 10 or more days late.
- Your periods are painful or you have PMS that has not responded to self-care treatment.
- You do not know how to perform a breast self-exam.
- You have not had a pap smear in the past year.

If you are a man, see a health care provider if:

- You do not know how to perform a testicular self-exam.
- You are experiencing sexual functioning problems on a recurring basis (at times other than when you are intoxicated).

Types of Help Available

Your campus health service may include or can refer you to a gynecologist for women's reproductive health issues or a urologist for men's reproductive health issues. Contraceptive counseling may be available from physicians, nurse-practitioners specializing in contraception, or peer counselors—students with special training in contraception and other issues related to sexuality. For some situations, psychological counseling is useful. If you prefer to see someone off campus, consult a family planning clinic in the community.

Beyond the Text

1. You have had sexual relations with two people in the past two weeks. You suspect that you now have an STD. What would you do? What would you say to your former partners?

2. Respond to the following statement: Contraception is a woman's responsibility.

3. After observing for several months, you are pretty sure your roommate is gay (or lesbian), but he/she hasn't mentioned anything. How do you feel? What do you do, if anything?

4. You suspect that your roommate is a victim of acquaintance rape. What should she/he do and why? What advice should you give?

5. Your roommate's sister says that she thinks she is pregnant and wants to have an abortion. What advice would you give her?

6. Respond to the following statement: If you don't have symptoms, you don't have a sexually transmitted disease.

Supplemental Readings

Every Women's Guide to Breast Cancer by Vicki Seltzer, MD. New York: Penguin Books, 1988. Up-to-date resource that answers questions concerning prevention, treatment, and aftermath of breast cancer.

How to Protect Yourself From STDs by Stephen H. Zinner, MD. New York: Summit Books, 1985. A practical "how to or not to" guide that gives authentic information essential for health for those who are sexually active.

Male Sexuality by Bernie Zilbergeld, PhD. New York: Bantam Books, 1978. An enlightened guide to sexual fulfillment for men. Deals with both physical and psychological aspects of sex for men.

New Our Bodies, Ourselves by Boston Women's Health Book Collective. New York: Random House, 1985. One of the best guides to female sexuality, with a comprehensive discussion on birth control.

Private Parts: A Doctor's Guide to the Male Anatomy by Yosh Taguchi, MD. New York: Doubleday, 1989. Explains how the body functions and answers questions about male sexual diseases and conditions generally not understood by most males.

The Complete Guide to Women's Health by Bruce D. Shephard, MD, and Carroll A. Shephard, RN, PhD. New York: New American Library, 1985. A comprehensive presentation with practical information on all facets of women's sexual health. Also covers many other health topics from acne to weight.

Key Terms Defined

abortion the premature removal or expulsion of an embryo from the uterus

AIDS acronym for acquired immune deficiency syndrome, a sexually transmitted disease that weakens the immune system

amenorrhea the absence of menstrual periods

contraception methods used for preventing pregnancy before conception

epididymis part of the seminal duct in which sperm collects until ejaculation

genitalia the reproductive organs

homosexuality sexual and emotional orientation toward someone of the same sex

hormones endocrine gland secretions of chemical substances into the body

impotence male sexual dysfunction; failure to achieve a penile erection, in spite of sexual stimulation

mammogram a film produced by roentgenogram of the breast

menstruation periodic discharge through the vagina of blood and tissue from the nonpregnant uterus

Pap smear test in which cells are removed from the cervix and examined under a microscope for signs of cancer

PMS a variety of symptoms that include physical and psychological distress occurring a few days before a woman's menstrual period

prostate gland gland surrounding the male urethra that secretes the primary fluid in semen

rape a violent act of coercion which results in forcible sexual penetration

sexually transmitted diseases (STDs) infectious diseases, such as chlamydia, gonorrhea, syphilis, herpes, and AIDS, that are spread by sexual contact

sterilization any procedure that renders a person incapable of reproduction

The AIDS Crisis

In 1981, physicians reported the first deaths of patients who suffered from a vast collection of disorders, all the result of an impaired immune system. This disease came to be known as AIDS, or Acquired Immune Deficiency Syndrome.

Since those early cases were recorded, the number of AIDS cases has grown exponentially. United States' statistics are chilling: over 100,000 reported cases of the disease, of whom 68,000 have died. Deaths have more than doubled since 1987.

No one is immune to AIDS. Nevertheless, the virus has not yet spread widely outside the two major risk groups of homosexual (or bisexual) men and intravenous (IV) drug abusers. These two groups make up 91 percent of all AIDS cases.

This chapter is presented in a unique format—a series of questions and answers. Over 25 of the most commonly asked questions about AIDS are discussed clearly and concisely so that you can obtain factual data about this disease. Researchers continue to search for a cure for AIDS, but positive results are not expected in the immediate future. Meanwhile, education programs attempt to help individuals make informed choices based upon accurate and current information.

Key Terms

AIDS	Helper T-cells	Opportunistic infections
Antibodies	High-risk behavior	*Pneumocystis carinii pneumonia*
ARC	HIV antibody test	Safe sex
AZT	Immunity	Virus
Carrier	Kaposi's sarcoma	

Contents

AIDS Overview

Though everyone refers to the AIDS virus, in fact the virus responsible for AIDS is officially known as the HIV-I, or human immunodeficiency virus, type I. Researchers in France and in the United States discovered isolates of the virus and gave the virus different names. To simplify this multiple nomenclature, the International Committee on the Taxonomy of Viruses has recommended the name HIV-I, or just HIV. Most people, however, continue to call it the AIDS virus.

The AIDS virus attacks the immune system. The body's immune system usually fights infections from foreign invaders, such as bacteria, viruses, and even ragweed pollen, by producing T-helper cells to attack these invaders. The AIDS virus can suppress these T-helper cells, creating a deficiency, so that the body cannot fight off infections. People with AIDS are then vulnerable to "opportunistic infections" that are not a problem for someone with a normal immune system. They develop numerous and massive infections. Even common parasitic and fungal infections that pose no threat to healthy individuals become lethal in immunosuppressed individuals. People with AIDS die of these infections, not of the AIDS virus itself.

Acquired Immune Deficiency Syndrome is an acquired disease. Scientists do know how AIDS is acquired. The HIV virus is primarily transmitted by sexual secretions (such as semen and vaginal secretions) and by blood transfer (as in blood transfusions, sharing IV needles, or across a placenta to a fetus). From the information currently available, AIDS is not transmitted by casual contact, food or air. The good news is that the HIV virus is very delicate. It thrives in blood and dies quickly when in air, water, urine, Vitamin C, alcohol, or even insect blood (which is a different temperature than human blood). Though the virus has been isolated in tears and saliva, there have been no cases documented of AIDS transmission through either substance.

You can limit your exposure. In terms of sexual transmission, abstinence is a sure prevention; condoms and spermicides are a close second. To avoid transmission through blood, do not share blood or blood products; especially avoid sharing IV needles. Blood transfusion products are now screened for the AIDS virus in the United States, so risk of contaminated blood from such sources is much lower than previously.

In no previous human "plague" could an individual take effective personal protection action; the individual could do little to ensure that he or she would not be infected. Earlier outbreaks of disease were airborne, waterborne, and insectborne; for these, isolation and quarantine were necessary and effective, though harsh, measures. Unfortunately, many people are advocating such public health measures as a means of combating AIDS in spite of the fact that such strategies are not effective with this type of disease.

Once infected with the HIV virus, the body develops antibodies to the virus over the next several weeks up to 24 months (results of a recent Fin-

1989 Federal Spending for Major Diseases	
(Estimated totals, in millions of dollars, including research, education and prevention.)	
Cancer	$1,449
AIDS	1,306
Heart disease	1,008
Diabetes	267
Stroke and hypertension	182
Alzheimer's disease	127

Source: *New England Journal of Medicine*

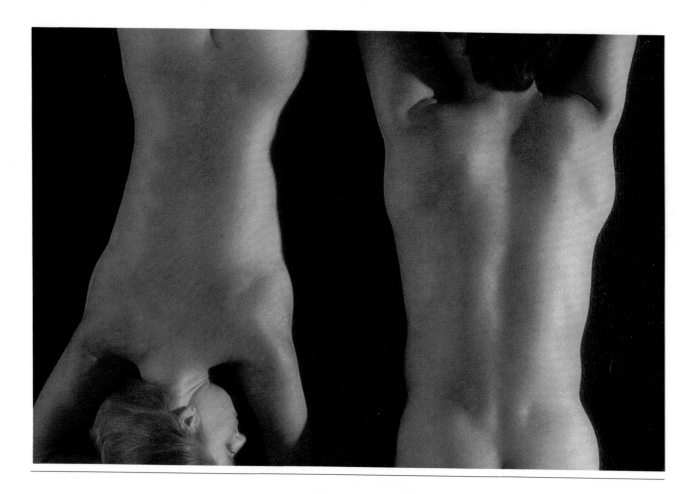

nish study). These antibodies can be detected in a blood test. The blood test does not diagnose AIDS; it simply measures exposure to the virus. Researchers developed this test to insure that the nation's blood supply was safe, not to diagnose AIDS in humans. At the present time the health care community assumes that people with positive antibody tests are shedding the virus and are "contagious" via sexual secretions and blood. Current predictions are that a large percentage of the people who test positive on an antibody test will go on to develop AIDS, though the incubation period of the virus can be several years. Once infected, there is no "cure," and any vaccine researchers may develop will be useful only for those not yet infected. Several companies are testing drugs that appear to "strengthen" T-helper cells in an attempt to bolster the immune system of infected patients.

What is your risk for AIDS? The national Centers for Disease Control indicate that by the end of 1989 the total number of confirmed cases of AIDS in the United States will exceed 115,000. Of those, over half have already died. The CDC estimates that by 1991 AIDS will have struck 270,000

The AIDS Crisis

C H A P T E R   13

Heterosexually-transmitted AIDS is already a serious and rapidly growing threat; there have been 780 documented cases as of 1988, but the CDC estimates that 30,000 heterosexuals are carrying the AIDS virus. Other researchers warn these numbers may be low, and that as many as 200,000 may be infected.

people in the United States. Though these are significant numbers, they are only people actually suffering from AIDS. Most of these people with AIDS are not only identified, but are sick enough that they are not a major risk to the general population through sexual contact or sharing of needles.

More frightening is the estimate of 2 to 3 million currently infected with the virus in the United States (as of early 1988) who are HIV positive but don't know it because they have not been tested. As many as 1 in 30 men between 20 and 45 years of age are infected. It is not known how many people have AIDS Related Complex (ARC), in which an individual shows only one or two of the AIDS symptoms, but not a full-blown case of AIDS. People with ARC greatly outnumber actual AIDS cases and are of potentially more risk to the community because they are capable of spreading the virus and yet still have a relatively healthy appearance. Because they have no symptoms, and the vast majority do not even know they are infected, they unknowingly subject others to the risk of AIDS.

As of 1989, the largest group of infected people is gay males, followed by IV drug users. The nonwhite portion of the population is overly represented. However, though the rate of infection is slowing in the gay community, it is growing in the heterosexual community. There are now twice as many heterosexuals being infected as there were homosexuals being infected just five years ago. Assuming that almost all of the estimated three million people who are HIV positive are in the age range of people who are sexually active, public health officials believe that anyone who engages in a high-risk activity with someone who has been sexually active with other people risks exposure to the AIDS virus.

High-risk activities are those in which sexual secretions/fluids or blood are exchanged. The only way you can tell whether a potential sexual partner is infected or not is a blood test (but not always; more on testing accuracy later in this section). If you are sexually intimate with a new partner, you are not only sleeping with that individual but with all of the people with whom he or she has slept, and with whom those people have slept, and so forth, for the last five to seven years—something on the conservative average of 10,000 people. Think about it.

A great deal of controversy surrounds the issue of AIDS testing. Usually, health professionals recommend testing for a particular medical problem among all people at high-risk for that condition. However, discrimination against people with AIDS is already high, and some people believe that AIDS testing will only further this discrimination without offering medical help or hope. The opposing argument is that people who know they are HIV positive will be more careful to avoid spreading the virus.

Should you be tested? This complex issue requires at least an hour of counseling before making a decision. The first important consideration is whether you have been exposed to the virus by engaging in a high-risk behavior or through contaminated blood products. AIDS counselors can help you identify high-risk behaviors. For example, even though the

The AIDS Crisis

media has indicated that male homosexual contact is a high-risk behavior, not all homosexual contact puts one at risk. It is estimated that as many as 40 percent of young males engage in at least one episode of mutual masturbation with another male. If the resulting semen came into contact with unbroken skin and did not enter a partner's body, then the risk of HIV exposure is minimal.

Second, the HIV antibody test does not show meaningful results for several weeks or sometimes months (over 24 months in one study) after exposure, because the body needs time to produce enough antibodies to be detected. Therefore, a test taken a few days after engaging in a high-risk activity would not tell you if that behavior exposed you to HIV. This "gap" is disturbing for another reason. A negative test indicates only that a partner has not been exposed before some unknown window in time. A person could have had sex or shared a needle with an infected person in the intervening time but not test positive.

Third, you might want to consider anonymous testing at a state designated site until issues of discrimination, including health insurance, are settled.

Personal prevention involves practicing safer sex, limiting the number of your sexual partners, avoiding exposure to sexual secretions, using condoms during all sexual activity in which sexual secretions can be shared, and not sharing IV needles. Avoid combining sexual activity with intoxication. Intoxication does not cause AIDS, but it does interfere with your ability to make rational decisions including choice of partners, type of activity, and whether or not you use condoms.

This has been a general overview of the AIDS crisis. The following sections answer in more detail questions you may have about AIDS: how it is transmitted, your risk of contracting AIDS, what you can do for protection, and so forth.

How You Can Get AIDS

Blood

- Through open cuts, wounds, gum abrasions
- IV drug use
- Blood transfusions before March 1985
- Placental transfer

Semen, Vaginal Secretions, Urine, Feces

- Penis-vagina
- Penis-rectum
- Penis-mouth
- Vagina-mouth
- Mouth-rectum
- Artificial insemination

NOT from saliva, tears or casual contact

What Is AIDS?

AIDS stands for Acquired Immune Deficiency Syndrome. By definition, this means that the disease is acquired; you are not born with it or even born with the genetic predisposition to acquire it. Immune deficiency means your body's defense system is not working properly. Syndrome simply refers to a group of signs and symptoms that reflect the disease process.

AIDS is caused by a virus, now labeled the HIV-I virus. If this virus enters your bloodstream, it attacks the T-cells in the immune system. People with AIDS are vulnerable to serious illnesses, opportunistic infections which would not usually be a threat to life, but which may result in death in a person whose immune system is not functioning adequately. The two most common opportunistic infections associated with AIDS are Pneumocystis carinii pneumonia (PCP) and a form of cancer, Kaposi's sarcoma (KS).

The AIDS Crisis

Is AIDS a Contagious Disease?

Yes, AIDS is a contagious disease, but it does not spread the way a common cold or measles does. It is contagious in the same way that sexually transmitted diseases, such as syphilis, gonorrhea or herpes, are contagious. According to current research, AIDS is NOT spread by common, everyday contact. It is only spread by the exchange of body fluids.

How Is AIDS Transmitted?

Current research indicates that AIDS is transmitted several ways. AIDS is transmitted through exposure to semen infected with the AIDS virus. Intimate sexual contact that involves an exchange of body fluids is considered a high-risk behavior. Minor, even imperceptible tears in the lining of the vagina or rectum may allow entry of the virus during insertion of the penis or fingers. Even without the presence of blood, the virus can enter a recipient's bloodstream through this tear in the tissue. Certain sexual activities are considered more risky than others: anal intercourse for both male and female recipients; vaginal sex when either the male or female is a carrier of the virus; oral-genital sex on a male is considered less risky. Oral sex is, in general, less risky if it is stopped before ejaculation. There may be a slightly higher risk when oral sex is performed on a female who is menstruating.

AIDS is transmitted by exposure to blood infected with the AIDS virus. Skin provides an effective barrier to prevent infection or invasion of agents that could result in disease. If this protective barrier is broken by an injury or needle puncture, fluid containing the AIDS virus may enter the body. Sharing needles for IV drug use is considered extremely high-risk behavior.

Can I Catch AIDS from Saliva, Tears or Casual Contact?

AIDS is not spread by casual contact, and it is not an airborne disease. Even though AIDS has been found in saliva, as yet there is NO evidence that saliva can transmit the disease. Many studies have confirmed that AIDS has not been transmitted by kissing. If any risk exists, it would be from prolonged, deep kissing where a carrier of the AIDS virus could transmit it through a break or tear in the tissue of the lips or mouth. Though the AIDS virus has also been found in sweat and tears, there is absolutely no reported instance of the virus being transmitted through exposure to tear or sweat fluid.

There is also NO evidence that casual contact with a person who has AIDS will result in contracting the disease. Activities such as touching, hugging, holding hands, sharing food or drinks, swimming in the same pool, or using the same toilet seat as an AIDS carrier will not transmit the AIDS virus. Your intact skin provides an effective protective barrier against transmission of this virus. It has also been determined that mosquitoes cannot transmit the virus.

Who Is Most at Risk for Catching AIDS?

The two major risk groups are homosexual or bisexual men (66 percent of known AIDS cases) and IV drug users (17 percent). Homosexual and bisexual men who are also IV drug abusers account for 8 percent of cases. These two groups account for 91 percent of all AIDS cases. Thus those most at risk are:

- Males, 20 through 24 years old; homosexuals head the list within this age group
- Anyone who has unprotected sex with someone who has contracted or been exposed to the AIDS virus
- Anyone who has shared a needle with an IV drug user
- Women most at risk are IV drug users who share needles; next are women who have more than one sexual partner. (Women account for 7 percent of all AIDS cases. The number is small, but growing.)

As a Woman, Am I at Risk?

Yes, women are at risk, as are men. Of all AIDS cases to date, 10 percent are women. The evidence (in spite of recent articles to the contrary) supports transmission of the HIV virus during normal unprotected intercourse. Though half the women with AIDS contracted the virus from IV

AIDS Linked to HIV

A CDC-sponsored study released in 1988 showed that 99% of a group infected with the HIV developed AIDS—within an average period of eight years. The AIDS patient can expect the disease to be fatal.

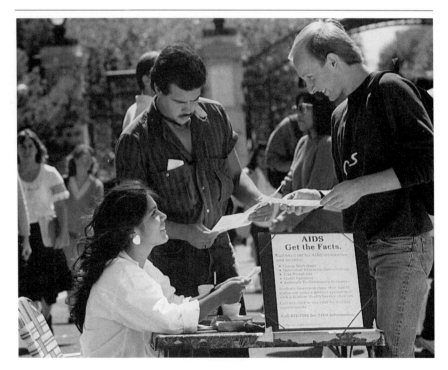

The AIDS Crisis

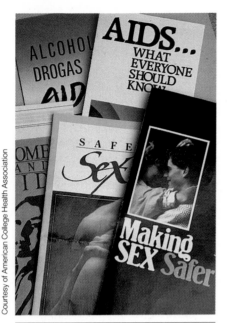

drug abuse, half contracted it from intercourse, either anal or vaginal. In 1981 the ratio of women to men with AIDS was 1 in 10; since that time, the ratio has increased. Men caught AIDS first; women are now catching up, just as the number of infected heterosexuals is increasing.

Heterosexual sexual activity can carry risk of AIDS virus transfer. Researchers have documented several hundred cases of transmission of AIDS virus from men to women and women to men. Transmission may not occur immediately, but chances are good it will occur sooner or later.

Women may face even greater AIDS risk in heterosexual contact than do men. Since most estimates indicate that more men than women are carriers, a woman is more likely to receive the virus from a male partner than the other way around. Second, the AIDS virus is more concentrated in semen than in vaginal fluid. In fact, women account for 79 percent of the cases called "heterosexual AIDS" from the Centers for Disease Control.

How Can I Protect Myself from AIDS?

AIDS can be transmitted through the exchange of body fluids. So, even though homosexual and bisexual men are at greatest risk for AIDS, heterosexuals should also limit sexual contacts and use the precautions of protected sex when active sexually. Specifically:

- Avoid the exchange of all body fluids including semen, vaginal secretions, blood, urine, and feces.
- Avoid multiple sex partners.
- Always have protected sex, using condoms, since any sexual contact with an infected person puts you at risk.
- Use latex condoms correctly and understand their limitations.
- Choose your partners carefully. The numbers indicate that one night of unprotected sex with a person who has been sexually active could expose you to thousands of sexual contacts. Particularly risky partners are men who have had homosexual or bisexual experience (bringing them in contact with a group having a higher percentage of AIDS carriers) and men who have sex with a prostitute (not only do prostitutes have many sexual partners, but they are more likely to be IV drug users and to have had sexual relations with IV drug users).
- Practice safe sex for whatever sexual activities you choose.
- Never share an IV needle with anyone.
- Do not share razors or toothbrushes because these items may expose you to small amounts of blood.
- Get required immunizations before you go overseas because sterilization techniques are not always adequate.

Can I Safely Enjoy Sex or Should I Abstain Totally?

Total abstinence is certainly the safest way to avoid exposure to any sexually transmitted disease, including AIDS. But you don't have to give up

The AIDS Crisis

sex, just play it safe. Use your own good judgment, be very clear about your beliefs and choices, convey them to every potential partner, act on what you believe, and maintain your immune system. You can reduce the risk of AIDS by following certain guidelines.

- Make careful, considered choices about your sexual partners. Feel confident that if you are in a long-term monogamous relationship, and neither of you has engaged in sexual activity with others, the risk is extremely minimal that either of you could contract AIDS. However, if either of you has been or chooses to be more sexually active, you have to take responsibility for your own health. Unprotected sex is unsafe sex. Unprotected sex with one or two partners is more dangerous than safe sex with several partners.
- Don't engage in casual sex. Know your sexual partners well enough to discuss how you both feel about sex. Talk openly about the need for safe, protected sex. Ask your partner about his or her sexual history, knowledge of STDs, and awareness and practice of safe sexual measures.
- Be committed to using condoms for sex. At this point in our knowledge of safe sexual practices, the use of the condom is critical for protection.
- Avoid any injury to body tissues during sexual activity. Remember that minor tears in anal or vaginal tissue could expose you to transmission of the AIDS virus, because it is transmitted through body fluids (semen) into the bloodstream.
- Do not use intravenous drugs or share needles, even if you know the person.
- Avoid using amphetamines (speed), recreational drugs such as poppers (inhaled nitrite drugs), or any drugs that would weaken your immune system. Since the AIDS virus attacks the immune system, you want to keep as healthy as possible.
- Do not mix alcohol or other drugs with sexual activity; this behavior impairs your judgment and may contribute to engaging in sexual practices that you would not ordinarily do. Also, alcohol weakens your immune system.

Wisconsin Students Say Fear of AIDS Alters Sex Lives

Undergraduates at the University of Wisconsin in Madison are altering their sexual practices because of AIDS, according to a recent survey. Fifty-one percent reported that they had changed their sex practices in some way because of AIDS; 40 percent reported they were using condoms more often and about 30 percent said they were decreasing their number of sex partners. One educator warned that no one wants to come across as foolish, so the pressure is to respond that sex practices have changed in some way.

Which Sexual Practices Are Considered Safe, Probably Safe, and Not Safe at All?

Sexual practices that are considered safe:

- Massage
- Hugging and touching
- Social (dry) kissing
- Rubbing bodies together
- Masturbation, alone or with a partner
- External watersports
- Talking about sex, verbal fantasies

The AIDS Crisis

CHAPTER 13

Sexual practices considered probably safe:

- There should be no exchange of semen, vaginal secretions, blood, urine, or feces, or the practice is considered unsafe.
- Vaginal intercourse with a condom (must be latex, used properly, and not break)
- Anal intercourse with a condom
- Finger-to-genital contact with a glove or finger cot
- French kissing (unless practice draws blood or partners have open sores on mouth). Researchers are now questioning the safety of open-mouth kissing with strangers (who may unknowingly be infected with HIV).

Sexual practices that are possibly unsafe or risky:

- Mutual masturbation on broken skin
- Speed, poppers, alcohol contribute to unsafe sex
- Prolonged deep kissing
- Oral-genital sex without a barrier
- Finger-to-genital contact without a barrier

Sexual practices considered definitely not safe:

- Vaginal intercourse without a condom
- Anal intercourse without a condom
- Oral-anal sex
- Semen or urine in the mouth
- Sharing objects that have had contact with body fluids
- Internal watersports

What Items Do I Need for Safe Sex?

- Condoms, particularly those made from latex
- Spermicides; nonoxynol 9, the active ingredient in most spermicides, has been found to kill the AIDS virus in laboratory situations (although there is no proof it kills the virus in the body)
- Disposable latex or rubber gloves or finger cots
- Latex or rubber barriers to prevent body-to-body direct contact

Should I Use Condoms? Do They Really Provide Safe Sex?

The absolutely validated answer is yes; use condoms to protect yourself and your partner. They are very effective in preventing the spread of STDs (sexually transmitted diseases) including AIDS. Condoms prevent the spread of gonorrhea, chlamydia, syphilis, and hepatitis-B. Recent studies show that they do prevent the spread of AIDS. In the AIDS condom study commissioned by the San Francisco AIDS Foundation and conducted by Dr. Marcus Conant and Dr. Jay Levy, the AIDS virus was not transmitted through five brands of commercially available condoms. The condoms, filled with fluid containing a high concentration of the AIDS virus, completely stopped the passage of the AIDS virus, even when tested over a three-week period. (Of the condoms used in the study, three were latex, one was of natural lambskin, and the last was synthetic skin.)

How Do I Choose a Condom?

At any drug store you'll see many varieties of condoms. They are not all the same size, color, feel, or even taste or smell. Finding the right condom for you is important. Buy several brands and try them on (if you're a man); experiment with them until you find one that feels right, fits right, and even smells right. The most expensive condoms are not necessarily the best. In fact, one connoisseur prefers Gold Coin condoms (manufactured by Circle Rubber Company of Newark, New Jersey), which cost a mere 10 cents, over brands that cost $2. In general, a latex reservoir-end condom lubricated with a nonoxynol-9 compound is considered the safest.

In an article published in *Condom Sense* during 1987 National Condom Week, one expert shared personal preferences that you might consider in your own choices. He liked an inner wrapper that is easy to open; no rubber smell (especially if it smells like petroleum); no tongue-curdling taste; latex as nearly transparent as you can find; texture that is not sticky; and one that is form-fitting and gripping. He prefers latex over the more natural sheep or lamb material, and it is less expensive. (Adapted from "The Buyer's Guide" by Buzz Bense.)

Don't be embarrassed to buy condoms; STDs and unplanned pregnancies are much more embarrassing. Find out where your friends buy condoms, or look for dispensing machines in restrooms.

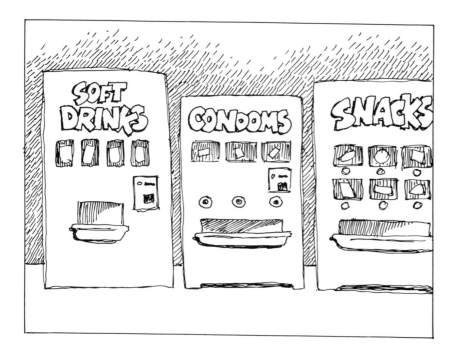

The AIDS Crisis

CHAPTER 13

How Can I Be Sure My Condom Will Be Effective?

There is no guarantee that a condom will work 100 percent of the time. In fact, condoms can fail; studies indicate that they do fail as much as 10 to 17 percent of the time. You can take precautions and behaviors to minimize the risk of your condom breaking.

- Use only new condoms.
- Some practitioners suggest that latex is safer, but in study results, both lambskin and synthetic skin were effective barriers.
- Put the condom on before intercourse; pre-ejaculatory fluid can transmit STDs, including the AIDS virus.
- Open the package carefully, don't rip it open. Be extra careful if you have long nails.
- Put a generous dab of water-based lubricant in the tip of the condom; it increases sensation without slippage.
- Gently press the end out of the condom tip to remove air bubbles; if present they can cause the condom to break. Plain-end condoms need a half-inch free in the end.
- Put the condom on carefully, unrolling it all the way onto the penis; cover the entire, erect penis with the condom.
- Use water-soluble lubricants, not oil-based, for extra lubricant on the outside of the condom before entry.
- During withdrawal, the condom should be held at the base so that leakage does not occur.
- Throw away the used condom; wash your hands.
- Do not store condoms in a car glove compartment or your wallet for weeks, near excessive heat, or in direct sunlight; the heat will deteriorate latex; if the condom is old or if the package appears old, don't use it.

Are Lubricants Safe?

Many sexually active people use lubricants with condoms because they reduce the discomfort associated with dryness. Water-based lubricants, such as KY Jelly, Ortho Lubricant, or Probe, are considered safe. Oil-based lubricants, such as vegetable oil, Crisco, mineral oil, or Vaseline petroleum jelly, are not safe; they do not dissolve and may weaken the condoms, reducing or eliminating their protective capacity. When you use any lubricant, make sure it comes in sealed tubes or packets so that germs are not spread with repeated use.

What Makes IV Drug Use So Dangerous as Far as AIDS Is Concerned?

- Shared needles and syringes permit blood-to-blood contact. This is the most direct method of transmitting the AIDS virus.
- Transmission of AIDS virus via IV drug use then permits further transmission to sexual partners of IV drug users through body fluid contact.

- Transmission of AIDS virus via IV drug use then permits further transmission to fetus of IV user during pregnancy.
- Use of alcohol or another other drug suppresses the immune system.
- Drugs impair judgment while you are under the influence.

Is There a Connection Between Alcohol, Other Drugs and AIDS?

Yes, there is a connection between alcohol, other drugs and AIDS. Abuse of these chemicals causes a variety of health problems. They also damage the immune system, leaving the individual vulnerable and increasing the risk of contracting AIDS.

- A moderately high intake of alcohol decreases the white blood cell count, which directly affects immune system functioning.
- Alcohol affects the liver; liver impairment can inhibit the body's ability to form T-cells, white-cell components critical to fighting disease.
- Chronic abusers of alcohol are found to have an inadequate nutritional intake; they lack essential nutrients necessary for a healthy body and a well-functioning immune system.
- A moderately high intake of alcohol interferes with the body's assimilation of vital vitamins and minerals, critical to maintaining a healthy immune system.

Other drugs also have a deleterious effect on the human body. Their use and abuse can result in numerous health problems—all of which may increase risk of contracting AIDS.

- *Amphetamines (speed, crank)* Use of these drugs, whether by injection or not, can result in severe damage to the immune system. Using and sharing needles increases the risk tremendously. Speed use causes liver damage, which in turn suppresses white blood cells. Malnutrition from appetite suppression also deprives the body of essential nutrients.
- *Marijuana* Though this drug is often believed to have few negative effects on the individual, in fact current research suggests that frequent use of this drug lowers the body's resistance to infection. Recent studies have yielded results that show a decrease in antibodies circulating in the bloodstream (thus limiting the person's ability to fight off invading organisms) and abnormalities in the T-cell function that closely resemble abnormalities found in AIDS victims.
- *Nitrites (poppers, Amyl)* Effect on the immune system remains unclear, but many researchers believe these drugs lead to general immune system depression. There is evidence that using poppers during anal intercourse expands the blood vessels of the rectum, increasing the risk of receiving the AIDS virus. There is also speculation that they may be a co-factor in the development of Kaposi's sarcoma, an opportunistic disease responsible for the deaths of many AIDS victims.
- *Other drugs such as cocaine, heroin, and Quaaludes* These have not been the subject of specific research studies. However, most scientists believe that they generally depress the immune system and make one vulnerable to the AIDS virus.

In addition to having physiological effects on the human body, alcohol and other drugs also impair judgment. They reduce your ability to make wise decisions, and they limit your awareness of choices; they also make you more prone to engage in high-risk sexual activities that place you at risk for contracting AIDS.

Can an AIDS Carrier Transmit AIDS?

Statistics show that not everyone infected with the AIDS virus will actually develop AIDS. Many of those infected will test positive and develop antibodies to the virus but not develop any of the symptoms of AIDS. These people will look and remain healthy—but the long-term outcome is unknown.

Up to three million people fall into this category. They are known as AIDS "carriers." It is estimated that 50 percent of these carriers will develop AIDS. The danger is that most of these millions do NOT know that they carry the virus and thus may more likely transmit the AIDS virus to others. A smaller group develops AIDS-Related Complex (ARC). These individuals have some but not all of the AIDS symptoms. ARC is secondary to HIV-caused immunodeficiency, but is not AIDS.

An even smaller percentage of people develops AIDS. AIDS includes a range of symptoms that are observable and can take anywhere from a few months to several years to manifest. Many of the symptoms that are present with AIDS are also found in more common illnesses such as the flu, colds and upper respiratory infections. With AIDS, however, these symptoms are persistent, recurrent and last for months. They also cannot be accounted for by any other diagnosis. Finally, with the damaged immune system, the person develops what is called an "opportunistic" infection that may be life-threatening.

What Will the AIDS Antibody Test Tell Me?

At the present time, the best way to determine if you have been exposed to the AIDS virus is to have a special test called the HIV antibody test or the ELISA test. This test is NOT a test for AIDS, however. It simply tests for the presence of antibodies (substances produced in the blood to fight invading organisms) to HIV. This test can give false positive or false negative results. A substantiated positive test indicates that a person has been exposed to the HIV virus. It does not indicate whether or not that person will develop ARC or AIDS. At this time, health professionals have no way of predicting if or when a person who has been exposed to the AIDS virus will, in fact, develop the disease.

If you decide to get tested, check the confidentiality of the test results. Many people are concerned that a positive test result, if it becomes part of your medical record, could jeopardize future employment or even insurance coverage. There are locations where you can obtain anonymous testing. Contact the county health department in your county to locate these specific sites.

Taking the test is not the only consideration. It is important to obtain counseling about the results and the implications of the blood test. Even if you think you can handle the results no matter what they may be, supportive counseling during this time of stress can be very helpful. Also, if the results are positive, you may benefit from expert help to assist you in considering available options.

In January, 1988, the National Cancer Institute announced a new test for the AIDS virus. According to researchers George Pulakis and Barbara Felber, this test, which measures the presence of the virus directly, is faster and more accurate than tests currently being used. This test may become available in the near future.

What Should I Do If I Get a Positive Antibody Test?

A positive HIV test result means you should be retested. If the second test is positive, the Western Blot Test is given for confirmation. If all three tests are positive, you must assume that you are infectious. You should take precautions in order to protect those with whom you will be in intimate contact. Remember, even if you develop no symptoms, you are a carrier and, as such, could transmit the virus to others. To protect others:

- Never have unprotected sex with a partner.
- Inform your past sexual partners or anyone with whom you have shared needles that they may have been exposed to the HIV virus.
- Inform your current or any future sexual partners of the positive HIV results so precautions may be taken.
- Learn and practice the behaviors that are considered to be safe sexual practices.
- If you are a woman with a positive test result, you will need to consider protection against pregnancy.
- Do not consider donating blood, organs or semen.
- Don't share razors, toothbrushes or other items that could be contaminated with blood.
- If you use drugs, enroll in a drug treatment program.
- Inform your doctor, dentist and eye doctor of the positive HIV results so that they may take proper precautions.

Someone who tests positive should do everything possible to minimize their chance that they will develop ARC or AIDS. Obtain regular medical evaluation and follow-up. Adopt measures that promote health (poor health habits are considered a co-factor in the development of AIDS). Though no action can definitely prevent such developments, certain health-promoting activities help your body to fight off infection; they support a healthy immune system.

Confidentiality and Anonymity

Confidential means access to your medical record is limited only to the clinicians and personnel taking care of you. That may, however, include lab technicians, secretaries and your insurance company.

Anonymous means no one ever knows your real name. You may be John or Jane Doe, or give a fictitious name. Some people never really feel anonymous because someone might know or recognize them.

The AIDS Crisis

What Are Basic Health Maintenance Measures to Prevent Immune System Depression?

You can keep your immune system in the best possible condition if you:

- Avoid alcohol and other drugs, especially immunosuppressive drugs (marijuana, speed, cocaine, alcohol). If you don't seem to be accomplishing this on your own, obtain counseling to assist in living your life without dependence on alcohol or other drugs.
- Maintain an adequate, nutritionally sound diet.
- Engage in stress-reducing activities such as exercise, meditation or removing self from a stressful situation (living with others who routinely use drugs).
- Obtain regular medical and dental care.
- Follow a lifestyle that provides adequate rest and exercise.
- Practice safe sex (to protect yourself from exposure to others STDs).

What Are the Symptoms of AIDS?

- Rapid, unexplained weight loss of 10 percent of body weight or 15 pounds.
- Persistent and profound fatigue.
- Recurring fever, chills, night sweats that continue for several weeks.
- Swollen lymph glands in the neck, armpits or groin that last longer than two months.
- Diarrhea that lasts longer than one week.
- White spots or unusual blemishes in the mouth or throat or on the tongue.
- New, persistent cough that may be accompanied by shortness of breath.
- Pink or purple-type bruises that seem to be under the skin, inside the mouth or nose. Though they seem like bruises, they do not disappear.

If one or more of these symptoms appear and do not go away in two or three weeks (or appear as indicated in the list above), please see a health care provider and request a complete physical examination. Don't hide from finding out what's wrong. Only by confiding in a medical professional can you learn what is causing such symptoms; remember, most of these symptoms may also indicate conditions other than AIDS.

If I Am Worried, Where Can I Get Help?

- Your college or university health service; they will arrange for you to have an antibody test and provide counseling.
- The public health department or community STD or family planning clinic in the city where you live or attend school.
- The women's health center or clinic, if one is available at your school.
- Private physicians.

How Is AIDS Diagnosed?

Even after someone tests positive for HIV, significant symptoms may first appear only years later. The person may be tired or suffer frequent, lingering colds and flu, perhaps a nagging cough. Perhaps he or she seems to get ill easily and stay ill longer than other friends. The symptoms of AIDS (discussed earlier) may appear singly or together. If not before, the individual may at this point go to a doctor to find out what is wrong.

A physician may diagnose AIDS if a patient has one of the opportunistic diseases commonly associated with AIDS, such as Pneumocystis carinii pneumonia or Kaposi's sarcoma. Either of these diseases indicates that the immune system is not functioning effectively. Certain blood tests that evaluate the white blood cells are done as part of the diagnostic process. The presence of opportunistic diseases plus a positive test for antibodies to HIV allows a positive diagnosis of AIDS.

A New Drug for AIDS

A new drug, dideoxyinosine (DDI) looks so promising in the war against AIDS that researchers are rushing DDI into expanded tests on 2000 patients. This drug is said to be the best new antiviral drug available and may prove to be the drug of choice over AZT.

Can AIDS Be Cured or Treated?

At this time there is no cure for AIDS. Although incredible energy and money have already been utilized to find a cure, medical science has not found any agent that kills the AIDS virus. Nor have they discovered any way to restore the immune system to viability so that it can kill the virus. AZT, the only drug approved by the FDA for treatment of AIDS, has significant inhibiting effects on the HIV virus in the body. However, recent reports of drug-resistant viruses in patients taking AZT are concerning scientists who fear mutant strains.

Studies have noted clinical improvement, overall diminished symptoms, and even an increase in neurological functioning with AZT, but serious adverse reactions have also occurred; the primary one is depression of the bone marrow. Because of these side effects, AZT should be used only by someone with AIDS, not a person with ARC. Also, this drug is expensive; the average cost is $1,000 per month.

Though supportive medical measures can assist AIDS patients to recover from opportunistic infections so that they may continue to live for reasonably healthy periods, eventually the person's condition deteriorates. He or she is very ill virtually all the time, and may require intermittent hospitalization. At this stage in the illness, a person with AIDS needs tremendous support from everyone in their world.

In time, the body is overwhelmed, and the person dies of one or more infections. There have been only one or two documented cases of AIDS recovery, and these have involved alternative therapies not generally accepted in the medical community.

Worldwide research is underway to find both a cure and a vaccine for AIDS. The first human trials for AIDS vaccines have just begun; scientists predict that no vaccine will be commerically available for five to ten years. A cure is even more remote.

The AIDS Crisis

Don't Pay for AIDS

"Treating" a friend to a prostitute for his 18th birthday or visiting the red light district with a group of buddies may seem like a lot of fun, but it could have deadly consequences, because of AIDS. Prostitutes have many sexual partners, who may have had all types of sexual or drug experiences. Even though many prostitutes now require that their customers use condoms, you have no way of really knowing whether a prostitute earlier did business without condoms, or how careful she and her customers are about safe sex.

Perhaps even more important, prostitution and IV drug use are often interlinked. Many young women who develop IV drug habits eventually turn to prostitution to support their habits. Others support the drug habits of sexual partners. In terms of AIDS, having sex with a prostitute is one of the highest-risk sexual activities a heterosexual man can choose.

If My Partner Tested Positive for AIDS, Can I Trust That He or She Will Tell Me?

We all would like to believe that a sexual partner would be truthful and honest in an intimate relationship. The facts indicate that this might not be so. In a study of 300 men conducted by the AIDS Prevention Studies Center at University of California in San Francisco, though a large percentage agreed that they would tell their partner if they tested HIV positive, in the homosexual group 12 percent indicated that they would NOT tell their "primary" partner and 27 percent said they would NOT tell their "nonprimary" partner. For the heterosexual group, 25 percent of the non-monogamous men said that they would NOT tell their "nonprimary" partners. The fact that many men do not intend to tell their sex partners if they are infected with the AIDS virus reaffirms the necessity to protect yourself by using safe sex practices. In this case, the old adage applies: "Better to be safe than sorry."

Is There Really a Danger of Getting AIDS from Other College Students?

As much as you might like to believe that the AIDS virus will or does not affect you, AIDS is a very real danger on college campuses today. In May, 1989, the American College Health Association and the CDC announced the results of a nationwide 19-campus study of the rate of HIV infection among college and university students. The study found 2 of every 1,000 students tested were infected with HIV. Dr. Richard Keeling, chairman of the American College Health Association AIDS Taskforce, said "Beyond any doubt HIV is established on college campuses." This could mean that 25,000 college students carry HIV, although this figure generalizes results nationwide. Estimates are that between 20,000 and 30,000 students on American college campuses carry a contagious form of the AIDS virus. These young people have or carry the AIDS virus in their blood but are asymptomatic and in good health. Though many of these carriers may not develop AIDS, they are able to transmit the virus to others.

U.S. campus life is a center for sexual activity. Various studies throughout the country estimate that between 40 and 70 percent of students are sexually active. Of these a frightening number know little about AIDS. Though the trend to publicize AIDS information is increasing, in the end each individual must take responsibility for learning about the disease, its transmission, and prevention. Don't lull yourself into feeling invulnerable or immune to AIDS because of your potential long life ahead. NO ONE IS IMMUNE. Don't let ignorance or apathy determine your future. Begin now to learn about AIDS and take the appropriate safe sex precautions to preserve your life.

How Can I Be Helpful If a Friend Has AIDS?

When a friend or family member develops AIDS, it is especially important that you continue the relationship. They may feel isolated, unloved, un-

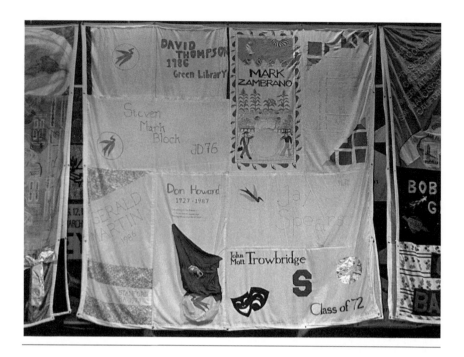

wanted, and undesirable. You may feel uneasy and uncomfortable about continuing the relationship. Please remember that casual contact will NOT transmit the AIDS virus. This is a critical time in the life of an AIDS victim, a time when he or she needs loving and supportive friends. Isolation simply adds yet another stressor to an AIDS victim's life; stress damages the immune system, which, if one has AIDS, is already severely impaired. So, here are ways you can help this friend or family member:

- Be available: try not to avoid your friend. Be there, the loving friend you have always been. The only thing that is different is that your friend has contacted a deadly disease and now needs your love and support more than ever.
- Don't put distance between you and your friend. Use touch, hugging and holding hands. This warm and loving behavior will let your friend know nonverbally that you still care and that you aren't disgusted by the disease. (Again, remember you cannot catch AIDS from touch, hugging or closeness; transmitting the AIDS virus requires intimate sexual contact.)
- Respond to your friend's emotions; allow your friend to weep if necessary. Show empathy by feeling with your friend: cry when they do, laugh with your friend. Sympathy is not useful and blocks communication. Empathy is simply feeling with your friend and allowing the expression of honest emotions.
- Encourage your friend not to give away his or her power; encourage your friend to make his or her own decisions. Giving up the ability to

make decisions takes away control and leaves one feeling powerless—a negative state.

- Offer to help your friend take care of problems, correspondence, or any activities that he or she cannot do alone.
- Encourage your friend to take care of his or her health. Suggest building up the immune system by eating nutritionally balanced meals. Help him or her explore alternative treatments such as stress-reduction or vitamin and mineral supplements. Help your friend comply with the treatment he or she is now receiving. If medications have been prescribed, support this medical regimen and encourage your friend to continue to seek medical guidance.
- Encourage your friend to avoid alcohol and other drugs, which damage the body and the immune system. Join your friend in exploring other ways of feeling good such as group therapy, counseling and activities with others.
- Offer to accompany your friend to see the doctor.
- Be supportive of friend or family member if other family members are unable to be supportive because of anger, fear, denial, or shame.
- Finally, take care of yourself. Recognize how you are feeling and find ways of meeting your own needs—to cry, to grieve, to express anger that your friend may be dying. And keep yourself and your immune system healthy.

How Can I Tell My Partner That I Want Safe Sex?

Talking about sex has always been more difficult than doing it. Even with the sexual revolution of the 60s, many people found open communication about intimate sexual details difficult. Today, when sex, safe sex and sexual protection are on everyone's minds, it is still difficult to talk about such subjects directly. But the times demand that you must do exactly that—be direct, honest and determined.

How do you begin such a conversation with an exciting, new potential lover (when what you would like to do is simply enjoy lovemaking in a natural way and not even deal with the subject of safe sex)? Well, one way to begin talking is to open up the conversation in general by saying, "I have been reading a lot about safe sex and how important it is. I'd like to know what you think." Or, you may try, "I'm concerned about having safe sex, but I'm not sure how you feel about it. Can we talk about it?" The more openly and directly you begin the interaction, the more easily your partner will be able to respond. Encourage your partner to say what he or she really thinks. If you both can discuss the subject objectively, placing no blame or suspicion on the other, then using safe sex methods will seem natural when the time arrives. You might even suggest that you examine safe sex alternatives together. If you create a comfortable, loving atmosphere during these intimate conversations, the physical intimacy will follow naturally.

Avoiding the subject, hoping it will never come up, or delaying the subject until it is too late to handle comfortably are not viable solutions. They don't work. To gain the confidence to actually discuss the issues, think ahead of time about how you are going to approach the subject, even role-play conversations with a friend. This is not just a remedial course in intimate conversation; the end result of not dealing with safe sex may be deadly. Remember, the AIDS virus (as well as many other STDs) is transmitted through the exchange of blood or body secretions—including semen and vaginal fluid. One mistake could mean the difference.

To handle this delicate subject with finesse, you have to be very clear about your own belief system. What do you believe? What are your own personal goals regarding sexual partners? Are you clear enough about where you stand on the subject to suffer rejection by your partner if he or she does not agree to safe sex? These are essential questions for you to consider before you have to deal with them in an actual relationship. If you are clear, unencumbered by ambivalence, you will send a clear message. Your partner can handle clear communication, even if he or she doesn't like it. If you are a man, you might say, "I have a condom with me. I believe that safe sex is important for both of us, so I plan to use it." Or, if you are a woman, you might say, "I think that safe sex is necessary. I have a condom with me and I would like you to use it." Both of these statements should be said before intimate contact—remember clear communication. What if your partner is not in favor of safe sex—for any number of reasons? The sample dialogue in the nearby box will give you ideas for effective responses if your partner objects to using a condom. After reading the responses, choose some that fit you; practice saying them until you feel comfortable.

Seeking Professional Help

Information on professional help is incorporated throughout this chapter. The answers to the questions will direct you to specific resources.

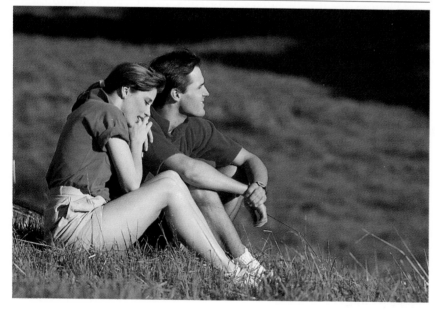

The AIDS Crisis

Communication about Safe Sex

Dialogue for Safe Sex

"I've been thinking a lot about safe sex—what do you think?"

"I disagree—I think everyone has to be careful today."

"No, I don't. But, for both our sakes, we need to use good judgment."

"Yes, using condoms is safe sex."

"Well, a condom may slightly decrease the feeling but we can still create romance."

"We can make putting on a condom part of the romantic process."

"Let's try it and see and we'll both be glad we had (protected) sex."

"I think this AIDS scare is overdone. We don't have to worry."

"Do you really think I carry around this AIDS virus?"

"I suppose good judgment means using a condom?"

"I don't like using a condom—it takes away all of the romance and feeling."

"How romantic is it to stop everything and worry about a condom?"

"I'll try it but I'm not sure I'll like it."

How to Handle Attempts at Manipulation

First Partner	Possible Response
"It makes me uncomfortable to discuss condoms and safe sex. Let's not talk about it."	"If we are going to be intimate sexually, it seems as if we ought to be able to talk about an intimate subject like safe sex."
"I think you're being unfair. You are implying I'm a diseased playboy (girl)."	"I didn't say that and I don't think that. I just think safe sex is better for both of us."
"I know I don't have any disease. Don't you believe me?"	"Yes—and I don't have any disease either, but for both our sakes let's protect ourselves."
"Using a condom is awkward and takes all the romance out of making love."	"It doesn't have to be awkward—especially if we make it part of the romance."
"Using a condom is like kissing through a glass door. There's no feeling."	"I'm sorry you feel this way. I believe safe sex is important for both of us."
"You mean you carry condoms—you were planning to have sex all along?	"Only if we both want to. I always carry condoms because I believe in protected sex."
"If you insist on using a condom, it means you don't trust me."	"That is not true—it only means I care about both of us and I want us both to be protected."
"Let's forget using a condom—and really enjoy our lovemaking."	"Let's not forget. We can still enjoy each other and be protected."
"I really want to make love but I don't have a condom."	"Luckily I do have one." Or, "Let's wait, then, until we are prepared for love making."
"Well, if you insist on us using a condom, I want to forget it."	"I'm sorry you feel this way. I also feel strongly about having safe sex."
"Well, I'm choosing not to use a condom—if you love me, you'll trust me."	"I do care about you but I don't care enough to die."

What Is Forecast—Really—about AIDS?

Right now the outlook is scary. The CDC predicts that the number of AIDS patients may exceed 365,000 by 1992, and at least 263,000 of these will have died. These numbers reflect primarily people already infected. San Francisco health experts estimate that 75 percent of all those now infected will develop AIDS unless new drugs can block its progress.

The projected worldwide statistics are also frightening. The World Health Organization has estimated that cases of AIDS in the world were more than 182,000 by October, 1988. WHO estimates that at least 1 million new cases will occur worldwide by 1993 and that between 5 and 10 million are infected with the virus now. Outside the United States, an estimated 1 million Brazilians may be infected, but only 1,200 Japanese. The AIDS epidemic continues to rage in Africa.

AIDS or the HIV-I virus is a dangerous infectious agent that is contagious. This virus does not respect person or gender; if it is present in the bloodstream of an individual, it can potentially be passed on to anyone with whom this individual is in intimate contact. If there is an exchange of blood or body secretions, the AIDS virus can be transmitted.

In the long run, the damage AIDS causes in our society will be determined by the will of all of us to implement educational programs and protect ourselves. Prevention is the key element to containment of this world health epidemic. It is clear that if a total, worldwide effort is not developed, AIDS will have a devastating effect in the decades ahead. You need to do your part to learn about AIDS, communicate the information to others, and live a lifestyle that will protect you and your friends and partners.

> **We should all be concerned about the future because we will have to spend the rest of our lives there.**
>
> **Charles F. Kettering**

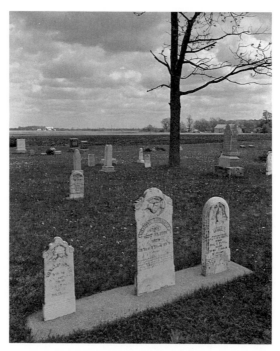

The AIDS Crisis

CHAPTER 13

Beyond the Text

1. Respond to this statement: AIDS is an equal opportunity virus.

2. Your roommate is infected with the HIV-I virus. What precautions do you need to take? Is there any reason for you to move?

3. Your best girlfriend is dating a man you know to be bisexual. She doesn't know. What would you do?

4. During a routine premarital blood test you find out your partner is infected with the AIDS virus. What would you do?

5. You are dating a man who feels uncomfortable talking about safe sex. What would you do or say to him?

6. Respond to the statement: Men are at higher risk for AIDS than women.

Supplemental Readings

AIDS in the Mind of America by Dennis Altman. New York: Anchor Press, 1986. Discusses the political and social implications of AIDS.

AIDS: A Self-Care Manual by AIDS Project, Los Angeles. Santa Monica, CA: IBS Press, 1989. Comprehensive guidebook that covers all aspects of AIDS management from exposure to treatment to educating others.

And the Band Played On: Politics, People, and the AIDS Epidemic by Randy Shilts. New York: St. Martin's Press, 1987. Written by an AIDS victim, this book exposed the political aspects of the AIDS disease and its treatment.

"Surgeon General's Report on AIDS" by C. Everett Koop. *Journal of the American Medical Association*, November 28, 1986. A detailed description of what AIDS is and how to cope with it.

The Biology of AIDS by Hung Fan, Ross Conner, and Luis Villarreal. Boston: Jones and Bartlett Publishers, 1989. Presents the biomedical aspects of AIDS and discusses the social issues raised by the disease.

Key Terms Defined

AIDS acronym for autoimmune deficiency syndrome; suppression or deficiency of the immune response caused by exposure to the HIV-I virus; leaves individual susceptible to a variety of "opportunistic infections"

antibodies also called immune bodies; proteins produced in the blood that respond to foreign invaders

ARC acronym for AIDS-related complex —characterized by a prolonged history of fever, unexplained weight loss, swollen lymph nodes, and/or fungus infections of the mouth; a certain but unknown percentage of persons with ARC will develop AIDS

AZT also called compound S, antiviral drug currently being used and evaluated for potential effectiveness against HIV virus

carrier virus-infected individuals with no symptoms, but capable of transmitting the HIV virus

helper T-cells type of lymphocyte, or white blood cell, affected by the HIV-I virus; helper T-cells interact directly with foreign substances to combat infection in healthy individuals

high-risk behavior behaviors that lead to the transmission of the HIV virus, such as sharing contaminated needles and unprotected anal or vaginal sexual intercourse

HIV antibody test test used to determine the presence of HIV antibodies in the blood

immunity state of resistance to infection due to the presence of antibodies that combat foreign invaders

Kaposi's sarcoma a type of cancer that causes purple or brown lesions on the skin or in the mouth; often seen in AIDS patients

opportunistic infections any infection that occurs when the body's immune system has been weakened; frequently present in AIDS patients

Pneumocystis carinii pneumonia parasitic infection of the lungs, one of the two rare diseases that affect 85 percent of AIDS patients

safe sex practices that need to be taught to the population at large in order to prevent transmission of STDs including the HIV virus; practices refer to the use of a condom and spermicidal foam for all sexual activity and preventing any exchange of blood or body fluids

virus minute parasitic organism that depends on nutrients inside cells for its metabolic and reproductive needs

Pregnancy, Childbirth and Parenting

Choosing to have a child is one of the most important decisions that a couple makes during their lifetime. The resulting changes in the couple's life are dramatic, and the impact of pregnancy on the relationship can bring the prospective parents much closer together or can alienate them to the point of ending their relationship. Pregnancy for unmarried women raises many issues ranging from her ability to support herself and her child to her decision whether or not to continue the pregnancy.

This chapter covers many topics important to pregnancy and childbirth: pregnancy decisions; the prenatal, delivery, and postpartum periods; and parenting. The section on parenting discusses the critical issues prospective parents should consider, preferably prior to the occurrence of pregnancy.

Key Terms

Abortion

Alpha-fetoprotein

Amniocentesis

Artificial insemination

Chromosomes

Conception

Dominant trait

Ectopic pregnancy

Fetal alcohol syndrome

Genes

Genetic diseases

Heredity

In vitro fertilization

Infertility

Midwife

Ovulation

Recessive trait

Sonography

Contents

Being Pregnant

- *Pregnancy was the happiest time of my life. When I found out I was pregnant, I was elated. It seemed like it took forever. We had only been trying for about six months but I expected it to be instantaneous. I mean, I knew you could get pregnant in the back seat of a car your first time, so I thought it would happen that way for me. Afterwards, though, I had a lot of difficulty adjusting. I was young and I wasn't used to having to put someone else's needs above mine.*

  45-year-old married woman with two children

- *All during my wife's pregnancy I just kept thinking, I wish I could do more because the mother is doing all the work. I wished I could share it with her. And when you see the baby come out it's like the conclusion of a great novel, something you have waited and hoped for and wondered about for a long time. It becomes the major watershed of your whole life.*

  35-year-old man two weeks after the birth of his first son

- *When I found out I was pregnant I was stunned and just began to cry. I was in a new relationship with a man who ultimately didn't want to be with me. I ended up having an abortion and I felt at the time like I lost everything—the man, the baby, and my innocence.*

  25-year-old single woman who became pregnant at age 20

- *I was extremely sick during most of my pregnancy and I was used to having a career and a full life with my husband, going hiking and doing the things we enjoyed. I really felt I had to give up a great deal to have the baby. Don't get me wrong, I'm very happy to have this bundle of joy, but it's a lot of work and my life has completely changed. Plus I was sick for five months and for six weeks I wasn't supposed to move around much.*

  32-year-old new mother

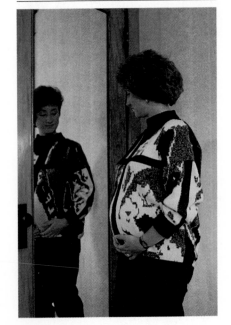

Whether pregnancy is the most thrilling moment of a woman's life or one of the hardest depends upon many factors: her emotional and financial readiness, her relationship with her partner, her age, her emotional support system, and her willingness to place herself in the background so she can care for her child. The same goes for the father or the woman's partner.

Pregnancy is nine months of new experiences followed by a lifetime of new experiences. Although having a baby inevitably causes upheaval in the mother's or the parents' lives, babies challenge mothers and couples to grow. Turning the challenges into successes requires thoughtful planning and knowledge. With adequate preparation, pregnancy can be an enriching, joyful prelude to caring for a child.

The Reproductive Process

Heredity may be thought of as the capacity to pass on characteristics to offspring. As recently as the early eighteenth century, scientists thought that the female egg consisted of a tiny, ready-made man or woman, or homunculus, which eventually grew into a male or female baby. Since then, particularly as a result of the pioneering work of Gregor Mendel, the nineteenth-century Austrian monk who experimented with hybrids of sweet peas, scientists know much more about heredity. The study of heredity and the laws governing it are now a separate branch of biology called genetics.

Heredity is determined by genes. Genes certainly determine your more obvious characteristics, such as the color of your hair and eyes and your height, but scientists now realize that genes influence much more, including weight, mental illness, musical and athletic ability, personality, moods, predisposition to certain diseases—even baldness and the inclination to squint.

Every single cell in the human body has 46 chromosomes, or cell structures that carry genetic information. The only exceptions to this rule are sperm and egg cells, which have 23 chromosomes. Each pair of chromosomes contains genetic material contributed from the male and female that make you simultaneously like your parents and distinctly individual. It takes thousands of genes to produce all the characteristics embodied in one single human being. The particular set of genes present in DNA is your genotype.

When the egg and sperm unite, the 23 chromosomes arrange themselves into matched pairs. Genes are arranged in linear order on the chromosomes; each gene has a specific place on a specific chromosome. Of the 23 sets of chromosomes, 22 sets are exactly alike. Only set 23 is different: it determines whether the baby will be male or female. A female has two X chromosomes, inheriting an X chromosome from both her mother and father. A male has one X chromosome and one Y chromosome.

Genes are either dominant or recessive. When genes for a particular trait differ, one gene will be dominant. For example, the gene for brown eyes is dominant, while the gene for blue eyes is recessive. If the genetic material for eye color in the egg is coded for blue eyes and the genetic material in the sperm is coded for brown eyes, the baby will have brown eyes. However, because the baby now carries a recessive gene for blue eyes, it can pass on the gene for blue eyes to the next generation.

Numerous genetic problems can occur at conception. Genetic material may be absent or too plentiful. In either case, the defective genes will produce their characteristic deformities in the child. Autosomal recessive genetic diseases are caused by defective recessive genes. If both parents contribute the same defective recessive gene, the child will be born with that particular disorder. If only one parent has the defective gene, the child will not have the disorder. However, even though the child is free of

Is Genetic Counseling Appropriate for Every Family?

Genetic counseling is appropriate only for families who have a medical history that reveals one of the following conditions:

- Congenital abnormalities including mental retardation, congenital malformations
- Familial disorders such as diabetes
- Known inherited disorders
- Identified carriers of metabolic biochemical or chromosomal disorders including sickle cell disease and Huntington's Chorea
- Multiple miscarriages or stillbirths
- Advanced maternal age (35 and over). The risk of Down's Syndrome in a mother age 25–29 is 1 in 1175; a mother who is age 36–40 is 1 in 250; and over age 46 is 1 in 25.
- Parental exposure to environmental agents (drugs, radiation, infections, environmental pollutants)

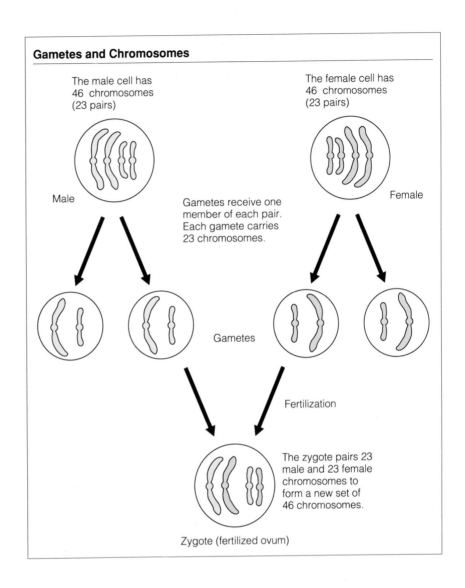

Gametes and Chromosomes

The male cell has 46 chromosomes (23 pairs)

Male

The female cell has 46 chromosomes (23 pairs)

Female

Gametes receive one member of each pair. Each gamete carries 23 chromosomes.

Gametes

Fertilization

The zygote pairs 23 male and 23 female chromosomes to form a new set of 46 chromosomes.

Zygote (fertilized ovum)

the disease, he or she will be a carrier, which means he or she will pass on the defective gene to the next generation. Cystic fibrosis is an example of an autosomal recessive disease. Carriers of defective recessive genes can transmit the gene for several generations without a problem until two recessive carriers have a child.

About one third of all pediatric hospital admissions involve genetic disorders. Genetic screening before having children is wise. Some genetic diseases cluster within certain ethnic groups, such as sickle cell anemia among blacks, thalassemia among Italians and Greeks (sickle cell and thalassemia are both types of anemia), and Tay-Sachs disease among Eastern European Jews.

X – Linked Inheritance Most Common Form

Female sex chromosome of an unaffected mother carries one faulty gene (X) and one normal one (x). Father has normal male x and y chromosome complement.

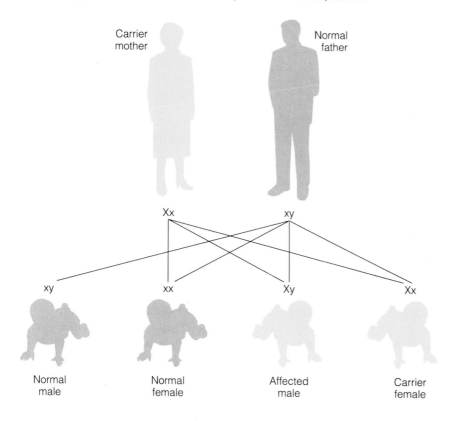

The odds for each *male* child are 50/50:
1. 50% risk if inheriting the faulty X and the disorder
2. 50% chance of inheriting normal x and y chromosomes

For each *female* child, the odds are:
1. 50% risk of inheriting the faulty X, to be a carrier like mother
2. 50% chance of inheriting no faulty gene

Source: Department of Health, Education, and Welfare: *What Are the Facts About Genetic Disease?* Washington, DC, 1977

Many genetic diseases, such as Tay-Sachs, can be tested for during genetic screening, giving parents sufficient information to make an informed choice before having children. Genetic screening and counseling are available at university health services, clinics, and medical centers.

A woman should seek genetic counseling before deciding to become pregnant. In situations where a family has a history of genetic disorders

Infertility is attributed to men about 35 percent of the time, to women about 35 percent of the time, and to a combination of male and female factors about 30 percent of the time. Ten to 20 percent of the time the specific cause cannot be determined.

The Odds on Infertility

Incidence   Two people marry. What is the probability that they will be unable to conceive a child? 12 in 100 (*This figure may be increasing, partly due to an increase in the spread of venereal disease.*)

Cause   A couple is infertile. What are the chances that the main cause is the male's low sperm production? 2 in 5

Prognosis   A couple is infertile. What are the chances that the problem can be corrected? 44 in 100

Source: *The Odds Almanac*, A. James Fix and David Daughton

or where the parents fit certain high risk categories, genetic counseling will help them understand their risks and make informed choices about becoming pregnant or seeking other options. When a child is born with certain defects, genetic counseling may be appropriate to help with future childbearing choices.

Infertility

Statistics indicate that 65 percent of the couples who are having unprotected intercourse regularly will conceive within six months; 80 percent will conceive within one year. Couples who have been unable to conceive after engaging in unprotected sexual relations longer than one year are diagnosed as infertile.

Infertility can be either primary or secondary. Primary infertility means the woman has never conceived or that the man has never impregnated a woman, despite routine unprotected sexual relations. Secondary infertility means that the couple has previously been pregnant, but is currently unable to conceive.

Male infertility is caused by anatomical or physiological abnormalities that include reduced sperm quality or quantity, problems in discharging the sperm during ejaculation, nutritional deficiencies, substance abuse, or psychological problems. Semen analysis is the most common test for male infertility. The sample is taken and examined for quality and quantity of sperm. Attempts at correcting male infertility have been disappointing. Treatment includes changing the diet, limiting frequency of intercourse to allow number of sperm to build up, and switching from jockey briefs to boxer shorts. Tight jockey briefs are thought to cause heat buildup around the scrotum, which reduces the number of sperm.

Anatomical problems in women can prevent the egg and sperm from uniting, the fertilized egg from implanting, or prevent the uterus from maintaining the pregnancy. Repeated infections of sexually transmitted diseases, especially gonococcal infections, can cause scarring of the fallopian tubes, which leads to infertility or sterility. Physiological or hormonal problems can prevent the woman from ovulating or can prevent her body from sustaining an implanted ovum. Additionally, nutritional deficiencies, psychological factors, and substance abuse have all been shown to cause infertility in females.

The following tests are used to diagnose infertility in women:

- Basal body temperature charts
- Cervical mucous records
- X-ray of the reproductive tract (hysterosalpingogram)
- Vaginal fluid tests after intercourse (postcoital test)
- Rubin's test (patency, opening of the tubes)
- Biopsies of the uterine lining
- Sperm allergy testing
- Laparoscopic examination of the abdomen

Treatment for female infertility varies according to the cause. For example, it may include surgery for correction of anatomical defects and drug therapies for hormonal deficiencies, inflammation, and infections. Changes in diet or emotional counseling may also be recommended.

When other treatments fail to produce a pregnancy, newer technologies may be used. These include artificial insemination and in vitro fertilization. Artificial insemination is the process of inserting a sperm specimen into the woman's vagina or uterus. This method is tried in situations where the partner is sterile, the woman is allergic to her partner's semen, or her partner's semen is weak.

In vitro fertilization, which produces so-called test-tube babies, begins by giving the woman drug therapy to stimulate her ovaries to produce eggs. These eggs are then surgically removed and placed in a sterile laboratory dish of culture media. Sperm are added to the dish and the specimen is incubated for 24 to 48 hours. If the eggs are successfully fertilized, they are surgically planted in the woman's uterus with the hope that one or more of the embryos will implant themselves into the uterine lining.

Infertility can produce intense feelings of anger, helplessness, desperation, and loss. Treatment for infertility is highly individualized and can be lengthy, frustrating, and costly. In addition, couples may have moral and ethical concerns about the specific treatments. Couples who experience infertility may need additional support or information. Support groups such as Resolve (P.O. Box 474, Belmont, MA 02178) offer help to infertile couples who wish to have a child.

Pregnancy Decisions

Pregnant women in the United States are getting younger. In 1985, 9.4 million unmarried minors under the age of 15 gave birth, 27.1 million unmarried adolescents between 15 to 19 years of age, and 30 million unmarried women between the ages of 20 to 24 gave birth. No one knows how many of these young women chose to become pregnant.

Choosing to have a child is one of the most important decisions we make during our lifetime. Couples who bear and rear children without giving enough thought to the direction they intend to take for themselves and for their children may become disappointed and discouraged, or they may suffer later in disruptive family situations.

Although this chapter does not imply that merely by thinking through the issues you will live happily ever after, it does suggest that the difficulties of pregnancy can be diminished with good planning. Studies show that families who plan are more satisfied in their child-rearing experience than those who do not. Planners will have a better sense of control and will be better prepared to deal with difficult situations as they arise.

The focus of this chapter will be on the woman's experience, whether or not the pregnancy occurs within a traditional family unit.

In-Vitro Fertilization: New Hope for Infertile Couples

In 1978, Louise Brown became the first baby to begin life outside a mother's womb. Since then, in-vitro fertilization has resulted in more than 5,000 births. In the future, test-tube babies may provide new hope for 2.3 million infertile couples in the United States. However, while this high-tech approach appears to be a viable solution to the infertility problem, in fact, it is a very expensive technique (about $7,000 per attempt) and has achieved only a 15 percent success rate. Although the chances of conceiving are slim, desperate couples continue to frequent the 200 in-vitro fertilization clinics that have sprung up across the country. The best clinics boast a 17 percent success rate. If you are considering in-vitro fertilization, check out more than one clinic and validate their success rates before you pay the high fee.

Source: *Time*, March 13, 1989

Pregnancy, Childbirth and Parenting

CHAPTER 14

Deciding to Become Pregnant

In times past it was considered a woman's duty to bear children. In rural and agrarian economies children were seen as extra hands to get the work done. However, in today's high-tech society children are no longer needed as laborers; now people who consciously choose to have children do so primarily because they want to raise them and love them. Having children is now a choice, and as new economic and ecological pressures begin to influence people's decisions to have children, many people are now choosing to limit the size of their families.

But many parents make the decision to become pregnant hastily or for the wrong reasons. If you are thinking about becoming or making someone pregnant, ask yourself if you want to do it for any of the following reasons.

- So he (she) will marry me
- So I will have someone to love me
- So my parents will be proud or stop nagging me
- Because my partner wants a child
- To prove I am a woman (man) or a sexual person
- To have someone to care for me when I am old
- To carry on the family name or tradition
- Because my friends are having children
- Because I did not think I (she) could get pregnant

If any of the above reasons fit your situation, you may want to explore your readiness for parenting. However, if you can answer the following questions affirmatively, you are probably ready to have children.

- Do I really want to have and raise children?
- Am I ready at this time in my life for the responsibility of a child?
- Have I done the things I really want to do?
- Do I have or will I be able to secure the financial resources necessary to raise a child? (Estimates range from $150,000 to $200,000 per child over a lifetime.)
- Do I have the social and emotional resources necessary to bear and raise children?
- Have I checked my partner's and my (or sperm donor's) genetic background to find out if it might be a problem for my children?

Women have more options now in choosing to have children than they did in previous generations. In addition to opting for the traditional husband-and-wife scenario, women are choosing to become single mothers or are having children with same-sex partners, generally by artificial insemination. In 1987, 34.1 percent of women under 35 were single parents, a 16.4 percent increase since 1960. For many of these women, the decision to raise a child alone was a personal preference. However, when deciding to have a child, the rights and responsibilities of the biological parent who will not be raising the child should also be considered.

Another issue to consider is discontinuing birth control. If a woman has been on birth control pills, she should talk with a doctor to see how long she needs to be off them before trying to conceive. Doctors recommend taking some time between stopping the pill and attempting to conceive; during this interim phase an alternate method of birth control should be used while the body is readjusting its hormone levels.

Because pregnancy makes great additional demands on a woman's body, someone contemplating childbearing may want to prepare by losing 20 extra pounds or giving up alcohol, tobacco, and nonprescription drugs before attempting conception. She might also begin to eat a more well-balanced diet or a special diet. Insulin-dependent diabetic women need to be sure their blood sugar is under control before attempting to conceive.

Testing to Confirm Pregnancy

Confirming a pregnancy is possible in the first several weeks. Home pregnancy tests are available and can be useful for early information. There are two main problems with using the home tests. First, the diagnosis is not always accurate. Accuracy depends on the quality of the test itself, as well as the user's ability to perform the test and to interpret the results. A false negative might cause the woman to delay seeking proper health care. A false positive may cause a woman to seek unnecessary medical care. In either case the outcome could be costly.

Second, if a woman's test is positive, she may decide that she feels well enough to delay initiation of prenatal care until much later in the

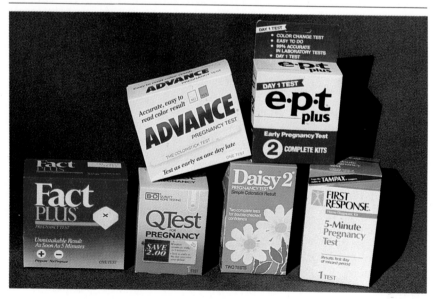

Am I Pregnant? I'll Know in 5 Minutes!

Home pregnancy test kits are now widely available as anyone watching television commercials is aware ("Are we pregnant, yet?" after five minutes in the bathroom). These tests are sold in drugstores and they are about 85–95 percent reliable.

- A positive test is based on the secretion of chorionic gonadotropin (HCG) in the woman's urine. It is usually detectable ten days after the first missed period. This test is 95 percent effective.
- A radioimmunoassay (RIA) test is the most sensitive but not readily available test. The test requires 24 hours to complete. Pregnancy can be detected before the first period is missed.

All tests may give false positive readings due to protein or blood in urine, neoplasms, ingestion of certain drugs (aspirin, methadone), if the woman has recently been pregnant or she does not complete the test or read the results accurately.

Pregnancy, Childbirth and Parenting

pregnancy. Delaying prenatal care can be harmful and expensive because some complications that develop in pregnancy can be diagnosed and treated early.

It is important to confirm a suspected pregnancy as early as possible so that appropriate actions can be taken. The woman who chooses to terminate a pregnancy will have less risk if the procedure is done early (less than 12 weeks). The woman who continues the pregnancy should seek prenatal care as early as possible to assure the best possible outcome for herself and her fetus.

Unwanted Pregnancy

Only abstinence and sterilization provide complete protection against pregnancy; every other form of birth control, including birth control pills, contains some risk of unwanted pregnancy.

A pregnant woman who did not choose pregnancy finds herself faced with a difficult decision: to continue the pregnancy and raise the child, to continue the pregnancy and give up the child, or to have an abortion. She must make a choice, even though her decision may produce anxiety, fear, guilt, and anger.

The arguments for and against abortion tend to be emotional and polarized. Despite the arguments, abortions are common in the United States. In 1987 there were 1,360,000 abortions and the number increases every year.

When a women is in the midst of considering how to resolve this issue, many questions must be considered. What are the role and rights of the father? How much involvement should the father and the parents of the pregnant girl have if she is an adolescent? Other aspects to consider are the emotional problems that result from a decision to abort or to give the baby up for adoption, how long these emotional stresses impact on the woman's life, and what problems result for the child and the parent if the woman chooses to have and raise the child.

For a broader perspective on these issues, please refer to the literature that describes women's different feelings about abortion, adoption, single parenting, and child abuse.

Fetal Development

Conception marks the onset of pregnancy. It occurs when a sperm fertilizes the egg. Generally, conception occurs after the penis has ejaculated into the vagina. However, pregnancy can occur at other times. The lubricating fluid produced by a sexually excited male can contain live sperm, so even sperm deposited into the vagina without ejaculation can cause pregnancy. Pregnancy is also possible if the man ejaculates in the vicinity of the moist vagina. Sperm travel fast and can make their way from the

Multiple Pregnancies

Double Ovum	Single Ovum
Dizygotic or fraternal twins	Monozygotic or identical twins
Ova from same or different ovaries	Union of a single ovum and a single sperm
Same or different sex	Same sex
Brother or sister resemblance	Identical genetic pattern
Two placentas but may be fused	One placenta
Two chorions and two amnions	One chorion and two amnions

edge of the vagina into the uterus and fallopian tubes, where they can fertilize the egg.

The egg and sperm have life spans that are more than momentary. An unfertilized ovum lives for 24 hours after ovulation; sperm live 48 to 72 hours in the female reproductive tract after ejaculation. Sperm deposited into the vagina within three days of ovulation can result in fertilization.

Pregnancies caused by these methods are rare, but they can happen. Once the ovum (egg) is fertilized, it begins to divide and develop in the fallopian tube as it makes it way to the uterus. The embryo implants itself in the uterine lining after six to seven days and elaborate hormonal mechanisms are established to support the developing embryo.

The fetus develops in three 13-week trimesters, or approximately nine months. During the first trimester, the placenta develops. Its two primary functions are being a conduit for maternal blood to bring oxygen and nutrients to the developing fetus, and providing for the removal of fetal waste products. The amniotic sac surrounding the fetus is filled with amniotic fluid, which protects the fetus against injury during the pregnancy.

The first trimester is critical for fetal development. All the organs and systems differentiate, and because the embryo develops so rapidly during this time, it is extremely vulnerable to environmental agents such as viruses, x-rays, and chemicals. By the end of the first trimester, the fetus is about three inches long and weighs about one ounce.

In the second trimester, the fetus gets longer and the skeletal features develop. By the end of this trimester, the fetus is approximately 14 inches long and weighs two pounds. At about the eighteenth week a woman begins to feel the fetus moving. In the beginning, this feeling is described as butterflies in the stomach or intestinal gas. At about 18 to 20 weeks the fetal heartbeat can be heard with a fetoscope (a large stethoscope). Hearing the fetal heart rate and feeling the fetus move are important landmarks used to determine the age of the fetus.

During the third trimester the fetus and the mother both gain weight, and the organs and systems continue to develop. After 40 weeks of pregnancy a normal fetus is about 20 inches long and weighs 7 to 7½ pounds.

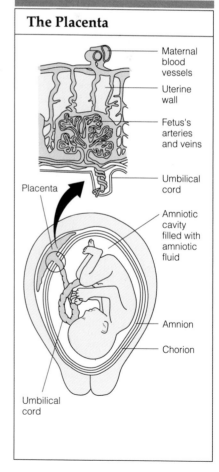

The Placenta

Maternal blood vessels

Uterine wall

Fetus's arteries and veins

Umbilical cord

Placenta

Amniotic cavity filled with amniotic fluid

Amnion

Chorion

Umbilical cord

First Trimester

Weeks 1–13

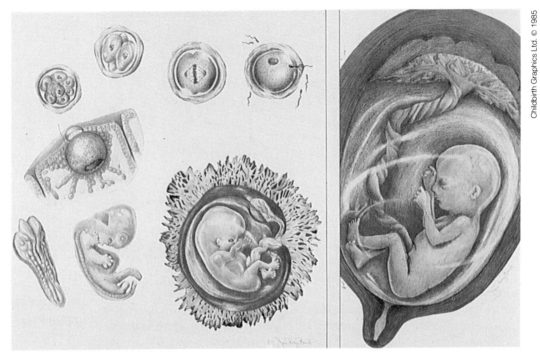

| Day 22 | Day 36 | 8 Weeks | 12 Weeks |

Second Trimester

Weeks 14–28

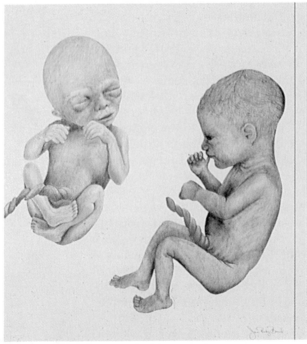
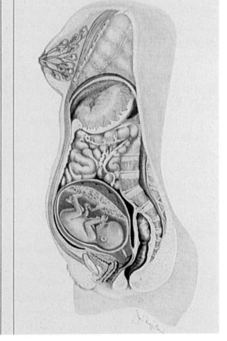

| 15 Weeks | 26 Weeks | 5 Months |

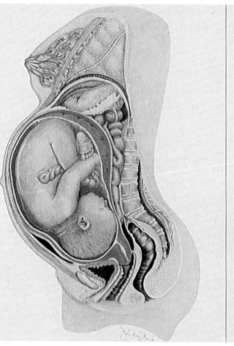

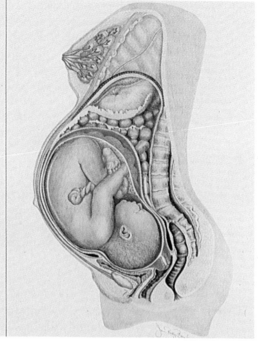

Fetus at Term

Lightening

The Prenatal Period

Technology has boosted medical science's ability to evaluate the fetus early in pregnancy, hastening the diagnosis of actual and potential problems. The most common prenatal procedures and tests done early in pregnancy include sonography, amniocentesis, and alphafetoprotein.

Prenatal Testing

Sonography establishes the presence of the fetus or multiple fetuses as well as the gestational age of the fetus. The test is a painless procedure in which sound waves are bounced over the uterus, giving a picture of what is inside.

Amniocentesis is done at about 15 weeks to diagnose genetic problems by removing a sample of amniotic fluid from the uterus. Amniocentesis is recommended for women with a family history of genetic disorders, women in risk groups for certain genetic problems, and women over 35.

A positive test indicates the woman is carrying a fetus with a genetic disorder. Because the test is done early, the woman has time to reassess the pregnancy. She may choose to abort the fetus, or she may continue the pregnancy and make special arrangements for the baby's care.

Pregnancy, Childbirth and Parenting

C H A P T E R   14

But there is a caveat: amniocentesis cannot be done before 14 weeks—and it takes three to four weeks to get the results. This means if the test is positive and the woman chooses to abort, she will have a riskier second trimester abortion.

Alpha-Feto-protein tests are done from a sample of the mother's blood at 15 weeks of pregnancy. The results are used to diagnose fetal problems. In many areas of the country, this test is being done routinely (before amniocentesis) as a screening procedure for such neural tube defects as spina bifida or hydrocephalus (which occurs in every one or two births/1000 in the United States).

When a diagnosis of a genetically defective fetus is made, the woman should be referred to a genetic counselor. Counseling provides the woman with facts and statistics about the expected outcome for the life of the fetus, as well as probabilities of problems during subsequent pregnancies. This information helps the woman make a decision about the current pregnancy while also planning for the future.

Prenatal Care

Once the choice to continue a pregnancy has been made, the mother-to-be will face many decisions about health care during her pregnancy. Prenatal care is health care for the woman and her fetus. The primary goal of prenatal care is to produce a healthy baby.

Prenatal care includes two basic components: physical assessment of mother and fetus, and education/counseling. Mother and fetus should be physically assessed because, although many pregnancies progress without difficulty, some women develop complications. Sometimes these difficulties threaten the life or well-being of the mother and the fetus. If problems are identified early, steps can be taken to eliminate or control the danger to the mother and fetus. Unfortunately, many of the complications related to pregnancy develop without any obvious symptoms. Noticeable symptoms often develop only after the problem has progressed and poses a significant threat to both the mother and fetus. Early and continued prenatal care is necessary to help decrease complications of pregnancy.

The second major component of prenatal care, education and counseling, provides the woman with important information and support, and helps her adjust to and plan for the changes. The expectant mother needs information early in her pregnancy about her nutritional needs, use of tobacco, drugs, alcohol, and body changes. The pregnant woman may need counseling concerning financial resources and living arrangements as well as about the emotional and social issues of pregnancy.

Although the fetus develops rapidly throughout pregnancy, it is most vulnerable during the first eight weeks, when all major organs and systems are differentiating. If the woman is aware of her pregnancy and is receiving care, it is less likely she will inadvertently be exposed to something harmful. (Refer to the section on fetal development.)

Pregnancy, Childbirth and Parenting

Psychosocial-Physical Changes During Pregnancy

Psychosocial-Emotional Changes

Pregnancy may be viewed as a period of increased susceptibility to crises due to the dramatic changes that occur in all aspects of life.

- Emotional reactions to pregnancy may vary from early rejection to elation.
- The woman may be puzzled by changes in her feelings. Quick mood changes are common; some emotional instability usually occurs.
- The woman may have fears and worries about the baby and herself.
- Dependency-independency conflict may be experienced as the pregnant woman realizes this new baby will be totally dependent.
- The first perception of fetal movement, called quickening, occurs between the sixteenth and eighteenth weeks.

Socialization for Parental Role

The pregnant woman and the father may fantasize or daydream to experience their role as parents before the actual birth.

- The woman will take on adaptive behaviors that are best suited to her own personality and situation.
- She will experience a "letting go" of her former role (e.g., as a career woman). There may be ambivalence about letting go of her old role to take on the new one. The desire to have a baby influences adjustment.
- During the first and second trimester there are concerns about body changes; fears of labor and delivery and the health of the baby; beginning conceptualization of the baby as a separate individual.
- By the third trimester the woman is more confident about labor and delivery. She shows readiness to assume care of the infant. She is now able to view the baby as a separate individual.
- The father may also experience ambivalence at taking on a new role, assuming increased financial responsibility, and sharing his wife's attention with the child.
- The father may experience physiologic changes, such as weight gain, nausea and vomiting, and a general malaise.

Initial Physical Changes

Early recognition of pregnancy is often made by the physical changes in the woman's body.

- Amenorrhea (cessation of menstruation) is one of the first signs of pregnancy.
- Breast changes occur—increased size and feeling of fullness, nipples more pronounced, areola darker.
- Nausea and vomiting (morning sickness) occur in 50 percent of pregnant women and usually disappear at the end of the third month.
- A frequent desire to urinate usually occurs in the first three to four months. Pressure on the bladder from an enlarged uterus gives the sensation of a distended bladder.
- Periods of fatigue, drowsiness, and lassitude are often present during the first three months.
- The first perception of fetal movement, quickening, occurs between the sixteenth and eighteenth weeks.
- Increased pigmentation of the skin, sometimes called the mask of pregnancy, often occurs.
- Vaginal changes such as discoloration and thickening of vaginal mucosa occur.

Continuing Changes

- Enlargement of the abdomen usually occurs after the third month when the fetus rises out of the pelvis into the abdominal cavity.
- The fetal heart rate may be heard at ten to twelve weeks by listening with a stethoscope or ultrasonic equipment.
- There are changes in internal organs. For example, a change in shape, size, and consistency of the uterus and softening of the cervix occur in the second month.
- The heart increases in size and cardiac output increases by 25 to 50 percent.
- The thoracic cage is pushed upward as the uterus enlarges—oxygen consumption increases 15 percent.
- An increase in body weight occurs—usually up to 25 pounds.
- Contractions begin in the early weeks of pregnancy and continue, but they are usually not felt by the mother until seven months. These are called Braxton-Hicks contractions.
- Active fetal movements are felt by the mother.
- X-ray or sonogram examination will show the fetal outline. Outline by x-ray is not visible until the fourteenth week or later, when bone calcification occurs.

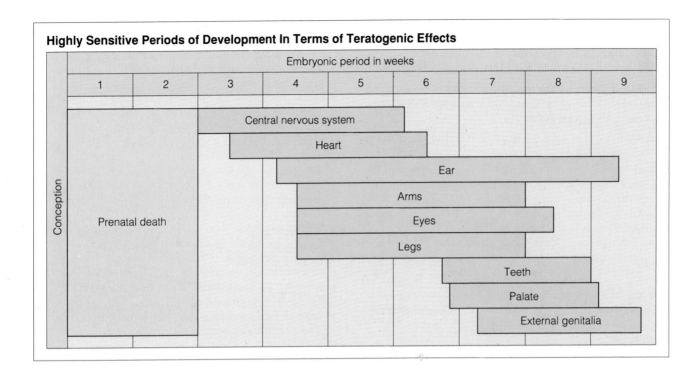

Highly Sensitive Periods of Development In Terms of Teratogenic Effects

	Embryonic period in weeks								
	1	2	3	4	5	6	7	8	9

Conception

Prenatal death

Central nervous system

Heart

Ear

Arms

Eyes

Legs

Teeth

Palate

External genitalia

Prenatal care is available from a wide range of providers. Women are encouraged to seek care from approved licensed providers in their local area. The primary types are private OB/GYN physicians (single or group practices), health maintenance organizations, hospital or public health clinics, nurse midwives, and nurse practitioners. Each type has advantages and disadvantages, but all provide basic physical assessment and educational and counseling services.

Issues to consider when selecting a provider are the cost of care, the number of practitioners you would see during pregnancy, the location of the service, the physical surroundings, the rights and responsibilities of those participating in the care, and the caregiver's philosophy on pregnancy.

Nutrition in Pregnancy

The idea that a pregnant woman is "eating for two" is prevalent but only partly true: the mother-to-be is not eating for two adults. The woman's dietary intake must be sufficient to maintain her health and to nourish the growing and developing fetus. An increase in caloric intake of 300 calories a day is recommended initially. Additionally, changes are recommended in the number of servings from each food group. Although it is currently recommended that women gain at least 24 pounds in pregnancy, eating a properly balanced diet that contains all the necessary nutrients requires active planning and effort on the part of the women. Although many people are trying to decrease salt and sodium in their diets, sodium is not usually restricted in a normal pregnancy. Weight reduction diets are discouraged until after a woman has weaned the baby from breast to bottle (or after delivery, if she chooses to bottle feed).

Iron supplements are often necessary during pregnancy. Because iron is hard for the body to absorb, foods rich in Vitamin C should be eaten along with iron-rich foods to enhance iron absorption. Eating an orange with your hamburger or half a grapefruit with your morning eggs will increase iron uptake.

Exercise and Hygiene in Pregnancy

Women are encouraged to exercise moderately throughout pregnancy, although taking up a strenuous new sport at this time is discouraged. Walking and swimming are ideal. In any case, the woman should discuss her plans for exercise during pregnancy with her care provider.

Frequent periods of daily rest are encouraged during pregnancy. Rest helps prevent fatigue, promotes blood return from the legs, and increases blood flow to the uterus and fetus. Lying on the left side is particularly beneficial in promoting blood flow to the uterus. Pregnant women may choose not to lie flat on their backs if they feel dizzy, nauseous or faint because of decreased blood flow to the baby.

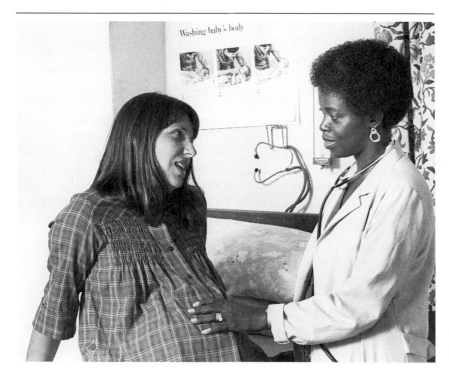

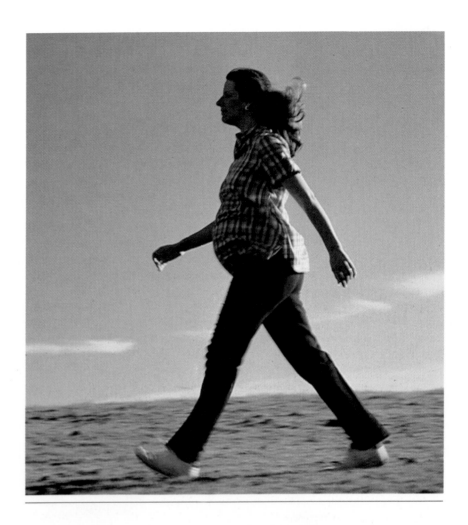

Higher metabolism during pregnancy produces an increase in body secretions, which calls for more frequent cleansing. Tub baths may be taken if membranes are intact and there is no vaginal bleeding. If the woman takes tub baths later in her pregnancy, she may need support getting in and out of the tub to guard against falling.

Drugs, Tobacco, and Alcohol in Pregnancy

All drugs should be avoided in pregnancy unless they are necessary to sustain the life of the mother. Even vitamins, aspirin, and Tylenol should be taken only under the supervision of the pregnancy caregiver.

Cigarette smoking is considered a risk behavior during pregnancy. Nicotine causes constriction of the blood vessels, which decreases the blood supply to the baby. Babies born to women who smoke during pregnancy have lower birth weights than infants born to nonsmoking mothers.

All women are encouraged to abstain from drinking alcoholic beverages while pregnant. Alcohol consumption during pregnancy has been linked to the development of the fetal alcohol syndrome, which causes mental retardation and a severe reduction in the child's growth rate.

Sexual Relations in Pregnancy

Sexual intercourse may continue throughout pregnancy unless the woman has ruptured membranes, vaginal bleeding, or premature contractions. As a woman who recently delivered said, "My husband said it's like having sex with a whale, but if you can contort yourself into a position that's comfortable, it's great. You learn to make do with what you can do." When in doubt the woman should seek clarification from her caregiver.

Changes in sexual desire can occur for both women and men and, while desire for sex during pregnancy increases for some people, it decreases for others. Couples are encouraged to discuss their feelings and to develop methods for satisfying their needs.

Serious Problems of Pregnancy

As pregnancy progresses, women experience normal changes that cause minor discomforts. Others develop changes that may indicate more serious problems, even though initially the symptoms are minor.

The primary major problems of early pregnancy are spontaneous abortion and ectopic pregnancy. Vaginal bleeding early in the pregnancy may signal abortion. Although a pregnant woman may experience vaginal bleeding that does not lead to miscarriage, she should report any vaginal bleeding immediately to the health care provider.

Ectopic pregnancy is generally accompanied by pain in the lower abdomen. Women often think it is normal to have abdominal discomfort in pregnancy and do not seek care immediately. Allowing this problem to progress without diagnosis or treatment can be fatal.

Two possible problems that can develop later in pregnancy are vaginal bleeding and pregnancy-induced hypertension (PIH).

Vaginal bleeding later in pregnancy may be a sign that the placenta is improperly situated. This can range from a minor problem to a serious and potentially life-threatening one. Women who experience vaginal bleeding at any time in pregnancy need to seek care immediately.

PIH is more problematic because in its early stages the condition develops without the woman realizing she is ill. PIH is a combination of complex symptoms that include rising blood pressure, spilling protein in the urine, and swelling. As this disease progresses, the nervous system and liver become involved. Untreated, the disease can lead to seizures and death for the mother and fetus. Detection of PIH in its early stages is another reason women should be strongly encouraged to seek prenatal care throughout their pregnancy.

Medical Hazards When You're Pregnant

You will want to avoid all drugs and x-rays whenever possible. Physicians even advise against taking aspirin because it tends to promote bleeding. The most common medications that are known or believed to damage unborn infants are

Accutane, acne medication

Anticonvulsant drugs

Aspirin, especially in the 3rd trimester

Asthma and cough medications

Barbiturates (Phenobarbital)

Hormones (oral contraceptives)

Painkillers (Darvon, codeine)

Tagamet (ulcer medication)

Tetracycline (antibiotic)

Tranquilizers (Valium or Librium)

Source: *Nutrition Action Healthletter*, April 1987

Pregnancy, Childbirth and Parenting

Sexually Transmitted Diseases in Pregnancy

Early initiation of prenatal care allows the woman to be tested and treated for any sexually transmitted diseases she may have already contracted. When left untreated, these diseases may adversely affect the fetus and newborn, as well as the mother. Since reinfection can occur when she has intercourse with untreated men, a pregnant woman is wise to limit her sexual exposure to a single partner whose sexual practices she knows; otherwise she may want to be retested later in pregnancy.

Gonorrhea (GC)   Women with gonorrhea may not have symptoms. Untreated GC in pregnancy can cause premature labor, infections in the amniotic sac, or low birth weight. GC affects the newborn primarily during birth when the baby passes through the infected vagina. The GC organism may cause an eye problem called *opthalmia neonatorum*. This occurs infrequently but it can cause significant problems for the newborn. To prevent infection, all infants are treated prophylactically at birth with antibiotic eye drops.

After the third month of pregnancy, GC rarely gets into the mother's fallopian tubes; however, after pregnancy, untreated GC can cause acute inflammation in the tubes, dermatitis, and arthritis.

Chlamydia   Like GC, chlamydia is also often without symptoms in the female. During birth, the organism can get into the baby's eyes as the infant passes through the infected vagina, causing *inclusion conjunctivitis*. If left untreated, this can lead to more serious eye problems. Eye treatment with an antibiotic ointment at birth generally prevents complications from developing. In addition, chlamydia infection in the newborn can also cause pneumonia.

Syphilis   Untreated syphilis in pregnancy is one of the major causes of second trimester (13 to 24 weeks) abortion in the world. After the fourth month of pregnancy, the syphilis organism crosses the placenta, causing congenital syphilis in the fetus. The infection can result in bone deformities, problems with the central nervous system, teeth, and eyes. Syphilis transmission to the fetus is best prevented by early diagnosis and treatment of the pregnant woman.

Herpes   Herpes is not usually a problem for the developing fetus. Problems occur when the baby passes through the vaginal canal at birth. If the mother has an active lesion at the time, the baby can be infected. The herpes virus can be lethal to the newborn; therefore, cesarean section is recommended. Fortunately, infection in the newborn is rare, although when it does occur it is often fatal. Survivors have significant eye and neurological problems. Because there is no cure for herpes, women who are known to have genital herpes infections need to tell their caregivers so that they may be followed closely during pregnancy and birth.

Theories of Childbirth

Most theories of childbirth view it as a natural occurrence. The more knowledge and information a woman has in preparation, the more this understanding dispels fears and tension about the birth experience. The purpose of adhering to a specific method of childbirth is to promote relaxation, allowing the mother to work with, rather than against, the labor process.

Many factors influence pain in labor, one of the most important being preconditioning by "old wives' tales." These stories and superstitions generate fear that accurate information will help to alleviate. Another factor that influences the actual level of pain is the individual's reaction to and interpretation of it. Pain produces stress, which in turn affects the body's tolerance level. These reactions can be altered by assisting the woman to refocus her attention. Feelings of isolation also influence pain; if the woman has support during this process, she is less fearful and more able to cope with the experience.

Education and training for both partners helps change both perceptions of birth and actual coping resources. Education includes anatomy and physiology of the reproductive system, the labor and delivery process, as well as nutrition, discomforts, expected signs, infant care and, in general, replacement of misinformation, fears, and superstition with facts. The training may include relaxation methods, controlled breathing and neuromuscular exercises.

The childbirth methods most in vogue focus on the theory that pain in childbirth increases with fear. In fact, the first natural childbirth method, introduced by Grantly Dick-Read in England, was based on the belief that pain in childbirth was psychological rather than physiological. Of course, any woman who has given birth is very aware that the pain is more than psychological. His method, however, began a trend toward a natural, participating delivery, rather than a passive, medicated one. Women learned that if they conquer the fear, the tension is less and the pain is modified. Other natural methods still used today are Lamaze and Bradley. The most common practice is not actually a method, but a series of labor classes.

Labor Classes

Women do not need to go to school to learn to give birth. Giving birth is utterly natural. Babies just pop out, right?

Wrong. Labor classes are now believed to be an important part of pregnancy. Classes teach women and their partners about labor, delivery, and care during pregnancy and childbirth, including specific exercises and procedures that can be used during labor to reduce pain and to increase a sense of control and well-being.

Most courses offer a series of classes for women who are at least 30 weeks pregnant. If you are going to be choosing a class, consider whether you want to have a natural birth (without the use of any drugs or anesthesia) or be assisted in the labor with some pain relief. Additionally, you need to think about who will be with you during labor so you can bring him or her to class with you. Once these decisions are made, explore classes in your area to see what is offered and select one most appropriate for your needs.

The Delivery Period

Signs of approaching labor are usually experienced with relief by a pregnant woman. After carrying this weighty package for nine months, she is usually more than ready for delivery.

Labor and Delivery

She may experience lightening—the uterus descends as the fetus moves down into the pelvis to prepare to be born. Suddenly, the mother can breathe easier because the baby is no longer pressing on her diaphragm. This discomfort, however, is replaced by feelings of urgency to urinate, requiring frequent trips to the bathroom as pelvic pressure increases. False contractions may start, continue and become quite regular, but often stop when the woman walks around or changes position. This is why they are called false labor. A sign indicating impending delivery is when the woman's "water breaks." Technically, this is the rupture of the amniotic sac holding the fluid that protects the fetus. This can happen any time before delivery and often it occurs in embarrassing circumstances. You've heard the story of the woman who realizes her water has broken in the grocery store and quickly drops a jar of pickles on the floor.

True labor begins when contractions increase in frequency, intensity, and duration. Walking does not relieve them and, as they become very regular and strong, the woman begins to make plans to enter the hospital or the birthing center. The purpose of labor—and it is just that, hard work—is to dilate the cervix or opening, propel the fetus down the birth canal, and expel the baby into the world. Regular contractions of the uterine muscles with secondary help from the abdominal muscles, push the baby along. Contractions do not last forever—even though to the woman experiencing them it may seem so. They have three stages: increasing intensity, peak or full intensity, then decreasing intensity. They can last from 10 to 30 seconds in the beginning to 50 to 90 seconds in the last or transitional phase.

The duration of labor varies. For a first pregnancy, labor may take 18 hours or longer; some labor has been known to last days. A woman who has had several children has a much more rapid labor; it may only take six to eight hours. Traditionally, the more children you have, the easier it gets. Someone, somewhere, has planned well, because no one in their right mind would continue having children if the length of labor increased with every child.

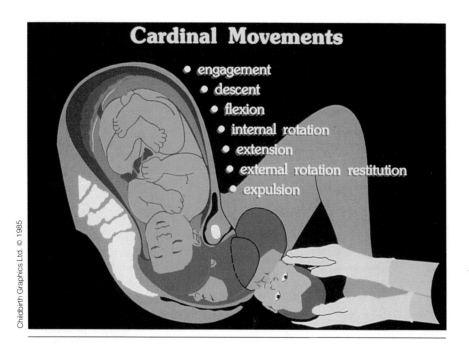

Cardinal Movements

- engagement
- descent
- flexion
- internal rotation
- extension
- external rotation restitution
- expulsion

In the final phase of labor, the woman is working very hard to withstand the intensity of the contractions and, at the end, to control her incredible urge to push the baby out. As the baby enters the vagina, the health practitioner will instruct the mother when to push so that neither she nor the baby is damaged. This is the phase of delivery when breathing

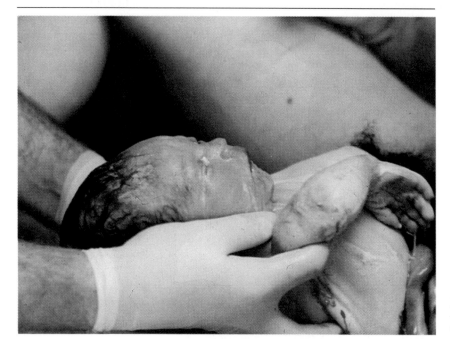

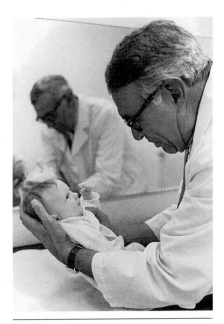

techniques learned in labor classes, and minimal fear really do assist the woman to have a positive delivery experience.

It may be that the woman cannot have a natural delivery. For a variety of reasons—a baby that is too large, a pelvic canal that is too small, fetal distress and other complications—a cesarean delivery may have to be performed. This is a surgical procedure that involves an incision into the abdominal wall and the uterus to remove the fetus. Recovery for the woman is the same as for any major surgery.

Special Delivery

Frederick Leboyer, a physician from France, introduced a radically different method of delivery—one that uses the environment of the delivery room to reduce stress on the infant. The room temperature is increased to a comfortable level for the infant (instead of near freezing), lights are dimmed, and the noise is controlled. The infant, immediately upon delivery, is placed in skin-to-skin contact on the mother's abdomen and gently stroked. The infant is submerged up to its head in a bath of warm water until it appears to relax, then it is dried and wrapped snugly in a warm blanket. What a marvelous contrast to an infant arriving in the world to a bright, cold, noisy room, held up in the air until he cries, then, totally stressed out, given to the mother.

It is common nowadays for the father or partner to attend the labor and delivery. However, if the woman's partner faints at the sight of blood, he may prefer not to be there. These feelings should be discussed openly and frankly so that an agreement can be reached before labor begins.

Some places allow the siblings and grandparents to attend the labor and birth. If this option is available, everyone involved should discuss it and be prepared well in advance of the event.

Before the 1960s, the delivery process was much more rigid and conservative. The woman was placed in a passive role and often not presented with alternatives to the standard delivery procedure. Usually, the father of the baby was not allowed into the delivery room. The mother was admitted to the hospital as soon as contractions began, anesthetized or medicated for pain, and after delivery remained in the hospital for several days.

Later in the 1960s, more couples began to control the delivery by choosing to deliver their babies at home. In response, the health care community examined its care and has become more flexible in the options it offers. Today there is a much greater emphasis on the woman's being in control of her labor. Fathers now attend labor and delivery, women walk around during labor, try alternative delivery positions such as sitting, squatting, or water deliveries, siblings watch, and delivery rooms are homier than they used to be. All these changes help make the woman feel more comfortable and the delivery more positive.

Although the amount of flexibility in care provided varies, things are generally better now than they were in the early 1960s; nevertheless, there is still room for improvement in attitudes of personnel and in the hospital environments across the country. Changes will occur more quickly if pregnant couples are clear about how they want their delivery experience to proceed, and if they are willing to take the responsibility to request and negotiate for what they want.

Many women choose to deliver in birth centers that are affiliated with hospitals in case emergency transfer is needed. To deliver in a birth center, women are usually first identified to be at low risk for complications. Women who do not meet the low-risk criteria are usually referred to hospital settings that are equipped to deal with any potential emergencies or problems.

The decision to deliver at home is being made less frequently today as more hospitals, health care facilities, and health caregivers are becoming more responsive to the needs and desires of pregnant women.

The Postpartum Period

The actual postpartum period lasts from four to six weeks following delivery. During this time, the reproductive organs revert from a pregnant to a nonpregnant state. After about six weeks the woman's body is back to normal but she still may not have lost the weight she gained during the pregnancy, especially if she is breast-feeding the baby.

In the 1940s, women remained flat in bed for 10 to 14 days after a normal vaginal delivery. Now, health care professionals know it is important to get the woman out of bed and back to normal routines as soon as possible after delivery. As a rule, hospital stays now average two to five days for a delivery, but the length of time a woman stays in the hospital will depend on her condition, her preference, and the advice of her caregiver.

Breast Feeding versus Bottle Feeding

The saying "Breast milk is the best milk for the baby" is true. However, it does not mean that breast milk is the *only* adequate method of nourishing a baby. Prepared formulas can provide nourishment that allows the baby to grow and thrive.

The advantages of breast feeding are as follows: breast fed infants do not get ill or have diarrhea as frequently as those that are bottle fed; they have fewer allergies; and breast milk provides maternal antibodies and immunological cells that stimulate the infant's immune system.

When deciding whether to breast or bottle feed, the mother should consider her desires and preferences. Women need to remember that either option will nourish the infant adequately, and that strong psychological relationships are not built upon the method by which the infant is fed.

Rh Negative Blood Type

About one in seven women has Rh negative blood type. This is not a problem unless the woman develops antibodies to the Rh positive blood factor. This can occur if she delivers an Rh positive baby or if she receives a blood transfusion of Rh positive blood. The presence of antibodies in the mother will cause problems for her fetus if she becomes pregnant with an Rh positive baby.

There is a drug called RhoGam that Rh negative women can take after pregnancy to prevent the development of antibodies. RhoGam must be given after each abortion, ectopic pregnancy, or full-term pregnancy when the baby is Rh positive.

Another benefit of early prenatal care is to determine blood type and plan for appropriate treatment to prevent the development of antibodies in Rh negative women. Knowing one's blood type and carrying a card to indicate it ensures that a person does not receive the wrong blood type in a situation requiring an emergency transfusion.

Pregnancy, Childbirth and Parenting

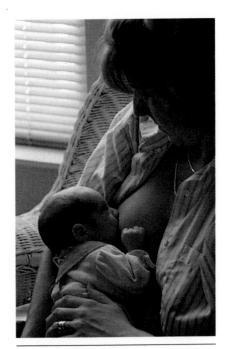

Solid Foods for the Infant

Solid foods for the infant are best introduced under medical supervision. Because of allergies and other problems, solid foods are usually not introduced until the infant has reached the age of six months—very different from past years.

Some parents choose to make their own food for their infants because they feel it is more natural and has fewer contaminants. These parents are willing to take the extra time required for food preparation. Others elect to feed their infants foods prepared especially for children of certain ages. They like the convenience of store-bought baby food and the fact that it is properly balanced for the specific age of the child.

Medical and Health Care for the Infant

Health care for the infant includes well baby checkups and arranging for care if the baby gets sick. The caregiver should be selected before delivery so that care and evaluation is available from birth. Major sources for pediatric health care include private physicians, group health care organizations, and health department clinics.

Infants are seen regularly by a nurse practitioner or doctor who evaluates their growth and physical status. Many babies need to receive periodic immunizations. Some parents do not want their children to be immunized because they feel it is not "natural," or because they think the incidence of certain diseases, such as German measles, is low. In fact, the incidence of these diseases is low because of immunizations.

A child who is not immunized is at high risk for developing the disease as it normally and cyclically swings through a population. Recent measles epidemics in this country are an example of what can happen to a group of children who have not been vaccinated. Also, many school districts will not admit children without evidence of immunization.

Parenting

Deciding to become a parent is one of the most difficult decisions you will have to make. Raising children has always been difficult, but changes in the social landscape has made it even more so. Several factors combine to make raising children a serious undertaking: the decline of the extended family, high divorce rates resulting in single parent or blended families, reinterpretation of the roles of men and women, heightened social pressure to achieve, overpopulation, and environmental pollution.

Good parents are made, not born. Parenting does not just come naturally—it is learned. Traditionally, parenting skills were grasped through the context of the extended family. Because the different generations lived together, child-rearing experience was passed from one generation to the next. Younger children were able to gain first-hand knowledge

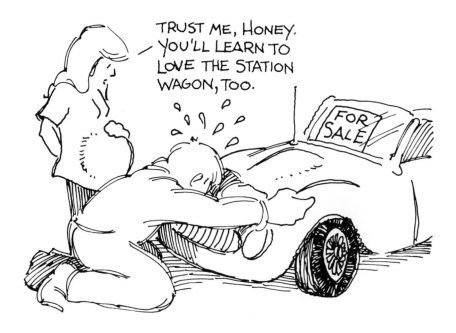

through direct observation and experience. Now, few new parents live close enough to their families to be able to learn from them.

The Decision Process

Parenting is a simultaneously joyful, creative, exhilarating, exasperating, and challenging experience. People want children for many reasons, among them generativity (or wanting to pass on their hopes and values to the next generation), love and emotional security, proof of adulthood, challenge and creativity, and being able to influence someone. Many factors need to be considered before having children, such as financial readiness, both for having a child and caring for a child during the early years.

If you work, it is important to ascertain the benefits you are entitled to if you choose to become pregnant. Does your insurance pay for the delivery, and if so, how much? How long is the pregnancy leave you are entitled to? Will you receive full or partial salary during the leave? Many employers offer only limited benefits to pregnant women and, therefore, women may feel they are being forced to choose between a baby and a career. Men, too, face resistance: it is the rare company that grants pregnancy leave to men who wish to be at home with their wives and newborns during the first months of the infant's life.

Does your company provide on-site child care or a stipend to help you cover the costs? Many working parents wait until the baby is born before they arrange for child care. Keeping up with work and children's schedules requires complex time management skills and needs to be

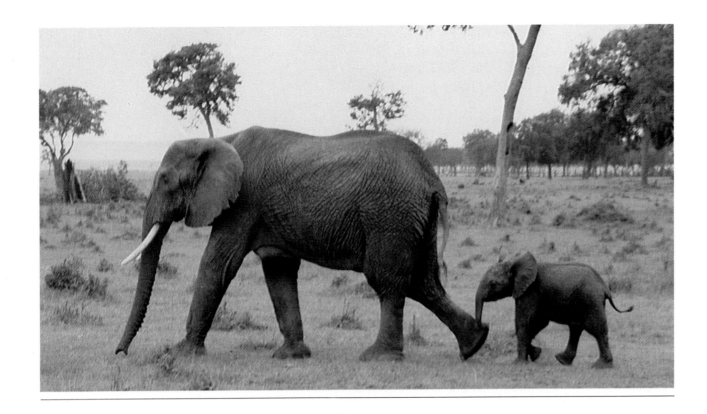

worked out in advance. How much sick time and vacation time are you entitled to? How would your company feel if you had to take time off because your child or child care worker was sick? These are all questions better asked and answered before the decision to continue working and have a family is made.

Emotional readiness is also important to consider; for example, your willingness to share your life with a baby, the political and social climate, and the reasons for wanting a child. Although the addition of a baby may bring couples closer together, it may also create stress and require numerous changes. Careers are interrupted or abandoned, leisure time is lost, and couples no longer have as much time for just each other. The joy and rewards from children make all of this stress easier to bear but it remains an important decision that should be consciously made.

Joan Ditzion and Dennie Wolf of the Boston Women's Health Book Collective (1978) state:

The decision to parent cannot be taken lightly. As soon as we've decided to become parents through pregnancy, adoption, or step-parenting, we find ourselves confronted with new emotional decisions. We want to develop a strong bond with our child and at the same time maintain our partnership, our adult friendships, as well as our involvement with the outside world. What we discover even before we have a baby is that our lives are thrown off balance once we become parents and we need time to establish a new equilibrium.

Pregnancy, Childbirth and Parenting

If you are thinking about becoming a parent, ask yourself the following questions.

- Why do I want a child?
- Am I willing to devote myself to a child twenty-four hours a day, seven days a week?
- Am I financially capable of supporting a baby?
- Am I willing to give up or interrupt my career?
- Do I have adequate support from my partner, spouse, family, friends, social network?
- Am I responsible enough to care for a baby? Have I responsibly cared for myself?
- How does my partner feel about becoming a parent?
- Do I drink alcohol, take drugs, smoke cigarettes, or have any destructive habits that might interfere with the health of a baby?

Following Through

Once you have decided to become a parent the real work begins: rearing a child. Much can be learned informally through interacting with other parents and children, or more formally through reading and talking to health professionals, teachers, and child specialists. However, most of the knowledge comes from on-the-job training. Even your mistakes (and what parent does not make mistakes) are teachers. You must be willing to admit your mistakes, reevaluate them—and carry on. The most important points to remember are to support and love the child.

Parents need to remember that children are neither clones nor the property of their parents: they have minds, wills, personalities, and interests of their own. Children are separate, unique, independent beings who simultaneously resemble their parents yet differ from them in important ways. Parents can foster self-esteem in their children by recognizing and appreciating them for who they are.

According to Erikson, the tasks of a parent are to instill trust, foster autonomy, encourage initiative, and demonstrate industry. Parents who recognize their children's individuality and separateness, and who encourage them to be who they are, help them become responsible, independent heirs of the future.

Child Care

Child care is a major concern of modern parents. Whether someone is hired to come into the home or the child is taken to some other place for care, there are several things you should look for when selecting someone to care for your child. What are the caregiver's attitudes toward children, past experience with youngsters, ability to function in an emergency, decision-making skills, and trustworthiness? If the child is older, then an important consideration is his or her level of comfort and contentment

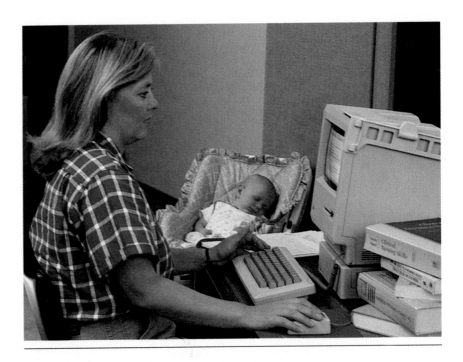

with the caregiver. Factors to consider when evaluating day care centers are the traveling distance, cleanliness, and state approval or licensing.

The cost of child care varies widely; for many families cost is a major consideration. Cost is not always a direct measure of quality. Often, however, good child care is expensive. Parents should explore their options early and widely. It is possible to find good quality for reasonable cost.

Family Relationships

The birth of a new baby introduces a new member into an already formed relationship. Before the birth of the first baby, there are often two people in the relationship who are accustomed to being with each other exclusively. The baby will cause an alteration in the relationship as it shifts to accommodate a new member. For many couples, this may result in some stress.

It is common for one of the members of the couple to be jealous of the amount of time, energy, and attention the partner gives the baby. The couple can ease the discomfort of this transition by discussing their feelings openly with each other, and by being aware that their feelings are normal. A strategy for maintaining a close bond between the couple is to plan regular times when the couple can be alone together, so they can devote that time to maintaining and nurturing their relationship.

Another consideration in expanding family relationships is the introduction of a new being into a family that already has children. The baby may cause the other children to experience feelings of loss, displacement, anger, or jealousy. Parents can help children decrease the impact of these feelings by recognizing and discussing them in a caring, accepting way. Also, providing regular, special time for siblings can help reinforce their feelings of being cared for and secure.

Seeking Professional Help

Because pregnancy and childbirth involve significant physical change, stress, and responsibility, the circumstances under which a woman should seek professional care in this area are numerous.

Seek Help If:

- You are sexually active and have a late or missed period ("late" depends on your normal cycle)
- You have a diagnosed sexually transmitted disease or suspect you may have one
- You are pregnant or planning to become pregnant in the near future. Some problems are easier to correct if a woman is not pregnant; others threaten the woman or her unborn child if they remain undetected. Certainly visit a physician before becoming pregnant if:

1. Your blood is Rh-negative, you have had a previous pregnancy and never had RhoGAM
2. You know or suspect your mother took DES while pregnant with you
3. You have a family history of genetically linked diseases, such as diabetes, epilepsy, Down's syndrome, Tay-Sachs, or sickle cell anemia
4. You are using birth control pills or an IUD
5. You are 36 years or older and this is your first pregnancy
6. You have health problems that may be complicated by pregnancy, such as hypertension, heart disease, anemia, Hodgkin's disease, or diabetes
7. You are using tobacco, alcohol, or other drugs (including OTCs) and would continue to do so while pregnant and nursing
8. You have had a voluntary abortion, miscarriage, ectopic pregnancy, or other reproductive-related problem

- You are pregnant and experience bleeding, fainting, dizziness, blurred vision, fluid retention, persistent vomiting, severe abdominal pain, or any other unusual and/or persistent symptom
- You suspect or know you are experiencing an unwanted pregnancy
- You are emotionally upset about a miscarriage, voluntary abortion, stillbirth, or other reproductive or parenting problem
- Every expectant parent should talk with their care provider before birth about signs of illness in babies and children.

Types of Help Available

If you are pregnant with an unwanted or unplanned baby, you may seek counseling from a family planning clinic, sexual health counselor, or private physician. For assistance with pregnancy, either an obstetrician, nurse practitioner, or certified midwife will counsel and provide care throughout pregnancy, labor, and delivery. Consult your care provider or family physician for a referral.

Beyond the Text

1. A single college friend of yours says she's pregnant (by a man she is no longer involved with) and that she's considering keeping the baby. What would you say?

2. Respond to the statement: Having more than two children just isn't socially responsible.

3. Respond to the following: Childbirth in hospitals is often unnecessarily invasive, stressful, restrictive, and actually increases some risks to mother and child.

4. A pregnant friend reports that a former sexual partner has been diagnosed as having an STD. What dangers could she have been exposed to?

5. Respond to the following statement: Parenting is a process that just comes naturally when children are born.

Supplemental Readings

Ideal Birth by Sondra Ray. Berkeley, CA: Celestial Arts, 1986. Presents a spiritual approach to conception, pregnancy, and childbirth.

Taking Care of Your Child by James Fries, MD, et al. Healdsburg, CA: Medical SelfCare, 1986. A classic guide to pediatrics for parents. Easy to use and reassuring.

The Biological Clock: Balancing Marriage, Motherhood, and Career by M. McKaughan. New York: Penguin Books, 1987. Written for women aged twenty-five to forty-five who are concerned about when, and if, they should have children.

The Maternity Sourcebook: 230 Basic Decisions for Pregnancy, Birth, and Baby Care by Wendy and Matthew Lesko. New York: Warner Books, 1984. Written for first-time mothers. Topics covered include nutrition and health, the hospital experience, legal rights, and others.

When Men are Pregnant by Jerrold Lee Shapiro. San Luis Obispo, CA: Impact Publishers, 1987. Discusses pregnancy and childbirth from a male perspective.

Key Terms Defined

abortion premature expulsion from the uterus of the embryo or of a nonviable fetus

alpha-fetoprotein test done from the mother's blood to diagnose fetal problems, such as spina bifida

amniocentesis medical test in which a small amount of fluid is drawn from the amniotic sac to test for Down's syndrome and genetic diseases

artificial insemination deposit of seminal fluid within the vagina or cervix by artificial means

chromosomes structures in the cell nucleus that carry the heredity factors (genes) composed of DNA and protein

conception fertilization of an ovum by a sperm, marking the onset of pregnancy

dominant trait a specific trait, determined by a gene that prevails over another, recessive trait

ectopic pregnancy fertilized ovum in the tube rather than the uterus—cannot develop to viable embryo

fetal alcohol syndrome condition distinguished by specific physical and mental abnormalities in infants born to mothers who ingest moderate to large amounts of alcohol during pregnancy

genes located on the chromosomes, these biologic units transmit hereditary information

genetic diseases specific diseases known to be inherited

heredity genetic transmission of traits from parents to offspring (determined at the moment of conception)

in vitro fertilization fertilization of an egg in a test tube, followed by transfer to a nutrient medium and subsequent transfer to the mother's body

infertility inability to conceive viable offspring

midwife specially trained women who administer prenatal care and assist at low-risk deliveries

ovulation release of a mature ovum from an ovary approximately 14 days prior to the onset of menstruation

recessive trait specific trait, determined by a gene on a chromosome, that will not occur in offspring unless matched at fertilization by an identical gene on the pairing chromosome

sonography recording of sound waves passed through body parts, such as a pregnant woman's abdomen, showing the image of the fetus

Alcohol and Other Drugs

Today, 85 to 95 percent of college students consume alcohol routinely. According to polls by the Gallup organization, "no other U.S. population has a larger proportion of drinkers than college students." Studies suggest that approximately 20 to 25 percent of college students have drinking problems, and over two-thirds of college students in one survey reported they had a friend with a drinking problem.

Alcohol is the most prevalent drug on campus, but it's not the only one. The marijuana and psychedelics of the sixties have been joined by cocaine, amphetamine "study drugs," and a constantly proliferating array of synthetically produced "designer drugs."

Knowing about alcohol and other drugs won't keep them from having negative consequences in your life. But you can make informed choices about what to do and what to avoid. You can learn to recognize when you or someone else is in trouble and know how to get help. The aim of this chapter is to help you keep problems with alcohol and other drugs from interfering with your college experience.

Key Terms

Addiction	Drug abuse	Opiate
BAC	Ethanol	OTC drugs
Codependent	Hallucinogen	Overdose
Crack	Intoxication	Psychoactive drug
Dependency	Marijuana	Recreational drugs
Depressant	Narcotic	Stimulant

Contents

Defining "Alcohol and Other Drugs"

If you take prescription medications, even in dosages that exceed therapeutic levels, maybe you say, "I don't use drugs; my doctor prescribed this medication." A friend might say, "I just drink and smoke cigarettes. They're legal; they're not drugs." In fact, all mood-modifying substances are drugs. In this chapter, "drug" refers to chemicals used to alleviate a medical condition, for social or recreational purposes, to change a mood, to facilitate a relationship, to solve a problem, or to produce a feeling of euphoria (being high). This definition includes prescription medications, over-the-counter (OTC) medications that can be purchased without a prescription, alcohol, cigarettes, and the caffeine in coffee and tea, as well as all the illegal substances we generally think of when someone says "drugs."

In our culture, you can easily forget that alcohol is actually a drug. After all, alcohol is legal (at least for those over 21), and you can buy it almost everywhere. Most people's parents use it. It may be served to students and faculty at the college president's home. In spite of this aura of social acceptability, more people are now recognizing that alcohol is a drug. Drinking alcohol alters mood, has complex physiological effects, and can create physical and psychological dependence and damage as powerful as any narcotic or other illicit drug.

Alcohol, Drugs and College

You learn about alcohol and other drugs from many sources: society, including television and other mass media, your ethnic and community surroundings, your family, and your friends. Each source teaches and urges certain drug-related attitudes and behaviors.

For centuries, people have used alcohol and opiates for relief; contemporary pharmacology offers college students literally thousands of pain-relieving drugs. The use of drugs for pain relief also includes seeking relief from emotional pain—conflict, alienation, stress.

At college, recreational use and social bonding use often overlap. Many campus parties include at least alcohol, if not other drugs as well. Sometimes alcohol and other drugs are adjuncts to the main social interactions, but sometimes they become the focus. Though you may make decisions about using alcohol or other drugs based on what your friends are using, you—not your friends—are really responsible for the choices you make.

The desire for intoxication, whether for spiritual purposes or pure enjoyment, is part of human nature. Native Americans in a sweat bath, Sufi dervishes whirling in religious ecstasy, and student drinkers at a Friday night kegger or passing a joint of marijuana are all seeking an altered state of consciousness. Alcohol and other drugs are the most common ways people achieve intoxication because they are easily available and require no physical exertion or mental concentration.

The trouble with life in the fast lane is that you get to the other end in an awful hurry.

John Jensen

I've never been drunk, but often I've been overserved.

George Gobel

Alcohol and Other Drugs

You may hear particular drugs promoted as a route to enhanced sexual, athletic, artistic, or academic performance. Various substances have had such reputations for centuries. Many impoverished Indians in Bolivia and Peru chew coca leaves to be able to keep working in the tin mines for 12 to 16 hours a day. For generations, "Spanish fly" (actually a ground-up beetle) had a reputation for sexual arousal; its users overlooked that its physical sensations actually resulted from damaging irritation of the bowel and urinary tract. Contemporary American drug forms are often more concentrated than in other times and cultures, increasing the likelihood of unwanted side effects. Though some drugs may make you feel more physically powerful, they don't actually create power or strength; a drug and its side effects also can rob you of strength and concentration just when you need them most. The one type of drug that does build muscle mass, steroids, does so at significant physical and psychological cost.

Truth and Consequences of Alcohol

On most campuses, between 87 percent and 93 percent of students drink, with female drinkers coming close to or equaling the number of male drinkers. If you drink, college is a critical time to learn to become conscious of and responsible about your drinking. Researchers report that heavy drinking on campuses has increased substantially in the past decade. Alcohol is the largest drug problem on college campuses; it is involved in the highest proportion of substance-related campus problems—injuries, property damage, unwanted pregnancies, STDs, auto and motorcycle accidents, and so forth. Problem alcohol use in college also interferes with interpersonal relationships, good health, and academic performance.

How Much Alcohol Is in Your Drink?

Alcoholic Beverage	Alcohol Content
Ale	5%
Malt Beverage	7%
Regular Beer	4%
Wine and Champagne	12%
Liqueurs	40%
Wine Cooler	4%
Distilled Spirits*	45%
Mixed Drinks**	
Strong	30%
Medium	15%
Light	7%

*Scotch, rum, vodka

**Martini, manhattan, daiquiri

Source: National Highway Traffic Safety Administration

How Alcohol Levels Affect Behavior

BAC	Behavioral Effects
0.02	No measurable effects
0.05	Decreases in reaction time; elevated mood
0.10	Loss of some motor coordination; greater decrease in reaction time; some impairment of judgment
0.15	Clearly identifiable impairment of motor coordination and reaction time; slurred speech patterns
0.20	Noticeably intoxicated; severe loss of motor coordination
0.30	Conscious, but minimal control of faculties
0.40	Unconscious, lethal dose to 50 percent of population (LD 50)
0.60	Lethal dose for 99 percent of the population (LD 99)

Source: Drug Abuse and Mental Health Administration

Drinking and Levels of Intoxication

Drinks (Two-Hour Period)
1.5 ozs. 80-Proof Liquor or 12 ozs. Beer

Weight												
100	1	2	3	4	5	6	7	8	9	10	11	12
120	1	2	3	4	5	6	7	8	9	10	11	12
140	1	2	3	4	5	6	7	8	9	10	11	12
160	1	2	3	4	5	6	7	8	9	10	11	12
180	1	2	3	4	5	6	7	8	9	10	11	12
200	1	2	3	4	5	6	7	8	9	10	11	12
220	1	2	3	4	5	6	7	8	9	10	11	12
240	1	2	3	4	5	6	7	8	9	10	11	12

Be Careful Driving BAC to .05%	Driving Impared .05%-.09%	Do Not Drive .10% & Up

The chart shows average responses. Tests show a wide range of responses even for people of the same age and weight. For some people, one drink may be too many. Source: NHTSA

The Basics of Drinking and Drunk

Because alcohol is legal and heavily regulated, dosage is predictable from drink to drink—drinking any particular amount has a fairly predictable effect. The amount of alcohol in one beer is equivalent to the amount in one five-ounce glass of wine or the one and one half ounces of liquor in a typical mixed drink. You can get just as drunk on beer as on hard liquor; beer just contains more water per gram of ethanol, the active ingredient in alcohol. The alcohol level in your blood gives a relatively accurate indication of your level of intoxication. Your body can metabolize approximately one drink (two ounces of ethanol) per hour. Drinking more than that increases blood alcohol level; drinking less lowers it. Because this metabolic process proceeds at a steady pace, the more you drink, the longer time it takes to become sober. The less you weigh, the more any particular amount of alcohol affects you. Having a full stomach postpones alcohol's effects somewhat, but it will not keep you from becoming drunk.

Alcohol has powerful effects. Though you begin to feel the effects of alcohol at a blood alcohol concentration (BAC) level of 0.05 (measured in

States Legislate to Reduce the Allowable BAC Level

Three states—Maine, Oregon, and Utah—already have lowered the allowable blood alcohol content (BAC) to .08 percent. At least five other states, including California, Illinois, Minnesota, North Carolina, and Rhode Island, have introduced legislation to reduce the BAC from .10 to .08 percent.

Common Costs of College Drinking

Results of a student survey at the University of California, Santa Barbara, showed that students reported the following negative consequences of alcohol use at least once during the preceding quarter. Many of these behaviors and consequences were reported as having occurred up to five or more times during the preceding quarter.

Hangover and nausea/vomiting	68%
Loss of memory while or after drinking	46%
Driving a car after several drinks	41%
Cutting class or work after drinking	22%
Giving someone a drink they said they didn't want	22%
Being involved in a violent argument, damaging property, or similar behavior after drinking	18%
Being involved in an accident after drinking	10%

Source: *Setting the Right Course: Alcohol and Drug Education on the College Campus,* University of California, Santa Barbara

How Alcohol Works

Alcohol's chemical structure consists of a carbon, oxygen and hydrogen atom. A common form of alcohol is made from grains—ethanol—and is the type we drink.

Alcohol enters the bloodstream quickly and directly from the small intestine. Once in the bloodstream, it is fairly uniformly distributed throughout all tissues and organs. Alcohol acts as a depressant to the central nervous system, but can cause structural damage to several major organs.

- *Stomach and intestines*: alcohol can cause bleeding; it has been linked to cancer.
- *Brain*: cells are altered and when subjected to increased amounts of alcohol, many die. Over long-term use, alcohol can cause irreversible deterioration.
- *Heart*: deterioration of the heart muscle can occur; blood pressure increases.
- *Immune system*: infection-fighting cells are prevented from functioning properly.
- *Reproductive system*: both men and women's reproductive systems and hormone levels are affected. Birth defects can occur, and alcohol is a major cause of mental retardation.
- *Liver*: this organ suffers more than any other because the liver is where most of the ethanol is broken down. The high calorie content of alcohol results in the liver metabolizing calories, not nutrients; it also causes fat to build up in the liver causing scarring. As the liver cells die, the result is cirrhosis, an often fatal degeneration of the liver (cirrhosis kills at least 14,000 alcoholics a year).

tenths of one percent of blood volume), at 0.1 you're already legally drunk, and at 0.4 you might be dead—at a concentration of just 4/10 of one percent. The effects of various BAC levels and the approximate amounts of alcohol needed to produce certain BAC levels at various body weights are indicated in accompanying charts.

Used responsibly, alcohol can have desirable consequences, such as pleasant taste, relaxation, and socialization. In the wrong amount or the wrong circumstances, alcohol may cause you or your friends harm.

Physical Costs of Alcohol

In extreme cases, alcohol leads to physical damage that is serious, sudden, and sometimes irreversible, such as comas, brain damage, or even death. However, even if you never pass out, alcohol could still be damaging your body. Some effects you would notice as they happen; others may occur without your even being aware. Here are some of these toxic effects:

- *Brain*—hangovers, memory lapses, blackouts
- *Digestive system*—nausea, vomiting, ulcers, liver diseases, other organ corrosion
- *Cardiovascular system*—high blood pressure, heart failure, respiratory distress or failure
- *Nerves and muscles*—loss of muscle coordination
- *Reproductive system*—sexual impotence, irregular periods
- *Overall*—malnutrition, increased cancer risk, weakened immune system, injuries due to falls as well as to violent behavior

The Costs of Drinking and Driving

Estimates are for a first-time offense for drinking and driving. Second or third convictions would result in much stiffer penalties, and include time in jail. Legal costs are based on research by attorney Robert W. Larin.

Fines	Including court costs and alcohol assessment	$ 700
Legal Fees	From arrest through trial	1,000
	To appeal conviction, includes transcript costs	2,500
	For administrative hearing to challenge driver's license revocation	300
	To appeal driver's license revocation	400
Insurance-Rate Increase	Based on a previous annual premium of $500 and for a period of three years	3,000
Total		$7,900

Source: *Friendly Exchange*

Though some of these problems, such as liver disease, take years to develop and are usually seen only in college students who have been drinking since early teen years, others happen quite frequently to college students—not only hangovers and vomiting, but injuries, blackouts, even respiratory failure. You are not too young to suffer significant undesirable physical consequences from alcohol.

Drinking and Driving

Motor vehicle accidents involving intoxication are the leading cause of death among people of college age. Driving While Intoxicated (DWI) (known in some states as Driving Under the Influence, or DUI) occurs with considerable frequency among college students. Not only does alcohol impair driving skills by reducing motor coordination and reflexes, but individuals with inhibitions lowered by alcohol are more likely to disregard traffic safety laws, such as speed limits and red lights. A BAC of 0.05 impairs your driving. At BAC 0.10 you are legally drunk and should not drive under any circumstances. For information on how to estimate whether your drinking exceeds these limits, refer to the chart Drinking and Levels of Intoxication.

In any accident involving DWI, someone may be injured or even killed—driver, passenger, friend, or total stranger. If you are the driver responsible for that injury or death, you may suffer guilt and other mental burdens for years.

If you drink and drive, you may be arrested even if you haven't been involved in an accident. DWI arrests are expensive. The total cost of a drunk

Drinking and Driving

On a national basis, total alcohol-related traffic deaths have averaged nearly 24,000 per year for the past five years. Alcohol-impaired driving is the leading cause of death and injury among those under 25 years of age.

driving conviction for a college-aged student often approaches $8,000, as the accompanying box details. The loss of a license, a fine, and a couple of days in jail are only part of the penalty. About 60 percent of drunk drivers are ordered to undergo mandatory substance abuse treatment, which can cost up to $5,000. In addition, once you get your license back, your insurance rates skyrocket for at least three to five years. Such lessons seem hard to learn: research has shown that 60 percent of those with one conviction for DWI repeat within two years.

If you (or friends) drink and drive, you may do so because you feel invulnerable—nothing can happen to you. Even if you (or your friends) have never had any accidents while driving after drinking, the next time may be different. Driving involves many variables beyond your control, such as road hazards and other drivers; you may encounter a driving situation in which being sober behind the wheel makes a life-or-death difference.

Alcohol and Sex

Intoxication lowers your ability to make safe decisions about sex, including with whom you will have sex and what precautions you will take. Intoxication distorts judgment, diminishes your ability to perceive danger, and reduces even your awareness of choices. A major way to prevent AIDS and other STDs is to minimize the degree of intoxication so you can make and carry out careful decisions about sexual activity. (For more information, see **AIDS** chapter and **Sexual Health** chapter.)

In almost all unplanned pregnancies, acquaintance rape cases, and incidents of pressured sex involving college students, one or both of the participants were intoxicated at the time of the occurrence. Students often report later, "We were drinking and didn't think of using protection." Imagine trying to put on a condom or insert a diaphragm properly while drunk; that's why responsible sexual relationship choices and responsible alcohol use cannot be separated. Avoiding intoxication, particularly in unfamiliar surroundings or with people you do not know well, is an effective technique in avoiding acquaintance rape.

Alcohol and Academics

A University of Minnesota study found that students with lower grades tended to be heavier drinkers than higher achievers. Though no one has proven that drinking causes poor academic performance, this study supports the possibility. Forty percent of 20 year olds had missed a class, work or appointment because of drinking; 9 percent said they got lower grades because of drinking.

Alcohol affects memory and concentration, so it makes studying effectively and understanding lectures more difficult. Students who drink a lot may skip class or studying, not just when drunk, but also when sleeping it off or suffering from a hangover. Some miss academic work because of

---

Is a Drink a Drink?

Each of these contains approximately the same amount of alcohol:

12 oz. beer mug = 5 oz. wine glass = 1½ oz. shot glass

According to research by John McKillip, a psychology professor at Southern Illinois University, a fifth of the university's 20,000 students test poorly or skip class at least once a month because of heavy drinking.

The Wall Street Journal

Categorizing Drugs

Congress passed the Comprehensive Drug Abuse Control Act in 1971. A law enforcement bill stemming from this act divided drugs with actual or relative potential for abuse into five categories called schedules.

- Schedule I   No accepted medical use and high abuse potential.
- Schedule II   Some currently accepted medical use but availability is tightly restricted. High potential for abuse, with severe physical dependence potential.
- Schedule III   Current medical use with less potential for abuse than drugs in Schedule I and II. Low to moderate potential for physical addiction but a high potential for psychological dependence.
- Section IV   Has a currently accepted medical use, a low potential for abuse, and limited potential for psychological or physical abuse.
- Section V   Has a currently accepted medical use and low potential for abuse relative to drugs in Schedule IV.

Did you know? Coca-Cola contained cocaine for 17 years until it was replaced by caffeine in 1903. Things must have really gone better in those days.

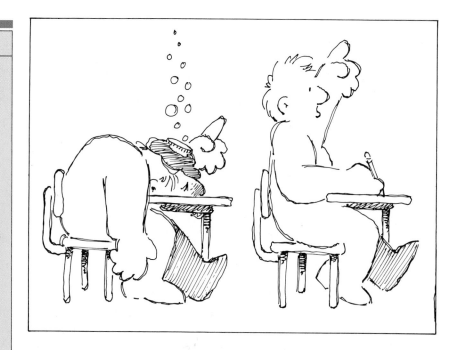

injuries sustained while drinking, or because of increased illnesses that result from the effect of alcohol on the immune system.

Uses and Risks of Specific Drugs

Drugs are usually classified according to their major physical effect: stimulant, depressant, narcotic, and hallucinogen. Each drug has specific effects and risks. However, diluting drugs with impurities, or mixing them, can cause very unpredictable results.

Stimulants

A central nervous system stimulant speeds up a major body function—heart rate, respiration, and so forth. It raises blood pressure, which increases risk of cardiovascular damage. All major categories of stimulants—amphetamines, cocaine, nicotine, and caffeine—are used in significant quantity on college campuses.

Amphetamines   First synthesized by a German pharmacologist in 1887, amphetamines have been popular as an "energizer" almost since that time. Their use has increased to between 10 and 12 billion doses yearly, and, as the use has increased, so has the abuse. Estimates are that 50 to 80 percent of this product is diverted for illicit use. On the street, these drugs are known as speed, dexies, bennies, cross tops, crank, and blackies.

Students who want to stay up late studying may take amphetamines to keep going. Dr. Katheryn McIntyre, a psychiatrist at the University of Texas Counseling and Mental Health Center, warns that "tasks that are creative are not enhanced" by chemical stimulants. A recent article in *Newsweek on Campus* added that "students who pull all-nighters with speed may end up having an even harder time absorbing and retrieving the information they're trying so desperately to master."

The most common methods of taking amphetamines are orally and by injection, either under the skin or directly into a vein. Several additives are used to "step on," or water down, amphetamines; these may provide a rush to make up for the absence of the drug.

Amphetamines act as adrenaline-like agents and cause a massive "fight or flight" response in the body. The signs and symptoms include dilated pupils, high blood pressure, and rapid pulse. The user has a feeling of euphoria and self-confidence and may be extremely talkative or irritable. Overdose with this drug can produce stroke, cardiovascular collapse, seizures, or even coma.

Amphetamines are not addictive in the true definition of the word because users build a tolerance level but do not suffer withdrawal symptoms when they discontinue use. Frequent users, however, must take increasingly higher doses to obtain the same effect.

Ecstasy, or MDMA, a drug analog of an amphetamine, is becoming more and more popular on college campuses. Though a stimulant, this drug has some of the properties of an hallucinogen. More about this drug is included in the section on "Designer Drugs."

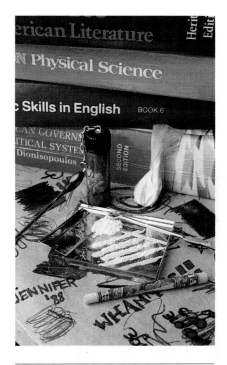

Cocaine   Now the most abused major stimulant in the United States, it is estimated that 5,000 people begin using cocaine every day. The typical user is male, 18 to 35 years old, with a history of prior abuse of alcohol or marijuana. Cocaine use among women is increasing, just as it is among teenagers. In one recent study, cocaine was the second-most prevalent nonalcoholic drug among college students (after marijuana). Although less than 4 percent of the students in this study reported currently using cocaine, almost 17 percent had tried it.

Cocaine users represent all socioeconomic groups and come from all occupations. The increased availability and subsequent lower cost has transformed this drug from an upper-class activity to a country-wide form of recreation. Cocaine appears to be the leisure-time drug of choice for many Americans.

Cocaine is most commonly used as a fine, white crystalline powder. Street names for the drug include coke, snow, toot, lady, blow, flake, happy trails, gold dust, green gold, and star-spangled powder. Purity of cocaine can vary from 25 to 90 percent, as it is mixed with different substances such as glucose, lactose, mannitol, cornstarch, and even flour or talc. Frequently it is used with other drugs; for example, a "speedball" is a combination of cocaine and heroin administered intravenously, and when cocaine is mixed with alcohol, it is called "liquid lady."

Although powdered cocaine can be taken by injection into a muscle or

New Facts About Cocaine

Cocaine produces long-lasting, if not permanent, effects on the brain. It damages the brain's ability to respond to neurotransmitters involved in control of movement.

Crack, the smokeable form of cocaine, is far more addictive and dangerous because it goes directly to the brain in much larger amounts than cocaine.

From 1983 to 1986, there was a 167 percent increase in hospital emergencies and a 124 percent increase in deaths related to cocaine.

How Cocaine Kills

Cocaine works by intensifying the normal physiologic effects of nerves that help regulate many of our internal organs, especially the heart and the brain. When these nerves are activated, they release a chemical called norepinephrine (pronounced nor-eppy-NEF-rin). This chemical causes a change in the activity of the organ served by the nerves (for example, it speeds the heart and causes it to beat more vigorously).

Ordinarily, the effects produced by norepinephrine last only a very short time because the nerves recapture much of the released norepinephrine and pump it back inside the nerve. There it can be stored and released again. By releasing and reclaiming the norepinephrine, the nerves can finely influence and control the organs.

Cocaine disrupts this control by preventing the return of norepinephrine to the nerve. As a result, the effects produced when the nerve is activated become prolonged, intensified and exaggerated as norepinephrine accumulates in the tissue served by the nerve. The brain and other organs may be harmed by too much norepinephrine-induced stimulation.

The peak effect of cocaine on the brain is long gone at a time when much of the drug still remains in the blood and is distributed throughout the body. Consider what happens when a person decides to take a second dose of cocaine one hour after the first. The second dose will add to the amount remaining from the first, and intensify the ensuing effects. If additional doses are taken more rapidly than they can be eliminated, the drug will steadily accumulate in the blood, with potentially disastrous consequences.

High doses of cocaine produce much more serious effects in the heart and the brain. These organs generate subtle electrical currents. Small amounts of norepinephrine released from nerves alter these currents and influence the function of the organs. Cocaine can cause the accumulation of enough norepinephrine to disrupt these currents and throw the delicate electrical balance of the organ into disarray. In the brain, such a disruption can cause convulsions and may lead to death from respiratory failure. Disruption of the electrical activity of the heart may stop the heart muscle completely—producing immediate death—by forcing it to beat so quickly that it becomes exhausted, like any other muscle when overused, and loses its power to beat further.

L. R. Willis, PhD
Indiana University

With a volume of $300 billion a year, the drug trade is the world's biggest business.

intravenously, it is usually taken intranasally, while freebase is generally smoked. Most users in the United States prefer nasal inhalation or "snorting." They arrange the powder in a line, about 10 to 35 mg, on a smooth surface, then breathe it in through a straw. The substance is rapidly absorbed through the nasal mucous membranes with peak effects occurring 15 to 60 minutes later, and a half-life duration of one to two hours.

Crack, or freebase, is a form of cocaine that has become increasingly popular. It is prepared by mixing powdered street cocaine with an alkaline solution and a solvent, such as ether. The combination separates into two layers; the solvent evaporates, leaving pure cocaine crystals, or the freebase form, which is usually smoked. It is called "crack" because of the cracking sound that occurs when the crystals are heated.

The primary effect of cocaine is stimulation of the central nervous system. It enhances the release of norepinephrine and dopamine which increase levels of circulating catecholamines causing sympathetic stimulation. This results in increased blood pressure, pulse, and respirations which accompany the feeling of euphoria, the first phase of cocaine intoxication. This lasts for only a few minutes and is characterized by intense pleasure and exhilaration. The more rapid the intake of cocaine, the greater the intensity of euphoria. About 20 to 30 minutes after the drug is ingested, the dysphoric phase occurs—a letdown and depression. The person becomes irritable, withdrawn, and at times antisocial. Repeating this cycle of up and down is called a "cocaine run." Some users get on this run and snort at 10 to 40 minute intervals over a period of several hours or even days. Finally, the user crashes and experiences deep exhaustion and depression.

Complications from cocaine use are devastating to the body and may result in death. They range from cardiac complications, which can lead to death from heart arrhythmias, and central nervous system problems, such as seizures, to cerebrovascular accidents and psychiatric disturbances. Cocaine can also lead to respiratory arrest, gastrointestinal symptoms, and severely impaired sexual drive and impotence. For pregnant women, it can result in major birth defects. It is one of the most addictive drugs known to man. According to emergency physician Dr. Charles E. Stewart, "Cocaine related death and emergency department visits have skyrocketed some 200 percent since 1976, while admissions to treatment programs have increased by more than 500 percent."

Nicotine and Caffeine Two drugs commonly found on college campuses, nicotine and caffeine, are easily obtained, relatively inexpensive, and very legal. For as long as colleges have existed in the United States, nicotine has played a role in daily life as the addictive ingredient in cigarettes, pipe tobacco, cigars, and smokeless tobacco. Since the mid-1960s, when the Surgeon General's report linked smoking to cancer and heart diseases, smoking has declined among the college educated segment of the population. A full description of nicotine's addictive qualities and effects is included in the **Health Hazards of Tobacco** chapter.

Caffeine is one of the most prevalent drugs on campus because it is an ingredient in popular beverages, such as coffee, tea, and many soft drinks. Caffeine is also found in chocolate and in several over-the-counter medications designed for weight control, fighting cold symptoms, or staying awake. You can develop a true physical addiction to caffeine which, like other stimulants, raises blood pressure. Significant long-term effects of caffeine include high blood pressure, gastrointestinal disorders, and certain forms of cancer. By gradually decreasing your intake to two servings per day and by shifting to caffeine-free beverages, you can minimize your risk of addiction and minimize threats to your overall health. Additional information on caffeine is included in the chapter on **Nutrition Awareness**.

The Crack Problem

Crack, a major problem in many sections of urban America, is beginning to spread to the suburbs. This highly-addictive form of cocaine (it is reported that 1 out of 3 crack users become addicted to cocaine) has more than tripled the number of cocaine addicts in New York City, just to cite one example. According to New York State statistics, the 182,000 regular cocaine abusers in 1986 grew to a total of 600,000 in 1988.

One reason crack is so addictive is that it delivers its most powerful effects with the first dose. Dr. Sidney Cohen, clinical professor of psychiatry at the UCLA Neuropsychiatric Institute, has said, "It is probably impossible to remain a 'social' crack user if crack is available. All who try the drug are liable to become crack dependent. Crack users try to recapture those first moments with every subsequent use. But it is never quite as good as the first time . . . the feelings of euphoria are followed inevitably by a 'crash,' a state of deep depression and sadness. Crack users attempt to relieve these bad feelings by returning to the drug that took them up before."

DWS—Driving While Stoned

The effect of marijuana on the smoker's ability to drive is harder to gauge than that of alcohol. Rather than affecting the simple motor skills involved in driving, marijuana seems to interfere with perception and attention processes. In combination with alcohol, it can have extreme effects on judgment and performance. And these effects may even be delayed and unpredictable.

Source: *University of California, Berkeley Wellness Letter*

Barbiturates   Abuse of barbiturates in America is well known. Either sedatives or hypnotics, these drugs have medical value and use. They are prescribed as anticonvulsants, they relieve anxiety, and they have helped to alleviate sleep disorders, although they are no longer the drug of choice. Overdependence on these drugs is dangerous, for even though physical dependence happens slowly over weeks or even months, it does occur.

Barbiturates are grouped on the basis of duration of action: the first group are short-acting, used primarily for anesthesia induction—Pentothal® is the primary drug in this category. The second group are short- to intermediate-acting and these are used as sedatives. Seconal® and Nembutal® are in this group; they have a 15 minute onset time and last two to three hours. The third group are long-acting barbiturates, and these drugs are used to control seizures, especially in epilepsy. This category is rarely abused. Some of the street names associated with barbiturates are blues, blue angels, blue birds (Amytal®); Nebbies, yellow bullets, yellow dolls (Nembutal); F-40s, Mexican reds, red devils, red dolls (Seconal).

Barbiturates produce depression of the central nervous system, creating a state in which one can be mildly sedated or almost in a coma. Abuse of these drugs results in intoxication, causing a person to act almost drunk, as if they had taken alcohol. This state reduces a person's ability to make good judgments. Those in the middle to upper socioeconomic group, between 30 and 50 years of age, are the most common abusers. In 1971, 40 million barbiturate prescriptions were issued, 22 million of them refills.

Barbiturates are usually taken orally, but they can be mixed with water for intravenous injection. The latter method is the most hazardous because the tolerance level is reached much more quickly. Barbiturates are also often used in conjunction with stimulants; a person uses "uppers" to keep going during the day and "downers" to sleep at night. Signs and symptoms of overdosage include slurring speech, unsteady gait, slowed reactions, and lethargy leading to respiratory depression and coma.

Tranquilizers   Introduced in the 1950s, these drugs are now more often referred to as antianxiety agents. They also function as muscle relaxants. In 1960, both Librium® and Valium® entered the marketplace and rapidly became one of the most abused drug groups. An estimated 5 billion doses of these so-called mild tranquilizers (to distinguish them from the major tranquilizers or antipsychotics used in severe mental illness) were sold in 1979.

These minor tranquilizers are used for patients who suffer from prolonged anxiety, stress, and insomnia. They are also used for any muscular or structural disorder, such as low back pain, stiff neck, and so forth. Those who have become dependent on these drugs for everyday survival find that they cannot function without them. Their tolerance level goes up and they find themselves taking more and more to have the same effect. Both physical dependence and withdrawal symptoms are dangers with these drugs.

Phencyclidine Usually called PCP, or angel dust, this was developed as an animal anesthetic and tranquilizer but is now used by some as a cheaper, more powerful marijuana. However, PCP causes much less predictable reactions than marijuana, reactions that are often very dramatic, even violent or psychotic. Psychologist Stephen J. Levy, who has served as director of the Division of Drug Abuse at the New Jersey Medical School, says, "Even experienced users cannot be certain how it will affect them each time." Young people zonked on PCP frequently wind up admitted to county psychiatric units. More than occasionally, these users do not return to reality; they suffer permanent psychosis.

Narcotics

Morphine and Heroin The term narcotic often refers to a central nervous system depressant. Looking back, we find that the opium poppy was cultivated 6,000 years ago in Sumeria, moved on to Egypt and by the first century AD, the technique to extract opium from the poppy pods was perfected. Today, opium is still harvested as it was centuries ago—gashes are made in the green pod and the next day the white sap, now brownish in color, is scraped off and shaped into opium balls. In the early 1800s, the active ingredient in opium was extracted. It was named morphine, after Morpheus, the Greek god of dreams. This discovery stimulated work on opium, and in the next few years, many different alkaloids were isolated. In 1832, codeine was purified. These compounds became more and more popular, and by the early 1900s, one million Americans were addicted to opiates. In 1898, a new form of opium was concocted and placed on the market as a cough suppressant. It was to be a heroic drug, so it was named Heroin.

Morphine and the other opiates are narcotic sedatives. They depress the central nervous system and interact with specific receptor sites in the brain to inhibit the release of dopamine, norepinephrine, and other neurotransmitters. Heroin also has an analgesic effect.

In 1914, the Harrison Narcotic Act was passed to regulate the sale of opium, coca leaves, and their products. The typical addict during these years was a middle-aged, Southern, white housewife who ordered her supply of opium or morphine from Sears and Roebuck. She used it orally, was probably very nice to her husband and children, and caused very few problems. However, as the addictive properties became more apparent— even many physicians were addicted—pressure was put on Congress to pass the narcotic regulating act. This was followed by the banning of heroin in 1924 from American medicine due to its severe addictive properties. It is now a Schedule I drug with a high potential for abuse and no currently accepted medical use. Because of illegality, a narcotics habit is also

---

Names on the Street

Amphetamines speed, dexies, bennies, cross tops, crank, uppers, wake-ups, lid poppers, cartwheels, blackies

Alcohol booze, white lightning, 3.2 (beer), suds, vino (wine)

Barbiturates barbs, reds, red devils, blues, bluebirds, blue devils, nimbys, yellow jackets, yellow dolls, tuies, double trouble, rainbow

Methaqualone ludes, Qs, love drug, 714s, sopers, quays

MDMA ecstasy, XTC, X, ADAM, love drug

Marijuana grass, weed, smoke, tops, pot, maryjane, hemp; hash, hashish

Heroin H, horse, junk, smack, scag

Morphine M, morph, Miss Emma

Opium O, Op, black stuff

Cocaine coke, crack, rock, snow, toot, lady, blow, flake, happy trails, gold dust, green gold, star-spangled powder

---

The total yearly revenue from narcotics sales in the United States alone is estimated to be between $60 and $120 billion.

quite expensive. Many of the most serious physical complications of these drugs result from their illegal status, such as overdose from inconsistencies in preparation, allergic reactions to contaminants, AIDS or hepatitis from a shared needle. Chronic injection can lead to abscesses, blood poisoning, and vein and lung infections.

Narcotic addiction has gone steadily up since the Harrison Narcotic Act was passed—it is now estimated that between 400,000 and 600,000 persons are narcotic addicted in the United States. Without federal regulation, it would probably be much higher.

Marijuana

The nation's most popular, but perhaps least understood, psychoactive substance is marijuana, or pot. It is illegal, but a great number of Americans do not seem to agree that it should be. They categorize it as harmless as sipping wine. Consisting of dried leaves and flowering tops of the hemp plant, the mixture is usually smoked (or occasionally baked into brownies).

At this time, there is not enough known about the dangers of smoking marijuana except for those who are at particular risk—young people, pregnant and nursing women, heart patients, and the emotionally unstable. Dr. Norman Zinberg, a Harvard psychiatrist says, "Nothing's been proved, but there's reason to worry."

Marijuana use peaked in 1978, but it continues to be popular, especially with the babyboomers who first tried it in the '60s and '70s. It is estimated that 18 million Americans smoke pot regularly and another 62 million have tried it.

Marijuana is not a single drug. In fact, scientists have discovered over 400 chemicals in the cannabis plant, some of which do not contribute to the "high," but others definitely have a psychoactive effect. Delta-9-THC (tetrahydrocannabinol) is the most significant potent hallucinogenic component. The average concentration of THC has increased from about 1 percent in the 1960s to 4 to 10 percent in the 1980s. Hash is the dried resin from the tops and leaves of the female plant. It contains more THC and is more potent than marijuana. When marijuana is smoked, THC enters the lungs and passes into the blood stream. From there it is carried to the brain. Since THC is fat-soluble, it may remain in the fatty tissues of the body—brain, adrenals, gonads, and so forth—for three or more days. These chemicals can be detected in the urine for several weeks; it is not known exactly how long the body stores them in fatty tissue.

People who smoke this drug feel a "high," which lasts for two to four hours. They feel relaxed, dreamy, and pleasant. Often they start craving food, especially sugary snacks. While this may be a problem for some, an even greater concern is that many pot smokers feel sober and continue to function as if they were. One California study showed that one-third of the drivers in fatal car crashes had been smoking marijuana. There is a wide range of reactions in people. The strength of the drug, frequency of

---

A teenager who tries pot has a 10 percent risk of becoming a daily smoker.

Alcohol and Other Drugs

CHAPTER 15

398

use, and basic physiological differences may be responsible for this variation.

The conclusion about marijuana seems to be that for the vast majority of smokers, pot is not physically addictive. It does rank far below the other drugs we have discussed, including alcohol and tobacco. However, used daily and heavily, marijuana could present a serious health problem for the individual.

It is wise to remember that it took decades to research and publicize tobacco's serious threat to health. Recent reports conclude that lung damage from smoking one marijuana joint equals that of smoking five tobacco cigarettes. Marijuana contains more tar and carcinogens than tobacco. Lung tissue of long-term marijuana smokers shows elevated levels of precancerous cellular changes.

Another possible danger of marijuana is to the mind. For those who take it to cope with stress, depression, or anxiety, it may only add to their psychological problems. There also is a recognized connection between smoking pot and poor motivation.

The effects on the reproductive system are unproven but seem ominous. The drug lowers the level of testosterone in men and decreases sperm, but the effect on infertility is unknown. Women who smoke heavily may experience a failure to ovulate and irregular menstrual cycles.

Many facts and, therefore, conclusions, about marijuana use are, as yet, incomplete. In spite of considerable research, the long-term psychological and biological effects continue to elude scientists. However, since marijuana is a drug, you can be sure that it has at least some deleterious effects on the body—the question is, to what extent.

Hallucinogens

Thousands of plants and synthetic chemicals contain hallucinogenic compounds that alter perception. For centuries, various cultures have used most of the "poisonous" mushrooms, several species of cactus, strains of morning glory seed, and many other substances as hallucinogens. More than 10 million Americans have tried hallucinogens, with more than one million stating they are regular users, according to the National Institute on Drug Abuse. Any drug that intensifies perception, cognition, or feelings of being disengaged from reality may be classified as hallucinogenic.

Hallucinogens are extremely powerful; they can affect the mind more dramatically than virtually any other drug. These effects vary widely in individuals, depending on one's individual personality traits, the setting in which the drugs are taken, and unknown determinants. Perceptual changes, the most dramatic effects, range from pleasant to horrifying. Persons exhibit euphoria, fear, alterations of space and time, pain, nausea and vomiting, as well as cardiovascular changes.

Potency differs significantly among hallucinogens; LSD (lysergic acid diethylamide) is 100 times stronger than the mushroom-derived hallucinogen psilocybin and 4000 times as powerful as cactus-derived mescaline. The LSD experience begins slowly, within an hour of ingestion; it

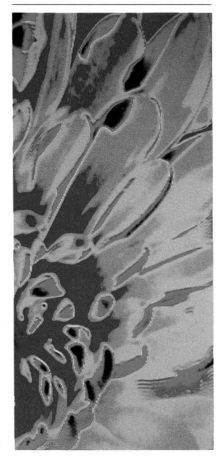

lasts for 2 to 12 hours. Psilocybin has a much shorter cycle, and a mescaline experience may last from 10 to 18 hours.

LSD The days of Timothy Leary in the '60s and the "turn on, tune in and drop out" gang who left academia and their professions to trip out on LSD are over. LSD is not the popular drug it was then, primarily due to its potentially powerful destructive effects.

LSD is usually taken orally, often on a sugar cube. It begins to work within an hour and the person may experience a variety of hallucinogenic effects—changes in perception, thought, and mood. Visual hallucinations may occur and one's sense of time is altered. People have reported bizarre experiences and also the feeling of oneness with the universe. There can be "good trips" and "bad trips." Bad trips are frightening, with paranoid perceptions and even psychotic reactions. Flashbacks may occur, when the user suddenly has a spontaneous recurrence of an LSD experience. These can be unpleasant, even dangerous, especially if you happen to be driving a car.

Magic Mushrooms Many plants, especially certain mushrooms, have LSD-like effects. The active ingredient is psilocybin. A person who consumes a few dried mushrooms may begin to feel the effects in half an hour and they last several hours. Changes in perception, the feeling of relaxation, and a pleasant mood are the predominant reactions. Like LSD, negative reactions can occur: dizziness, numbness in the mouth, nausea and vomiting, flushing, and fatigue. While these side effects may not seem dangerous, if psilocybin is bought on the street, it can contain other dangerous ingredients—for example, PCP, which is cheaper and easier to make. This is a potentially lethal drug, and while it may cause hallucinations, it is not classified as an hallucinogen.

Designer Drugs

A designer drug is a drug analog, a complex copycat of a controlled substance. Synthesized in clandestine labs, this drug will differ slightly from another drug already classified by law as illegal. There are many designer drugs available on the street. They are often significantly more powerful and much less predictable in their side effects than their prohibited chemical cousins.

China White and Ecstasy Well known examples of designer drugs are china white and ecstasy. Fentanyl, or china white, is structurally only a molecule away from heroin, but has proven to be 1000 to 2000 times more powerful. When this drug analog hit the streets, it killed users with one shot. While the Drug Enforcement Agency (DEA) processed the paperwork to have this drug listed as a controlled substance, its manufacture was still technically legal and users continued to die.

Ecstasy, or MDMA, another designer drug analog, was hailed as a key to helping mankind find peace and tranquility. Also called ADAM, X, the love drug, it was the LSD of the 1980s. Ecstasy is a modification of the hallucinogenic amphetamine, MDA. In its legal form, MDA has been used as an adjunct to psychotherapy. This drug has been very popular on college campuses throughout the United States. Its popularity was based on a euphoric effect, low cost, and lack of serious side effects. However, every person who tries this drug is at substantial risk because its potential side effects have not been sufficiently researched. At one southwestern university, surveys revealed that 20 percent of the students had tried ecstasy.

Dangerous Dilemma   The dilemma designer drugs present is the conflict between research and development of new drugs for medical purposes on one hand and the potential harmful effects of black market drugs on the other.

Dr. David Smith, of the nationally-known Haight-Ashbury Medical Clinic in San Fransisco, advocates legal controls but also would like to see allowance made for legitimate research and medical use. For example, if there was an opportunity to study ecstasy under controlled, legal conditions, either the potential dangerous side effects might be identified, or a medical application might be found. So far, legal restrictions have been unable to encompass policies that allow legitimate medical research on an illegal drug. And, any illegal drug remains dangerous to the user.

Designer analogs are all risky. First is the unknown aspect of side effects—you never know exactly how you will respond to the drug, nor will you have knowledge of a potential range of reactions because this drug has not been studied under controlled research conditions. The second risk inherent in buying a designer drug on the street is that you will never know exactly what is in it. A study of 1,000 doses of a substance being sold as ecstasy in San Francisco found that none of the tablets contained the actual drug, MDMA.

Designer drugs are dangerous—they can and do kill. Just because they are inexpensive, available, and make you "feel good" is not enough reason to take a chance. Choose to not make drugs, either designer or others, a part of your life.

Ice, a New and Deadly Drug

Ice, a smokeable form of methamphetamine (speed), is more addictive, potent, and destructive than crack. Ice gives a direct jolt to the brain that can cause hallucinations, paranoia, and violent behaviors. Experts are concerned that Ice may replace crack as the nation's number one problem drug.

Physical Costs of Drugs

Without medical supervision, drugs are more likely to result in negative physical effects. These effects may be significant or even fatal. Following are examples of untoward effects of certain drugs.

- hangovers (depressants)
- nausea and vomiting (narcotics, hallucinogens)
- tremors (cocaine, other stimulants, tranquilizers)
- sexual impotence (depressants, narcotics; also amphetamines and inhalants, which exist in drug folklore as sexual enhancers, but which can actually cause impotence and temporary loss of erections)

■ cardiovascular damage, including high blood pressure, deterioration of heart muscle, heart failure—can be fatal (depressants, narcotics, cocaine, amphetamines)
■ respiratory failure—can be fatal (depressants, narcotics)
■ injury through loss of motor coordination resulting in automobile accidents, tripping, falling, drowning, and so forth (depressants, cannabis, hallucinogens, narcotics)
■ injury through violence or deliberately self-destructive behavior (PCP, cocaine, other stimulants)
■ depressed immune system (marijuana, narcotics)
■ memory impairment (cannabis)

Drugs and Sex

As with alcohol, the behavioral and psychological effects of many drugs can place you at greater risk for AIDS, STDs, unwanted pregnancies, and acquaintance rape. Additionally, because shared intravenous (IV) needles are one very effective means of transmitting the AIDS virus, everyone should avoid needle use (those who do use needles should never share needles). (For more information, see the **AIDS** chapter.)

Drugs and Academics

If you are under the influence of drugs, you may participate less effectively in academics. Tranquilizers and marijuana affect memory and concentration; intoxication may reduce intellectual motivation. You may also miss study and class time trying to obtain drugs or recovering from their effect. Drug-depressed or overstimulated nerves may decrease your ability to effectively handle acute or ongoing academic stress.

Social and Psychological Effects

Some students may choose drugs as a way to enhance social bonds; in the end, this benefit is illusory. Bonds based exclusively on shared drug use become destructive as the user develops psychological, financial, and sometimes physical needs to trust someone with whom he or she may have little in common other than drugs.

Drug abuse can have social and psychological effects similar to those found with alcohol abuse—heightened interpersonal conflict and avoidance of problem resolution. Drugs also often affect your emotions directly—depressants contribute to depression and lethargy. Coming down from stimulants such as cocaine may also bring on depression. Amphetamines, cocaine, and hallucinogens can produce paranoia. Cocaine and PCP may trigger psychosis. Hallucinogens may expose underlying psychological problems. Some of these effects last only until the drug wears off; on occasion they may become chronic.

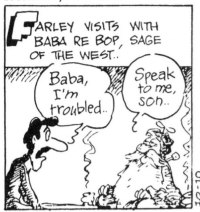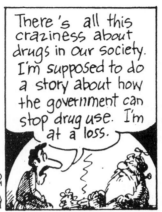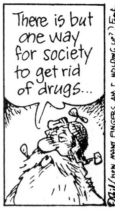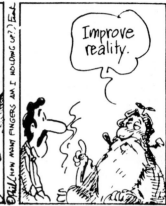

Identifying Alcohol and Drug Problems

Since so many people on campus drink, you may wonder how to tell whether someone is OK, at risk or chemically dependent. Perhaps one member of your group always seems to be the one who suggests getting hammered. Or you wonder whether a friend's alcohol or drug use contributes to his or her relationship troubles. Maybe someone has suggested that alcohol or drugs are negatively affecting your life. The following material will help you discern whether you (or a friend) are at risk for substance abuse problems, engage in acts regarded as warning signs of abuse or dependency, or have a risky pattern of use.

Who Is at Risk?

One in ten people who drink alcohol becomes chemically dependent. Though not all college problem drinkers become alcoholics, according to a report from University of California at Santa Barbara, "Students who are classified as 'problem drinkers' in college are more likely to be problem drinkers later in life." Researchers and drug counselors have devoted much effort in recent years to learning how to identify the individual who has a potential for substance abuse and dependence. They are examining genetics, learned behavior, and social and psychological circumstances as sources of risk.

Addiction definitely runs in families. According to the American College Health Association, "50 percent of all alcoholics have an alcoholic parent; there is strong evidence to suggest that there is a fourfold risk of becoming an alcoholic if one parent has the problem. Research indicates that there may be genetic factors that are related to differences in alcohol metabolism and the susceptibility to some forms of alcoholism." Some researchers believe that your social environment is a much more significant

> **The United States now has an estimated 1.2 million drug addicts, and 23 million more are "recreational" drug users.**

Alcohol and Other Drugs

CHAPTER 15

403

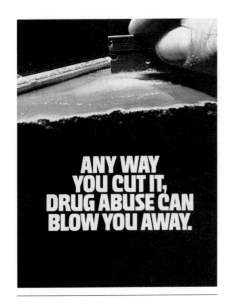

ANY WAY
YOU CUT IT,
DRUG ABUSE CAN
BLOW YOU AWAY.

risk factor than genetics. That is, if you're around people who drink heavily and then get rowdy, you're more likely to as well. If your friends drink lightly, you're more likely to. Of this unresolved debate, Mim Landry and Dr. David E. Smith have commented, "Environmental factors can be very powerful, but a family history of addiction is perhaps the most important single element in determining who may have a pathological reaction to psychoactive drugs such as cocaine or alcohol."

Your family background and social setting may also play roles. Parents' behavior regarding use of prescription drugs, cigarettes, alcohol, and other "recreational" drugs becomes a critical model for their children. If you have poor self-esteem, you may feel anxious and insecure about your own abilities to solve life's problems; you may find that alcohol or other drugs temporarily replace those disturbing feelings with a sense of calm or capability. Neglect, stress, excessively punitive patterns, and other major disturbances in the growing-up years can leave you susceptible to alcohol and other drugs. Turning to drugs when faced with social problems may lead to abuse and dependence. As one educator explains, "The more the drugs are used, the more the person believes they are necessary. Each use confirms the belief that with drugs it is possible to get by; without drugs it is not."

Warning Signs

Signs that you or a friend may be having problems with alcohol or other drugs may be dramatically obvious or rather subtle. The individual who overconsumed alcohol at a party and passed out appeared to have a "drug problem." Such an incident, while potentially very dangerous, may have been a isolated event and not clear evidence of a problem. Repeated occurrences provide more signs that a problem may exist. Some of the more subtle signs include attitudes and verbal statements, such as, "I can't get out of bed in the morning until I've lit up a cigarette," indicates a specific attitude. Abnormal behaviors, such as consistently missing classes due to hangovers, are warning signs. Quantity consumed often is less important than the psychological or physical dependence on a particular substance whether it be caffeine or cocaine. Sometimes the individual's strongly worded denial of dependence is a key signal. What really matters is whether drug use interferes with how you really want to conduct your life.

Though no printed lists of warning signs can replace talking with a counselor in determining whether you or someone you care about has an alcohol or drug problem, they can give you a sense of whether you should check out the possibility more thoroughly. The questions that follow are adapted from material used for self-diagnosis and study of college students and other young adults who may have problems with alcohol or other drugs. Answer the questions for yourself (or in terms of someone about whom you are concerned).

CAGE

The following four-item questionnaire, known as CAGE, has become recognized as one of the most efficient and effective alcohol dependency screening devices.

Have you ever felt you should . . . . **C**ut down on your drinking?

Have people . . . . **A**nnoyed you by criticizing your drinking?

Have you ever felt . . . . **G**uilty about your drinking?

Have you ever had a drink first thing in the morning to steady nerves or to get rid of a hangover? . . . . **E**ye-opener

Two or more *yes* answers means you may have an alcohol problem. Four *yes* answers is an almost certain diagnosis of alcoholism. If you give two or more positive answers, counseling may be appropriate. Self-help hotlines and suggestions for seeking professional help are presented at the end of this chapter.

Source: *Journal of the American Medical Association*

Warning Signs of Alcohol and Drug Use Problems

- Do you drink or do drugs to overcome shyness and build up self-confidence?
- Do you usually take a drink or do drugs before going out on a date?
- Do you drink or do drugs to avoid academic or personal problems?
- Have you ever had memory loss from drinking or drugs?
- Have you driven while intoxicated (DWI)?
- Do you miss classes or lose time from studies because of drinking or drugs?
- Do you often borrow money in order to purchase liquor or drugs?
- Do you deliberately hang out with friends where your style of liquor or drugs is easy to get?
- Have you dropped certain friends since you've started drinking or doing drugs?
- Do you drink more or do drugs more than your friends?
- Is drinking or doing drugs affecting your reputation?
- Do you hide the amount you are using from others?
- Do you sometimes drink or do drugs alone?
- Do you drink until the bottle is empty or the drugs are all gone?
- Does it bother you if somebody says maybe you drink too much or do too many drugs?
- Do you get annoyed with classes or lectures on drinking or drugs?
- Do you think your use has caused difficulties with (or helped) your social life, family life, or friendships?

> In the last two years, we've had students at (one fraternity) who have had to leave, who became psychologically disabled and had to be hospitalized, who became socially and academically dysfunctional. Put quite simply, the consequences of drug abuse were high.
>
> James W. Lyons
> Dean of Student Affairs,
> Stanford University

If you answer more than a few questions affirmatively, you may be taking serious chances with your alcohol and drug use. Talk with your health care provider or an alcohol and drug counselor at your college health center. Consider your pattern of use in more detail. As you read the following material, keep in mind your answers to the questions. Try to identify which type of usage pattern most closely resembles yours (or your friend's).

Know Your Pattern of Use

Abstinence, using no alcohol or other drugs, is certainly the most risk-free choice. If you abstain, you may do so for a variety of reasons—religion, morality, taste, or concern for health and safety.

Responsible use is a pattern of drug and alcohol consumption appropriate to your culture and setting that does not interfere with your personal health or the rights of others. Much, though not all, prescription drug use falls into this definition, as does most caffeine use in this country. Such attitudes sometimes shift over time. The increasing segregation of smokers in restaurants and airplanes illustrates the dramatic narrowing of our culture's definition of responsible nicotine use.

Marginal abuse is use that has the potential, if continued, to lead to problems related to alcohol and other drugs. Marginal abuse includes fairly frequent or regular use solely with the intent to get highly intoxicated, facilitate a relationship, or reduce stress. Because binge use or spree use—using large amounts of alcohol or other drugs in a short time—can lead to acute physical or behavioral problems, it is also a type of marginal abuse.

Abuse indicates a level or pattern of alcohol or drug use that seriously interferes with a person's physical, psychological, or emotional functioning. Chemical dependence includes not only a pattern of drug use that causes significant problems in your life, but also a psychological or physical craving that you can satisfy only by repeating the drug experience. In today's drug-oriented society, this broader term is more useful than addiction or alcoholism, and less emotionally loaded. Either physical or psychological dependency can be sufficiently powerful to take over an individual's life. Physical dependence occurs with some but not all drugs. If you are physically dependent on alcohol or another drug, your body has become so accustomed to that substance that if you discontinue the substance, you suffer painful withdrawal symptoms. Withdrawal from heroin and other opiates is challenging and uncomfortable. Withdrawal from alcohol, barbiturates, or tranquilizers can be dangerous or fatal if not done carefully under medical supervision.

Psychological dependence refers to a learned response in which you desire again and again the feeling the substance produces. Alcohol and other drugs create psychological dependence in various ways. The behavior of taking a particular drug produces a response that an individual may find rewarding, such as the "mellowing" effect of marijuana, or the decreased inhibitions from alcohol. This psychological hook can be so great that a person can become drug-free, remain so for thirty years and still crave that drug experience every day.

Preventing Alcohol and Drug Problems

If you think of yourself or a friend as only occasionally involved in marginal abuse, taking preventive measures now can be critical in avoiding abuse or dependency. A recent article by two professors of clinical psychiatry said, "The critical question is not whether or not alcohol dependence, as opposed to alcohol abuse, is present. The central question is, 'Is this student at substantial risk if the present alcohol-use pattern persists?' " If you recognize yourself or a friend as already involved in substance abuse or dependency, prevention may not suffice; you probably need counseling, support, and treatment.

Colleges Work on Prevention

For decades, many colleges followed a laissez-faire, "boys will be boys" attitude toward on-campus drinking. They wanted to avoid taking on the role of "parent." After beer busts and other parties, roommates put drunken buddies to bed to "sleep it off." Campuses that did not allow alcohol were surrounded by off-campus bars, liquor stores, and other places where students could get liquor easily.

Now, college administrations and living groups across the country are taking action to reduce the incidence of alcohol- and drug-related problem behaviors among students. College administrators active in alcohol abuse issues acknowledge that most college students do drink; what they are working for is responsible drinking. Harvard Assistant Dean Tom Dingman said, "Students are simply drinking too much and are sometimes out of control." Other college administrators point out that students should be expected to manage alcohol in a socially responsible manner. Arrival on a college campus is not license to go totally berserk over consumption of alcohol and other drugs, and students must be prepared to take responsibility for their actions.

Many colleges have strict alcohol codes and enforce them more than before, many in response to state increases in legal drinking age. However, recognizing that problem prevention requires more than laws and policies, most colleges have special programs set up to reduce the incidence of drinking problems on campus and identify and treat students at risk for problems with alcohol and other drugs. In fact, any college that receives federal financial aid must certify that it has a drug abuse prevention program accessible to any student or employee.

The size and style of programs vary, depending on school size, location, and specific campus issues. Some programs reach out to students,

The International Drug Scene

The United States is not the only nation experiencing major drug problems.

- Soviet Union has 131,000 registered drug users; 80,000 Soviet people had drug-related charges against them in the last two years according to the Soviet Weekly.
- Hungary is said to have between 30,000 and 50,000 drug abusers.
- Poland has an estimated 200,000 to 600,000 addicts and users of hard drugs.
- Western Europe is predicted to reach 3 to 4 million regular cocaine users by the mid-1990s.
- Spain already has an estimated 60,000 to 80,000 cocaine users.

When Drinking Kills; The Tragic Legacy of Ted McGuire

On October 26, 1986, Ted McGuire, a 19-year-old Yale University sophomore, was found dead in his room. The cause of death was established as alcohol poisoning. The incident was a shock to the entire Yale community, and attracted widespread attention in the press. Below, Frank Gibson, '49, a close friend of the McGuires, reflects on the tragedy and its implications for Yale, its students, and their families.

"Here's to good old Yale, drink it down, drink it down. . . ."

"Here's to good old Yale, she's so hearty and so hale. . . ."

Arms around each other, glasses raised on high.

"Drink it down, drink it down, drink it down, down, down!"

"Boy, did I get trashed last night!"

"Trashed? You passed out . . . Just before I did. What a night that was!"

Tradition. This is what our fathers did before us, what our sons and daughters unborn shall hail. This is what, as freshmen first, we learn. This is what college is all about, right?

Wrong!

On a Sunday morning last fall, the unthinkable happened. Ted McGuire, a Yale sophomore, didn't wake up.

"Yale student dies from drinking." The wire services picked it up. It became sensational news. But the emphasis was all wrong.

Who was Ted McGuire? Was he an alcoholic? No. Was he on drugs? No. Was he a loner? No. He was one of us.

Ted McGuire came from Falmouth, Massachusetts. He was in the top two percent of his high school class. He was also president of his class, co-captain of the basketball team, a varsity tennis player and a National Merit semi-finalist. He had his heart set on going to Yale. He was pre-med and worked at Yale-New Haven Hospital. He kept in shape at the gym, even though he didn't have time for varsity sports. He worked hard. He played hard. In other words, he was a typical Yalie, if there really is such a thing.

"He soaked up Yale like a sponge," said his mother. "He loved it." And was loved in return. In 1989, in what would have been Ted's senior year, there will be a new award, the Ted McGuire Cup, given to the senior in Silliman who best exemplifies the spirit and character of Ted McGuire.

So what happened? Why did this young, respected Yalie die?

Ted McGuire made a mistake. His roommates made a mistake. All of us made a mistake. None of us ever recognized that alcohol, pure and simple, all by itself, can kill. Sure, we all know that alcohol and driving don't mix. We all know that alcohol and drugs are deadly. None of us would ever be stupid enough to play Russian roulette. But just plain drinking? So you pass out. So what? It happens to everybody. You work hard, you play hard.

That's why the emphasis in the news stories was wrong. This wasn't a case of a college kid overdosing on drugs. This wasn't a case of an alcoholic finally succumbing to a debilitating disease. This was something that simply was not supposed to happen.

"I suspect every one of us, learning of Ted's death, has asked, 'Why does such a tragedy happen?' " said Ted's uncle, Donald Wilson, in his eulogy at the memorial service for Ted. To the packed pews of St. Anthony's, Don Wilson asked the question that had been unanswerable on the Yale campus for a month: "What killed Ted McGuire?"

I'd like to answer that question with some more questions:

Was it Yale tradition? One of the innumerable drinking games which go by so many names? The sheer idiocy of chug-a-lug?

Was it ignorance? "Gee, last Saturday night I passed out, too. But I didn't know that could happen," a young woman told her college dean the next day.

Was it fear? Are students afraid to call for help when one of their peers is in trouble? What will the campus police say if they are under the legal age? What will Yale say?

Was it benign neglect? I woke up on the morning of the Falmouth memorial service and said to my wife, "You know, as parents we don't know anymore than those kids know. Remember when Stevie came back to the house after his sister's wedding? And we all laughed when he was so spaghetti-legged and could hardly talk and his parents told his buddies to put him to bed; and to make sure they put a basin next to it. We all figured he'd feel like death warmed over the next day, but we never considered he actually might have been dead. Right?"

The answer, I think we have to admit, is, "all of the above."

After Ted's death, Dr. G. Douglas Talbott, '46, consultant to the Atlanta Falcons and the Atlanta Braves, discussed the issue with Yale students. If what he had to say—and it was plenty—had to be boiled down into one sentence, it would be this:

Alcohol is a drug.

Most undergraduates don't understand this. Neither, unfortunately, do most alumni.

"One of the things that bothers me tremendously, as I travel throughout the campuses," said Dr. Talbott, "is that I will ask somebody, 'Are you on drugs?' and they answer, 'No. All I do is to use grass and drink beer. I'm not on drugs.'

"My concern is that when we talk about alcohol, we are not looking at the issue that alcohol is a drug. Alcohol is probably the finest drug that there is in America today. If you take a bottle of wine, or a can of beer, or a bottle of bourbon, and just take off the color and the taste and drip off the water, what do you have? Ether. C_2H_5OH minus water is ether.

"Your brain has no more idea than a pussycat whether you're

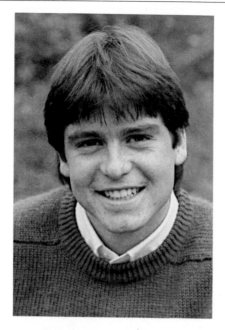

taking a six-pack of beer, or a glass of vodka . . . or if you have a mask over your face and you are inhaling ether. Alcohol is a drug . . . it's a sedative, a hypnotic drug; it's an anesthetic drug and, if you choose to OD on it, then there are some consequences which you must consider."

Ted McGuire OD'd on the drug alcohol. He didn't choose to do it. The terminology, "Choosing to OD on the drug alcohol," would have been as new to him as it was to almost everybody listening to Dr. Talbott. It may be a new terminology to most reading these words.

"There is something we can do," said Ted's uncle, concluding his eulogy. "The most significant thing of all. We can try to prevent other young people from dying in the manner Ted did. Ted was an exceptional young man in many ways, but his use of alcohol was typical of young men his age. He was not an alcoholic: he was an occasional drinker and in fact had a low tolerance for alcohol. If such a tragic mistake could be made by Ted it will certainly be made by others—unless we influence them to change."

But, as Dr. Talbott said, "We have learned more about alcohol in the last seven years than we had learned in the previous seven thousand years."

In memory of Ted McGuire, '89; for the future of all college students, past, present and future, it's time to put what we've learned to work.

"Here's to good old Yale, she's so hearty and so hale, save a life, save a life, save a life, life, life!"

Source: *Yale Alumni Magazine*

presenting on-campus and residence hall forums on such topics as responsible drinking, the role of alcohol in campus life, and alcohol and drug abuse prevention. Some schools have a counseling service available not only to students referred by administrators because of problem behavior, but also to students concerned about their own use or that of a friend.

Most programs on preventing alcohol and drug problems usually include information and assistance in several areas: first, recognizing and accepting responsibility for the role of alcohol and other drugs in your life; second, minimizing your emotional and psychological susceptibility to abuse and dependency; and third, taking practical actions that foster responsible use instead of problems in alcohol and drug situations.

Take Responsibility

Other people don't determine when, where, or how much you drink; these are always your decisions. Though you may find that alcohol and drug choices at college sometimes involve social conflicts, in the end you are responsible for what you put in your body and for the consequences of your choices.

Taking responsibility does not have to mean giving up alcohol or even drugs. It means using these substances so they don't impact negatively on the rest of your life. If you decide to drink or use drugs, take steps to keep yourself out of trouble. Begin by acknowledging your actions. You may say, "Alcohol and caffeine are my drugs of choice." The word "choice" tells you that you are responsible for these actions and that you can change your usage if you decide to.

If you discover you are particularly susceptible to alcohol or other drugs, cultivate behavior patterns that keep your susceptibility from developing into abuse or dependence. If your life (or a friend's) isn't going well and others attribute your problems to drinking or other drug use, don't blame parents, party hosts, friends, or alcohol or drugs themselves. If your life seems increasingly wrapped up in alcohol or other drugs, talk with someone. Take advantage of college resources that can give you perspective and support. If your college experience or your life (or a friend's) seems about to go down the tubes, take responsible action by getting help now.

Minimize Emotional and Psychological Susceptibility

Most people who are high-risk users have difficulty identifying feelings. Many have grown up in homes where expressing feelings was discouraged, dangerous, or absent. (This includes children of alcoholics, but is not exclusively limited to them.) Emotional pain is a symptom of something wrong; masking pain with alcohol or other drugs doesn't correct the source of pain. If you (or friends) are in chronic emotional discomfort, you need increased skills in handling the challenges of living—interpersonal communication, loneliness, conflict, and values clarification.

If you use alcohol or other drugs not because you feel bad, but rather to feel the high of intoxication, remember that the goal of abuse prevention is not to avoid intoxication or feeling good, but to seek a variety of safe, healthy ways that fit into your life and do not harm yourself or others. To avoid problems, consider not using mood-altering substances as your only way of getting high. Cultivate other non-chemical pathways to feeling high, such as music, dancing, running, meditation, nature, and love.

Strategies to Prevent Problems

Among almost 100 college students previously identified as high risk for chemical problems (because they had been picked up for alcohol or drug-related behavior problems on campus), only one could name a strategy he might employ that would minimize his chance of developing a chemical problem—other than stopping use, and no one was going to do that. This single student said he might drink only with his girlfriend because he observed that he didn't get quite so drunk when he was with her. On the other hand, each of several undergraduate classes on the same campus came up with more than 50 suggestions in less than 15 minutes. High-risk users seem unaware of strategies that would lower their risk, but you can learn these skills.

If you develop and use a personal alcohol and drug use plan, you are less likely to encounter trouble related to alcohol and other drugs. As you read the techniques presented in the material that follows, consider which ones would most help your circumstances. The material includes techniques that cover most college alcohol situations, including social gatherings, party hosting, driving, fraternity and sorority rush, and bars. It also provides some techniques that pertain specifically to drugs other than alcohol.

Consider How Much and When   The amount of alcohol or other drugs you take is vitally important, but often ignored, in determining appropriate choices. If you take one or two alcoholic drinks, you'll probably feel relaxed and less inhibited. If you take ten drinks in two hours, you are stuporous and at risk for respiratory arrest or suffocation. Set limits on the amount of drinking or other drugs you ingest. Dosage makes a big difference between a pleasant experience and a dangerous, or at least uncomfortable, one. Many people, including college students, learn how to adjust the dosage of caffeine or alcohol to produce a desired effect. For example, if you get hangovers after a certain amount of alcohol, you may abstain or limit consumption the night before an exam. With illegal drugs, dosage can be a more hazardous variable, because street drugs have no standard of quality. Unknowingly using drugs of a significantly higher purity than you are used to can cause serious overdose or even death.

Avoid taking a large amount of alcohol or other drugs in a short period of time. This creates a maximum, and sometimes risky, effect. The same dosage taken over a longer period has less risk because the body has an opportunity to detoxify or metabolize some of the earlier doses.

A survey of University of Minnesota students revealed that 17 percent of students had "driven a car when drunk" at least once during a one-month period.

Alcohol and Other Drugs

No Drinking with These Drugs

Many drugs interact with alcohol to cause serious health damage; some interactions may even cause death. Don't drink alcohol if you are taking any of these drugs:

- Barbiturates (most frequent fatal interaction)
- Major tranquilizers
- Sedatives, tranquilizers, sleeping pills
- Pain killers, narcotics
- Antihistamines
- Antidepressants
- Acetaminophen (Tylenol, Anacin-3, etc.)
- Aspirin (Anacin, Excedrin, etc.)
- Arthritis medicine (Indocin, etc.)

Source: *Medical Self-Care*

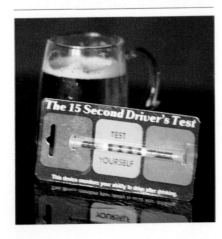

Any drug that intoxicates—whether alcohol, caffeine, cocaine, or narcotics—may first lift the mood but eventually acts as a depressant. A pattern of drug use to repeatedly alter your mood can lead to larger and more frequent dosages, as well as chemical dependency. To avoid developing these problems, begin by recognizing that any substance you take to get you high will eventually bring you down. If you do choose alcohol or another drug, plan to do something else to bring yourself back into balance—listen to music, go for a walk, sleep, eat.

Avoid alcohol and other drugs if you are not feeling well, have some other health problem, or are taking contraindicated prescription or over-the-counter medications. If you are tired or ill, you may react more intensely (particularly in negative ways) to drugs or alcohol. Certain health situations can be made much worse by drinking or taking other drugs. And some medications can have deadly effects when combined with alcohol or other drugs. The most frequent deadly combination is alcohol and tranquilizers. Others are listed in the accompanying chart.

Learn to Drink in Moderation   You are more likely to consume moderate amounts of alcohol if you are partying with others who are moderate. Studies have also shown that males drinking with females are at lower risk than males drinking with males. Women, on the other hand, tend to drink less with other women and more when they are with men. Risk is greater when alcohol or other drugs are the only reason for socializing rather than simply part of a number of activities. Whether you're at a fraternity party, a friend's apartment or a public bar, here are some actions that you can take to avoid drinking too much.

- Consume alcohol with food; don't drink on an empty stomach.
- Set a reasonable limit on the total number of drinks in an evening.
- Pace yourself (remember, your body can only metabolize one drink per hour).
- Count your drinks or ask someone else to count them for you.
- Alternate a non-alcoholic drink with an alcoholic one.
- Never drink straight shots.
- Use large amounts of mixer or water in drinks.
- Ask for feedback from friends about your use and its effects on you.
- Focus on goals that motivate you to limit consumption of alcohol (such as weight management, academic goals, and physical fitness).

If you choose other drugs besides alcohol, similar strategies can help you develop patterns of moderation.

Prevent DWI   The two most famous mottos about DWI are "Don't drink and drive" and "Friends don't let friends drive drunk." You can take practical steps to avoid DWI situations. One increasingly popular solution is to use the designated driver system. One person in your group agrees to drive but not drink for the entire event. You can rotate this responsibility among friends in your group. This idea is becoming more popular on campus. In one university poll, 75 percent of students indicated that they were willing to take their turn being designated driver. Numerous bars now participate by providing free soft drinks for the designated driver in a party.

Another solution is to choose places to party that do not involve driving or that allow guests to stay overnight. Or use alternative transportation such as taxi, bus, walking (perhaps with other people), or call a sober friend to pick you up.

Limit your own drinking through the event to stay below 0.05 BAC by drinking no more than one drink per hour (or use the chart earlier in this chapter). If you drink at that rate and do not drink in the last hour before driving, you are at low risk for DWI.

If you are in a situation in which someone else wants to drive while intoxicated, take away the keys, or slip them away and say they're lost. Try to talk the person into another alternative, such as letting you drive. In any event, take responsibility for your own health and safety; avoid riding in a car driven by someone who is intoxicated. This is particularly an issue for women, though certainly not exclusively so. Almost 95 percent of those arrested for drunk driving are males. A woman who considers ahead of time what to do—what to say, how assertive to be, what options are available—is prepared to act in her own best interests if a potential DWI situation arises. If you feel your date for an event is likely to become intoxicated, agree that you will not drink and that you will drive home, or arrange alternate transportation.

Responsible Party Hosting When you give a party, you and your fellow hosts are responsible for deciding what to serve, including alcohol. You want your guests to have a good time and to be protected from harm. As the person (or persons) in control of the property on which the party takes place, you are also legally responsible for the safety and well-being of guests; you can be sued in the event of damages or injuries that could have been avoided by reasonable party planning. In addition, in almost every state, if any money exchange takes place that can be traced to the purchase of alcohol served at the party, you are also responsible for any damages your guests commit while intoxicated, even after they leave your property. Many states include all "illegal furnishing of alcohol" in such legislation; this would include providing alcohol to someone under legal age. You can take several practical steps to keep yourself and your guests from getting into such trouble. Stop serving alcohol at least one hour before the end of the party if people will be driving home. Replenish the coffee and food at this time. Set up designated driver arrangements or have people sleep over and serve them breakfast.

Dry Rush, an Increasingly Popular Alternative Studies on heavy college drinking have linked many unfortunate incidents to the system of fraternity rush. On too many occasions, candidates unaccustomed to drinking have consumed several alcoholic drinks at each of many visits

Avoiding and Treating Hangovers

- Drink only in moderation.
- Drink only one kind of drink (for instance, don't have both beer and wine).
- Eat before and while you are drinking.
- Have one to two glasses of water while you're drinking, and again before going to bed (this minimizes dehydration and the resulting headache).
- Take a B-vitamin supplement before going to bed (if you remember—otherwise, take one in the morning).
- The next day, eat foods that are easy on the liver, such as fruits and vegetables, bread, cereals, and pasta.
- Don't sleep in too late; get up and have something to eat. The low blood sugar brought on by alcohol processing can contribute to headaches.
- If you drink coffee every morning, get up in time to have your first cup of coffee not more than a couple of hours after your usual time. Don't force your body to go through caffeine withdrawal as well as the alcohol effects.

Alcohol and Other Drugs

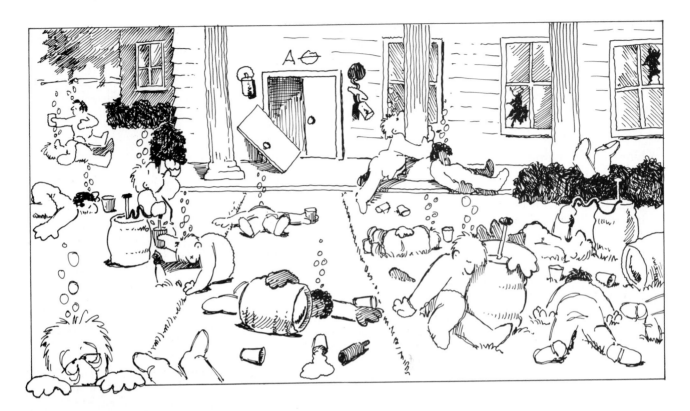

during the same evening. The resulting intoxication has been the cause of automobile crashes, falls, drowning, and other injury or fatal accidents. Fraternities at over 150 colleges now feature a non-alcoholic, dry rush. Many groups are creating social environments that encourage responsible drug-and-alcohol patterns among their members.

Alternative Bars   On many college campuses, the "alternative bar" is becoming popular at social functions. An alternative bar serves a range of non-alcoholic drinks. The idea started among a group of students who complained that sometimes they went to a bar to be with friends but didn't want to drink alcohol. They surveyed bars near campus about alternatives to a "Shirley Temple" or a two-dollar soft drink. In addition to the various popular "designer" mineral waters, they found a Screwless Driver and a Virgin Punch.

Preventing Problems with Drugs

Many of the keys to avoiding potentially troublesome situations with drugs are the same as with alcohol, such as passing up parties whose primary focus is intoxication, avoiding DWI situations, and responsible party hosting. The illegality and culturally disapproved nature of much drug use makes certain other cautions particularly important.

Find out about any drug you or a friend may use. Be aware of side effects and lethal dosages. Check with the Physician's Desk Reference (PDR) in your college library or health service, with other publications, and with your college alcohol and drug treatment program or community drug program. You can usually make these inquiries anonymously if you like.

Don't mix drugs or drugs and alcohol. This unpredictable practice can be fatal. College-age adults are a likely group to engage in polydrug use—using more than one drug (including alcohol). Researchers found that virtually everyone under thirty in a Los Angeles alcohol treatment program also used other drugs. Certain alcohol and drug combinations are particularly common. For instance, because cocaine makes users anxious, agitated and unable to sleep, they often use another drug to depress those overstimulated nerves; typically, that drug is alcohol. The combined effect of two drugs may be synergistic, far exceeding the sum of their individual effects. Polydrug use contributes to some of the most dangerous and deadly consequences of alcohol and other drugs. Alcohol and Valium (the most commonly prescribed tranquilizer) are a fatal combination even when the individual dosages are not problematic.

Acknowledge the special risks of illegal drugs. In addition to the risks inherent in the chemical composition of many drugs, any drug that is illegal poses additional risks just because of its illegal status. In the first place, illegal drugs are often quite expensive. Dealers need to cover costs of secret manufacture and processing, smuggling, payoffs, distribution networks, and extravagant lifestyles. Getting money for drugs can be difficult or cause you to scrimp on basics. Students sometimes deal drugs as a way to support their own usage or earn lots of money fast, but the risks for dealing are even higher than for users (both legal consequences and proximity to serious criminals).

Because you're buying from dealers, you may encounter criminals, unsafe environments, other illegal actions, and, of course, not know whom you can trust. The government does not supervise and regulate manufacture of illegal drugs, thus they may contain dangerous impurities.

If convicted of certain drug charges, students may be ineligible for several career paths, including law and medicine. In fact, as Judge Donald Ginsberg discovered in 1987, even occasional moderate use came back years later to block his appointment to the U.S. Supreme Court.

Do not assume a substance is safe just because it's legal. A drug's legal status and social acceptability are not good indicators of risk potential. Alcohol is the major drug problem on campus and in our country, yet it is the cause of many deaths, injuries, health problems, and interpersonal anguish. Tobacco contributes to 350,000 U.S. deaths annually. According to the General Accounting Office, "Millions of Americans abuse prescription drugs, often with tragic results." In 1980, 75 percent of drug-related problems brought to hospital emergency rooms resulted from misuse of prescription drugs. Even OTC drugs have potential for harm—many cold medications contain alcohol—including Nyquil and other cough medi-

Drug Tests—Not Just for Athletes Anymore

Urinalysis drug testing at college is not limited to athletes involved in intercollegiate sports. Career planning and placement personnel report that such tests are part of the application process of a growing number of business firms. The constitutionality of such testing has not yet been resolved; however, the reality is that many firms consider only applicants who pass drug tests.

There are many kinds of drug tests; some screen for only a few substances; others are more thorough. If you are being tested, find out specifically what the test is designed to show. Many tests can yield false positive results from certain foods and legitimate medications. If you get a positive result but have not been using banned substances, find out more information about what could cause such false positive results before resubmitting another sample for testing.

cines. Diet pills and study drugs can overstimulate the nervous system. Many OTCs contain caffeine, such as Accutrim, Contac, and Actifed. Read the ingredient list and directions for any OTC you consider taking.

Treating Alcohol and Drug Problems

Sometimes prevention is too late or insufficient. If you are ever in a situation in which someone has taken too much or the wrong stuff, you'll probably be very scared. You'll feel more confident and take more effective action if you know what to do, what kind of treatment to seek for long-term improvement, and how to help a friend with a substance problem.

Overdose—Too Much Alcohol or Drugs

In spite of the folklore that recommends putting a drunk to bed to "sleep it off," such behavior can lead to fatal results. Alcohol comas and deaths often involve individuals who on one particular occasion drink more than their normal amount. Many drugs can induce overdoses: any depressant (alcohol, barbiturates, tranquilizers, methaqualone), cocaine, narcotics, and hallucinogens. Taking more than one type of drug during the same period of time, especially mixing alcohol with other depressants such as barbiturates or tranquilizers, can result in life-threatening medical emergencies.

Prompt first aid for overdose can mean the difference between life and death. For any of the following symptoms, *get medical assistance immediately*.

- Difficulty breathing (depressants, narcotics)
- Rapid breathing (cocaine, other stimulants)
- Heart attack or irregular rhythm; chest pains (depressants, narcotics, cocaine, nicotine, amphetamines)
- Seizures (barbiturates, methaqualone)
- Unconsciousness; cannot be awakened (depressants, narcotics)

While waiting for help to arrive, here's what to do:

- Keep the individual warm with clothes and blankets
- Do not give person any alcohol or other drugs
- Do not put person to bed
- Try to ascertain what substances the person may have taken (including prescription and OTC medications)

Don't let the involvement of illegal drugs in the situation make you hesitate to go directly to the emergency room. Most health centers have significant experience with treating drug overdose victims; their first concern is to protect that individual's life, not report patients to law enforcement officials. College health centers usually inform parents or college

What To Do with a Drunk

Do

Keep the person still and comfortable. Keep calm. Don't let your anxiety transfer to the individual in trouble.

Stay with the drunk person who is vomiting. When laying him/her down, turn head to the side to keep the tongue from falling back into the throat. Protect the person from swallowing vomit.

Monitor the person's breathing. **If you detect unconsciousness or respiratory problems, get immediate medical help.**

Keep your distance. Before approaching or touching, explain what you intend to do. Drunks may be unpredictable and violent.

Speak in a clear, firm, reassuring manner.

Don't

Don't try to walk, run or exercise the drunk person; don't try to keep the person awake. Any abrupt or unnecessary movement might cause the drunk person to fall or faint, with resulting injury. Above all, don't permit the person to drive.

Don't administer anything orally—food, liquid or drugs—to sober the person up. This might induce vomiting and result in choking. The only thing that will sober a drunk person is time.

Don't give the person a cold shower—the shock may cause him/her to pass out, with resulting injury.

Don't attempt to constrain the person without (sober) assistance.

Don't laugh, ridicule, provoke, anger, argue, or threaten.

Source: *Dealing with Alcohol at Dartmouth*, Dartmouth College

---

administrators only if the student is gravely ill, in danger, or must undergo surgery.

Complications of Alcoholism

The long-term consequences of alcohol abuse are many and varied. Because people develop a tolerance for alcohol, they have to drink greater and greater amounts to feel the same effect. As the intake of alcohol increases and intake of essential nutrients decreases, the body becomes more and more depleted. Increased amounts of alcohol over the years cause considerable damage to the body—the brain, heart, blood vessels, gastrointestinal system, and of course, the liver. In addition to the damage to internal organs, an alcoholic is more susceptible to such illnesses as infections, gout, and diabetes. Psychiatric problems, central nervous system damage, lapses of memory, and gastrointestinal damage may occur. The way alcohol damages your body is unpredictable, and what may occur in one person may be different in another. Long-term alcohol abuse may decrease a person's alcohol tolerance, and because the liver is so damaged, it can no longer produce the amount of enzymes necessary to metabolize the alcohol.

Withdrawal symptoms occur when an alcoholic stops drinking. These symptoms may be merely unpleasant (feeling shaky or jittery, nauseous) or life-threatening. Delirium tremens, an acute condition that manifests

Statistics on Alcoholism

- Alcoholism is the third greatest health problem in the United States (heart disease and cancer rank first and second).
- Alcoholism affects almost 15 million people in the United States.
- Alcoholism is involved in approximately 30,000 deaths and 500,000 injuries (primarily auto accidents) every year.

Fetal Alcohol Syndrome

Women who abuse alcohol during pregnancy experience many problems. They have a higher rate of spontaneous abortion, which suggests that alcohol is toxic to the fetus. Infants born to alcoholic mothers have a high probability of developing fetal alcohol syndrome (FAS). These children may have facial deformities, growth deficiency, or mental retardation. The severity of FAS appears to be dose-related; the more alcohol the mother consumes, the more damage to the unborn child. A safe level of alcohol has not been established for pregnant women, but even two drinks per day may decrease birth weight. Research on FAS has determined that any alcohol ingested during pregnancy has potential consequences for the unborn embryo.

Founded in 1935, AA is a fellowship of recovering alcoholics dedicated to helping others recover.

Alcohol and Other Drugs

C H A P T E R   15

Assessment, Treatment and Aftercare

If you (or a friend) are ready to explore and acknowledge how alcohol and other drugs are contributing to rather than solving life's problems, you can voluntarily ask for help at your health center, campus alcohol program, an alcohol and drug treatment clinic, or a self-help program. You may come to discuss alcoholic family members and learn more about your own susceptibility to chemical problems.

If an assessment determines that you have problems related to alcohol or other drugs, counselors will work out a treatment plan with you. Because several hundred treatment options are available, it is important to match each individual's treatment to his or her situation.

One-to-one counseling with a therapist   For minor problems, a few sessions with a counselor can help you chart out new actions and directions for your life. Some changes may relate specifically to chemicals, others to learning to handle emotions constructively and improving social skills.

Groups   The most effective treatment program for chemical dependency has been developed by Alcoholics Anonymous. Groups usually work better than one-to-one treatment. All members are individuals who have been dependent, who really know how it feels to lead a life focused on alcohol or other drugs.

Outpatient treatment   Outpatient treatment is designed for people who still have some control over part of their lives. For instance, an individual might go to treatment on an outpatient basis five evenings per week, while still living at home and attending school.

Inpatient treatment   Inpatient treatment is necessary when an individual's life does not have enough structure and support to keep that person sober long enough for outpatient or group work to be effective. The individual leaves his or her harmful environment for three to four weeks to live in a total treatment setting.

Treatment succeeds only if an individual acknowledges that something is wrong and is willing to consider that alcohol (and other drugs) could be important factors in those problems. Honesty, open-mindedness, and a willingness to work and change are important to success. Many students find it helpful to work with counselors and programs experienced with the specific drugs involved in their particular situation, though this is not necessary. Seek medical supervision for any health problems related to alcohol or drug use.

Withdrawal is just the beginning. The individual must learn chemical-free solutions to pain, social dilemmas, emotional and communication needs. Sometimes the individual must build new sets of friends, family relationships, even academic and career goals. The director of the Alcohol Assistance Program for Students at Rutgers University says, "The student in recovery from a chemical dependency not only has to stay abstinent from mood-altering drugs, but also must reconstruct his or her life away from chemicals. During the student's active addiction, many aspects of daily living became subtly involved in chemicals."

The important issue in treatment and recovery is not just to become temporarily "dried out," but to maintain a healthy new lifestyle. Most people need intense reinforcement of new behaviors for at least a few months; some stay in contact with support groups or counselors permanently, or at least in times of stress. If you have had chemical abuse or dependency problems, you remain susceptible to dependency for the rest of your life.

Drug Therapy   Alcoholism may be treated by drug therapy. The drug of choice is called Antabuse® (disulfiram). When this drug is taken, it blocks the enzymes of alcohol metabolism so that the chemical acetylaldehyde builds up. When a person who has taken Antabuse drinks alcohol, the symptoms are very unpleasant—headache, nausea, vomiting, and a severe hangover. As long as the person is taking Antabuse, he or she will not be likely to drink because of the uncomfortable consequences. The drug, itself, without the alcohol, has no side effects.

Alcoholics Anonymous   Alcoholics Anonymous (AA) is a worldwide, nonprofit, nonprofessional organization that assists alcoholics to recover from the illness of alcoholism. This self-help program has assisted millions of people to handle their problem with alcohol and begin the road to recovery.

The basic tenet of AA is that alcoholics are powerless to stop their drinking pattern as a way of coping with life. AA members provide an atmosphere of support and caring. In a relaxed environment, members share their stories, experiences, strengths, and failures, and give practical tips on how to stay sober. Each new member is offered a person-to-person sponsor who provides support for remaining sober.

AA has meetings in almost every city in the country as well as abroad. Anyone can attend these sessions. You can be any age, race, have any educational background, or political persuasion. Anonymity is respected; members do not even use last names. There are no dues or fees. The only requirement is that you wish to do something about your drinking problem—to have a desire to remain sober.

AA does not recruit members. A basic assumption is that the desire to stop drinking must come from the individual. The AA program is built around a process called the Twelve Steps to Recovery. According to research, AA is the most effective program available to treat alcoholism and maintain sobriety.

Alcoholics Anonymous has several auxiliary groups to help family and friends of the recovering alcoholic. Al-Anon is a group that helps family

---

Twelve Steps of Alcoholics Anonymous

1. We admitted we were powerless over alcohol—that our lives had become unmanageable.
2. We came to believe that a Power greater than ourselves could restore us to sanity.
3. We made a decision to turn our will and our lives over to the care of God, as we understood Him.
4. We made a searching and fearless moral inventory of ourselves.
5. We admitted to God, to ourselves, and to another human being the exact nature of our wrongs.
6. We were entirely ready to have God remove all these defects of character.
7. We humbly asked Him to remove our shortcomings.
8. We made a list of all persons we had harmed and became willing to make amends to them all.
9. We made direct amends to such people wherever possible, except when to do so would injure them or others.
10. We continued to take personal inventory and when we were wrong promptly admitted it.
11. We sought through prayer and meditation to improve our conscious contact with God, as we understood Him, praying only for knowledge of His will for us and the power to carry that out.
12. Having had a spiritual awakening as the result of these steps, we tried to carry this message to alcoholics and to practice these principles in all our affairs.

Source: Alcoholics Anonymous World Services, Inc.

Codependency

Problems of substance abuse affect not only the abusing or recovering individual, but also family and friends who become embroiled in the chaos of that person's life. Within the past decade, professionals have begun using the term "codependent" to describe a person obsessed, tormented, or dominated by the behavior of others. Codependents often feel helpless, miserable, hopeless, and angry as they accept the victim role.

A person may be codependent in a relationship with a parent, lover, spouse, or friend. This person may be an alcoholic, drug abuser, gambler, compulsive eater, sex addict, batterer, or have any other compulsive disorder. Once codependent behaviors and attitudes are established in one relationship, the pattern may continue in other relationships.

A codependent typically feels responsible for the behavior and mood of another; when a person's alcohol or drug use causes problems, the codependent cleans up the mess and gives excuses. The codependent sees herself or himself as a victim, constantly giving time, energy, and support to others. Inside, the codependent may feel like a little child, desperate to be loved and wanted. But the situation is not resolved by solving someone else's addiction.

The codependent must learn to separate his or her own life from that of the addictive person's needs and feelings.

Similar to recovery from substance abuse, only the codependent can take the necessary steps toward his or her own recovery. Many codependents have received useful encouragement and guidance from the Twelve-Step Program of Al-Anon, a support group for family and friends of alcoholics. More than 28,000 Al-Anon groups exist in 100 countries worldwide. Other organizations exist for codependents of people with many types of addictive problems. Specific clinics also deal with these problems.

One of the most important techniques recovering codependents learn from these groups, and from professional counselors, is to detach their lives from those of others. They develop a perspective on their childhood so they can complete "unfinished business." They also learn not to try to control someone else's life and to stop playing the victim role. If the codependent person sets personal goals for life, then lives one day at a time, with a positive and realistic, rather than perfectionist attitude, he or she will be able to break the codependent pattern.

and friends understand the illness, support the alcoholic as he or she struggles to remain sober, and support themselves as they learn to live with the recovering alcoholic. Al-a-Teen is a related organization that helps children cope with a parent who is an alcoholic. In the last few years, it has become apparent that many children of alcoholics suffer severe personality damage. Al-a-Teen helps support these children to learn that they are not responsible for their parents' problems and to cope with guilt, sadness, and anger.

Children of Alcoholics (COA's)   During the past ten years, researchers have begun to focus on the problems of alcoholism in our society. There are approximately fifteen million alcoholics in the United States. One out of eight adults, or almost 30 million people, have grown up in an alcoholic family.

In addition to being victims themselves, alcoholics negatively affect those with whom they associate, especially their children. Only during the last few years have therapists begun to recognize that children of alcoholics have special needs and problems that manifest later in life. A 1987 Gallup poll found that one in four families reported a problem with liquor in the home, the highest level since 1950. Problems within an alcoholic household include family violence, battering, and incest. Fifty-five percent of reported family violence occurs in alcoholic homes. Fifty percent of the children of alcoholic parents marry an alcoholic, and children of alcoholics are four times more likely to become alcoholics. While these statistics are dramatic, they do not reveal the intense psychological damage that occurs to children of alcoholics.

A psychological handicap and a common thread with these children is that they have very low self-esteem. Stanley Coopersmith and Morris Rosenberg studied self-esteem among children and teenagers and found that individuals with high self-esteem perceive themselves as competent, successful, free of anxiety, self-reliant, outgoing, accepting of others, and generally well-rounded. Those with low self-esteem, on the other hand, feel isolated and unloved. They suffer from anxiety, self-consciousness, and a lack of capacity for joy or self-fulfillment. Children from alcoholic homes experience their lives from the perspective of low self-esteem. They manage to survive, but not to live, and they displace a great deal of energy into denial.

Warning signs of denial are important to recognize in yourself. First, listen to how you defend your parents' behavior and perhaps even excuse their drinking. Next, ask yourself if you can admit that your parent(s)' alcoholism has had a major effect on your life. Do you have difficulty acknowledging your feelings about growing up with an alcoholic parent? Finally, do you exercise superhuman willpower to "rise above it all, take control of your life, or not let this affect you?" This is the third level of denial. If you recognize yourself in any of these levels of denial, you may decide to change your life and pursue treatment. Every child of an alcoholic deserves to experience healing.

Many therapists and counselors who are concerned with these problems have established special groups to aid adult children of alcoholics. One therapist, Dr. Janet Geringer Woititz, wrote a best-selling book, *Adult Children of Alcoholics*, describing personality characteristics that appear time after time among these individuals. If you are an adult child of an alcoholic, and determine that several of the behaviors listed below apply to you, you may choose to seek help. Rebuilding a shattered self-esteem, learning to establish warm, loving relationships, and developing trust in others takes time in addition to professional and peer support.

Certain perceptions seem to characterize adult children of alcoholics. If you are a child of an alcoholic, you are likely to

- guess at normal behavior.
- have difficulty following a project through from beginning to end.
- lie when it would have been just as easy to tell the truth.
- judge yourself without mercy.
- have difficulty having fun.
- take yourself very seriously.
- have difficulty with intimate relationships.
- overreact to changes over which you have no control.
- constantly seek approval and affirmation.
- usually feel that you are different from other people.
- be super responsible or super irresponsible.
- be extremely loyal, even in the face of evidence that your loyalty is undeserved.
- be impulsive, and tend to lock yourself into a course of action without giving serious consideration to alternative behaviors or possible consequences of your actions.

If you are an adult child of an alcoholic parent, what can you do? Perhaps the first step is to realize that you are not alone; thousands of others also have suffered similar experiences. Once you acknowledge this awareness—that is, admit that you are the child of an alcoholic and that you may have emotional problems because of it, you have begun the healing process. Honesty with yourself is the first step. The next step is to seek support. Yes, it requires courage and discipline, but this is called recovery.

If you do choose to seek help, telephone your local Alcoholics Anonymous or Al-Anon and request a referral to a counselor or group that works with adult children of alcoholics in your area. You may also write the Children of Alcoholics Foundation, 540 Madison Avenue, New York, NY 10022, or call (212) 351-2680.

How to Help a Friend

You may wonder what to do if a friend or family member has a problem with alcohol or drugs. The issue may not be how much that person is using. You may feel he or she is using for the wrong reasons, or that his or her usage is having disturbing effects on health, relationships, or academics. Whether or not you're experienced with alcohol or drugs yourself, helping someone in trouble with alcohol or other drugs is often quite difficult.

If you're concerned about someone, first inform yourself about substance abuse and dependency. Discuss drinking (or drugs) with your friend. The American College Health Association (ACHA) reports that "many recovered alcoholics attribute their initial awareness of their drinking problem to the intervention of a friend or relative." Don't be accusatory; try to get your friend to talk about the situation. Rather than say, "You have a problem," ask, "How do you feel about what happens when you drink," or "Does drinking ever seem to complicate your life?"

If your friend becomes defensive, don't push. Just leave it at, "I like you. I care about you. And I just brought up the subject because I thought some of what happens when alcohol (or drugs) are involved was hurting you (or others around you)." Knowing you care may mean more to your friend than anything else. Let him or her know you are available if he or she ever wants to talk or do something about it. At a later time, you may find your friend more open to discussing how alcohol (or drugs) might be contributing to problems in his or her life.

Denial is a frequent barrier to treatment. If your friend doesn't acknowledge having problems, discuss the situation with mutual friends or family members. Try to work out a unified strategy. One positive limit is to create alternatives to drinking and drugs. Spend time with your friend in social settings that don't include alcohol. Let your friend know when you see him as funny, sexy, witty, or otherwise valued even when he hasn't been drinking. Tougher limits may include ignoring him if he has been drinking, saying he can't drink in your room, or not loaning him notes if he misses classes on account of hangovers, or not loaning him your car if he drives after drinking.

You may want to ask a professional counselor or a support group for some advice. Al-Anon is a nationwide support group for family and friends of alcohol-dependent individuals, with chapters in many communities. These groups provide information and guidance about responsibility for alcohol consumption.

If your friend agreed that some of his problems result from drinking (or drugs), ACHA suggests that you help him consider four questions:

- Why do you think you are having a problem with alcohol?
- What do you think you can do about it?
- What are you going to do about it?
- What kinds of support do you need from me in order to discontinue or curtail your drinking?

Support your friend's efforts to solve problems, whether or not such efforts include getting outside help. If quitting drugs or alcohol seems too much for your friend, help explore other alternatives. You and your friend can find help on campus and in the community. Visit a counselor or treatment center together and both ask what's involved. Sharing this experience may give your friend the needed incentive to really get help. Facilitate contact with others who have recovered from similar problems with alcohol (or drugs).

Seeking Professional Help

When to Get Help

Get help if:

- You or a friend display more than a few of the problem warning signs described earlier in this chapter.
- You wonder if you or a friend are involved in marginal abuse, abuse, or dependency patterns with alcohol or any drug.
- You or a friend have suffered overdose or other medical crisis involving alcohol or other drugs.

Types of Help Available

Most college campuses have counseling offices or health service professionals who either can deal with alcohol and drug problems or are aware of the community referral agencies available to students. Phone books in most cities list an "inter-group" number under Alcoholics Anonymous. Even if the primary problem is not alcohol, AA is often helpful to individuals with chemical dependency problems or who are dealing with someone who is chemically dependent. The AA office can usually tell you if there are self-help groups in your area for other specific problems, such as Al-Anon for family and friends of chemically dependent individuals, Narcotics Anonymous (which often deals with all drugs, not just narcotics), and Cocaine Anonymous.

Drugs Commonly Used/Abused on College Campuses

Central Nervous System Stimulants

Drugs	Immediate Effects	Most Common Complications	Potential for Dependence
Amphetamines (Benzedrine, Dexedrine, methadrine, diet pills, MDMA)	Euphoria, increased alertness, talkativeness. Stimulates heart, increases adrenaline. Insomnia, restlessness.	Nervousness, paranoia, hallucinations, dizziness, tremors, decreased mental abilities, sexual impotence, seizures. Death from OD.	Psychological, physical, withdrawal
Cocaine (cocaine powder, crack, freebased coke)	Brief euphoria, increased energy and sense of power. Restlessness. Surface anesthetic, suppressed appetite.	Tremors. Nasal bleeding, inflammation, perforation. Toxic psychosis, seizures. Depression (particularly afterwards), confusion. Death from OD (heart or respiratory failure) or impure supply.	Psychological
Nicotine	Relaxation, increased confidence, increased metabolism. Stimulates heart and nervous system.	High blood pressure, emphysema, bronchitis, heart disease. Cancer of lungs, lips and mouth.	Psychological, physical
Caffeine	Increased mental alertness. Increased blood pressure and respiration rate.	Nervousness, insomnia, dehydration, stomach irritation, fatigue after use, heart palpitations.	Psychological, physical

Central Nervous System Depressants

Drugs	Immediate Effects	Most Common Complications	Potential for Dependence
Alcohol (beer, wine, liquor, some medications for coughs, colds, and congestion)	Muscle relaxation, intoxication, depression, impaired motor control, impaired memory and judgment.	Dehydration; hangover; long-term liver, heart and brain damage. Overdose or mixing with other depressants can cause respiratory failure.	Psychological, physical
Tranquilizers (Valium, Librium, Equanil, Miltown)	Relief of tension and anxiety, drowsiness.	Hangover, menstrual irregularities, increase or decrease effect of other drugs. Mixing with alcohol or other depressants can be fatal.	Psychological, physical
Phencyclidine (PCP)	Loss of inhibition, excitement, muscle rigidity, loss of concentration and memory.	Visual disturbance, delirium, feelings of isolation and paranoia, violent behavior, psychosis.	Psychological
Barbiturates (Nembutal, Amytal, Seconal, phenobarbital)	Euphoria, relief of anxiety, loss of inhibition, muscle relaxation. Loss of motor control, drowsiness.	Lethargy, hangover, blurred vision, nausea, depression, seizures. Mixing with alcohol or other depressants can be fatal.	Psychological, physical

Narcotics

Drugs	Immediate Effects	Most Common Complications	Potential for Dependence
Heroin, morphine, opium, codeine, methadone, Demerol	Euphoria, drowsiness, pain killer.	Respiratory and circulatory depression, dizziness, vomiting, sweating, dry mouth, lowered libido, complications from injection.	Psychological, physical
Methaqualone (Quaalude)	Euphoria, sedation, loss of inhibition, muscle relaxation. Loss of motor control, drowsiness.	Hangover, nausea, seizures. Mixing with alcohol or other depressants can be fatal.	Psychological, physical, withdrawal

Cannabis

Drugs	Immediate Effects	Most Common Complications	Potential for Dependence
Marijuana, hashish, tetrahydrocannabinol (THC)	Relaxation, altered sense of hearing, time, vision; euphoria, increased heart rate and appetite; dilated pupils, memory impairment.	Impaired driving ability. Possible lung damage. Reduced sperm count and sperm motility. May affect ovulation cycles. Damage from impure doses.	Psychological

Hallucinogens/psychedelics

Drugs	Immediate Effects	Most Common Complications	Potential for Dependence
LSD, psilocybin, MDA, mescaline (peyote), DMT, STP	Hallucinations, altered sense of time, space and visual perception. Nausea, disorientation, panic.	Depression, paranoia, physical exhaustion after use, psychosis ("freaking out"); exaggerated body distortion; fears of death, flashbacks, adverse drug reactions.	Psychological

Other

Drugs	Immediate Effects	Most Common Complications	Potential for Dependence
Inhalants (amyl nitrate, butyl nitrate, nitrous oxide, glue and paint	Lowered blood pressure, relaxation of sphincter muscles, feeling of heightened sexual arousal.	Nitrates: headache, dizziness, accelerated heart rate, nausea, nasal irritation, cough, lost erection. Solvents: bone marrow, liver, kidney, heart, CNS impairment.	
Steroids	Not usually taken for mood modification but by athletes for muscle mass increase.	Blood disorders, liver problems, cancers, aggressive behavior, possibly psychosis.	

Note: Because of the burgeoning designer drug phenomenon and variations in drug use patterns in different geographic areas, this list cannot be all-inclusive. For information about any drug consult your college alcohol and drug treatment program.

Beyond the Text

1. Your friend consumes at least two or three beers *every day* but insists that daily drinking in moderation is not a problem.

2. Respond to the statement: Marijuana use always leads to harder drugs.

3. Children of alcoholic parents frequently experience low self-esteem. Why does this occur and what are some steps they can take to reverse this?

4. Your roommate's girlfriend becomes highly intoxicated at every party. What risks is she taking by such behavior?

5. Alcohol is a drug that kills, and it's legal. Therefore, marijuana and other drugs should be legal, too. What is your position?

6. A very drunk friend lies down on the couch saying he wants to take a little nap. What are the risks and what should you do if he passes out?

Supplemental Readings

Adult Children of Alcoholics by Janet Geringer Woititz, EdD. Deerfield Beach, FL: Health Communications, Inc., 1983. Written for the alcoholic's family members who suffer emotionally from their parent's affliction.

Beyond the Booze Battle by Ruth Maxwell. New York: Ballantine Books, 1986. Guidelines for what to do when alcoholism or chemical dependency hits close to home.

Codependent No More: How to Stop Controlling Others and Start Caring for Yourself by Melody Beattie. New York: Harper & Row, 1987. A guide for co-dependents who wish to heal themselves. Includes helpful advice for victims.

Drugfree by Richard Seymour and David Smith, MD. From Facts on File, New York, 1987. The authors, who manage the Haight-Ashbury Free Medical Clinic, address a wide range of addictive substances, from chocolate to cocaine, and how to eliminate them.

The Emotional Pharmacy: How Mood Altering and Psychoactive Drugs Work by Roberta Morgan. Los Angeles: Price Stern Sloane, Inc., 1988. Describes therapeutic uses, dangerous abuses, dependencies, and addictions associated with little-understood psychoactive drugs.

Key Terms Defined

addiction physiologic or psychologic dependence upon a substance, with a tendency toward increased use of the substance

BAC acronym for blood alcohol concentration, or amount of alcohol in the blood; expressed as tenths of one percent (e.g., .10%)

codependent a person in a continuing relationship with a chemically dependent person and whose actions enable the addiction to continue

crack highly addictive, smokeable form of cocaine

dependency state in which there is a compulsion to take a drug in order to experience its effects or to avoid the discomfort of its absence

depressant drug that acts on the central nervous system to slow down activity at all levels, for example, barbiturates

drug abuse excessive use of a drug (or drugs) for a purpose other than that for which they are prescribed or recommended

ethanol derived from grains, the main ingredient in alcoholic beverages

hallucinogen chemical agent capable of producing hallucinations or false perceptions; LSD and mescaline are examples

intoxication condition produced by excessive use of alcohol

marijuana preparation made from the leaves and tops of Cannabis sativa, which is known for its euphoric properties

narcotic a substance that produces insen-

sibility or stupor; morphine and heroin are examples of narcotics

opiate any sedative narcotic containing opium or any of its derivatives

OTC drugs acronym for over-the-counter drugs, those available without prescription, such as aspirin

overdose excessive dose of any drug; may be fatal

psychoactive drug a chemical substance that affects one's mind or behavior

recreational drugs any drugs used nontherapeutically in social situations or as a pastime

stimulant substance capable of exciting the central nervous system

Health Hazards of Tobacco

Tobacco has been commercially grown in the United States since 1612. By the middle of the twentieth century, 42 percent of American adults were consuming tobacco in the form of cigarettes, pipe mixtures, cigars, and smokeless. Convinced that tobacco posed significant health threats to smokers, the U.S. Public Health Service launched a campaign in 1964 to educate the public on the health hazards of tobacco. Since the mid-1960s, smoking among adults has dropped dramatically, but tobacco continues to impair the health of adolescents and adults who persist in using it or are exposed to environmental tobacco smoke.

This chapter describes why people smoke and how tobacco can adversely affect the user's health, such as cancer, cardiovascular disease, respiratory disease, and other conditions. Involuntary smoking hazards are discussed as well. The section on progress toward a smoke-free society puts today's antismoking programs, such as the ban on airline smoking, into perspective. Finally, smoking cessation programs are briefly discussed.

Key Terms

Aversion therapy

Behavior modification

Carbon monoxide

Carcinogenic

ETS

Nicotine

Smokeless tobacco

Tobacco tar

Contents

True scientific understanding of how tobacco affects health has been achieved only in the twentieth century.

Historical Perspective on Tobacco

Depicted in ancient Mayan art as early as 600 AD, the tobacco plant was native to the New World and was smoked in pipes by American Indians long before Europeans discovered our shores. The diaries of Christopher Columbus and other explorers make reference to tobacco. English colonist John Rolfe initiated commercial tobacco production in Virginia in 1612, and tobacco soon became an important export item from the Colonies. From the time of its introduction to Europeans, use of tobacco was controversial. European physicians declared that tobacco should be confined to medicinal purposes, but members of the royal courts believed that it should also be used for pleasure.

This conflict continued through the seventeenth and eighteenth centuries with neither side able to produce sufficiently convincing arguments to win over its opponents. In the early nineteenth century, scientists isolated the main active substance in tobacco and named it "Nicotianine," after Jean Nicot, a French diplomat who sent tobacco seeds to the French court in the late 1500s. The chemical formula was determined in the 1840s and "nicotine" was first synthesized in the 1890s.

For several hundred years, tobacco was primarily used for cigars, pipe mixtures and chewing. Cigarette smoking did not become widespread in the United States until the late 1800s, when the first efficient cigarette-making machines were perfected. As cigarette smoking gained in popularity, medical researchers began to study the effects of nicotine on the central nervous system. The smoking of tobacco as a means of administering nicotine was compared to the smoking of opium as the means of administering morphine. Meanwhile, use of tobacco flourished as a wider segment of the U.S. population consumed more cigarettes every day. The popular practice of giving free cigarettes to military personnel during World War II resulted in substantial numbers of relatively young adults becoming addicted to nicotine. By the 1950s, conclusive evidence established cigarette smoking as the largest single preventable cause of premature death and disability in the United States. As early as 1964, a federal government report on the health hazards of smoking set the stage for a monumental education effort to convince the American public of the dangers of smoking.

Landmark Report Ignites Public Concern

On January 11, 1964, Luther L. Terry, MD, Surgeon General of the U.S. Public Health Service, released the report of the Surgeon General's Advisory Committee on Smoking and Health. That landmark document was America's first widely publicized official declaration that cigarette smoking is a cause of cancer and other serious diseases. The committee stated, "Cigarette smoking is a health hazard of sufficient importance in the United States to warrant appropriate remedial action." While specific remedial actions had not been identified, the report and its conclusions

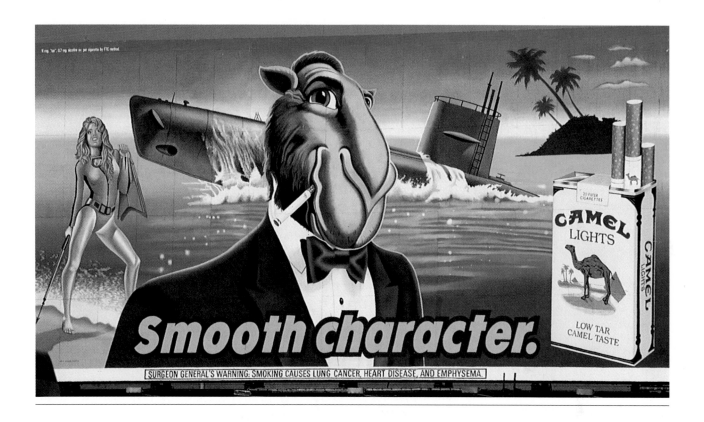

SURGEON GENERAL'S WARNING: SMOKING CAUSES LUNG CANCER, HEART DISEASE, AND EMPHYSEMA.

acted as catalysts for action on the part of government, public agencies, private organizations, and individual citizens. During the next 25 years, smoking among adults dropped dramatically from 42 percent in 1965 to 29 percent in 1987. Despite this sharp decline in smoking, one in six preventable deaths in the United States, a total of 390,000 in 1985, were attributed to tobacco use. Young men and women continue to take up smoking, and many individuals who have become chemically dependent on nicotine still experience difficulty or failure in their attempts to quit the habit.

Battle Lines Were Drawn   Soon after publication of the surgeon general's 1964 report, the Federal Trade Commission recommended adding warning labels to cigarette packaging and printed advertisements. The Federal Cigarette Labeling and Advertising Act, which was passed by Congress in 1965, prohibited cigarette advertising on television and restricted the content of advertisements in the print media. The battle lines were drawn between the health care advocates on one side and the tobacco industry and defenders of one's right to smoke on the other. Tobacco companies developed and promoted "healthier alternatives" in the form of filter cigarettes and brands with low-tar content. Total U.S. sales peaked at 640 billion cigarettes in 1981, then declined to 547 billion in

Health Hazards of Tobacco

1987. In 1985, the tobacco industry spent $2.5 billion for advertising, free samples, and other promotional activities. Cigarettes continue to be the most heavily advertised product category on outdoor billboards, second in magazines, and third in newspapers. 1988 revenues from the sale of all tobacco products were $37.8 billion.

The Perils of Tobacco

The most common method of subjecting the body to the effects of tobacco is to inhale the smoke from burning cigarettes, cigars, or pipe mixtures. A person can also experience the effects of tobacco by using smokeless tobacco (chewing tobacco and snuff).

Nearly 4,000 substances have been identified in tobacco smoke; among them are 43 chemicals labeled as carcinogenic (capable of producing cancer), a potentially lethal gas (carbon monoxide), and an addictive psychoactive drug (nicotine). When inhaling, the smoker draws a combination of hot gases and particles into the lungs, where harmful substances are absorbed into the bloodstream. Individuals who smoke but who do not inhale, or who use smokeless tobacco, absorb dangerous ingredients into the bloodstream via the mucous lining of the mouth or the digestive system. It is not surprising that a multitude of illnesses and causes of premature death are linked to smoking, including cancer, heart and respiratory diseases.

Nicotine Nicotine is a powerful chemical agent, and its harmful effects on the human body have long been suspected and researched. When carried by the bloodstream to the brain, nicotine activates various receptors to produce a variety of responses. Initially, nicotine acts as a stimulant triggering the release of neurotransmitters (including norepinephrine) and creating a euphoric feeling or "high." Eventually, high levels of nicotine will depress the central nervous system. Due to nicotine tolerance that individuals build up, a lethal dose is difficult to predict; about 60 milligrams is considered sufficient to kill most adults. A cigar contains 120 milligrams of nicotine, which, if inhaled as cigarette smoke, could kill the smoker. The average cigarette contains 0.05 to 2.5 milligrams of nicotine. When inhaling, the smoker absorbs about 90 percent of the nicotine into the bloodstream, while the noninhaler receives 20 to 50 percent. In addition to producing a high, nicotine's effects include release of epinephrine and norepinephrine, increased heart rate, dilation of respiratory airways, constriction of peripheral blood vessels, and gastrointestinal hyperactivity.

Carbon Monoxide Carbon monoxide, a tasteless, odorless, colorless gas, is one of the most harmful components of tobacco smoke. When inhaled, carbon monoxide impairs the red blood cells' ability to transport oxygen and reduces the efficient functioning of the brain, heart and other

Health Hazards of Tobacco

organs. The smoker's physical endurance is diminished, so heavy smokers usually experience shortness of breath with little exertion.

Tobacco Tar   Tobacco tar consists of hundreds of chemicals that are evident in the sticky brown residue on ash trays and smoker's fingers. This same residue can coat your lungs. Carcinogenic substances in the tar are considered to be the cause of several types of cancer.

Health Hazards of Smoking Cigarettes

Medical researchers estimate that the average male who smokes two packs per day should expect to die seven to eight years earlier than his nonsmoking counterpart. Not only premature death but other costs—social, psychological, and economic—of illnesses and disabilities must also be considered.

Cardiovascular Disease   The relationship between tobacco use and cardiovascular disease has been the focus of intensive research for several decades. Smoking is a major risk factor for heart attack. Nicotine increases the heart rate, which, in turn, raises the blood pressure and causes narrowing of the coronary arteries. Nearly a third of all cardiovascular disease can be linked to smoking cigarettes. Cigarette smoking is a major cause of cerebrovascular disease (stroke), the third leading cause of death in the United States. Smoking contributes to about 170,000 deaths from heart disease each year. Further information on cardiovascular diseases is presented in the chapter on **Cardiovascular Disease and Cancer**.

Cancer   Cigarette smokers have a substantially higher (up to ten times) probability of developing lung cancer when compared to nonsmokers. Researchers estimate that 80 percent of all cases of lung cancer are related to cigarette smoking. The remaining 20 percent are caused by environmental factors (air pollution) or the inhaling of harmful substances (asbestos), or toxic chemicals (herbicides). The American Cancer Society estimates that deaths from lung cancer reached 135,000 in 1986; 85 percent were directly attributable to active cigarette smoking.

The probability of developing lung cancer is closely related to the duration of the smoker's habit (number of years smoking), number of cigarettes consumed per day, nicotine and tar content of cigarettes smoked, and the amount of smoke inhaled. The harmful effects of tobacco are linked not only to lung cancer but also to cancer of the mouth, esophagus, bladder, larynx, kidney, and pancreas. Further information on cancer is presented in the chapter on **Cardiovascular Disease and Cancer**.

Respiratory Disease   Smoking is one of several causes of chronic bronchitis, an inflammatory condition of the upper respiratory tract. When an individual gives up smoking, the symptoms of bronchitis are usually reversed. Tobacco smoking is also a contributing factor in emphysema, the

Surgeon General's Warnings

- Cigarette Smoke Contains Carbon Monoxide.
- Smoking Causes Lung Cancer, Heart Disease, Emphysema, and May Complicate Pregnancy.
- Smoking By Pregnant Women May Result in Fetal Injury, Premature Birth, and Low Birth Weight.
- Quitting Smoking Now Greatly Reduces Serious Risks to Your Health.

Health Hazards of Tobacco

destruction of tiny air sacs in the lungs. The resulting inability to exchange oxygen causes shortness of breath, which incapacitates many persons and kills others.

Smoking and Pregnancy   Pregnant women who smoke have more complications than their nonsmoking counterparts, including spontaneous abortion, fetal death, premature birth, and birth defects. A common effect of smoking is low birth weight, which adds stress to the infant's vital organs and systems during the early period after delivery. Smoking women are also at increased risk for cancer of the uterus and cervix.

Health Hazards of Other Tobacco Products

Although cigarettes are today's most popular method of tobacco consumption, most people smoked cigars or pipe mixtures, or chewed tobacco until the early twentieth century. The popularity of noncigarette tobacco products grew in response to the recent campaigns to reduce cigarette smoking.

Pipe and Cigar Smoking   This practice entails a substantially lower risk of lung cancer because the smoke is usually not inhaled into the lungs. However, cancer of the lip, mouth, larynx, and esophagus are linked to pipe and cigar smoking. Because some of the tar is swallowed, there is also risk of stomach and bladder cancer.

Clove Cigarettes   Introduced into the United States in the early 1980s, and known also as "kreteks," clove cigarettes are about 40 percent ground cloves and 60 percent tobacco. They contain twice as much tar and nicotine as U.S. manufactured cigarettes, so the claim that these are safer cigarettes is false.

Smokeless Tobacco   An estimated 12 million people in the United States used smokeless tobacco in 1985, and at least half this number used it weekly or more often. In the last year alone a shocking 16 percent of young men between the ages of 12 and 25 have used smokeless tobacco. One-third to one-half are regular users and use is increasing. Chewing tobacco, packaged either as a solid block (plug) or loose-leafed in a pouch, is placed between the user's cheek and gum. The tobacco juice and saliva are expectorated. Snuff, finely ground tobacco, is placed between cheek and gum (dipping) or placed on the back of the hand and sniffed through the nose. Users of smokeless tobacco avoid the effects of tar, carbon monoxide, and other gases. However, nicotine is absorbed into the blood via the mucous membranes in the mouth. Nicotine levels in the body from smokeless tobacco are similar in strength to nicotine levels from cigarette smoking. This form of tobacco use can be as addictive as cigarettes. Its hazards are numerous, including increased heart rate, elevated

> From 1964 to 1986 pipe and cigar smoking declined by 80 percent among men.

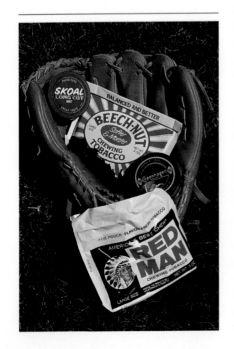

blood pressure, and a multitude of potential cancers located in the mouth, pharynx, esophagus, bladder, and pancreas. The user's teeth darken and mouth tissue is usually damaged. Additionally, the high sugar content of molasses and other tobacco's flavorings has potentially negative health effects on heavy users.

New Products to Counter Antismoking Campaigns

Tobacco firms responded to antismoking campaigns with an array of new products. Their overall strategy was to present the smoking public with products less hazardous to health, featuring filter tips, low-tar and low-nicotine content. Other new products include low-smoke and nicotine-free cigarettes. The "smokeless" cigarette consists of a carbon heat source at one end and a filter at the other with tobacco and flavorings in a compartment between the two. After lighting the carbon tip, the "smoker" draws hot air across the tobacco and into the mouth via the filter. The user does not inhale the hazardous gases given off by burning tobacco, nor are nonsmoking individuals irritated by sidestream smoke. However, tests reveal that the smoker ingests compounds and carbon monoxide at levels equal to those delivered from low-tar cigarettes—not a significant health breakthrough. Complaints about poor taste led the R. J. Reynolds Tobacco Company to end market acceptance tests of its low-smoke Premier brand in early 1989.

Two cigarettes are advertised as "ultra-low-tar" brands. In mid-1989, market testing began on a new cigarette featuring "ultra-low-nicotine." Critics point out that smokers will, as necessary, inhale low-nicotine brands more deeply and smoke more per day to maintain their nicotine high. The American Medical Association reports that the smoke of burning tobacco contains at least 40 to 45 carcinogenic substances regardless of its level of nicotine.

Involuntary Smoking

The Surgeon General's 1986 report, entitled "The Health Consequences of Involuntary Smoking," drew three main conclusions:

1. Involuntary smoking is a cause of disease, including lung cancer, among healthy nonsmokers.
2. The children of parents who smoke have an increased frequency of respiratory illnesses and infections including bronchitis and pneumonia when compared with the children of nonsmokers.
3. The main effects of irritants contained in environmental tobacco smoke (ETS) occur in the eyes and mucous membranes of the nose, throat and upper respiratory organs.

Because nearly two thirds of the smoke from a burning cigarette is released into the surrounding environment, a room crowded with smokers

Smokeless Catches on Early with Males

Sixteen percent of males between 12 and 25 years of age have used some form of smokeless tobacco within the past year. In certain parts of the country, as many as 25 to 35 percent of adolescent males indicated current use.

Involuntary smoking is a cause of disease, including lung cancer, in healthy nonsmokers.

Health Hazards of Tobacco

CHAPTER 16

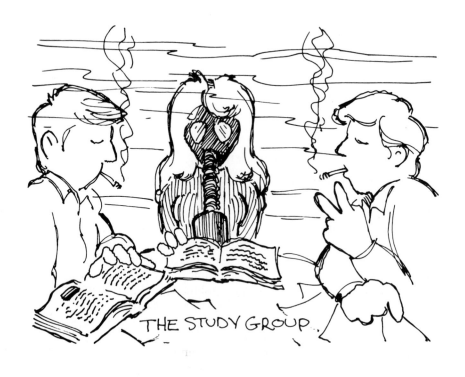

THE STUDY GROUP

contains considerable smoke, especially under conditions of less than optimal ventilation. In fact, in one hour under such adverse conditions, a nonsmoker can inhale the equivalent of one cigarette's nicotine, carbon dioxide and other harmful substances. Environmental tobacco smoke (ETS) is not only bothersome to many nonsmokers; it also presents health hazards. ETS is either smoke emitted from a burning tobacco product (sidestream smoke) or smoke that has been exhaled by another smoker (second-hand smoke). Sidestream smoke has higher concentrations of irritating and hazardous substances, such as carbon monoxide, nicotine and certain carcinogens, than does second-hand smoke. The amount of ETS breathed by the involuntary smoker depends on the concentration of smoke in the environment and the length of time he or she is exposed to it. Fresh air is the most effective remedy, but in classrooms, dining facilities, and bars, it is often difficult to maintain air circulation that will effectively disperse tobacco smoke.

In response to the findings regarding the health hazards of involuntary smoking, many states, cities and companies have restricted smoking, particularly in public places. Segregation of smokers from nonsmokers in restaurants and other public places has met with mixed results, because nonsmokers continue to detect tobacco smoke and smokers feel unfairly isolated. The ban of cigarette smoking on certain airline flights has pleased many nonsmoking travelers but frustrated the smokers.

Voluntary Smoking

About 30 percent of the American public continues to smoke in spite of acknowledging tobacco's potential health hazards. People give the following reasons for their use of tobacco:

- *Decreasing the effects of tension, anxiety, and anger.* Many people begin smoking as a way to handle stress and continue to smoke as a method of dealing with ongoing daily stress.
- *Relaxation and social interaction.* Cigarette advertising strongly associates smoking with relaxing situations and social success. Peer group acceptance is a powerful lure, especially among teenagers.
- *Craving.* As nicotine use increases, the body's tolerance level is raised, and the craving or addiction becomes a powerful influence. The discomfort of withdrawal leads to many failures for those who try giving up the habit.
- *Habit.* People become conditioned to smoke under certain situations: while drinking caffeine or alcohol, getting into a car, studying, or after a meal. Reaching for a cigarette becomes almost a reflex action.
- *Role models.* The sudden spurt in use of smokeless tobacco among many young men is directly related to its use by professional baseball players. Stars of the sports, fashion, and entertainment fields are seen smoking in magazine photos, portraying the habit as acceptable and even glamorous.

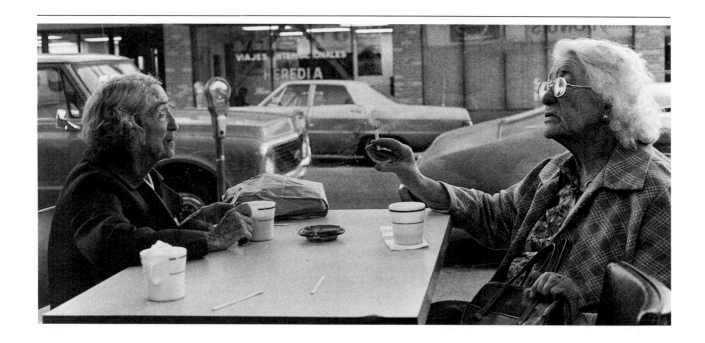

In 1985 about 56 million Americans 15 to 84 years of age were smokers. In the absence of an antismoking campaign, an estimated 91 million would have been smokers.

People start smoking and continue for many of the above reasons. Another factor is that many do not think *they* will become ill from tobacco. Someone else will contract the dreaded diseases. They believe the misconceptions surrounding filter cigarettes, smokeless tobacco and other "healthier" alternatives.

Toward a Tobacco-free Society

In his 1989 annual report, the surgeon general stated, "Nearly half of all living adults who ever have smoked quit." Of course, many who did not quit have cancer, heart disease and/or other illnesses that will reduce their life expectancy. The accompanying chart summarizes key results in the campaign to reach a smoke-free society by the year 2000. Continued progress depends on the effectiveness of public education programs, added legal restrictions on smoking, and economic incentives to influence the behavior of nonsmokers to abstain and smokers to quit.

Public Education Programs

Campaigns aimed at informing the American public about the health hazards of smoking include government-mandated warnings printed on cigarette packaging, prohibition of television advertising of tobacco products, and inclusion of health warnings in magazine and newspaper advertisements. The American Heart Association, American Lung Association, and National Cancer Society continue their antismoking programs. Since the late 1960s public awareness programs have been most effective among graduates; the probability of quitting smoking increases with the individual's level of education.

Government-sponsored education campaigns during the 1990s will focus on specific population groups whose tobacco consumption continues at hazardous levels, including minority groups, pregnant women, high school dropouts, military personnel, blue-collar workers, and the unemployed. The 16-year-old, unemployed, pregnant, high school dropout is very difficult to reach with an effective antismoking program, much less to convince her to give up what may be one of the few pleasures in life.

Adolescents—the New Smokers

About one million teenagers begin smoking each year. Sixty percent of these new smokers take up the habit by age 14, and by age 18, 80 percent of them are subjecting their bodies to the hazards of tobacco. Surveys conducted among high school students indicate increased rates of smoking during the past several years. Health educators are alarmed at this trend. Public health advocates charge tobacco companies with targeting young people with their cigarette advertising. Spokesmen for the tobacco firms

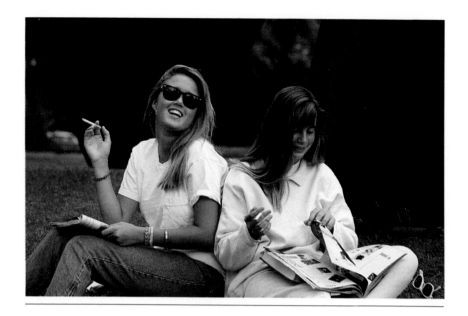

have denied these allegations. Although 43 states and the District of Columbia legally restrict the sale of cigarettes to minors, tobacco products are relatively easy to buy, particularly from vending machines.

Direct Restrictions on Smoking

Pressured by private enterprise and consumer health advocate organizations, federal, state, and local governments have enacted restrictions on smoking that were considered unthinkable in 1964. Of these, public spaces and workplace locations have been the most common targets. Over 40 states have passed laws restricting smoking in public, and airlines have banned smoking on flights of two hours or less within the United States. Newly released research concerning the health hazards of environmental tobacco smoke has encouraged consumer advocates to press for a complete ban on smoking on all airline flights and other public transportation, as well as in restaurants, other public buildings and all schools. Although restrictions on smoking are directed toward protecting nonsmokers and involuntary smokers, the impact on attitudes has influenced smokers' behavior and is probably reducing the total consumption of cigarettes.

Economic Incentives

Federal and state excise taxes add an average of 34 cents per pack to the price of cigarettes. Surveys indicate that increases in cigarette prices result in decreased consumption, especially among adolescent smokers. Nearly

The Smoking versus Nonsmoking Controversy

Since 1964, health advocates have vigorously pressed for a smokeless society. The controversy has taken on economic, political, social, and moral dimensions in addition to the basic health issue. The following statements reflect opinions that support the rights of tobacco users.

Sanctimonious Selfish Anti-Smokers

. . . "in accord with Federal Aviation Association regulations this is a nonsmoking flight." A large number of passengers cheered and applauded.

There was something so sanctimonious about this outburst that I spent the remainder of the flight trying to understand why. I concluded that I had witnessed a self-righteous exhibition of moral superiority. This is not something most people, in these days of subjective moral values, have much opportunity to do. However, smoking has now become a sin, so opposing it has taken on a sanctioned and religious quality.

There is a certain elitism in the antismoking movement, something that underlies most moral crusades. Undeniably, there are very serious health problems associated with smoking. Yet, for many people, smoking may be one of the few pleasures they experience. Increasingly, those people are members of the working class. Given the enormous amount of knowledge of the health risks associated with smoking, should people be denied the right to decide for themselves that the benefits outweigh the risks?

Editorial by sociologist David Scott Davis, *The New York Times*, January 27, 1989

Stop Picking on Me

You see, I'm a smoker. And smokers enjoy about the same status in the United States today that witches enjoyed in seventeenth century New England. I, for one, am tired of it.

I'm tired of the looks that come my way—looks of disgust and contempt and naked hostility, looks that leave me sorely in need of a bath—every time I walk into a restaurant or a theater or onto an airplane with my pipe in my mouth.

Why, then, should it be smokers who are invariably singled out for second-class citizenship? Why should those who drink coffee—or beer or wine or distilled spirits, for that matter—be left free to feed their drug habits in eateries, aboard planes or wherever without so much as a wink of disapproval, while smokers are treated like lepers for doing the very same thing in the very same places?

Editorial by Jeff Rigsenbach, *USA Today*, June 23, 1989

---

all life insurance companies offer lower premiums for nonsmokers. However, only a few insurers of health and disability provide premium discounts for nonsmokers. Unfortunately for those who wish to quit, health insurance policies rarely reimburse the costs of smoking cessation programs or treatment for nicotine dependency.

On-Campus Smoking Concerns

About 14 percent of college students are smokers; this is significantly lower than the estimated 29 percent of the U.S. adult population that uses tobacco products. Although students and administrators acknowledge the health hazards of tobacco, few colleges and universities have addressed the issue of on-campus smoking. In order to implement effective smoking restrictions in residence halls, dining facilities, and classroom buildings, college administrators have to deal with students, faculty, and

Health Hazards of Tobacco

staff. Fear of violating smokers' rights and the difficulty of enforcing smoking policies have inhibited effective control of smoking. Health educators urge that campus health centers offer education, prevention, and cessation programs for tobacco similar to those now provided for abuse of alcohol and other drugs. College women, who tend to smoke more than college men, are a particularly high risk group.

Quitting Smoking

The best way to avoid the health hazards of tobacco is to refrain from using it. For those who now use tobacco, the process of quitting can be uncomfortable and frustrating. The degree of nicotine dependency strongly influences one's ability to break the habit. An estimated 30 million individuals have successfully quit smoking since 1964. Statistics summarize the results, but they do not do justice to the anguish that many smokers experience during the process of quitting. Studies indicate that 95 percent of the people who quit smoking cigarettes do so by themselves. The remaining individuals obtain help from group programs or treatment clinics.

Smoking cessation programs are available in a variety of formats, including behavior modification (positive reinforcement), aversion conditioning (negative reinforcement), hypnosis, and acupuncture. Stop-smoking clinics are sponsored by nonprofit organizations such as the American Heart Association, American Cancer Society, American Lung Association, and Seventh-Day Adventists. Several commercial organizations offering programs for a fee are SmokEnders, Smoke Watchers, and Schick Laboratories. It is impossible to predict which approach or program would be most effective for a specific individual. Unfortunately, the better programs have only a 20 to 30 percent long-term (over one year) success rate. Preparation, quitting, and maintenance of a smoking-free life are the three phases of a typical cessation program.

Preparation The first step is to understand why you use tobacco (the most common reasons are summarized earlier in this chapter) and why you wish to quit. External pressure from friends, relatives, fellow workers, or physicians influences some users to agree to quit. But when the decision is generated internally (you want to quit), the process has a better chance for success.

Quitting Many alternatives are available. Some people are able to quit abruptly ("cold turkey"). This calls for strong determination and even stronger discipline. Certain individuals can tolerate the withdrawal experience more easily than others. Researchers recommend that heavy smokers try a reduction or tapering off regimen to reduce consumption to about seven cigarettes per day, followed by a complete stop.

Health Benefits of Quitting Smoking

- Greater energy
- Increased appetite
- Improved sense of taste and smell
- Reduced heart rate
- Improved circulation to hands and feet
- Lowered blood pressure
- Increased breath capacity
- Decline in "smoker's cough"

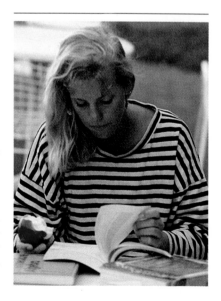

Maintenance   The key to maintaining a tobacco-free life is substituting other rewards for those previously gained from smoking. For some individuals, realizing how much better they feel is sufficient reward. Other people substitute healthy activities (physical exercise) or perhaps not-so-healthy reactions (snacking on junk food). The addictive quality of nicotine explains why many individuals experience difficulty and failure. Shaking a dependence on nicotine is similar to breaking a cocaine habit, and experts are just now recognizing how difficult it is to give up nicotine.

Nicotine Withdrawal and Nicotine Substitutes   As one's body develops a tolerance for nicotine, more cigarettes are required to achieve the same rewards of stimulation, euphoria, and so forth. The heavy smoker most likely has developed an addiction to nicotine. When the supply of nicotine to the blood stream ceases, withdrawal reactions may include headache, nausea, diarrhea, and general irritability. The strength of the craving and degree of irritability often trigger a resumption of smoking. Many individuals fail several times before finally reaching success.

Nicotine substitutes are now available to assist with the withdrawal progress. A gum containing nicotine resin has been reasonably successful when it is supported by behavior modification or other therapy. Available on a prescription basis, each piece of nicotine gum delivers about as much nicotine as one cigarette. Just as with chewing tobacco, the nicotine is absorbed into the bloodstream through the mucous membrane of the mouth. The smoker who is trying to quit avoids the health hazards of the gases and tar of normal cigarettes. The objective is to taper off the use of gum and nicotine over a prescribed period of time without becoming dependent on the gum.

In mid-1989, researchers reported that nicotine patches proved safe and effective in a preliminary study conducted at the Martinez, California, Veterans Administration Hospital. Of 80 smokers trying to quit, those using the nicotine skin patches were twice as likely to stay smoke-free for ten weeks as those who received unmedicated patches. Nicotine patches should be available for public use in about two years.

The long-term success of breaking any drug dependence rests primarily with the individual. Personal motivation and self-discipline play crucial roles. Support and continued positive reinforcement from peers, family, and co-workers can ensure that the program to quit continues and succeeds.

Seeking Professional Help

Seek Help If:

- You smoke or use other forms of tobacco and are even considering quitting
- You smoke and have been experiencing shortness of breath, coughing, or other respiratory problems
- You are smoking while pregnant or nursing
- You chew tobacco and have sores in your mouth
- You want to quit smoking but are worried about gaining weight if you do

Types of Help Available

Physicians can help assess physical effects and damage due to tobacco use. They can give you encouragement and tell you what to expect during the withdrawal period. They can usually recommend local programs and courses of treatment (such as prescription nicotine gum) to help you give up tobacco.

Many people have found success with stop-smoking clinics and programs; ask your physician or college health center for referrals. Refer to your telephone directory for local numbers for the American Cancer Society, American Heart Association, or American Lung Association; these organizations provide information about quitting smoking and smoking cessation programs.

Beyond the Text

1. Respond to the following statement: Since environmental tobacco smoke is potentially harmful to nonsmokers, the government should legislate antismoking laws for all public places.

2. Your younger brother joined a baseball team. He says he probably won't get any playing time if he doesn't take up smokeless tobacco like the other team members. What do you tell him?

3. The tobacco industry supports thousands of farmers and pays millions of dollars in taxes—the tobacco companies should be allowed to advertise their products on television. What is your position?

4. Your roommate's friend comes over frequently to study. This person's cigarette smoking bothers you but not your roommate. What would you do?

5. Respond to the statement: I'm under so much pressure; if I gave up smoking, I'd just start drinking or eating too much.

Supplemental Readings

The Cigarette Underworld—A Front Line Report on the War Against Your Lungs by Alan Blum, ed. New York: Lyle Stuart, 1985. An exposé of the tobacco industry.

How to Stop Smoking Through Meditation by Richard Tyson, MD. Chicago: Playboy Press, 1976. A common sense "how to" book based on scientific principles to relieve the anxiety of giving up smoking.

If You Love Somebody Who Smokes by Cynthia Morgan. Berkeley, CA: City Miner Books, 1987. Written by an ex-smoker with humor and compassion to help people understand, control, and then extinguish their nicotine addiction.

Smoking: Your Choice Between Life and Death by Alton Ochsner, MD. New York: Simon and Schuster, 1970. Discusses the connection between smoking and various diseases and offers a ten-point program to help the smoker break the habit.

Switch Down and Quit: What Cigarette Companies Don't Want You to Know About Smoking by Dolly Gahagan. Berkeley, CA: Ten Speed Press, 1987. Offers a program for the smoker to switch to a different, lower nicotine content brand every three weeks. This allows the body to adjust to lower levels of nicotine until the smoker can voluntarily quit.

You Can Stop by Jacquelyn Rogers. New York: Simon and Schuster, 1977. Written by the co-founder of SmokEnders, this book focuses on self-awareness and a strong commitment to take responsibility for quitting.

Key Terms Defined

aversion therapy   treatment that attempts to help a person overcome a dependence or a bad habit by making the person feel disgusted or repulsed by the habit

behavior modification   an approach to changing behavior through the application of principles of learning theory (reinforcement)

carbon monoxide   colorless, odorless gas; a byproduct of burning tobacco that displaces oxygen in the hemoglobin molecules of red blood cells

carcinogenic   substance that produces cancerous cells or enhances their development and growth

ETS   acronym for environmental tobacco smoke; consists of second-hand smoke (previously exhaled by another person) and sidestream smoke (from a burning cigarette, cigar, or pipe mixture)

nicotine   major addictive chemical found in tobacco

smokeless tobacco   tobacco products, such as chewing tobacco and snuff, that are chewed or sucked rather than smoked

tobacco tar   thick, brownish substance condensed from particulate matter in cigarette smoke

Cardiovascular Disease and Cancer

The two leading causes of death in the United States, cardiovascular disease and cancer, should command our attention. Although they tend to affect older adults much more frequently than young adults, cardiovascular disease and cancer often are the long-term results of various lifestyle behaviors commenced in the early adult years. Recent health promotion programs link cancer to tobacco use and heart disease to overindulgence in high-cholesterol foods. Genetics and environment influence our risk of contracting heart disease and cancer, but diet, exercise, and other behaviors that we can control are usually the most determining factors.

This chapter discusses the major risk factors that apply to cardiovascular disease and cancer. The emphasis of this presentation is prevention—what you can do to minimize your chances of developing either disease and develop healthy lifestyle behaviors.

Key Terms

Angina

Bronchitis

Cancer

Carcinogenic

Cardiovascular system

Congestive heart failure

Coronary arteries

ECG

Hypertension

Malignant

Melanoma

Metastasize

Myocardial infarction

Radiation

Sigmoidoscopy

Stroke

Contents

Overview of Cardiovascular Disease and Cancer

Cardiovascular disease and cancer are the two leading causes of death in most developed countries, including the United States. Although the two diseases are quite different from a medical point of view, they share a number of common characteristics, such as the tendency of both diseases to affect older adults more often than young adults. Factors over which we have little or no control, such as our genes and our environment, influence the risk of developing heart disease or cancer. However, health choices made in adolescence and young adulthood also have a major impact on the risk; in fact, many of our personal health decisions are linked to both heart disease and cancer. This chapter discusses the major risk factors that apply to both diseases as well as those specific for one disease or the other. The major emphasis of this section is prevention—how you can minimize your chances of developing either heart disease or cancer.

Physiology of the Heart

The heart, a muscular organ that functions as a pump, has four compartments or chambers: the right atrium and right ventricle and the left atrium and left ventricle. Blood returns from the body to the right atrium through veins. It flows into the right ventricle, which pumps the blood into the lungs, where it exchanges carbon dioxide for oxygen. The blood then flows into the left atrium and to the left ventricle. From there, blood is pumped into the aorta and smaller arteries, and is carried to all parts of the body. One-way valves control the flow of blood into and out of the ventricles. The ventricle relaxes and fills with blood during diastole; it

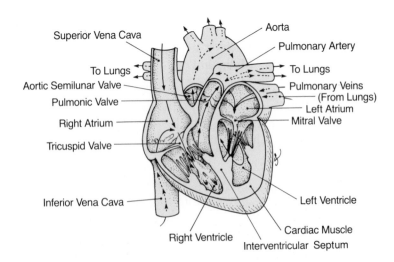

Blood flow pattern through the right and left side of the heart.

Cardiovascular Disease and Cancer

contracts and pumps the blood out during systole. The ventricles contract, or beat, at about 70 beats per minute. The pacemaker, a specialized group of cells, tells the heart when to contract and sends the signal to the atria and ventricles. The heart muscle itself gets its blood supply through the three coronary arteries.

Heart Disease

The term heart disease refers to a group of illnesses, about 2 percent of which are congenital and the remainder are acquired. Congenital heart disease is a group of structural abnormalities of the heart and large blood vessels due to abnormal development of the embryo and fetus. These abnormalities can cause heart failure and/or delivery of oxygen-poor blood to the body.

Coronary Heart Disease   Acquired heart diseases are characterized by a variety of causes, symptoms, and outcomes. A combination of genetic and other risk factors determines the likelihood of developing coronary heart disease. The most common cause of cardiac disability and death, this disease results from narrowing coronary arteries with ultimate blockage of blood flow to the heart muscle. This process can cause angina (chest pain due to coronary heart disease), heart attacks, and sudden death. The term heart attack is a lay term, and usually refers to a myocardial infarction. The interruption of or insufficient blood supply to the heart causes severe oxygen deprivation and death of some of the heart muscle.

Hard Heart Facts

Every day the average heart beats 100,000 times and pumps close to 2,000 gallons of blood. If you live 70 years, your heart will have expanded and contracted more than 2.5 billion times.

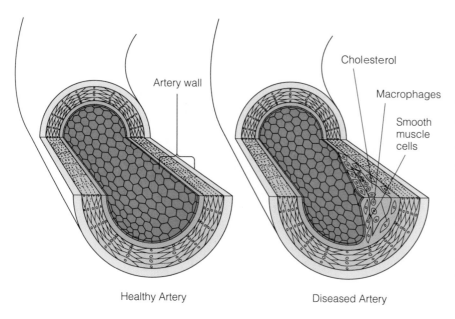

Healthy Artery   Diseased Artery

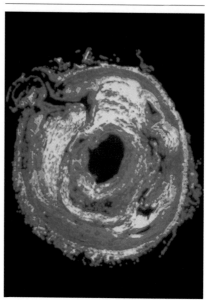

Most of the same risk factors also apply to stroke, which results from a blockage of blood flow to a part of the brain, and to peripheral vascular disease, which affects arteries in the rest of the body. While we cannot control some of these risk factors, others are possible to both control and eliminate. These will be discussed in the following section.

Valvular Heart Disease   Rheumatic heart disease results from complications of streptococcal infection (e.g., "strep throat"). This infection can lead to destruction of the heart valves.

Other disease processes can also cause valvular heart disease. The most common type of valve problem usually identified in young adults is called mitral valve prolapse (MVP), in which the mitral valve (located between the left atrium and left ventricle) bulges back into the atrium during systole. In more severe cases, blood leaks back into the atrium. Some people with MVP, or with other types of valvular heart disease, need to take antibiotics before dental work and other procedures in order to prevent endocarditis, another form of heart valve infecton. Most people with MVP do not develop significant valve leakage or blockage.

Hypertensive Heart Disease   Hypertensive heart disease can be caused by hypertension, or "high blood pressure." The elevated pressure in the arteries makes the left ventricle work harder and, if not treated, the left ventricle ultimately fails. This condition is common. It occurs in 10–15 percent of white adults and 20–30 percent of black adults. Congestive

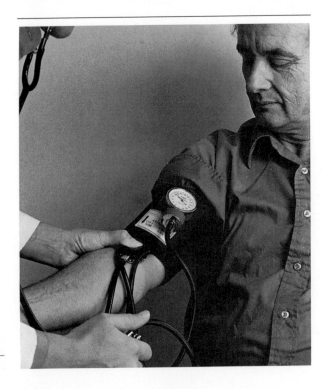

Cardiovascular Disease and Cancer

heart failure is the end result of many of these heart diseases. It is characterized by swelling of the legs, shortness of breath, and difficulty exercising.

Cancer

Cancer, like heart disease, is also a group of illnesses, which are classified by the organ in which they originate (e.g., lung cancer, colon cancer, breast cancer). Although cancer is often thought of as a rapid growth of cells, in the vast majority of cases the cancer cells are growing more slowly than other cells in the body, but they are not maturing normally. Cancerous collections of cells are often called malignant tumors. They can spread to other parts of the body (metastasize), and they can interfere with vital body functions. Cancer develops over a period of years as a result of genetic, environmental, and behavioral factors.

Risk Factors for Heart Disease and Cancer

Both heart disease and cancer result from a combination of factors, but not everyone exposed to one or more of these will develop a disease. Some risk factors are very powerfully related to disease, whereas others are weak or only operate in concert with other variables. Three factors important in both diseases are smoking, diet, and stress. Risk factors pertaining only to cancer or only to heart disease will be reviewed after these, followed by recommendations for prevention, early detection, and treatment.

How Cancer Spreads

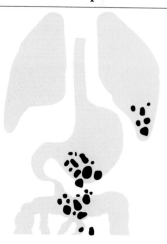

Within a body cavity

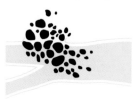

Via blood vessels

447

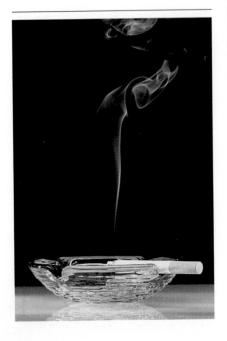

Smoking

It is difficult to overemphasize the importance of smoking as a direct cause of heart disease, cancer, and several other major health problems, such as stroke, peripheral vascular disease, and emphysema. Tobacco smoke contains carbon monoxide, which blocks the availability of oxygen; nicotine, which accounts for the physical addiction that smokers develop; and numerous carcinogens, chemicals that cause cancer. Oral, laryngeal, and lung cancer are the most closely associated with tobacco use, since these organs receive the most intense exposure to the carcinogens. Use of smokeless (chewing) tobacco is linked to high rates of oral cancer. Other types of cancer are also more common in smokers. For example, bladder cancer occurs more frequently in smokers because some of the carcinogens are absorbed into the bloodstream and excreted into the urine. Overall, tobacco use accounts for at least 25 percent of all cancer deaths in this country each year.

Smokers have a much higher risk of developing coronary heart disease prematurely and a higher risk of sudden death from heart disease. Thousands of scientific studies have demonstrated that smokers have a shorter lifespan, higher rates of disease and disability, higher medical care costs, and more pregnancy-related problems. Besides these risks, smokers' skin ages more rapidly and wrinkles much faster than the skin of nonsmokers. The good news is that smokers who quit decrease their risk of heart disease over a period of only a few months, and decrease their risk of cancer over the next few years.

While fewer Americans are smoking today than in the mid-1960s, a significant number of young people start smoking each year. Obviously, the best way to avoid the dangers associated with tobacco use is never to start. Although curiosity, peer pressure, and advertising can all be temptations to start smoking, it is also important to consider the short-term and long-term consequences. Individuals with a family history of cancer, lung disease, or heart disease and those with high blood pressure, high cholesterol, diabetes, or lung problems have additional reasons to avoid tobacco.

People who have already started to smoke should stop. While that is easy to say, it is hard for most smokers to quit. Nicotine is an addicting drug, and many smokers develop withdrawal symptoms within hours of trying to stop. Just "cutting down" or switching to a low-tar, low-nicotine cigarette may not reduce the health risks of smoking, since most smokers inhale deeply or smoke the entire cigarette to maintain their nicotine (and carbon monoxide and carcinogen) intake. Smokers also develop a strong psychological dependence on tobacco, making it difficult to quit. Therefore, it is not surprising that many attempts to quit smoking are unsuccessful. However, help is available for smokers who wish to quit. Several organized smoking cessation programs are available in most communities, and many health care professionals can help. Medication can reduce nicotine withdrawal symptoms. Finally, remember that one's chance of quitting permanently increases with repeated attempts. Further information on this topic is contained in the chapter on **Health Hazards of Tobacco**.

Diet

The food we eat is a second important factor related to our risk of developing heart disease and certain types of cancer. Several types of cancer, including breast, colon, and prostate cancer, as well as coronary heart disease, have been linked to diet in studies done in many countries around the world. Diet may turn out to be as important a determinant of cancer risk as smoking, but much more research is needed. Fortunately, a diet that minimizes one's risk of heart disease also lessens one's chance of developing cancer. The principle dietary components correlated with increasing or decreasing risk of heart disease and cancer are saturated fat, cholesterol, fiber, and certain vitamins and minerals. In addition, a few food additives have been linked to certain types of cancer.

Intake of fat, especially saturated fat, is a major determinant of the blood cholesterol level, which is one of the three major reversible risk factors for heart disease (the other two are smoking and high blood pressure). The mechanism whereby fat intake influences the development of cancer is less clear. Saturated fat comes from animal sources and from a few tropical oils, notably palm and coconut. Fat provides about 40 percent of calories in the typical American diet. Reducing that figure to 30 percent is recommended for everyone. Some individuals with high blood cholesterol levels need to reduce their fat intake to 20 percent of their total calories. Cholesterol intake is generally correlated with saturated fat intake, since it is found exclusively in animal origin foods. Most Americans consume too much cholesterol; even though the body needs cholesterol, the liver can make all it needs. For further discussion on cholesterol, refer to the chapter on **Nutrition Awareness**.

Dietary fiber intake is inversely related to fat intake. Dietary fiber appears to decrease one's risk of heart disease and colon cancer through complex mechanisms. Fiber in the diet can replace fats or sugars; fiber helps to lower cholesterol levels, and it decreases the length of time it takes feces to transit through the colon, thus reducing the time that any cancer promoting substances are in contact with the bowel lining. Most Americans eat too little fiber, an important substance for preventing various bowel diseases. Both soluble (oat bran) and insoluble (wheat bran) fiber help bowel activity, but only soluble fiber has a significant effect on cholesterol levels and heart disease.

Several vitamins, especially A and E, and minerals, such as selenium and magnesium, have been shown to protect against cancer and/or heart disease. The exact mechanisms by which these micronutrients exert their beneficial effects are not fully understood. Vitamin A is known to play an important role in cell maturation, and vitamin E is an antioxidant, which may prevent some carcinogenic substances from being formed inside the body. Studies have shown magnesium, an important component of the

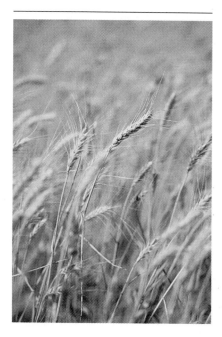

The Framingham Heart Study

A famous twenty-year study of the causative factors in heart disease, The Framingham Study, examined many aspects of heart disease. At a cost of over fifty million dollars, the U.S. Public Health Service revealed that males who were classified as Type A developed chest pains three times as often as their more peaceful Type B counterparts. Another fascinating conclusion was that those who remained calm and serene (Type B personalities) rarely developed high cholesterol levels regardless of what they ate. The study did confirm that a combination of three major risk factors (cigarettes, cholesterol, and high blood pressure) can increase the likelihood of a heart attack.

Risk Factors for Heart Disease

- Age
- Genetic predisposition
- High blood cholesterol
- Gender
- Hypertension
- Diabetes
- Smoking
- Other less important factors
  Obesity
  Physical fitness
  Personality type

heart's muscle cells, to be associated with lower rates of heart disease. While these micronutrients probably have less impact on disease development than do some of the other risk factors discussed, eating a balanced diet with a variety of foods is a worthwhile goal. Not all micronutrients are necessarily good; for example, a toxin which can form in decomposing peanuts can cause liver cancer. Excess salt consumption can increase the likelihood of certain individuals' becoming hypertensive. The old adage "all things in moderation" is a good rule to live by.

Stress

Stress and an individual's method of handling it have been associated with the risk of developing heart disease, cancer, and other illnesses. While stress is an inevitable part of life, excessive amounts of it can contribute to poor health. When one goes through a very stressful period, it is important to work through that stress, rather than ignore it.

The mechanisms by which stress leads to disease may differ for heart disease and cancer. Perceived stress leads to a release of adrenaline, cortisol, and other hormones within the body. These substances, in turn, increase the heart rate, blood pressure, cholesterol level, and platelet stickiness. When stress becomes chronic, these physiologic changes can accelerate atherosclerosis, the process that causes coronary heart disease. Individuals with Type A behavior are known to be at increased risk of heart disease; Type A behavior is defined as having a constant sense of time urgency and feeling a freefloating anger at the world in general. These behavior patterns can be seen as a maladaptive way of dealing with chronic stress.

The immune system may be the stress–cancer connection. Chronic stress causes changes in the immune system which can interfere with its ability to recognize and destroy cancerous cells. Several researchers have shown that cancer patients have a characteristic personality pattern years before their cancers are diagnosed. Part of this personality pattern involves difficulty dealing with stress and turning conflict inward instead of confronting it directly.

Other Risk Factors for Heart Disease

Aside from an inherited predisposition to heart disease, advanced age, and being male, one of the strongest risk factors is high blood pressure, or hypertension. It is important to realize that stress and tension are not direct determinants of blood pressure. Most individuals with uncomplicated hypertension do not feel sick in the early phases of the disease. In the absence of effective treatment, hypertension can lead to heart failure, heart attack, kidney failure, and stroke. In most cases, the cause of hypertension is unknown. It commonly starts in young to middle adulthood, and close relatives of people with hypertension are more likely to develop the disease themselves.

450

An individual's blood pressure varies from minute to minute, depending on activity level and other factors. Therefore, a single elevated blood pressure reading is not always an indication of hypertension. Usually several blood pressure readings over a period of a few weeks are used to diagnose hypertension. Blood pressure is expressed as two numbers: the systolic pressure is the number recorded when the heart has contracted, and the diastolic pressure is the number recorded when the heart is relaxed. Generally, blood pressures below 140/90 (systolic/diastolic) are considered normal, although people in their late teens to early twenties usually have readings below 135/85.

Lack of exercise and obesity are interrelated and also correlate with heart disease. Strictly speaking, obesity means an excessive amount of body fat. People who weigh more than 130 percent of their ideal body weight are at increased risk of heart disease. Recently, two different patterns of obesity have been described. Male pattern obesity, where the excess fat is concentrated in the abdomen ("beer belly"), appears to carry a

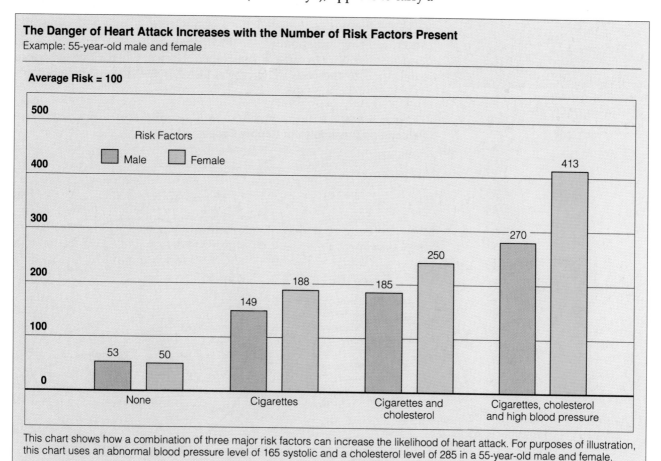

The Danger of Heart Attack Increases with the Number of Risk Factors Present
Example: 55-year-old male and female

Average Risk = 100

This chart shows how a combination of three major risk factors can increase the likelihood of heart attack. For purposes of illustration, this chart uses an abnormal blood pressure level of 165 systolic and a cholesterol level of 285 in a 55-year-old male and female.

Source: *Framingham Heart Study* (Aug. 1987)

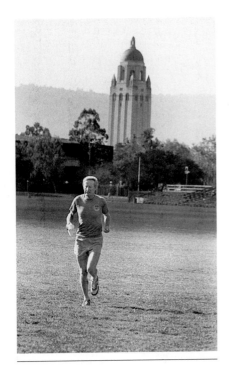

greater risk of heart disease than does the female pattern, where the excess fat is more evenly distributed. (Women can have male pattern obesity, and vice versa.)

Many studies have shown that people who get regular aerobic exercise have lower rates of heart disease than do sedentary people. The real effect of exercise is somewhat controversial because the people who exercise regularly also tend to be nonsmokers, medium-to-lean build, and eat a low-fat diet. Nonetheless, aerobic exercise (rhythmic sustained activities that keep the heart rate elevated) performed for about 30 minutes three times per week probably lessens the risk of heart disease. Part of this effect may result from an increase in HDL cholesterol, which protects against heart disease. Exercise probably has other beneficial effects as well. It may help with stress management, and most people who exercise regularly feel better and think they look better.

Other Risk Factors for Cancer

Various forms of electromagnetic radiation are well-known causes of cancer. Ionizing radiation, whether from natural sources, medical x-rays or nuclear fission, can cause several types of cancer when a sufficient dose is delivered to the body. The critical factor is the dose of radiation re-

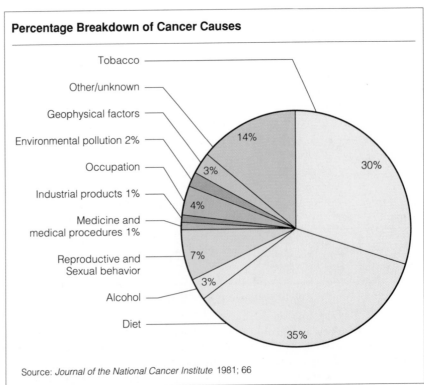

Percentage Breakdown of Cancer Causes

Tobacco — 30%
Other/unknown — 14%
Geophysical factors — 3%
Environmental pollution 2%
Occupation — 4%
Industrial products 1%
Medicine and medical procedures 1%
Reproductive and Sexual behavior — 7%
Alcohol — 3%
Diet — 35%

Source: *Journal of the National Cancer Institute* 1981; 66

ceived. Everyone is constantly exposed to small amounts of natural radiation, an unavoidable fact of life. Even though small amounts of radiation are absorbed from medical and dental x-rays and scans, these diagnostic techniques can be extremely useful. People in certain occupations are also exposed to radiation. In these situations carefully monitoring is required. However, it is generally very hard to show any measurable increase in cancer rates due to low-level exposures. For example, it is estimated that for every one million women who have mammography done to test for early breast cancer, one will develop breast cancer as a result of that radiation exposure. Yet hundreds of these women will benefit by having breast cancer detected early, while it is at a curable stage.

Remember, though, that the critical factor is the dose of radiation absorbed by the body. Repeated exposures to low doses of radiation will, over time, create an increased risk of developing cancer. One such danger can come from radon, an odorless, colorless, radioactive gas that has recently been found in fairly high concentrations in homes and schools all over this country. If this gas has been found in your area or if you are concerned, it is appropriate to have your home tested for radon. Further information on radon is contained in the chapter on **Environmental Health Issues**. Likewise, unnecessary use of medical and dental x-rays can result in excessive radiation exposure. Patients should feel free to question their health care providers about the need for recommended x-ray tests before undergoing them.

Exposure to excessive amounts of ultraviolet radiation from natural and artificial sources causes damage to the eyes and skin, ranging from cosmetic problems, like wrinkling, to cancer. Most skin cancers are quite easily cured if detected early, but one type, melanoma, can be a very dangerous cancer. Melanoma can also occur inside the eye due to excessive UV light exposure. Most skin damage occurs as a result of sunburns, but even simple tanning may cause damage. There is no proof that going to a tanning booth will provide a "base tan" that will protect against skin damage from the sun. Using a sunscreen, wearing sunglasses that filter out UV light, and avoiding excessive sun exposure are the only good methods of minimizing the risk of skin and eye cancer.

Exposure to chemicals that cause cancer (carcinogens) has become a very controversial topic. In some cases, exposure can occur passively due to air or water pollution. In other cases, exposure results from improper use of a substance at home or in the workplace. For example, excessive use of alcohol is linked to cancer of the liver and esophagus, and androgenic steroids have been related to liver cancer. Daughters of women who received diethylstilbestrol (DES)—a medication administered to pregnant women in the 1950s and early 1960s to prevent miscarriage—have an increased risk of cervical and vaginal cancer. Also several powerful medications used to treat cancer have been associated with the development of secondary cancers. Asbestos is another well known health risk due to its association with lung and other cancers. Although at times it seems that "everything causes cancer," you should keep these reports in perspec-

Heart Disease and Cancer Prevention Summary

Following is a summary of ways to minimize the risk of developing coronary heart disease and cancer.

1. Don't smoke!
2. Follow a no-added-salt, low-fat, low-cholesterol diet with adequate amounts of fiber, vitamins, and minerals.
3. Know your blood pressure and cholesterol levels.
4. Exercise three times a week.
5. Keep stress under control.
6. Avoid excessive sun exposure.
7. Follow "safe sex" guidelines. (See the chapter on **Sexual Health**.)
8. Limit alcohol intake to no more than two drinks per day.
9. Avoid unnecessary exposure to x-rays.
10. Take proper precautions around potentially carcinogenic substances at home and at work.
11. Do breast or testicular self-examinations on a regular basis.
12. Follow standard recommendations for health checkups.

Cardiovascular Disease and Cancer

tive. Cigarette smoking still causes more cancer than all other known carcinogens combined.

Certain viruses have recently been implicated as a cause of various cancers in humans. For example, the virus that causes genital warts, human papilloma virus (HPV), is closely linked to cervical cancer in women. The AIDS virus, human immunodeficiency virus (HIV), is associated with Kaposi's sarcoma, a form of cancer that affects AIDS patients, but is otherwise very rare. In other parts of the world, viruses related to HIV appear to cause leukemia. Chronic Hepatitis B virus infection can lead to liver cancer. Avoidance of exposure to these viruses requires the use of "safer sex" practices.

Early Detection of Heart Disease and Cancer

While prevention is the best approach, some of us will develop heart disease and cancer despite our best efforts. Early detection allows the disease to be treated more effectively and with greater likelihood of complete cure. Several research groups and experts have made recommendations regarding methods of screening healthy people for early signs of cancer and, to a lesser extent, heart disease.

Detection of Heart Disease

The most effective approach to early detection of heart disease is early detection of the major risk factors. Blood pressure should be checked on a regular basis starting in the late teenage years. This is available quite commonly now. In fact, blood pressure is measured during visits to most health care providers, and blood pressure screening programs are frequently run in shopping malls and in the workplace. Everyone should know his or her normal blood pressure.

People with high blood pressure can manage it with diet and medication. Dietary control includes achieving and maintaining ideal body weight, following a "no added salt" diet (not using a salt shaker), and limiting the intake of saturated fat. An adequate intake of calcium and potassium may also be beneficial. Regular aerobic exercise has been found to help control high blood pressure. If medication is indicated, several types are available. Diuretics (drugs that eliminate excess fluid in the body) are often the first medication prescribed, although beta blockers (drugs that decrease myocardial oxygen needs) and calcium channel blockers are also used quite commonly as first-line antihypertensives. A combination of two or more drugs can be used if necessary. Your physician can make the best choice based on your age, gender, race, and other medical history.

It is wise to know your blood cholesterol level. Cholesterol can be measured in blood taken from an arm vein or from pricking a finger. The cholesterol level should be below 200 mg per 100 ml of blood, although

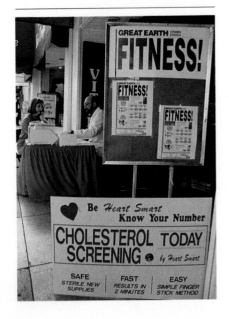

people in their late teens have less risk at a level below 180. If the test is under 200, it should be repeated within five years, since cholesterol levels tend to rise with age. If the result is over 200, the first step is to repeat the test, because cholesterol levels vary somewhat from day to day.

If the second test results are still over 200, a breakdown of the components of total cholesterol should be obtained. Cholesterol in the blood is carried on several different proteins: some proteins carry cholesterol to the walls of arteries, where plaque is formed; other proteins carry cholesterol from plaque back to the liver. The proteins are named according to their density: high-density lipoprotein (HDL) cholesterol is associated with a lower risk of heart disease; low-density lipoprotein (LDL) cholesterol is associated with a higher risk; and very low density lipoprotein (VLDL) cholesterol is weakly associated with a higher risk.

It is not necessary to fast to get an accurate measurement of total cholesterol or HDL cholesterol (the good kind), but fasting for 12 hours is necessary to measure the triglycerides, another fatty substance in the blood. The VLDL cholesterol level is equal to the triglyceride level divided by five. When these three values are known, the LDL cholesterol (the bad kind) can be calculated. With this information and knowledge of any other risk factors, your health care provider can outline a plan to bring your cholesterol level down. The first step is dietary modification. If this is not effective, sometimes medication is prescribed. Although certain over-the-counter dietary supplements (e.g., fish oil and niacin) can help lower cholesterol, it is best to consult with a health care professional first.

While certain tests do allow heart disease to be diagnosed early, none are practical for mass screening. The electrocardiogram (EKG), a recording of the electrical activity of the heart, is not helpful when the patient is resting. The stress test, usually done on a treadmill with electrocardiographic monitoring, can provide evidence of insufficient blood flow to parts of the heart muscle, but the results must be interpreted in light of the patient's symptoms and risk factors. Coronary angiography demonstrates blockages in the arteries of the heart, but the procedure is expensive and has a significant complication rate, so it is only done when medically indicated.

The use of low doses of aspirin to prevent coronary heart disease has been in the news recently. Studies have shown lower rates of second heart attacks in men who have had a previous heart attack and then started taking a small dose of aspirin (less than one tablet per day). Aspirin probably works by decreasing platelet stickiness, which is one factor in the atherosclerosis process. It is too early to say whether individuals with no known heart disease can benefit from this strategy.

One important fact concerning early detection of heart disease is that chest pain is a potentially serious symptom in high-risk individuals. Too many middle-aged and older adults have died within hours after the onset of chest pain that they attributed to indigestion or a pulled muscle. Chest pain in adolescents and young adults is almost never due to heart disease, but in older adults it must be taken seriously.

Cholesterol Levels and Heart Disease

Statistics show that 3 out of 1000 adults with a cholesterol level of 185 develop heart disease; 6 out of 1000 adults with a cholesterol level of 260 develop heart disease.

Just the presence of a high blood cholesterol level will double your chances of developing heart disease.

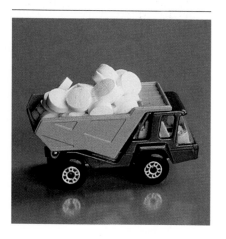

Cancer Detection

■ Women should start screening tests for breast and cervical cancer around age 20. Breast self-examination is easily learned and should be done by all women once a month, right after the menstrual period ends. (For a description of the procedure, see the chapter on **Sexual Health**.) Examination of the breasts by a health care provider should be done about every two years until age 40, and then annually.

■ Mammography (an x-ray of the breasts) should be done every one to two years beginning around age 40. Women with a strong family history of breast cancer may need to have these tests done at an earlier age and more frequently.

■ The Pap test is a very effective method of detecting early precancerous changes in the cervix. Women should start having regular gynecological exams, including the Pap test, when they become sexually active, or when they turn 20, whichever happens first. After two negative exams one year apart, subsequent checkups can be every one to three years, depending on the woman's individual circumstances. During the gynecological (also called GYN or pelvic) exam, signs of uterine and ovarian cancer can also be detected.

■ Although not as well publicized as breast self-examination, testicular self-examination is an equally important technique for men to learn. Testicular cancer is one of the more common malignancies in young men, but it is quite easily detected and is usually curable when found before it spreads.

■ Cancer of the colon and rectum can usually be detected in an early stage with a combination of several screening tests. Starting at age 40, both men and women should have rectal examinations annually. Rectal exams can also detect prostate cancer in men. After age 50 the stool should be tested annually for microscopic amounts of blood (which may be a sign of a tumor in the intestines), and sigmoidoscopy should be done every three to five years to look for tumors in the left colon. Sigmoidoscopy is performed by sliding a tube through the anus into the colon and examining the lining of the colon for abnormalities. It takes about 20 minutes and does not require anesthesia.

Certain other cancers can be detected through routine physical examinations. Unfortunately, no early detection is available for lung cancer. By the time it appears on a chest x-ray, it has usually spread too far to be cured. Likewise, neither pancreatic cancer nor leukemia can be diagnosed early in a way that allows for more effective treatment.

Treatment Options

Several forms of treatment are available for both heart disease and cancer. The physician's decision to use one type of therapy versus another depends on how advanced the cancer or heart disease process is, the patient's age, and general state of health.

The Seven Warning Signs of Cancer

As part of being aware of your body when it is healthy, you need to know what changes may indicate problems. Be aware of the warning signs and symptoms of illness discussed in earlier chapters. Also, if you observe any of the American Cancer Society's seven warning signs, check with your health care practitioner.

■ Change in bowel or bladder habits
■ A sore that does not heal
■ Unusual bleeding or discharge
■ Thickening of lump in breast or elsewhere
■ Indigestion or difficulty in swallowing
■ Obvious change in wart or mole
■ Nagging cough or hoarseness

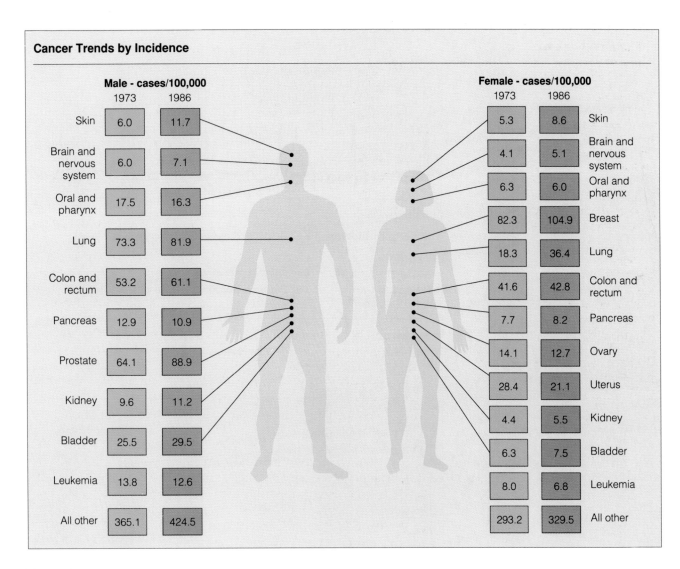

Cancer Trends by Incidence

	Male - cases/100,000				Female - cases/100,000		
	1973	1986			1973	1986	
Skin	6.0	11.7			5.3	8.6	Skin
Brain and nervous system	6.0	7.1			4.1	5.1	Brain and nervous system
Oral and pharynx	17.5	16.3			6.3	6.0	Oral and pharynx
					82.3	104.9	Breast
Lung	73.3	81.9			18.3	36.4	Lung
Colon and rectum	53.2	61.1			41.6	42.8	Colon and rectum
Pancreas	12.9	10.9			7.7	8.2	Pancreas
Prostate	64.1	88.9			14.1	12.7	Ovary
					28.4	21.1	Uterus
Kidney	9.6	11.2			4.4	5.5	Kidney
Bladder	25.5	29.5			6.3	7.5	Bladder
Leukemia	13.8	12.6			8.0	6.8	Leukemia
All other	365.1	424.5			293.2	329.5	All other

Heart Disease Treatment

Heart disease can be treated with medications or surgery or both. Nitrates (e.g., nitroglycerin) are used to relieve angina by dilating both veins and arteries. Betablockers (e.g., propranolol, Inderal) prevent angina by stopping the heart from beating too fast or too forcefully. Digitalis (e.g., digoxin, Lanoxin) is used to help the failing heart beat more forcefully, and can slow down abnormally fast heart rhythms. Diuretics (e.g., furosemide, Lasix) help the kidneys excrete excess salt and water. Antiarrhythmic agents (e.g., lidocaine, procainamide) help to control abnormal heart rhythms. When a heart attack occurs, drugs which dissolve the blood clot formed at the site of blockage can restore blood flow and decrease the extent of heart muscle damage.

Heart disease costs $88.2 billion a year.

Cardiovascular Disease and Cancer

CHAPTER 17

457

EKG Wave Form

Lead I

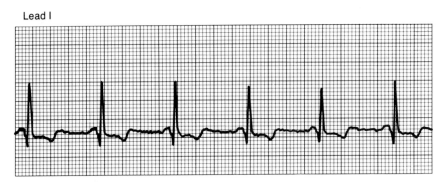

The electrocardiogram (EKG) displays the electrical energy of the heart.

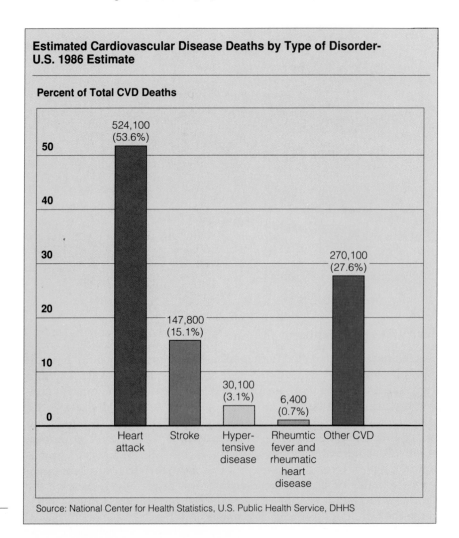

Estimated Cardiovascular Disease Deaths by Type of Disorder- U.S. 1986 Estimate

Percent of Total CVD Deaths

Heart attack	524,100 (53.6%)
Stroke	147,800 (15.1%)
Hyper-tensive disease	30,100 (3.1%)
Rheumtic fever and rheumatic heart disease	6,400 (0.7%)
Other CVD	270,100 (27.6%)

Source: National Center for Health Statistics, U.S. Public Health Service, DHHS

In some cases surgery is the preferred treatment for heart disease. The evaluation for surgery usually involves a diagnostic procedure called cardiac catheterization. Special plastic tubes (catheters) are advanced through veins or arteries into the heart to measure pressures or inject dye for x-ray pictures. Some heart problems can be treated at the same time; for example, a blockage in a coronary artery can be treated by blowing up a tiny balloon inside the artery, compressing the plaque against the wall of the artery. This procedure is called balloon angioplasty. More often the blockage must be bypassed using veins from the patient's legs to replace the damaged ones. Damaged valves can be replaced with either artificial or pig valves. When heart disease has damaged the heart's ability to regulate the heart rate, a pacemaker can be placed under the skin with a wire connecting it to the heart. Heart transplantation is undertaken when the heart is extensively damaged, but the patient should be relatively young and otherwise in good health. The artificial heart is useful only for short-term support of a patient until a transplant is available.

Cancer Treatment

In cases of cancer, surgery is usually the preferred method of treating solid tumors (lung cancer, breast cancer, colon cancer, and so forth). If the tumor can be completely removed and it has not spread even in microscopic amounts to other sites in the body, the patient can be cured of the disease. Other cancers, like leukemia and lymphoma, cannot be treated surgically, but they can often be cured with radiation and/or medication called chemotherapy. Chemotherapy drugs kill cancer cells to a greater extent than they kill normal cells, but they tend to have significant side effects: nausea, vomiting, and depressed blood counts are the most common. Radiation therapy uses very high doses of radiation to kill cancer cells, but it, too, can have side effects similar to those of chemotherapy. Some types of leukemia and other cancers are being treated with bone marrow transplantation. In this procedure, the patient's blood-producing bone marrow and the cancer are wiped out with large doses of radiation and chemotherapy. Bone marrow from a suitable donor (usually a close relative) is then transfused into the patient. If all goes well, the patient regains the ability to make blood cells and the cancer is cured.

Even when a cancer cannot be cured with surgery or other treatments, relief of pain or other symptoms (palliation) can be accomplished with radiation, medication, or limited types of surgery. A great deal of research is underway to find new ways to treat cancer. Immunotherapy—using the immune system to destroy cancer cells—is now being used with encouraging results in a few types of cancer.

The War on Cancer

Are we winning the war on cancer? The answer seems to depend on whom you ask. The National Cancer Institute (NCI) says yes because half of all patients diagnosed with cancer can now be cured (up from one third in the 1960s). If 580,000 people develop cancer in the year 2000, with these projections 290,000 would be cured. The opposing argument says these figures are not good enough. John Bailor, from the Harvard School of Public Health and long time critic of NCI, believes that we must focus our resources on prevention instead of hi-tech treatments and dramatic breakthroughs. Bailor points to the growing numbers of people contracting cancer (171/100,000 in 1985 as opposed to 157/100,000 in 1950) as evidence that we are losing the war.

Source: *Hippocrates*, January/February 1989

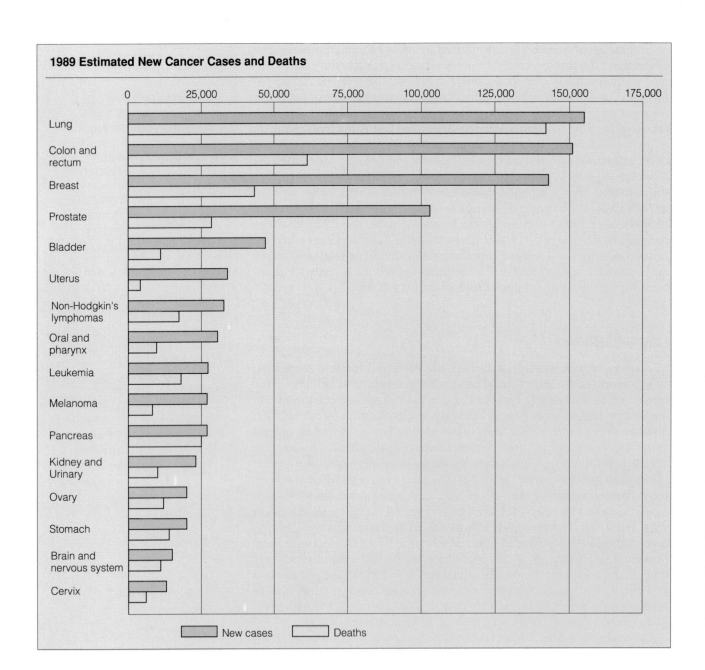

1989 Estimated New Cancer Cases and Deaths

Lung

Colon and rectum

Breast

Prostate

Bladder

Uterus

Non-Hodgkin's lymphomas

Oral and pharynx

Leukemia

Melanoma

Pancreas

Kidney and Urinary

Ovary

Stomach

Brain and nervous system

Cervix

0   25,000   50,000   75,000   100,000   125,000   150,000   175,000

☐ New cases   ☐ Deaths

Cardiovascular Disease and Cancer

Seeking Professional Help

Seek Help If:

- You smoke tobacco
- You are more than 20 percent overweight
- You have a poor diet, eat saturated fats, and have a high cholesterol level
- You use narcotics, hallucinogens, or stimulants without a prescription, such as cocaine, amphetamines, or LSD that can stress your heart muscles

Consult with your physician about the appropriate frequency of screenings that assess heart disease risk factors, such as blood pressure, cholesterol level, blood glucose, and cardiovascular stress tests.

If you experience any of the following potential signs of heart disease, seek help immediately:

- Excessive shortness of breath
- Unexplained sweating, dizziness, or fainting
- Irregular pulse or rapid pulse without known cause
- Heavy, squeezing pain or discomfort in the center of the chest that does not worsen with a deep breath or cough
- Pain radiating across your shoulder and down your arm

The American Cancer Society has identified seven warning signs of cancer. Seek help immediately if you observe any one of the seven listed in the chapter.

Types of Treatment

If your concern relates to lifestyle behaviors, the college health center or your primary care physician can usually give you advice and guidance. As discussed in earlier chapters, other resources such as nutritionists, weight management programs, and stop-smoking clinics can also give you information and support.

A physician who evaluates physical symptoms can order and evaluate appropriate tests. Your physician may then refer you to a cardiologist (heart specialist) or oncologist (cancer specialist).

For further information on preventative actions, warning signs, or treatment options, consult your telephone directory for local listings for the American Heart Association, American Cancer Society, or American Lung Association.

Beyond the Text

1. As a woman, you know you should perform a breast self-exam every month, but you just don't seem to get into the habit. What are your risks?

2. Respond to this statement: No one in my family has ever had heart problems, and I feel fine. So I've got a few years before I need to start paying attention to all this exercise and cholesterol stuff.

3. Your father has cancer and has been given an uncertain prognosis. A friend tells you, "If he just thinks positively, he can beat the cancer." What do you think?

4. Respond to the following statement: As long as you minimize your intake of cholesterol, your chances of heart problems are minimal.

5. Respond to the following statement: All of our fresh fruits and vegetables are contaminated with cancer-causing chemicals, so it's no longer safe to eat them.

Supplemental Readings

Choices: Realistic Alternatives in Cancer Treatment by Marion Morra and Eve Potts. New York: Avon Books, 1987. Answers questions concerning types of cancers, diagnoses and tests, treatments, and side effects—all with an array of available options. Very complete and informative.

How to Fight Cancer and Win by William L. Fischer. Canfield, OH: Fischer Publishing Corp., 1987. Summarizes results of recent research from the National Cancer Institute and other sources with special emphasis on preventative steps, especially dietary planning.

Love, Medicine and Miracles by Bernard Siegel, MD. New York: Harper & Row, 1986. Lessons learned about self-healing from a surgeon's experience with exceptional patient's who took control in order to heal themselves from cancer.

The Cancer Prevention Diet by Michio Kushi. New York: St. Martin's Press, 1983. Summarizes research on the relationship between nutrition and diet and cancer to offer macrobiotics, a cancer prevention plan.

The Healing Heart. Antidotes to Panic and Helplessness by Norman Cousins. New York: W. W. Norton and Co, 1983. The author shares his experiences of recovering from a massive heart attack as well as his strategies for summoning the regenerative processes needed to overcome illness.

You Can't Afford the Luxury of a Negative Thought by Peter McWilliams and John Roger. Los Angeles: Prelude Press, 1989. A book for anyone with a life-threatening illness. An amusing, informative, worthwhile book that can really make a difference in your life.

Key Terms Defined

angina chest pain that results from impaired blood supply to the heart muscle; symptoms of severe, steady pain and pressure in the region of the heart

bronchitis inflammation of the bronchi of the lungs as a result of irritation; often accompanied by a chronic cough

cancer a cellular tumor whose natural progression is fatal; cancer cells are invasive and tend to spread to new sites throughout the body

carcinogenic substance that produces cancerous cells, or enhances their development and growth

cardiovascular system pertaining to the heart and blood vessels

congestive heart failure broad term denoting conditions in which the heart's pumping capability is impaired

coronary arteries vessels that supply oxygenated blood to heart muscle tissue

ECG electrocardiogram (also called EKG) which is a graphic tracing of the electrical strokes of the heart

hypertension condition in which a person has persistently high arterial blood pressure

malignant tending to grow progressively worse and become life threatening; may result in death

melanoma virulent cancer of the melanin (pigment-producing portion of the skin)

metastasize process by which a disease, e.g., cancer, spreads to other tissue from a localized organ not directly connected

myocardial infarction condition characterized by dead tissue areas in the muscle of the heart, caused by interruption of the blood supply

radiation energy, in the form of rays or light, emitted from atoms as they undergo intermittent change

sigmoidoscopy direct examination of the interior of the sigmoid colon

stroke a sudden and severe loss of blood flow in the brain by vascular lesion of blocked vessel, e.g., hemorrhage, thrombosis

Aging through the Life Cycle

You probably do not perceive aging as an immediate personal health problem. However, older Americans now make up a larger proportion of the nation's population than ever before, and this number will continue to grow during the decades ahead. In order to respond to their unique emotional and physical needs, you should understand the process of aging and the health challenges with which older people must cope. Undoubtedly, you will be asked to help care for this rapidly growing population segment.

This chapter discusses our social perceptions of growing old and summarizes the physical, social, and emotional problems associated with aging. Because we all need to begin preparing for our own old age now, suggestions are presented on how to achieve a longer, healthier life.

Contents

Key Terms

Ageism
Aging
Alzheimer's disease
Arthritis
Dementia

Diabetes mellitus
Geriatrics
Gerontology
Glaucoma
Life expectancy

Menopause
Midlife crisis
Osteoporosis
Sandwich generation

America Is Graying

For many people, the mere thought of old age evokes fear, denial, and anxiety. Old age is linked in people's minds with illness, mental deterioration, nursing homes, loneliness—and death.

But despite these emotional responses, we cannot shut old people and old age out of our thoughts. Not only do the elderly live and work among us, but one day we will join them. When we stare at the face of old age, we are not just looking at strangers: we are looking into a prophetic mirror—at ourselves.

At present, America's social fantasies are at odds with its social realities. On the one hand, the youth culture, with its blind adoration of youth and beauty, predominates. On the other hand, America is graying—rapidly. With declining birth rates and rising life expectancies, older Americans now make up a larger proportion of the population than ever before—and they are the fastest growing segment of the population. By the beginning of the next century there will be 32 million Americans over 65 and by the year 2030, persons over the age of 65 will constitute 21 percent of the population.

Our graying America has catalyzed another new social reality—the transformation of the carefree Pepsi generation into the overwhelmed Sandwich generation. "Sandwich generation" is the new term for people and families caught between two generations—their young children and their aged parents—neither of whom can care for themselves.

We urgently need to understand what aging means, to see it clearly for what it is, to sift the truths from the mythologies, and to find ways to care for our aging population.

We also need to begin preparing for our own old age now, no matter how distant old age seems from our present lives. How we accept the challenges of living in an increasingly aged population—as well as how we accept our own aging—will determine whether our future, collectively and individually, is ruled by fear and misunderstanding or by acceptance and grace.

A Definition of Aging

When is a person old? The answer is as variable as the human race. Some people describe themselves as "ninety years young" and still happy to be here, whereas others look and feel years, even decades, older than their chronological ages.

Old age is as much a state of mind as a state of body. The answer to the question "What is old?" resembles the answer to the proverbial question "What is art?" We may not know what art (or old) is, but we know it when we see it (or feel it).

Aging is broadly defined as a progressive decline in an adult's body functions that reduces the capacity to adjust to the environment and

The Aging Population

Population	1950	1985	2020
Ages 65–84 (in millions)	11.7	25.8	44.3
85 and over (in millions)	0.6	2.7	7.1
65 and over as % of total population	7.7%	12%	17.3%
Life Expectancy			
Total (years)	68.2	74.7	78.1
Male	65.5	71.2	74.2
Female	71.0	78.2	82.0
Black	60.7	69.5	75.5
White	69.0	75.3	78.5

Source: *Time*, February 22, 1988

Aging through the Life Cycle

eventually ends in death. Aging is also defined as the decreasing ability to maintain homeostasis, or the state of stability and equilibrium within the body.

Senescence is a process of deterioration resulting in decreased survival capacity; generally senescence occurs after the reproductive period ends. Although the terms aging and senescence have similar definitions, aging has a more general meaning, referring to the progressive decline throughout a person's entire adulthood, while senescence has a narrower application, limited to changes occurring after the reproductive period.

Even though aging follows a broadly predictable course, the rate and extent of aging varies widely among people. Gerontology, or the branch of medical science that studies aging and senescence, still has not been able to pinpoint the cause of aging. Several theories have been offered, and the following theories are the most widely accepted.

The immunologic theory proposes that our immune systems weaken with age, lowering the body's resistance to disease. The somatic mutation and error theories state that coding errors accumulate in our genes over time. The errors supplant the normal genetic coding, and the genes begin to replicate the mutations. As these genetic errors increase, organ and tissue functions break down. The free radical theory suggests that certain substances, such as environmental pollutants and the oxidation of fat, protein, and carbohydrate, produce unstable free radicals in the body. These free radicals damage chromosomes and alter collagen. Vitamins A, C, and E, so-called antioxidants, are believed to inhibit the action of free radicals, thereby retarding aging.

Other theories cite hormonal imbalances, enzyme malfunctioning, and the accumulation of harmful waste products as possible causes. According to the programmed theory of aging, our cells can only reproduce a limited number of times. Once that number has been exceeded, cells die and organs deteriorate. The rate of aging is governed by a genetically programmed internal biological clock.

The "wear and tear" theory maintains that the body simply wears out from use. Actually, the opposite appears to be true: a well-used body is healthier and younger than an unused body. When it comes to the human body and brain, it is a clear case of use it or lose it. Research shows that we are much more likely to rust out than to wear out.

> ## The Many Ways to Say Old
>
> Older population—55+
> The elderly—65+
> The aged—75+
> Extreme aged—85+
> Young old—60 to 74
> Middle old—75 to 84
> Old-old—85+

> ## I represent the youth and hope of England.
> William Gladstone, 83, in a speech to
> the House of Commons

Social Perceptions of Aging

Many cultures of the world today, notably China and Japan, venerate older people and think of them as invaluable—as the living repositories of history and memory within a community or family. In cultures where the majority of the population die young, old people are not just venerated—they are thought to be magical. How else could such people have lived so long, if not by magic or extraordinary powers the other people do not

Aging through the Life Cycle

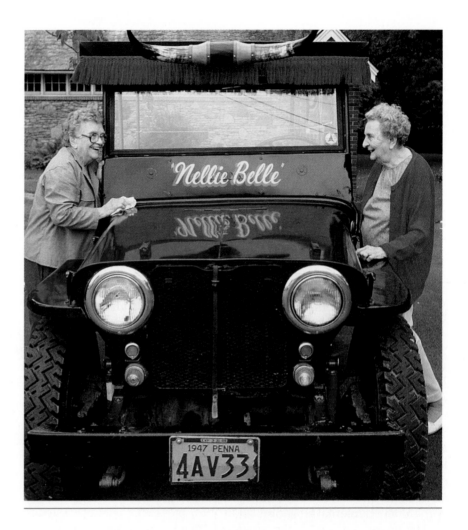

Aging through the Life Cycle

CHAPTER 18

possess? Even in this country, old age did not go out of fashion until the early 1900s—just about the time people started living longer.

Now, popular American culture often presents old age as horrible or tragic. "Ageism" is a recent coinage to describe age-based discrimination particularly against old people, including negative images based on prejudice and stereotypes. America's love affair with youth and youthful beauty contributes to the ageism so pervasive in this society.

Misconceptions about Aging

What is your image of older people? We get our perceptions of aging from stereotypes, romantic notions, misconceptions, hearsay, and truths. Many people assume the elderly are merely living on past memories of beauty or greatness. Miss Havisham, the terrifying fictional creation from Charles Dickens's *Great Expectations*, fulfills this stereotype: sitting in her room for decades in her faded wedding dress waiting for her dead lover, never reconciling herself to the present.

Others hold a more romantic view of old people, believing they are crusty sages like Katherine Hepburn and Henry Fonda in "On Golden Pond." Although these fictional creations may have some real life counterparts, the truth lies between these two extremes—older people, like people in other age groups, do not fit into tidy, preconceived categories.

A great discrepancy exists between younger people's assumptions about aging and the way old people themselves actually perceive aging. Many young people assume the majority of older people are sick and live in nursing homes. Not so. Only 5 percent of people over age 65, and only 6 percent of people age 75 to 84 live in nursing homes in the United States. Although older people do have the greatest number of health problems, most elderly people regard themselves as healthy, and this feeling is confirmed statistically: only 30 percent of older persons assessed their health as fair to poor.

America is finding a new way to grow old: with vitality, creativity, and enthusiasm. Reminiscent of the early days of our country when the pioneering spirit caught on and thousands left the safety of a known world to explore, expand, and grow in a new part of the country. Today, the elderly seem to be taking a new lease on life—they are not satisfied to fade away into nursing homes.

Many young people believe that the elderly must be unhappy because they have lost their youth. Not true, say the elderly. According to Gail Sheehy, author of *Pathfinders*, older people say they like being older better than they liked being younger and that they grow happier with age. At age 80, writer Paul Claudel still found life a celebration—despite the physical limitations: "Eighty years old! No eyes left, no ears, no teeth, no legs, no wind! And when all is said and done, how astonishingly well one does without them."

The elderly attribute their heightened sense of well-being to greater self-knowledge, greater wisdom and judgment, financial security, having the tempests and uncertainties of youth behind them, and not worrying as much about what other people think.

It is not just that the elderly are living longer and healthier lives—they are living them differently. They are retiring to islands, warm climates and Sunbelt states, involving themselves in the community, leisure activities, lessons to master new skills, even part-time jobs. McDonald's has created McMasters, a job-training program for people over 50. After four weeks, these elders can enter the job pool and avoid an idle old age. Younger married women who used to volunteer hundreds of hours are now entering the job market. There remains a strategic hole to fill and millions of elderly are now volunteering their time and expertise in schools, hospitals, prisons, and nonprofit organizations. They are also returning to the work force after trying retirement and finding out it is not for them.

Some Facts on Aging

- Retired people in the United States outnumber the entire population of Canada.
- For every 100 women over 85 there are 44 men.
- Most elderly people regard themselves as healthy.
- The largest gains in longevity are a result of a decrease in infant mortality, vaccinations, sewage treatment, and sufficient food.
- In 1986 the percentage of Americans over age 65 was 12.1 percent.
- By the year 2000, persons over 65 are expected to represent 13 percent of the population.
- Percentage of people over 65 who live in nursing homes: 1 percent of those 65 to 74, 6 percent of those 75 to 84, and 22 percent of those older than age 85.

Source: *A Profile of Older Americans*, AARP

Aging through the Life Cycle

Growing old does not always mean one has to grow up.

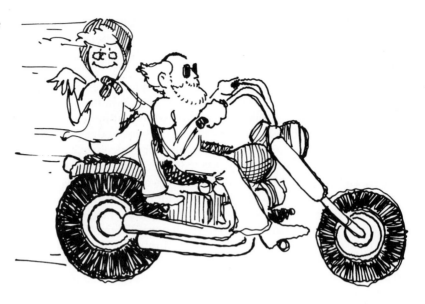

Corporations are beginning to recognize the fantastic potential of hiring back retired employees. For example, Travelers Insurance Company of Hartford hired back retired workers instead of hiring workers from temporary agencies and saved over $1 million a year.

Space-Age Aging

As residents in the space age, we are bombarded with technological breakthroughs that promise to combat and vanquish the ravages of age. There are antiwrinkle face creams, youth pills, revitalizing elixirs, bionics—even cryopreservation. A time may even come when you can walk into a doctor's office and say, "Beam me up, Scotty, and turn your blaster to full volume so you can warp-drive these wrinkles off my face. And while you're at it, set my phaser back a few decades; I feel old today."

Despite so much promising science and technology, the hope for a cure for old age and death is still just that—a hope. Aging and death are as inevitable now as they were when Ponce de Leon dreamed of a magical fountain of youth. Although medical science has eliminated some of humanity's ablest killers, we now face new ones—heart disease, cancer, diabetes, AIDS. It will be a long time—if ever—before we can get beamed up to have our biological clocks rewound a decade or two.

High-Tech Advances for the 21st Century	
Today's 40-Year-Old	**Tomorrow's Middle-Ager**
Eye's lens hardens	Drops will protect vision
Hairs shrink—balding	Hormone-based formulas will reverse balding
Muscles stiffen	High-tech fitness machines will optimize exercise
Skin thins and loses elasticity	Anti-aging compounds will rejuvenate the skin

Aging Means Changing

Legends about superannuated mortals and fountains of youth date back to earliest recorded human history. According to Biblical legend, Adam himself lived into his ripe old 800s. However, compared with the 900-year-old Methuselah, Adam was barely out of diapers when he died. Ancient Greek mythology tells of the Hyperboreans, a race of people whose full and vigorous lives ended abruptly at age 100, when they took it upon themselves to drop blissfully off into the sea.

Ponce de Leon, not Indiana Jones, was the most famous explorer in search of the Fountain of Youth. The Spanish conquistador died in 1591 having discovered Florida and Cuba—but not the magic brew.

Myths about Methuselah aside, people are living longer. When discussing age, we should distinguish the differences among the terms life expectancy, life span, and longevity.

In the United States, life expectancy, or the average number of years a person can reasonably expect to live, is 78 for males and 83 for females. At the turn of the century, it was 47 years, so this reflects a gain of more than a quarter of a century. Since the early 1900s, life expectancy in the United States has risen 30 years.

Life span is the maximum potential for longevity of a species. Longevity is the actual length of time a person or a group of people, such as a family or village, lives. Longevity is primarily influenced by heredity and tends to run in families, but environmental factors also play a role. People whose parents or grandparents lived to see their hundredth birthday are more likely to see their own as well.

Although average life expectancy for humans has increased, human life span remains remarkably stable. Even under the best of conditions, life span does not exceed 115 years of age. Although numerous claims of people living to 115 have arisen, many have proven false or unverifiable.

Age is not such an uncomfortable thing, if one gives oneself up to it with good grace.

Horace Walpole, 63

Aging through the Life Cycle

The oldest verified human was Shigechiyo Izumi of Japan who died June 29, 1984, at 119 years of age.

The Middle Years

People are no longer simply young or old. We now think of life as a progressive passage through different phases; we speak of childhood, adolescence, adulthood, middle age, old age, and old-old age. Each phase of life may last a decade or longer.

When is a person middle-aged? It is hard to pinpoint an exact number, but it is generally accepted that middle age begins in the early to mid-forties and lasts until the early to mid-sixties. Midlife is characterized by an increase in the physical signs of aging and by an increased awareness of death.

This growing awareness of one's own mortality causes people to feel a sense of haste about achieving their dreams and goals. The knowledge that time is limited prompts midlife adults to reassess their life goals. This period of reevaluation can either fill them with a more vigorous sense of purpose (valuing life more, feeling less concerned about outward manifestations of success, being more introspective, and living life more fully from day to day) or it can lead to depression (when they realize that they are running out of time to achieve goals of status, power, financial independence, and success).

This period of psychological readjustment in midlife is referred to as midlife crisis. According to Hollywood movies of the 60's and 70's, the midlife crisis goes something like this: men trade in their conservative grey suits for gold chains, wide plastic belts, and loud shirts with floral patterns, then they leave their wives and children to indulge in sexual sprees with women half their ages. The current-life version of midlife crisis probably involves an aging Casanova reversing the ravages of time by having a face lift, liposuction, tummy tuck, and hair implants. The Hollywood scenario for the midlife woman is much like the scenario for the midlife man—except that Hollywood is squeamish about pairing up a midlife woman with a much younger man.

The Hollywood version does have a small kernel of truth. People in the middle of life do seek change, but the changes they make usually have more to do with reevaluating one's life and planning for future happiness than they do with youthful attire and sexual prowess. Although all middle-aged people feel the need to reassess and redirect their lives, not everyone finds the transition from adulthood to middle age cataclysmic.

Part of the misconception about what happens to midlife adults arises from the term itself—midlife crisis—which evokes images of adjustment problems and negative psychological and emotional states. While this does occur, the term includes the entire process of midlife change, not merely the negative aspects. The definition of midlife crisis is "a normal state in the ongoing life cycle in which the middle-aged person reevalu-

---

How to Stay Healthy Longer

There may be no guaranteed method for staying healthy longer, but gerontologists have some recommendations that make sense.

- Stop smoking
- Drink only in moderation
- Stay out of the sun
- Eat a healthy diet
  Cut down on cholesterol and salt
  Eat more fiber and complex carbohydrates
  Eat more fruits and vegetables
- Do consistent aerobic exercise
- Handle stress before it handles you

---

ates his or her total life situation in relation to youthful achievements and actual accomplishments."

Erik Erikson, a student of Freud and a psychoanalyst and teacher, mapped the human life cycle into eight psychosexual stages of development. According to his theory of personality development, the developmental crisis of midlife adults is generativity versus stagnation.

Generativity is the willingness to contribute to the welfare of future generations or to society as a whole. The mature person chooses generativity over stagnation, becoming involved in establishing and guiding the next generation. A shift toward generativity leads to new interests, greater productivity, more satisfying relationships, and achievement of mature social and civic responsibility.

Stagnation results from an unresolved midlife crisis, in which the person refuses to assume power over and responsibility for the goals of middle age. Stagnation produces feelings of emotional impoverishment and boredom.

Having children of one's own is one way to achieve generativity in midlife, but people also contribute to succeeding generations through their art or their work—enriching the world with their music, painting, writing, and teaching, as well as other professional or volunteer work. In fact,

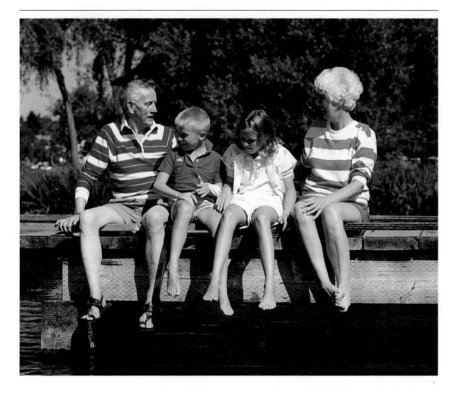

Aging through the Life Cycle

C H A P T E R   18

> Grow old along with me,
> The best is yet to be.
> The last of life, for which the
> first was made.
>
> **Rabbi Ben Ezra**

a study of the world's 400 greatest achievers in art, music, science, literature, and architecture reveals that 66 percent made their greatest contributions after age 60.

Great Expectations

As we age changes occur: internal, external, physical, and psychological. Finances and environment may be altered, and even relationships take on new aspects.

The Aging Face   When the first visible changes begin at approximately age 30, they are often so subtle as to go unnoticed: fine crow's feet appear at the corners of your eyes and faint smile lines form around your mouth. By age 40, grey hairs pop out and the once fine lines in your face deepen. By age 70, your skin has sagged and lost its tone, excessive pigment has caused age spots, fatty deposits have formed bags under your eyes, and your nose and earlobes have dropped as much as one-half inch.

The Aging Body   Internally your body begins to age around age 30, but once again the changes occur so gradually and in such small increments they may go unnoticed. With each passing year, your cardiovascular and respiratory systems slow down. Your aerobic capacity decreases, and your heart pumps less blood volume. Your metabolism slows; minerals leach out from your bones, making them weak and brittle; muscle mass declines and is replaced by fat; overall muscle strength drops; and your reaction time slows. The kidneys become less efficient at regulating sodium, concentrating urine, and filtering; urinary output drops.

Changes in the senses include hearing loss (particularly in the high-frequency range), loss of taste due to fewer taste buds and decreased salivary output, and an impaired sense of smell. The two primary vision problems among the elderly are blindness resulting from glaucoma (increased pressure within the eyeball sufficient to damage the optic nerve), and blurred vision caused by cataracts (clouding of the lens).

Doonesbury

BY GARRY TRUDEAU

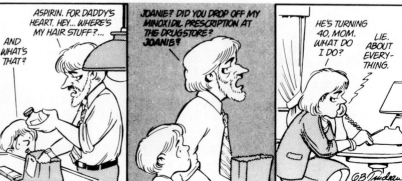

Aging After Thirty

Don't look now, but your physiological destiny is catching up. If you are under 30, you still have a while to go; over 30, you have already started falling apart.

- Your immune system starts to decline at age 30
- Metabolism begins to slow at age 25
- Lungs lose 30 to 50 percent of their capacity between ages 30 to 80
- Kidneys lose up to 50 percent of their efficiency between ages 30 to 80
- Blood vessels lose elasticity, but your heart remains amazingly strong and healthy

- Bone mass peaks at age 30, then begins to drop about 1 percent a year
- Shoulders narrow and your midsection bulges after age 40
- The ability to taste and smell begins to deteriorate at age 40
- Hair growth decreases and if you are male, an increase in testosterone is short-circuiting hair growth on the top of your head
- Impotence increases after age 50. Sexual events go from 1.91/week at age 30 to 0.90 at age 50. Erotic thoughts no longer result in arousal
- Vision begins to change after age 40 and continues downhill
- Hearing fades, especially in the high frequency ranges

- Vocal cords stiffen and you may speak in higher ranges
- Skin loses its elasticity and becomes dry after age 40
- Muscle mass is yielding to fat, as muscle cells do not repair as fast or as well
- Regulation of body temperature becomes less efficient with age
- By age 25 you will have begun to shrink; by age 45 you will have lost one-quarter inch
- The need for sleep decreases and the quality changes with age
- Reflexes slow because the brain takes more time to process information
- The brain loses about 20 percent of its weight, but essential abilities remain (thank God) unimpaired

Additionally, your spinal discs deteriorate, making you shorter than you used to be. If they had only four words to describe how being old feels different from being young, most older adults would say they felt stiffer, colder, slower, and drier.

The Aging Brain   As people age, the brain shrinks and the skull thickens and expands. However, research has shown that despite the reduction in brain size, intellectual capacity does not necessarily decline in old age. Reaction time, speed, and short-term memory all decline, but vocabulary, comprehension, and the ability to retain information remain stable—and, as if to balance the score—what the elderly lose in speed they may make up for in wisdom.

When an older person puts the cat dish in the refrigerator, he or she all too quickly assumes dementia is setting in, whereas a younger person would shrug the incident off as normal. Although some loss of memory is inevitable, simple forgetfulness or temporary lapse of memory does not justify an automatic diagnosis of dementia.

Perhaps all the older person needs to stimulate his or her memory is an effective strategy for reinforcing the information—such as writing down conversations, double-checking information, or leaving eye-catching reminders around the house. If the memory problem is persistent or frightening, or is accompanied by other symptoms, such as disorientation or a change in personality, seek medical attention.

The rule for preserving your intellectual ability is the same as that for preserving your physical ability: work it. The single biggest cause of intellectual decline in older people is the lack of intellectual stimulation and challenge. Stimulation and knowledge do not care how old you are—only you do.

The Aging Woman

Menopause   For women, aging eventually brings menopause, the cessation of menstrual periods, marking the end of a woman's fertility. Menopause occurs from ages 45 to 55, with an average age of 52. Menopause may be preceded or accompanied by hot flashes, weight gain, headaches, depression, insomnia, weakness, dizziness, and mood swings. Women's responses to menopause vary widely. Some women have a hard time during menopause while others find the transition easy and enjoy life more after their periods have ended. Many physicians are now advocating estrogen replacement therapy (ERT) as a way to cope with the symptoms of menopause and prevent osteoporosis.

Osteoporosis   Prior to menopause, estrogen prevents calcium from leaching out from the bones. As estrogen levels drop, the bones lose calcium and become brittle and fragile. This decreased bone density, called osteoporosis, puts women at risk for bone fractures. About 24 million Americans, the majority of them women, develop this disease. One fourth of all white women in the United States eventually develop osteoporosis, resulting in over one million bone fractures each year. Brittle bones fracture easily, even during routine activities like bed making. Fractures, particularly hip fractures, are extremely serious in the elderly, and can lead to crippling or death from infection or pneumonia.

Estrogen replacement therapy is one way to prevent osteoporosis, although this is not a solution for every woman. The best approach is to begin preventing osteoporosis well before it begins—decades before menopause—by increasing bone density. Regular exercise, particularly weight-bearing exercises such as running, walking, aerobics, and dancing, strengthen bones.

Also, a well-balanced diet high in calcium helps increase bone density. A high calcium intake in the teen to twenty-five years is the biggest factor in building bone density, and, once you have it, you will maintain the strong bones for years. Now is the best time to include calcium-rich foods in your diet and make exercise a habit—so you can store up bone density for later. Foods rich in calcium are skim milk, yogurt, broccoli, salmon with the bones, and low fat cheeses. Studies show that women who are athletes and regular exercisers have greater bone density than nonexercisers, thereby lowering their susceptibility to osteoporosis after menopause.

Sexuality   Older women also experience vaginal itching and a reduction in vaginal secretions. Vaginal dryness may make intercourse uncomfortable, although a woman can easily remedy this problem by using vaginal jellies or lubricating creams. Post-menopausal women do have some good news; one recent survey showed that a decrease in hormonal levels in women after menopause had no effect on their sexual desire. Most married women in their 60s, the study reported, had sex an average of five times a month, and that they enjoyed it just as much as they did when they were younger.

Is Old Age a Woman's Burden?   The average American woman lives eight years longer than her male counterpart. At every age, death rates for females are lower. Women need to bear in mind that the social security system only pays high benefits to women who have worked in the labor force. Surviving spouses will receive some benefits, but at a lower rate than if they worked themselves. Without some kind of financial preparation or pension plan, a woman could find herself in tragically reduced financial circumstances in her old age.

The Aging Man

No single event in men's lives marks the passage of time for them as distinctly as menopause does in women's lives. For want of a better term, the midlife changes men experience due to aging are frequently referred to as male menopause. The most common aging problems among men are impotence, prostate problems, and balding.

Impotence   As men age, their testosterone level drops, making it more difficult for them to get and maintain an erection. Men require more stimulation to get aroused. They also produce fewer sperm, and the muscles in the penis do not contract as frequently or as vigorously. These normal changes of aging can trigger concerns about impotence, often unnecessarily.

Despite these changes, some men remain fertile until their 80s. As far as sex itself is concerned, most men find their interest and desire in sex remains fairly constant from middle age on. Oliver Wendell Holmes's interest did not wane, even at age 92. "What I wouldn't give to be seventy again!" he exclaimed after seeing a pretty girl walk by.

Changes in the Prostate Gland   As men age, the previously unobtrusive prostate gland begins to make its presence uncomfortably known. Rare is the man who does not experience some problem with his prostate gland. The most frequent conditions, in order of most likely to most unlikely, are prostatitis, or inflammation of the prostate gland, benign prostatic enlargement, and cancer of the prostate.

Balding   The Biblical story that tells of Samson losing his strength after he cut his hair rings true for the balding man. Balding reminds men they are aging—and that they can do little about it. Although there are different patterns of baldness, it usually begins with a receding hairline at the

> These docs, they always ask you how you live so long. I tell 'em if I'd known I was gonna live this long I would have taken better care of myself.
>
> Eubie Blake

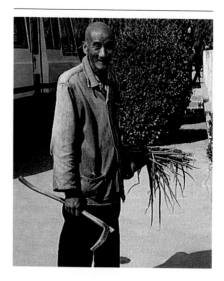

475

temples, then progresses over the top of the head. A new drug called minoxidil may retard balding in some men, but so far no lotion, pill, food, or injection can prevent balding or restore hair loss.

Health Problems of Aging

Most older people have at least one chronic health problem, and many have multiple problems. The most frequently occurring conditions for the elderly are arthritis, hypertension, heart disease, diabetes, visual impairments, stroke, dementia, hearing impairments, orthopedic impairments, and cataracts.

Arthritis Chronically swollen, tender, or painful joints accompanied by decreased mobility, signal arthritis (inflammation of the joints). From age 40, joints and cartilage degenerate and lose elasticity. Arthritis ranks first among chronic conditions in noninstitutionalized people over age 65; however, crippling disability is rare and treatment is available. The cause of arthritis is unknown. In fact, less than half of those 65 and over suffer symptoms of the degenerative, arthritic changes.

Hypertension Hypertension, or consistently elevated blood pressure, is a silent but deadly health problem affecting one in five Americans. It is the second (after arthritis) most common complaint of the 65 and older age group. Untreated hypertension increases the risk of heart disease, kidney failure, and stroke. The incidence of hypertension rises as people age, although neither symptoms nor warning signs may appear. Obesity, salt intake, and heredity all contribute to hypertension.

Heart Disease Heart disease is the number one killer of Americans. There are different types of heart disease: congestive heart failure, coronary artery disease due to atherosclerosis (hardening of the arteries due to accumulation of plaque, a combination of cholesterol and calcium), and mitral valve prolapse. Of the several types of heart disease, heart attacks are the most feared. Treatment for heart disease ranges from drugs and surgery to programs that stress changes in lifestyle habits, such as diet modification, exercise, and quitting smoking. Check the chapter on heart disease for more information.

Diabetes Although deaths from diabetes trail deaths from heart disease and cancer, diabetes is a potent killer of Americans. Diabetes is one word used to describe two diseases: Type I, insulin-dependent diabetes and Type II, noninsulin-dependent diabetes. Type II accounts for 90 percent of diabetes in adults. This disease is caused by an excessively high level of blood sugar that results from the body's inability to utilize glucose effectively.

The top four chronic medical conditions found in the 65-and-over age group are arthritis, high blood pressure, hearing impairment, and heart disease.

Uncontrolled blood sugar causes severe dehydration, hypoglycemia, or coma. Diabetes is a major cause of blindness in adults, and contributes to kidney, circulatory, and cardiovascular problems.

Type II diabetes occurs more frequently among overweight people, and obesity and lack of exercise are blamed for the rising incidence of diabetes in the United States. Treatment for diabetes begins with diet modification, weight management, and exercise, all of which reduce blood sugar. If these modalities are not effective, oral medication or insulin injections are given.

Visual Impairments Glaucoma, cataracts, diabetic retinopathy, and age-related macular degeneration are the principal causes of vision loss in the elderly.

Glaucoma occurs when internal fluid pressure in the eye increases to the point of damaging the optic nerve. Glaucoma need not lead to blindness; it can be prevented with medication or surgery. Early screening and treatment are recommended to prevent loss of vision and complications.

Over 90 percent of Americans over age 65 have some form of cataracts. A cataract is a gradual clouding of the lens of the eye until not enough light passes through to the retina, resulting in blurred vision and extreme sensitivity to bright light and glare. Surgery is an effective treatment for cataracts. Today this surgery is usually done with a laser or by freezing the lens and removing it. The surgery is performed on an outpatient basis.

Diabetic retinopathy is a progressive impairment of circulation in the eyes so that the blood vessels and eye fluid in the retina are affected. It is now the leading cause of new blindness in the United States among adults ages 41 to 60. Since this disorder is a chronic complication of diabetes, it is important that the disease be monitored and controlled.

Stroke Stroke is among the top killers of Americans. The medical term for stroke is cerebral vascular accident, or CVA. The accident, or event, is a temporary interruption or reduction of blood supply to the brain. Strokes result in tragic, often irreversible brain damage. Strokes are associated with hypertension: maintaining normal to low blood pressure is considered the most important factor in preventing strokes.

Dementia Perhaps the greatest fear people have about old age is not that they will lose their physical stamina, but that they will lose their minds. Although only 15 percent of those over 65 suffer from senility, everyone fears this serious mental impairment. Senility, or more precisely, dementia, is the progressive decline of intellectual abilities. Symptoms of dementia include loss of memory, disorientation, inability to concentrate, and a change of personality.

The most common form of irreversible organic brain syndrome is Alzheimer's disease, accounting for 50 percent of known cases of dementia.

> When one has reached eighty-one, one likes to sit back and let the world turn by itself, without trying to push it.
>
> Sean O'Casey

Health Care Costs Escalate for Elderly

$50 billion was spent on health care for the elderly in 1980. This is expected to reach $200 billion by the year 2000. Unless there is a major change, pension and health care costs will account for more than 60 percent of the entire federal budget by 2040. If the entire system is not revamped, the trust fund that supports the hospital insurance part of Medicare could be bankrupt by the year 2002.

Source: *Time*, February 22, 1988

This is a severe and progressive dementia leading to death within five to ten years. Small strokes are the second leading cause. Dementia caused by depression, physical disease, or drugs is partially or completely reversible. Dementia caused by Alzheimer's disease or stroke is not.

Emotional and Social Problems of Aging

Loneliness and Isolation   Older people suffer more losses than younger people. Their loved ones and friends die, and they cannot easily find new friends their own age. Also, because men die earlier than women, more older women than men are on their own. Half of all older women in 1986 were widows, five times more than the number of widowers.

Older people can take steps to lessen loneliness and isolation. Group retirement homes, day programs, religious groups, and common interest organizations all provide opportunities for older people to socialize and interact while retaining their independence.

Depression   Depression is the most commonly ignored disorder in the elderly population. About 15 percent suffer from this problem, double the percentage in the general population. Serious depression is characterized by loss of interest in life, a sense of hopelessness, difficulty sleeping, reduced sexual desire, weight loss, and fatigue. This condition can kill. All too frequently suicide is a misguided attempt at finding a self-cure for depression.

People over age 65 account for 20 percent of suicides in this country, the highest suicide rate of any age group. Mounting losses of loved ones, friends, work, poor health, or drugs can all trigger depression in the elderly. On the other hand, most older people weather life's sorrows and losses without experiencing serious depression. Trained professionals can successfully treat even serious depression with both therapy and medication.

Drug Abuse   Most people do not link drug abuse with the elderly, but it does occur. Although the elderly do not have drug abuse problems with illegal drugs, they do have problems with legal drugs—their own prescriptions and over-the-counter medications. Almost 80 percent of people 65 and over have at least one chronic medical problem that requires medication—one third have three or more.

Most people in this age group use more than five medications. Tranquilizers account for the greatest amount of drug abuse among the elderly; sleeping pills, pain medications, and laxatives make up most of the remainder of the problem.

Some older people juggle schedules of eight or more drugs per day—all prescription. Complicated schedules, coupled with symptoms that come and go, lead people to dismiss their doctor's orders and to fashion their own treatment plans, omitting medications they feel are unnecessary and doubling up on others. Older people need to be carefully educated about the medications they are taking; this includes their purpose, effect on the body, side effects and dangers, and schedule for taking the drugs.

Financial Problems   Retirement may increase leisure time, but it also reduces income. The poverty rate for persons age 65 and over is 12.4 percent, and women, blacks, Hispanics, and those who live alone are the poorest of the poor. Even though the major source of income for older people is social security (35 percent), not all seniors are poor. A recent addition to our slang vocabulary ("woopies"—well-off older people) indicates that this group is a financial force in our country.

Couples 65 and over have a median income of $22,000 (as of 1986) which goes a long way when children are on their own and the mortgage is paid. But, for many older people, social security payments simply do not provide enough income to meet expenses. Fortunate, indeed, is the older person of means, who either has saved enough to provide for a comfortable retirement or whose employer has set up a generous pension plan. But people of means are not the rule, or even the majority, and many older people may find themselves financially pinched. Additionally, rising health care costs, coupled with older people's greater use of the health care system, means many elderly people are just one health crisis away from financial catastrophe.

Nursing Homes   Only 5 percent of persons over 65 live in nursing homes. Nevertheless, as people's age rises, so does their chance of living in a nursing home: 22 percent of persons over age 85 live in nursing homes.

The Sandwich generation, those who are caring for both their children and their aged parents, may have to decide whether or not to place a parent in a nursing home. Although placing an aged parent in a nursing home can be one of the most agonizing decisions a child ever has to make, uniformly dismissing nursing homes as an option for care is unrealistic. A nursing home may not be a family's first choice, but it may be the right choice—and it does not have to be permanent.

If a nursing home is the right choice, sound information and thorough planning are the best ways to approach making the decision. Learn as much as you can about nursing homes in your area. National organizations like the American Association of Homes for the Aged and local organizations offer information on nursing homes, including how to select, residents' rights, and medical treatment.

Aging Wisely

So you want to live to be 100 and you want to be vigorous and healthy the entire time. These may not be impossible dreams. Although your genes play a significant role in determining how long you will live and the dis-

---

Demand for Nursing Homes

Between now and the year 2000, there will have to be a new 220-bed nursing home opened every day to keep up with the demand for these facilities as more of our population reaches 65 and over.

Who Will Pay?

The elderly consume almost one-third of America's medical resources and Medicare cannot begin to cover the costs of a long illness—who should pay?

Experts predict a 160 percent increase in physicians' visits by the elderly, a 200 percent rise in days of hospital care, and a 280 percent growth in number of nursing home residents by the year 2040—who will pay?

Aging through the Life Cycle

eases to which you are susceptible, factors other than inheritance also influence longevity. As one quip says, the human body, when properly cared for, will last a lifetime.

Active people who work hard and create new challenges for themselves live the longest. Vilcambamba, a small village in the Ecuadorian Andes, contains the longest-lived residents in the world. These villagers typically live into their hundreds—and many have reached 112 or 113 years old. Dr. David Davies, a gerontologist, studied the villagers to determine what accounted for their longevity. Men and women alike attributed their long lives to work—even in their nineties and beyond, they never stopped working or being active contributors to their community.

According to Dr. Davies, the key to long life is remaining physically and intellectually engaged in life, no matter how old you are: "It seems that those people who have the best chance of a healthy and active old age are those who use their minds and bodies much, even toward the end of their life span. . . . The people who seem to live the shortest lives are those who try in many ways to conserve their energy and their powers, using their brains and little else, and living a very sedentary life."

Long Life and Good Health

The dream of living for a century becomes a nightmare if it means a century of infirmity, pain, and lost vitality. Ask people if they would like to live to be 100 and they invariably say yes. Ask them if they would like to live to be 100 if they were chronically ill and they invariably say no.

In order to become better engineers of our own aging process, we need to learn to accept the things we cannot control and strive to change the things we can. We may not be able to alter our genetic makeup, but we can alter our habits and the way we live. Healthy habits not only improve the quality of our lives as we age, they actually slow down the aging process itself.

Researchers have determined that the following factors promote long life. (Warning: Some of these recommendations may sound just like those your parents have told you.)

- *Exercise.* The evidence is in—people who exercise live longer than people who do not. Many of the effects of aging are attributed to loss of vital organ reserves. Exercise has an anti-aging effect on the respiratory and cardiovascular systems; it also tones muscles, strengthens bones, reduces body fat, and increases people's vitality and sense of well-being. An elderly person can increase their physical function by 50 percent through exercise alone (a young person can only increase it 10 percent).
- *Eat a well-balanced, low-fat diet and maintain normal weight.* Research suggests that long-term calorie restriction may slow down aging and extend life. Some intriguing experiments on rats at Cornell University found that calorically (but not nutritionally) deprived rats looked younger and lived longer than their well-fed counterparts.

However, scientists have not done comparable studies on humans, and no evidence exists that severe calorie restriction is healthy in humans. In fact, as Dr. Davies points out in *The Centenarians of the Andes*, studies of undernourished human populations generally show the opposite effect: people on nutritionally inadequate or chronically low calorie diets age more rapidly than their well-fed counterparts.

Obesity, which increases in likelihood as people age, clearly contributes to health risks: higher incidences of heart disease, cancer, diabetes, and death. The best advice is to eat a low fat diet and to maintain normal body weight.

- *Do not smoke.* Smokers die earlier than nonsmokers and have a greater incidence of cancer, heart attack, and chronic lung disease. Smoking also causes premature aging of the lungs and—for those who are concerned about their appearance—the skin.

- *Wear seat belts.* Seat belts save lives. Accidents rank fourth among causes of death in the United States, and most accidental deaths result from automobile accidents. Many of those deaths could have been prevented with seat belts.

- *Use alcohol moderately.* The evidence on alcohol intake is contradictory at best. Shigechiyo Izumi of Japan, the world's oldest authentic centenarian, claimed he drank a half-pint of firewater distilled from brown sugar every night before his 8 p.m. bedtime.

However, Mr. Izumi's anecdotal information may not be the best basis for your own drinking behavior. Instead, concentrate on the facts: immoderate use of alcohol is a known health risk that leads to liver damage, nervous system damage, gastrointestinal problems, and traffic deaths. Alcohol contributes to one-half the traffic deaths in the United States. Current information suggests that alcohol, like most things, is safest if consumed in moderation.

- *Attend to your health problems.* Health problems such as high blood pressure and atherosclerosis are human time bombs if left untreated. As a precaution against cancer, which often has no symptoms in the early stages, women should have a Pap smear every year or as often as their gynecologists recommend. People should have yearly physical examinations as well as immediate examination of any unusual symptoms that appear. From the middle years onward, it is particularly important to be aware of the warning signs of cancer and heart disease, which often occur during this period of life. Since both heart disease and cancer, the major killers in our society, can be treated and even reversed, it is crucial to seek treatment early.

- *Learn to manage stress.* Stress—we can't live with it and we can't live without it. Stress is associated with increased incidence of heart disease, high blood pressure, cancer, and other diseases. You can use many techniques to reduce stress—yoga, a walk on the beach, exercise, listening to music, talking to friends—the important thing is to manage stress before it starts to manage you.

- *Find out what you love to do and keep doing it.* Billboards throughout the country should have a new warning label that reads: Warning: Retire-

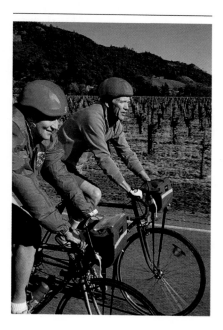

481

Influence of the Older Generation

Madison Avenue is beginning to note that the prosperity of America's retirees means big business. Americans over 50 earn more than half the discretionary income in this country. This group is also becoming a political force—one that future politicians will want to take into account. The American Association of Retired Persons (AARP) has 28 million members and is larger than most countries. This is a powerful group capable of influencing social issues, legislation, and even elections. The Gray Panthers are already on the move; 80,000 strong, they pressure Congress on issues such as health insurance, housing costs, and social security.

ment and inactivity may be hazardous to your health. Studies show that people who enjoy their work and their lives tend to live longer.

■ *Make friends for life.* Studies show that isolated people have more health problems and die earlier than people who are attached to others. Now is the time—when you are in the younger age group—to take the time, energy and determination to make friends for a lifetime.

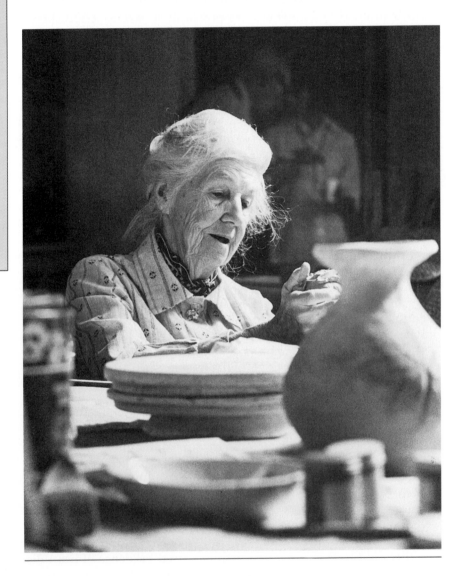

Aging through the Life Cycle

Planning for Your Future

Health is both individual and social. Healthy habits may lengthen your life, but how will you live when you are old? How will you support yourself? How do you want to be treated? How much obligation does the government have toward you as an individual? How are we all socially obligated to one another regardless of our age differences?

Everyone hopes for a long, peaceful, healthy life. Cultivating healthy habits helps you achieve that goal, but social and financial factors also influence your well-being.

With the collective aging of the baby boom population and life expectancies rising for the population as a whole, more people will need financial, social, and medical help in the near future. Their greater numbers will place a tremendous stress on the social security and health care systems. More of us may have to rely on ourselves and our own resources for support in our old age. But how much can we do alone? How much should we have to do alone?

Millions of elderly Americans travel, enjoy life, and lead satisfying lives—and you could be one of them. But millions of others have insufficient funds to meet the costs of their basic living and health expenses—and you could be one of them, too. Much depends on you as an individual; but equally as much depends on us as a society.

Meeting the needs of the elderly will require both private and public action. The time to consider these issues is now, while you are young. Public policies being made now will affect your future. We need to safeguard not just our personal health—but the health of our whole society. Educating yourself about issues affecting the elderly will give you a clearer picture of the future, which—one day soon—will be yours.

Seeking Professional Help

Health problems that strike seniors most frequently may also occur to adults at any age. Seek help in any of the following circumstances, but particularly if you are a senior:

- Persistent headaches or blurred vision
- Blood in the urine or feces
- Difficulty sleeping that you cannot resolve by using home methods
- Increased loss of balance resulting in falls
- Increased joint swelling, stiffness, or discomfort
- Increased memory problems
- Unexplained pain any place in the body
- Taking more than one prescription or OTC medication without your physician being aware of the multiple medications

Sometimes individuals who are experiencing memory problems and behavior shifts do not acknowledge the problem or take the initiative to seek help. If so, the spouse or other close family member should contact the physician.

Finally, if you or a family member is considering in-home or nursing home care for a senior, consult with outside resources before making decisions.

Beyond the Text

1. Your father has a hearing problem, but refuses to wear a hearing aid. What would you say (loudly) to him?

2. Your grandmother, recently diagnosed as having Alzheimer's disease, may move in with your parents. Is this a good solution? What can make this change as successful as possible for all concerned?

3. You know several single older people living in your neighborhood. They seem lonely, isolated, and depressed. What are some solutions to this problem?

4. Your grandparents cannot take care of their house, cook, or care for themselves. They resist moving to a nursing home. What would you suggest to help them?

5. Respond to the statement: Older people naturally get wrinkles. Face lifts are cheating and narcissistic. Just accept that you won't look as good anymore.

Supplemental Readings

Aging and Mental Health by Robert Butler and Myrna Lewis. St. Louis: Mosby, 1983. Focuses on the high rate of suicide among elderly white men in their 80s, perhaps because of depression over loss of status and good health. Points out the importance of treating depression as a preventative measure against risk of suicide for the elderly.

Healthy Aging: New Directions in Health, Biology, and Medicine by Joseph Bonner, PhD, and William Harris. Claremont, CA: Hunter House, 1988. Reports on recent advances in studies on the biology of aging. Discusses hormones, drugs, diet, and exercise in relation to the aging process.

How to Survive Your Aging Parents by Bernard H. Shulman, MD. Chicago: Surrey Books, 1988. Provides helpful insights into the aging process and the attending problems that affect relationships between elderly people and their middle-aged "kids" who love them and are responsible for their care.

Life Extension by Durk Pearson and Sandy Shaw. New York: Warner Books, 1982. An extraordinary and compelling approach to aging by two researchers who have spent years involved in aging studies. You may add "years to your life and life to your years."

The 35-Plus Good Health Guide for Women by Jean Perry Sprodnik, RD, and David P. Cogan, MD. New York: Harper & Row, 1987. Written by a general internist and a clinical dietitian, this comprehensive guide deals with preventing as well as treating the effects of aging.

Vital Involvement in Old Age: The Experience of Old Age in Our Time by Eric Ericson, et al. New York: W. W. Norton and Co., 1988. A refreshing look at the needs of the elderly in our society, taken from a long term study of octogenarians in Berkeley, California.

When Your Parents Grow Old by Florence D. Shelley. New York: Harper & Row, 1988. A practical, informative resource covering medical facilities, diseases of the elderly, money matters, agencies, and other topics.

Key Terms Defined

ageism prejudice against people because of their age

aging process of maturing and becoming older, usually causes decreasing ability of the body and mind to function optimally

Alzheimer's disease irreversible organic brain syndrome, a severe and progressive dementia

arthritis inflammation of the joints

dementia organic mental disorder characterized by general loss of intellectual abilities and personality changes

diabetes mellitus group of disorders in which an insulin imbalance causes failure of the body tissue to break down carbohydrates at a normal rate resulting in glucose intolerance

geriatrics branch of medicine dealing with the problems of aging and diseases of the elderly

gerontology scientific study of the problems of aging in all its aspects

glaucoma group of diseases of the eye characterized by increased pressure resulting in pathological changes, defects, and even total loss of vision

life expectancy average number of years a person is expected to live

menopause cessation of menstruation in the female, usually between ages 40 to 50; caused by physiologic factors when ovulation no longer occurs

midlife crisis period of emotional upheaval noted among middle-aged persons as they struggle with their past and reconcile themselves to the future, including death

osteoporosis condition common in older people in which loss of bone density results in easily broken, brittle bones

sandwich generation new term used to describe people who must simultaneously care for their young children as well as their aging parents

Death, Dying and Grief

Death and the dying process are difficult subjects to study and discuss. Most of us prefer not to think about death, especially our own. However, the sudden death of a relative or friend is a jolting experience that focuses our attention on the meaning of life, if only for a short time. Sometimes death is the expected conclusion of a long illness, and we can be somewhat prepared to accept the pending departure of a loved one.

This chapter discusses death, the stages of dying, and the individual's reaction to these processes (grief). The hospice movement is described and suggestions are provided to help the reader provide support for a dying person. The stages of grief are defined and guidelines for coping with loss are provided.

Contents

Key Terms

Analgesic
Brain death
Clinical death
Cremation
Death
Denial

Embalming
Ethics
Euthanasia
Grief
Hospice

Mourning
Near-death experience (NDE)
Reincarnation
Spiritual
Wake

Death and Dying

Death is the end of life. Every living thing, from plant to human being, eventually dies. When we are young, our own death seems far away, and probably it will be. But the death of a loved one may be closer—a beloved pet with whom we grew up, a friend, a grandparent, or even a parent. Ultimately, no one escapes having to face and cope with death.

What is this event we call death? Dr. Elisabeth Kübler-Ross suggests that perhaps it is only a transition from one form to another. If consciousness, like energy, can neither be created nor destroyed, then what is death?

This chapter discusses death, the stages of dying, and the individual's reaction to these processes (grief). Each of these topics revolves around the concept of loss, for when we lose a loved one or learn of our own impending death, we feel loss. Death is perhaps our most devastating experience of loss. We cope with loss through the grieving process.

Death and the dying process are more than difficult subjects—most of us find them very frightening. In the last few years, this subject has received increased attention, primarily due to the work of Dr. Kübler-Ross and her colleagues.

Twenty-five years ago, when a man's heart stopped beating and he stopped breathing, he was considered dead. Usually, under these circumstances, he stayed dead. However, the story goes that the original purpose of wakes was not only to speed departed ones on their way but also to keep watch in case they awakened before burial.

The United States has criteria that establish death, although no consistent state-by-state consensus exists. As our medical technology becomes more sophisticated, our ability to determine death becomes more complex, and we can no longer depend on the old definition. Since our current technology can often keep a person technically alive indefinitely, physicians, lawyers, and many religious leaders prefer a new definition of death called "brain death." A person is considered dead if an electroencephalograph detects no brain activity for at least 24 hours. This indicates a total lack of central nervous system function, including all reflex activity, and lack of responsiveness to the environment. Other definitions include clinical death (lack of heartbeat and breathing), and cellular death (tissues and organs stop functioning and rigor mortis occurs).

The brain death definition, though the most commonly preferred method of judging death, raises important questions. For example, when does brain death reach the point where it cannot be reversed? How long can a person remain in a coma?

Stages of Dying

Dr. Kübler-Ross, author of *On Death and Dying* as well as many other books about the dying process, describes the stages that a person experiences on learning of his or her own impending death.

She identifies the first stage as *denial* ("It can't be happening to me"). The denial may be partial or complete. Denial is usually a temporary defense that a person uses as a buffer until able to mobilize his or her defenses to face the inevitability of death.

The second stage is often *anger* ("Why is this happening to me?"). The person feels violent anger at having to give up life. This emotion may be directed toward specific persons or projected into the environment at random. Dr. Kübler-Ross reflects on the origin of this rage: "The problem here is that few people place themselves in the patient's position and wonder where this anger might originate. Maybe we, too, would be angry if all our life activities were interrupted so prematurely."

The third stage is *bargaining* ("If you'll only let me live, God, I will . . ."). The person attempts to strike a bargain for more time to live or more time to be without pain in return for doing something for God. The person often turns or returns to religion during this stage.

Depression is the fourth stage ("Oh, God. I'm going to die, and I see no way out"). Usually when people have completed the processes of denial, anger, and bargaining, they move into depression. Sometimes called reactive depression, this stage occurs when the person reacts against the impending loss of life and grieves for himself.

The final stage of dying is that of *acceptance* ("Yes, I am going to die and I am ready to leave"). This occurs when the person has worked through the previous stages and accepts his or her own inevitable death. With full acceptance of impending death comes readiness for it; however, even with acceptance, hope is still present and needs to be supported realistically.

Many factors influence how individuals accept death, from their personal values and beliefs about life to past experiences in coping with traumatic situations. Regardless of how prepared we think we are, we will not know our coping resources until the day comes when we must face impending death.

The Glaser-Strauss research team offered another conceptualization of the dying process in their now-classic works, *Awareness of Dying* and *Time for Dying*. The first research team to actually study the distinctive characteristics of terminal illness, Glaser and Strauss used the term "dying trajectories" to refer to perceptions about the course of dying. These trajectories may be either lingering or crisis oriented. The expectations of care providers (family or medical staff) about a patient's dying affect the level of care that patient receives. These expectations also affect the patient's own beliefs about his or her dying. For example, if care providers view the individual as being in a lingering death trajectory, that person may give up control over his care; and when that individual does die, the caregivers see that event as appropriate.

We need more sensitive research, more hospice-type centers, more publications on the dying process. The more aware our society becomes of the rights and needs of the dying, the more it can support and care for them. Many hospitals have a standard joke that once a patient is "terminal," the doctor does not come around. In fact, this unfair allegation crys-

> You are the mosaic maker. The rest is simple logic. You look at life and decide how it is. Then you pay the price or enjoy the benefits. The decision is yours alone.
>
> Hans Selye

Religious Archetypes

Every religion, as well as great myths and fables, connects change and growth with the archetypes of death and rebirth. Easter and Passover, symbolic of death and resurrection, reflect a theme of life as a process of growth.

tallizes the difficulty most health care workers have in relating to the dying patient. Somehow, this sensitive and supportive level of care is often missing in the hospital setting. The sophisticated technology is present, but the touching is missing. Where we do see sensitivity and nonjudgmental caring is in hospice centers and at home.

The Hospice Movement

The hospice movement, which originated in England, has done much to support the process of dying in this country. Many hospice programs provide both inpatient and home care services. The hospice emphasizes comforting rather than curative care. Control of pain is a goal, and the staff strives to support the patients' and the families' suffering. The essence of the hospice concept is that it combines high-level medical care with personalized attention and support in a setting conducive to caring for the terminally ill.

Rather than isolating the patient and pretending that death is not approaching, the hospice center creates a special environment to support the dying and provides specially trained counselors for the families. The hospice movement is really an attempt to humanize death. The high cost of hospitalization, together with its sterile, cold environment, leads many to consider this option. Even hospital physicians recommend this alternative to hospitalization for the terminally ill.

In the United States, the hospice movement has gained respectability and acceptance as a mainstream treatment approach. This change from the early days, when it was considered a fringe alternative, has been facilitated by the positive feedback from participants in the hospice program and by legislation that allows reimbursement for care given at certified hospice programs.

The Meaning of Death

Robert Kastenbaum, in his book *Is There an Answer to Death?*, gives us an excellent resource on the subject of death. He suggests that the meaning of death in our culture depends in part on the social setting. Since we are social beings who learn from experience, we determine the affective quality of death through learning. Do those around us believe that death is a natural process? Is it frightening? Is it fair or unfair? We absorb many beliefs concerning these questions while growing up; when the time arrives for us to face our own death or the death of a loved one, our reactions may, at least in part, depend on this socialization process.

Adults, in both young adulthood and middle age, often conceptualize death in a way that has individual meaning. For example, the greatest death-related fear of a person who cannot stand pain in life might be the fear of a painful death. Someone who is constantly trying to control persons and environments may have a major concern about the loss of con-

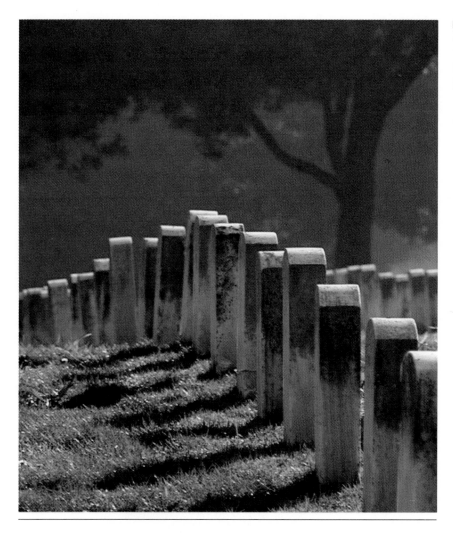

There is no cure for birth and death, save to enjoy the interval.

Santayana

trol that death implies. A person fearful of anything new may view the unknown territory of death as the paramount terror. Often the most intense fear and avoidance are caused not by the thought of death itself, but of how it approaches.

Though Kastenbaum's ideas about death do not conflict with Kübler-Ross's (in fact, they incorporate many of her stages) he does conceptualize differently the ways adults respond to death. He categorizes responses as "avoidance" or "authentic".

Avoidance responses include depression, or giving up, and displacement, a process that Kastenbaum discusses as translating death into something else. Direct avoidance may lead to fear. More authentic responses (and healthier ones from both a psychological and an existential point of view) include sorrowing, overcoming fear of death, and, finally,

Death, Dying and Grief

a desire to participate in the death. This last reaction is the most spiritually advanced. The person making this response views death as one of the most interesting events in life and chooses to participate in the process. Authenticity corresponds to the final Kübler-Ross stage of acceptance.

Views of Death at Different Ages

The age at which we encounter death affects how we handle it. Young children cannot grasp the concept of death; they may believe that the person is really sleeping and will wake up soon. When children are a little older, between five and ten, they are able to realistically understand death. At this age, death may be frightening, especially for a child who has grasped the finality of death. According to a study by Lansdown and Benjamin, all children studied understood death by the age of nine.

After the age of ten years and especially after twelve, children understand death fully. According to Piaget, a theorist of cognitive development in children, abstract, conceptual thinking takes place about twelve years of age. After this time, the teenager is able to intellectually grasp death, even though emotionally he may not have the maturity to deal with it. An adolescent will often not deal realistically with death in relation to self. The adolescent feels invulnerable; death happens to others. Even teenagers who have developed a philosophy of both life and death basically believe in their own immortality.

Aspects of Dying

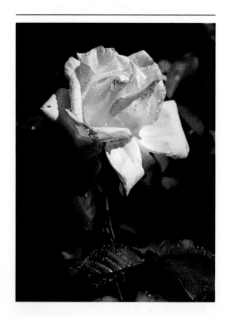

The Physical Aspects   During the dying process the patient is often in physical pain. This challenges not only that person, but family, friends, and care providers. Seeing a loved one in severe pain can be intolerable—perhaps that is why we so often try to escape the presence of death. In our culture, we most commonly deal with intractable pain by administering high doses of drugs, such as analgesics or pain killers. The problem, according to humanists and others concerned with spiritual growth, is that the most sophisticated painkillers alter consciousness. One solution is to give enough medication to make the person comfortable, but not unconscious. The central issue seems to be to prevent the dying person from suffering severe, unrelenting pain.

The Psychological Component   Even those who have faced death and completed the grieving process usually find the act of dying fearful and traumatic. If you have some awareness of the psychological aspects of dying, it will assist you to understand what a dying person is experiencing.

- The person who is dying faces three primary tasks: coping with physical symptoms, moving from a known to an unknown state, and coping with the impending separation from loved ones.

- This person faces the truth that this life is near an end; he or she approaches death in a way consistent with the manner in which life was approached—with bravado, acceptance, strength, procrastination, disdain, or fear. A dying person remains true to his or her personality, coping mechanisms, and general attitude toward life. Understanding this may help you to accept your loved one's response to dying.

The dying person's ability to cope depends not only on his or her own strength but also upon support systems: family, friends, and health care staff. The dying person often seeks identification and intimacy with someone, because closeness reduces the fear. The continued presence of a helping person and a meaningful relationship will provide necessary support for the family and dying patient.

The goal of care for a dying person is not to conquer disease but to provide comfort, ease pain and fears, and enhance whatever time is left. Those who care for and support someone during the dying process greatly influence the extent to which that person can experience this final life event to the fullest.

The Spiritual Dimension Everyone eventually dies. As Dr. Dennis Jaffe points out, death is not a failure of medicine. Once we accept death as real, then we ask simply, "When is death appropriate?" Translating the dying process to a spiritual question allows the caregivers and the dying person to discuss the purpose and meaning of life and death.

When we are considering the spiritual implications of dying, we may also have to examine our own beliefs about God—is there really one? Will she be there to meet me? What about heaven, hell, reincarnation, and so forth?

Many who believe that there is nothing beyond the grave find death very frightening. Perhaps this is why 75 percent of the world's religions incorporate the concept of reincarnation into their beliefs about death. (I hope I don't come back as a dog, but I'd rather be something than nothing.) Those of us who subscribe to the reincarnation theory believe that we get many chances to be reborn or to come back, so leaving is not quite so traumatic.

Dealing with the spiritual aspects of death is traumatic—both for the person experiencing the dying process and for the family and loved ones. Because we have spent most of our lives denying death, when it happens to a loved one, we are usually unprepared and ill-equipped to deal with it. According to Ram Dass, a former Harvard psychologist now working with the Hanuman Foundation's Dying Project, we can overcome this unwillingness by setting as our goal the creation of a relationship of respect, truth, love, and spiritual collaboration between a dying person and those around him or her.

The Hanuman project, though supporting the psychological aspect of dying, actually focuses on the spiritual nature of the dying process. It aims to assist people to use death as a vehicle for spiritual awakening.

> **Death is a reality which can't be avoided, halted, or altered. We all know that one who takes birth will surely die, but we don't want to see it, hear about it, or feel it. That is only because our mind dwells in the ignorance of 'I am this body.'**
>
> Baba Hari Dass

Death, Dying and Grief

This view of dealing with death gives us a more constructive perspective and is far more expanding than simply avoiding pain or ignoring the subject of dying. By accepting the belief that the experience of dying may offer our lives the most significant opportunity for awakening, we can face death with dignity and equanimity. We no longer regard it as the ultimate fear to avoid at all costs, but as the last physical stage of growth, a transitional process undertaken with conscious awareness.

Larry Dossey, former chief of staff at a Dallas hospital and author of numerous health publications, asserts that medicine has an outmoded, mechanistic view of reality that includes only physical aspects, a view based on atoms, molecules, and biochemical processes. Those studying and practicing medicine often learn this way of thinking, which makes it difficult to view life as many different levels of reality. This spiritual blindness or inner inertia, as Dr. Dossey calls it, precludes both a deeper spiritual understanding of death and alternative healing methods. Modern healers, or shamans, have introduced healing methods that have resulted in "miraculous recoveries" (as reported by Dr. Lewis Mehl, professor of Behavioral Medicine at Stanford University School of Medicine). They have also led to "miraculous deaths," in which loved ones encouraged, supported, and assisted the dying person to die with consciousness on his or her way to merge with the Supreme Being.

As a way of increasing our understanding of death, we might turn to the Buddhist tradition which incorporates different levels of reality. Buddhists discuss four natural states of existence: Birth, Life, Death, and Transit. *The Tibetan Book of the Dead*, a classic text of one form of Buddhism, is a treatise and almost a do-it-yourself text on achieving liberation at the moment of transit. For instance, it says:

> *The time of death is when you shed*
> *your physical body and individual ego and*
> *become one with the absolute Spirit of God.*

When a Loved One Is Dying

Almost everyone finds supporting and caring for a person who is dying desperately difficult. Becoming aware of your personal orientation toward the dying process helps you to care for the dying person effectively. Explore your own feelings about death and dying. Think about how you would react if you suddenly learned you had six months to live. Write your own obituary and experience how it feels to leave all of your loved ones. Consider your personal beliefs about dying: do you believe in a life beyond death? Do you believe in a heaven or a hell? Coming up with all the answers is not critical to the process—just the contemplation of death may be enough to make you sensitive to the needs and feelings of a person who is experiencing dying.

How can you be therapeutic and support a loved one who is dying? Here are some ways of caring that may demonstrate your love and support.

Death, Dying and Grief

- Spend time with the person, sharing thoughts, dreams, even fears. Try to verbalize your feelings; complete the relationship while you still have time.
- Stay physically close to the dying person, recognizing that touch and physical closeness help when we are frightened.
- Respect the person's need for privacy and withdraw with equanimity if he or she needs to be alone or to disengage from personal relationships.
- Be tuned in to the person's cues that he or she wants to talk and express feelings, cry, or even intellectually discuss dying. Also, remember to talk about the good times; laugh and bring light and love to the relationship.
- Accept the person at the level at which he or she is functioning, making no judgments. Do not force a discussion of dying or leaving loved ones.
- Recognize the grief pattern and support the person as he or she moves through the grieving process.
- Assist the person living through the experience of dying in whatever way you can. Support family and friends in discussing, accepting, and working through the loss.

Euthanasia For hundreds of years society has wrestled with the question of euthanasia, or "mercy killing." Euthanasia, literally meaning "good death," can be either active or passive. Active euthanasia refers to taking steps that hasten another's death out of the desire to end the loved one's suffering. Passive euthanasia involves withholding life-sustaining

> **Because I can no longer ignore death, I pay more attention to life.**
>
> Treya Wilber,
> **terminal cancer patient**

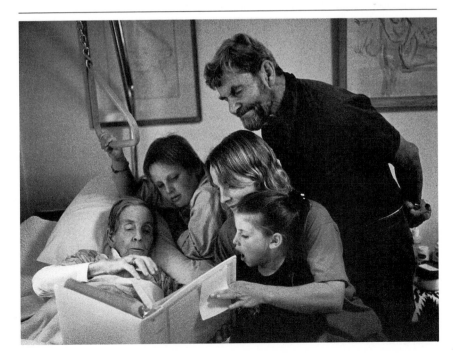

Death, Dying and Grief

procedures or providing the lethal drugs or weapons to end life. Though on the surface such actions may seem humane, our society questions whether one individual has the moral, ethical, or legal right to take another's life—even if that person wishes to die. There are persuasive arguments on both sides of this issue. In the United States we have yet to resolve it.

The question of euthanasia may arise in many different scenarios. In one, a person has remained in a deep coma for many months and is considered "brain dead." In another, a loved one is terminally ill, unconscious, and slowly losing physical function of body systems. Finally, a loved one may be terminally ill, suffering intolerably, with no hope of recovery.

Who makes the decision to end a life? Sometimes the court makes the decision; some settings allow the family, together with the physician and a hospital ethics committee, to decide. More often, no one makes the decision, even though both the terminally ill person and the family wish for death to occur.

Several years ago established medical organizations condemned the Netherlands for their policy of euthanasia. Today this country, as well as Canada and Britain, are much more open to this idea and considering the need for it to be accepted. The Dutch call it the gentle death. Every year in the Netherlands, doctors perform euthanasia on from 2,000 to 6,000 people. While technically illegal, it occurs when both the individual and the family desire it. The court system has developed criteria and guidelines under which a physician may aid a terminally ill patient to achieve death. The person receives a barbiturate to induce sleep, then another drug to terminate life.

In this country, the Supreme Court of New Jersey, in 1985, ruled that artificial feeding, like other life-sustaining treatment, may be withheld or withdrawn from an incompetent patient if it represents a disproportionate burden and would have been refused by the patient under the circumstances (Claire Conroy case). This ruling was consistent with a 1983 California Court of Appeals ruling that allowed health care providers to discontinue an IV feeding (Barber case).

Aside from the moral issue associated with euthanasia there are financial considerations. If someone is medically brain dead, should we maintain life at a cost of $100,000 a year? Should we expect families to absorb these costs? If insurance companies pay these fees, as they usually do, how do these expenses affect everyone else's premiums? Who should determine in what manner and for how long a person should remain in an irreversible coma?

At this time, the United States Supreme Court has not issued a ruling regarding who may make such decisions (medical personnel, family, or the courts). In 1988, a California right-to-die initiative failed to receive enough signatures to be placed on the ballot, but supporters say they will try again. National polls by the Roper Organization indicate wide support for the right to end a life when a terminally ill person requests that his or

> Birth is not one act; it is a process. The aim of life is to be fully born, though its tragedy is that most of us die before we are thus born. To live is to be born every minute. Death occurs when birth stops.
>
> Erich Fromm

her physician do so. Supporters argue that it is a basic human right for the person dying to choose when life no longer has meaning. Choosing to die is the ultimate act of self-determination. On the opposing side, many physicians' associations unilaterally oppose euthanasia. They argue that life in any form has meaning, that medicine's duty is to preserve life, despite pain and suffering and that official sanction of euthanasia will damage public trust in the medical profession. Physicians may also want to avoid any legal exposure they could experience for performing euthanasia. Others argue that euthanasia would tarnish the image of society as the standard bearer of life. For example, in the Hastings Center Report (1983), Steinbock asks, "If it is permissible to remove a feeding tube from a comatose patient, why not from a barely conscious, senile and terminally ill patient?"

The Right to Die   Those who administer lifesaving measures (paramedics, ambulance attendants, emergency room personnel) often must make life-and-death decisions. What seems right in one situation may seem wrong in another. Many states have instituted "right to die" legislation which provides legal guidelines for withholding resuscitative efforts from a patient. Even with legislation, medical personnel, parents, children, or family must judge whether to continue resuscitation efforts or allow the dying person to die.

The paramedics are called to a home where frantic parents have retrieved their comatose three-year-old from the backyard pool. No one knows how long the child was in the pool. The paramedics begin resuscitation. A little water is expelled, and one partner begins to blow puffs of air into the lifeless form. No signs of life appear. The child is transported to the hospital. Efforts at revival seem to be in vain—should they continue?

The same paramedics are called to the residence of an older couple, where they find a 78-year-old man who appears very ill and wasted. He has suffered a long bout with cancer and undergone numerous surgical procedures in unsuccessful attempts to stop the disease. As they assess his condition, his heart begins to beat unevenly. They detect arrhythmias, usually life-threatening. He pleads with them to let him die at home peacefully. Do they attempt to stabilize the heartbeat?

Ethics are defined as "the basic principles of right action." What ethics are involved in life or death situations? Knowing what the suffering person would want can ease such decisions. Millions of adults have used a "living will" to inform others concerning their preference about lifesaving measures. The Living Will, first devised in 1969 by the Euthanasia Educational Council (now called Concern for Dying), is a legal document. It states that the person does not wish to remain alive if artificial means or life-sustaining measures are required. The person must sign the living will while mentally competent. This document will assist the family and the doctors to abide by the wishes of the individual who, after all, has the right to make decisions concerning his or her own death.

A Legal Right to Die?

The U.S. Supreme Court has agreed to hear a case brought by the parents of a severely brain damaged 31-year-old woman against the state of Missouri. The parents are seeking to overturn a law that requires a patient in a comatose condition to be maintained on life support equipment indefinitely. The parents maintain that their daughter has no chance of recovery. State courts in Missouri have blocked the parents' attempts to have their daughter's feeding tube removed.

Two thirds of physicians surveyed by the American Medical Association in 1988 indicated that they had been involved in a decision concerning continued treatment for a comatose patient. This situation affects nearly 10,000 people in the United States today. Recently, the AMA and the American Association of Neurological Surgeons adopted guidelines that permit withdrawal of feeding tubes for persons in a "persistent negative state." However, physicians are still uncertain of their legal risks and responsibilities. The Supreme Court's decision may clarify this difficult dilemma.

Living Will

In case of terminal illness, Euthenasia Council's "Living Will" can clarify your wishes. (Copies can be obtained by writing the Council at 250 W. 57 St., New York 10019.)

Some people use a similar document, called the Durable Power of Attorney for Health Care. This document assigns a specific person the authority to make medical treatment decisions if the patient is incompetent or otherwise unable to make such decisions. Many people sign a living will with a durable power of attorney.

The living will has legal standing in a majority of states, but even with this legal sanction, individuals should take safeguards. First, have a discussion with your primary physician about his or her personal and professional philosophy about carrying out the intent of the document. If the doctor hesitates to carry out your wishes, you may decide to choose another physician. Second, determine that your hospital's policy does not preclude implementing such wishes of the patient.

Death, Dying and Grief

The Funeral—A Rite of Passage

Funeral customs are special ceremonies that take place after a person dies. These customs serve to honor the dead, comfort the living, and help survivors express grief and resolve the grieving process.

Sixty thousand years ago our prehistoric ancestors observed special customs when burying their dead. Neanderthal graves contain tools, weapons, and the remnants of flowers. Through time we have held onto the funeral ceremony, as it seems to meet a deep need to express sorrow at the passing of a loved one. In fact, this ceremony can be viewed as a "rite of passage": it is associated with the completion of one phase of life and the beginning of another.

In the United States, as well as other countries, funerals are "big business." A casket alone can cost hundreds of dollars; adding a cemetery plot, grave site care, embalming the body, use of the funeral home, a memorial service, flowers, clergy, and so forth, the total cost may run in the thousands of dollars. The average funeral costs the family $3,500, and many total two to three times this price.

When someone dies, we have several choices about how to care for the body. Embalming is one of the most common. This technique artificially preserves the body by injecting it with special fluid, often a combination of formaldehyde and alcohol. As early as 4000 B.C., embalming was a highly skilled profession in ancient Egypt. Egyptians believed that survival of the soul required preservation (mummification) of the body. Today, a slightly more practical rationale underlies the tradition of embalming: to preserve the body until it is buried. Many states require embalming if burial does not occur within 24 hours.

Today, many families cremate their loved ones instead of burying them. In cremation, a funeral home incinerates the body in a special furnace so that only the ashes remain. The number of those choosing this method has doubled in the last few years and now exceeds ten percent. Many funeral homes handle all of the services for cremation. Often families will hold a memorial service rather than a funeral for the deceased. Cremation may cost as much as a funeral.

Cultural beliefs often determine what families choose to do with the body. In Christian, Jewish, and Muslim faiths, burial is the most common method. Some faiths do not allow cremation; for example, Muslim beliefs do not allow cremation, donation of organs, or even an autopsy. Orthodox Jews believe that the body should be buried intact; thus cremation or embalming or even cosmetic additions cannot be done. Hindus often celebrate death, believing that it is a new beginning. In India and in Buddhist countries such as Japan, cremation is the method of choice.

Near-Death Experiences

Near-death experiences, affectionately called NDE's, have been reported by thousands of people who were close to death but somehow survived.

Old Mummies

In 1880 the body of King Mer-en-re was found in his pyramid, where it had lain undisturbed for 4,500 years. In 1881 archaeologists discovered the 3,200-year-old mummy of Ramses II at Dayr al Bahri.

I do not believe in an afterlife, although I am bringing a change of underwear.

Woody Allen

According to a Gallup poll, one in twenty Americans reports having had a near-death experience. As more and more people have these experiences and share them with others, a larger segment of the U.S. population is beginning to develop an awareness that something exists beyond death. Our knowledge of reality is expanding—an exciting if not exactly reassuring thought.

One of the first published accounts of these experiences was *Life After Life* by Raymond Moody, MD. Dr. Moody reported hundreds of stories of people who had been clinically dead, then resuscitated. He identified many common themes in their accounts, even the sensations they experienced. He and others identify three common stages in NDE's. The first, resistance, seems to reflect the person's struggle to remain in the present and avoid the fear of the unknown. In the second stage, after having moved beyond the body and the experience of pain or fear, the person reviews past-life experiences. When the last stage occurs, the person travels through a long, dark tunnel toward a warm, loving light, while experiencing incredible peace, joy, even ecstasy. Dr. Elisabeth Kübler-Ross has said that before she cared for many dying people she did not believe in life after death (or even reincarnation). However, being present time after time while patients described leaving the body and traveling toward the light, convinced her of the validity of these experiences.

People relate that in NDE's everything seems real; they have no pain—only awareness of a loving light that radiates total acceptance and love. Most reports indicate that once they reach the final stage, individuals do not want to return to their bodies. When they do, and many choose to return to meet commitments in this life, often their lives change permanently: they no longer fear death; many experience life more profoundly and with a deeper commitment than previously; and, they return much more forgiving of others, less judgmental, and more loving.

Grief and Loss

When we lose something or someone, we must cope with the loss in some way. We may have an actual loss (of a partner, limb, relationship) or imagined loss. How we experience, cope with, and resolve this loss affects our body and our life. We have all developed ways of responding to losses, some more effective than others.

Loss and grieving are inseparable. When loss cannot be resolved, research has shown that it may be a critical factor in the development of both psychological and physical illness. The following section presents grief as a natural reaction to loss.

Grief is a response to loss—not only the death of a loved one, but also the loss of a relationship, career, or family structure. Coping with grief varies in intensity and may take months or years. For some, it becomes a debilitating experience of pain; for others, it provides the opportunity for growth. Grief may affect people very profoundly, particularly those who have sustained many unresolved losses in the past. Those who have adequate coping and support resources and are able to complete the grieving process for a loss may handle a subsequent loss without being devastated.

Erich Lindemann shaped the classic description of the grieving process. Lindemann observed and treated victims and survivors of the 1940 great Coconut Grove fire in Boston. Through his skilled work with these people, he found that the emotion of grief accompanies and complicates all losses.

Lindemann concluded that when a loved one dies, we endure major loss and subsequent grief. He found that other forms of separation could also result in grief. A child going off to college or marriage, a loved one going to war, a relationship that disintegrates—all may result in grief. Lindemann described the process people go through when they cope with loss as the work of mourning or "grief-work."

Stages of Grief Following Lindemann's work, George Engle described the classic progression of the grief process in stages. These stages may occur in order, or an individual may skip a stage, become locked in a particular stage, or even return to an earlier stage already worked through.

The first stage is *shock and disbelief*. On first learning of the death of a loved one, a person may feel shock and refuse to accept or comprehend the fact. After this reaction, the person may have a stunned, numb feeling that keeps him or her from acknowledging the reality of death. This initial phase is characterized by denial—attempts to protect oneself against severe stress by blocking recognition of the death.

Developing awareness is the second stage. Within minutes or hours, the individual becomes acutely and increasingly aware of the anguish of loss. He or she may feel anger during this time and may direct that anger toward persons or circumstances the griever holds responsible for the death. Crying and regression to a helpless and childlike state frequently accompany this stage.

The third stage is *restitution*, in which the various rituals of the culture, such as funeral, attire, wake, folkways and mores, help to initiate the recovery process. Rituals emphasize the reality of death. The very act of experiencing rituals assists the mourner to face the loss.

As the person accepts the reality of death, coping with loss begins. This involves a number of steps. First, the mourner attempts to deal with the painful void. At this time, the deceased may occupy almost all the individual's thoughts. The mourner becomes more aware of his or her own body and bodily sensations. Finally, the mourner begins to talk about the dead person, recalling the dead person's attributes and personality, and reminiscing about the memories they shared. Resolving the loss is a long and painful phase.

Many people then experience the stage of *idealization*. They repress all hostile and negative feelings toward the dead person. As the process pro-

---

Examine Your Personal Experience with Loss

1. Reflect back over your life, and identify the most crushing losses you have experienced. Put them in descending order, from most to least devastating.
2. Describe the toll these events have taken on your life—your reactions, feelings, physical illnesses that occurred, and so forth.
3. Note how you coped with the losses—be specific.
4. Decide whether you have worked through and resolved these losses or whether you have unfinished business to complete. Understand that significant unresolved losses may surface again later in life if a new loss occurs. Which losses do you feel need more work?
5. Formulate a plan to deal with unresolved loss. Here are a few ways of helping yourself resolve a loss. Write a letter to a lost loved one (you don't have to mail it—so far, no P.O. boxes in heaven). Start a journal of expressed feelings related to the loss and keep journaling until the grief begins to lessen. Seek a therapist qualified to assist you, or attend a group designed to deal with the unfinished business of loss. Attend a psychodrama course in which you can act out the original loss and benefit from the support of the group members. Work with a regressive therapist to go back in time, under hypnosis, and deal with the loss. Do a series of meditations focused on your feelings about the loss and allow yourself to experience them thoroughly.

499

ceeds, two important changes are taking place. First, recurring memories of the dead person bring the more positive aspects of the relationship to awareness. At the same time, the mourner begins to assume certain admired qualities of the dead person through identification. The mourner may begin to dress, speak, or develop mannerisms or beliefs similar to those of the person who was lost. Experiencing this process often requires many months. As it dissipates, the mourner's preoccupation with the dead person lessens. At this point the person may begin to reinvest intimate feelings toward other people and activities.

Resolution, the outcome of the mourning process, usually takes a year or more. The clearest evidence of healing is the ability to remember the deceased comfortably and realistically, with both the pleasures and the disappointments of the relationship. By this stage, the obsession with the loss has ended, and the survivor accepts responsibility for living his or her own life.

Each individual who experiences loss goes through at least some of these stages as he or she attempts to cope with loss. The various stages of grief help us to move through loss to resolution. Several factors influence the eventual outcome of mourning:

- The importance of the person lost as a source of support.
- The degree of dependency on the relationship—the more dependent, the more difficult the task of resolution.
- The degree of ambivalence felt toward the deceased. When persistent hostile feelings exist, guilt may interfere with the work of mourning.
- The number and nature of other relationships on which the mourner can depend. Someone with few meaningful relationships may be less willing to give up attachment to the deceased.
- The number and nature of previous grief experiences. Losses tend to be cumulative in their effects; someone who has not successfully worked through previous losses will find that these experiences aggravate grieving for the current loss.
- The age of the person lost. The loss of a child has a more profound effect on the survivor than the loss of an aged parent.
- The degree of preparation for the loss. For example, in terminal illness, grief work may have begun long before the actual death of the person.
- Finally, the physical and psychological health of the mourner determine one's capacity to cope with loss. In circumstances of diminished coping resources, grief may become overwhelming. Sadness may shift into depression.

Coping with Loss Each person moves through the grieving process at his or her own pace, but as a friend, partner or family member, you can assist someone to cope more effectively with loss. The following guidelines may help you.

- Allow the person to deny grief so he or she can have time to move through shock and mobilize defenses.

- Accept the person's inability to face reality, and allow mood swings and reminiscences of happier times.
- Anticipate expression of anger toward others; allow tantrums or "acting-out" of feelings and verbalization of anger.
- Encourage the person to take as much control as possible over care and environment. Avoid criticism and negative feedback at this time.
- Support the person's self-esteem and understand that awareness of the loss will affect one's own self-image.
- Be aware of your own feelings of sadness and loss.
- Spend quiet time with the person, interacting on a nonverbal, non-demanding level.
- Encourage verbalizations about loss, its meaning in the person's life, and feelings about the loss.
- Show respect for cultural, religious, and social customs throughout states of mourning.

Failure to complete griefwork may lead to feelings of helplessness and depression. Rather than avoiding, denying or suppressing grief feelings, it is much healthier to face the loss, experience the emotions and move through the grieving process to resolution.

When we have successfully completed the grieving process, we can remember both the pain and the pleasures of the lost relationship. The memories and unique characteristics of the loved person remain intact. When we have fully resolved the loss, we will be able to form new intimate relationships with openness and commitment.

Seeking Professional Help

If someone close to you has died or is dying, or if you yourself are facing death, you will benefit from talking about your feelings. If you have a strong support system of friends and family, you may be able to care for this need informally.

If someone's death or dying is consuming most of the rest of your life, talk with someone. If such issues are a part of your life, seek help if you experience:

- Marked decrease (or increase) in appetite
- Avoidance of friends and family you used to be close to
- Increased drinking or drug use
- Difficulty sleeping that you cannot resolve by using home methods
- Lethargy and/or apathy
- Persistent feelings that life lacks meaning (depression)
- Guilt about your dying or someone else's

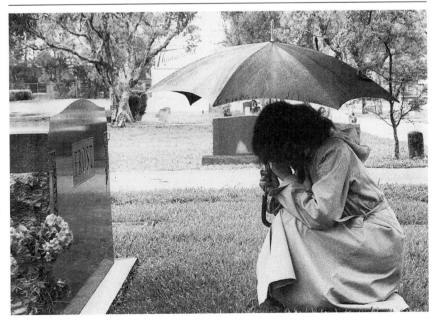

Healing
One thing I forgot:
after the
pain of parting
comes the
happiness of healing.
Rediscovering
   life,
   friends,
   self.
Joy.

Beyond the Text

1. What can you do to support your best friend whose younger sister is dying of leukemia?

2. A good friend recently had a near-death experience. He tells you about it and says it changed his ideas about death. How would you respond?

3. What have been your personal losses—loved ones, pets, and so forth? How have you grieved, and what did you learn about yourself in the process?

4. Since your uncle died a year ago, your aunt hasn't given away his clothes or changed anything in the house. She's been very withdrawn. What would you do to help her?

5. Your roommate has just learned that her "favorite" grandfather died suddenly. She says that she's too busy with her studies to go home for the memorial service. What advice would you give her?

Supplemental Readings

Death: Current Perspectives by Edwin Schneidman, ed. Palo Alto, CA: Mayfield, 1984. A comprehensive compendium of essays relating to many aspects of death and dying. This excellent edited book covers the dying process as well as personal statements of grief.

Death: The Final Stage of Growth by Elisabeth Kübler-Ross. Englewood Cliffs, NJ: Prentice Hall, 1975. A classic treatment of death, a subject that is largely evaded, ignored, and denied by our youth-worshipping, progress-oriented society.

Life After Life by Raymond A. Moody, Jr., MD. New York: Bantam Books, 1975. The author studied more than one hundred subjects who have experienced "clinical death" and been revived. He summarized many of their accounts in an interesting and informative manner.

Necessary Losses by Judith Viorst. New York: Ballantine Books, 1986. Describes how we grow and change through the losses that are necessary and inevitable parts of life. The loss of parents and loved ones due to death or separation helps us gain deeper perspective and true maturity, explains the author.

The Hospice Way of Death by Paul M. DuBois. New York: Human Sciences Press, 1980. Describes the growth of the hospice movement in the United States.

The Right to Die: Understanding Euthanasia by Derek Humphry and Ann Wickett. New York: Harper & Row, 1986. A clear, unbiased discussion of all aspects of euthanasia—legal, cultural, and historical.

Who Dies? An Investigation of Conscious Living and Conscious Dying by Stephen Levine. New York: Anchor Books, 1982. A sensitive discussion of how to die with dignity and awareness.

Key Terms Defined

analgesic drugs that relieve pain without causing loss of consciousness

brain death cessation of all brain function, determined by flat electroencephalograph reading

clinical death absence of a heart beat and the cessation of breathing

cremation reducing a dead person's body to ashes through burning

death cessation of all physical and chemical processes that invariably occurs in all living organisms

denial defense mechanism in which the existence of unpleasant realities is denied and kept out of conscious awareness

embalming chemical treatment of a dead body to retard decomposition

ethics rules or principles governing right conduct

euthanasia deliberately inducing death of a person in as painless a method as possible, for reasons intended as merciful; also called mercy killing

grief emotional response to a loss; intense mental anguish or sorrow

hospice a supportive environment to care for persons in the last stages of their life, with emphasis on spiritual and emotional, as well as medical, problems

mourning culturally defined manner of expressing grief

near-death experience (NDE) experience of a person who has been clinically dead, then resuscitated, and recalling having left their body at the point of death

reincarnation rebirth of the soul in a new body or form of life

spiritual relating to the essential philosophy or beliefs each of us has about the universe, human nature, and the significance of life and relationships

wake a group of loved ones together to watch over the body of a dead person prior to burial, sometimes accompanied by festivity

Accidents, Safety and First Aid

More than 90,000 people die from accidents each year in the United States, and only heart disease, cancer, and stroke rank ahead of accidents as causes of death. For individuals between the ages of 18 and 38, accidents are the primary cause of death. This means that accidents are the main health risk for college-age individuals. Of the various types of accidents, motor vehicle accidents account for the greatest number of fatalities among the 18- to 24-year-old population. Accidents often result in long-term pain and suffering from injuries, such as back or knee damage, impaired eyesight, loss of limb, and even partial or complete paralysis.

Most accidents are caused by carelessness, recklessness, ignorance, poor judgment, misconception, or a feeling of invincibility. However, these behaviors can be changed. The objectives of studying about accidents are to gain factual knowledge concerning this serious health threat, and to develop an awareness of how you can integrate accident prevention (safety) into your daily life.

Contents

Key Terms

Accident

CPR

Disabling injury

DWI

First aid

Injury

Risk

Safety

Suffocate

Types of Accidents

For purposes of reporting and analysis, the National Safety Council categorizes accidents in four main groups reflecting where they typically occur.

- *Motor vehicle* includes automobile, motorcycle, bicycle, and pedestrian accidents.
- *Work* includes job-related motor vehicle accidents, falls, electric shocks, burns, and overexertion.
- *Home* includes falls, burns, poisoning, suffocation, and firearm accidents.
- *Public places* includes recreational accidents and incidents taking place in public areas other than the highways, such as schools and parks.

Table 1 summarizes deaths and disabling injuries in the United States for each major category during 1987, the latest year for which complete reports are available. Table 2 summarizes how people died accidentally during the same year.

Motor Vehicle Accidents

Motor vehicle accidents account for approximately 50 percent of all fatal accidents and about 20 percent of all disabling injuries. These accidents involve collisions between motor vehicles, collisions with fixed objects (tree, guard rail, abutment), vehicle rollovers, pedestrian accidents, and collisions with bicycles and railroad trains. The age group at greatest risk for motor vehicle accidents is 16 to 25 years old. One fifth of the nation's licensed drivers (just over 160 million) are under the age of 25, but this group accounts for one third of all motor vehicle accidents. And 18,700 victims of fatal accidents in 1987 were age 25 or under.

Motorcycles When involved in an accident, a motorcycle operator's chances of being killed or injured are much greater than if he or she was driving an auto or truck, which provides a great deal more protection. Motorcycle fatalities have declined slightly in the 1980s, but nevertheless, deaths have exceeded 4,000 every year in the past decade.

Pedestrians and Bicyclists   Collisions between motor vehicles and pedestrians or cyclists are responsible for nearly 10,000 deaths and 130,000 nonfatal injuries per year. Three fourths of those injured or killed in bicycle accidents are between 5 and 24 years old. A recent study of bicycle injuries conducted in North Carolina concluded that bicyclists were at fault in more than 60 percent of the cases. Less than 5 percent of the riders reported wearing helmets. Motor vehicles have an exceptional advantage in collisions with pedestrians and bicyclists. Many pedestrian accidents occur during conditions of poor visibility when the driver does not see the pedestrian or on occasions when the pedestrian crosses the path of the auto in an unauthorized zone.

Causes of Motor Vehicle Accidents

Alcohol   According to the National Highway Traffic Safety Administration, alcohol is a factor in more than 50 percent of fatal automobile accidents and nearly 30 percent of serious injury accidents. In 1986, 39 percent of fatally injured drivers were legally intoxicated with blood alcohol concentration (BAC) levels of 0.10 percent or greater at the time of the accident. Alcohol affects specific functions of the body, especially muscle coordination and reflexes. Mental capacity is also reduced by alcohol, which contributes to carelessness, inattention, and sometimes a disregard for safety.

Alcohol-Related Traffic Deaths	
1987	23,632
1986	23,990
1985	22,360
1984	23,760
1983	23,650

Source: National Highway Traffic Safety Administration

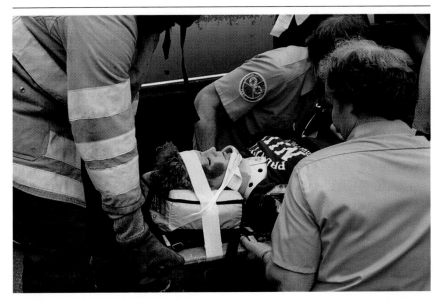

Accidents, Safety and First Aid

Improper Driving   Nearly three fourths of all motor vehicle accidents involve improper driving. Excessive speed is the primary factor in about 30 percent of fatal and 25 percent of injury accidents. Violating the right of way—failing to yield, passing stop signs, disregarding traffic signals—is another major cause of accidents. The number of motor vehicle fatalities on rural interstate highways increased by nearly 20 percent in the states that recently raised their speed limits to 65 mph, according to the Department of Transportation.

Fatigue   Many late night wrecks occur when the driver falls asleep. People driving long distances on relatively boring interstate highways often feel drowsy, especially if they don't break up the driving hours by periodic stops. The effects of alcohol and other drugs add to feelings of sleepiness. Some prescription and over-the-counter medications such as antihistamines cause drowsiness and can create a potentially dangerous situation if taken just prior to driving.

Preventing Motor Vehicle Accidents

Because so many motor vehicle accidents are the result of human error—DWI, excessive speed, fatigue—appropriate actions to reduce accidents are based on behavioral changes. The following recommendations, if heeded, will reduce the probability that you will become involved in a motor vehicle accident.

- Avoid driving under the influence of alcohol or other drugs. This advice is given continuously but ignored frequently. The enforcement of DWI laws (driving while intoxicated) and penalties for their violation are not as strict in the United States as they are in certain foreign countries, such as Sweden. The frequency of alcohol-related accidents and their resulting deaths and injuries has caused private groups such as MADD (Mothers Against Drunk Driving) to lobby for greater enforcement and harsher legal penalties. Refer to the chapter on **Alcohol and Other Drugs** for additional recommendations, such as the "designated driver" system.
- The axiom "Speed Kills" is very accurate. Excessive speed, when coupled with alcohol-impaired mental and muscular reflexes, creates a potentially fatal situation. Even without the influence of drugs or fatigue, excessive speed can cause drivers to lose control of their autos on curving or uneven road surfaces. At high speed, the distance required for an emergency stop is much greater than what is needed to stop at slower speeds.
- Warning signs are posted for your protection and for the safety of your passengers and other drivers. In addition, defensive driving techniques and compliance with all traffic rules will increase your chances of avoiding high risk situations, particularly those caused by other drivers.
- Avoid situations that require you to drive when you are likely to fall asleep. Team up with a designated driver, invite yourself as an over-

night guest, or sleep in your vehicle after parking it in a safe location. These and other alternatives are preferable to risking loss of control due to fatigue.

Work Accidents

The rate of fatal work accidents has dropped substantially during the past several decades. While the work force has grown in size, the total number of accidental work deaths has declined. Safety education and protective equipment, backed up by strict safety regulations and enforcement, have contributed greatly to this trend. Incentive for employers was originally created by the passage of the Workers' Compensation laws (in the early 1900s), which holds employers responsible for medical costs incurred by injured employees.

The shift in the labor force away from hazardous occupations such as mining and agriculture to less physically demanding jobs in wholesale/retail trade and service industries has decreased the accident rate. Today the construction industry leads in fatal worker accidents, while manufacturing, trade, and services account for the majority of disabling injuries.

About 35 percent of the 11,000 work-related fatalities are caused by motor vehicle accidents. Falls are the next highest cause of deaths, as well as the cause of a substantial number of disabling injuries. According to the Bureau of Labor Statistics, in 1987 about 28 percent of the 4.4 million work injuries resulted from lifting, carrying, pushing, or pulling objects. Injuries involving striking or being struck by another object accounted for another 26 percent.

Preventing Work Injuries

Employers have learned that providing and maintaining a safe work environment reduces accidents and injuries. Designing the work area ergonomically (so that employees never have to physically lift more than 30 pounds, bend over or twist and lift, or carry loads while walking) prevents accidents and injuries—and costs less than paying medical bills.

By following on-the-job safety requirements for footwear, hard hat, eye and ear protection, and other safety gear, you can minimize the risk of work injuries. Attention to job-site hazards that cause burns, falls, or other common injuries will help to reduce your chances of an accident. Requiring employees to use personal protective equipment—or be fired—is a major deterrent to accidents and injuries.

Proper lifting and moving procedures greatly reduce the risk of injury to the back, legs, or other parts of the body. Many injuries occur when the individual fails to use his or her legs to assist with lifting a heavy object, so the back absorbs the entire load. Operators of commercial vans and trucks are just as likely to experience accidents as drivers of automobiles. Use of seat belts and adherence to safe driving rules reduces the number of on-the-job motor vehicle accidents and injuries.

Youth Dominate Fatal Accident Statistics

During 1985, fatal accidents caused the deaths of 54,207 persons between the ages of 1 and 24 years. Young people accounted for 57 percent of all accidental deaths in the United States that year.

Electric shock, explosive materials, steam, and corrosive liquids account for more than 2,000 fatalities per year.

Accidents, Safety and First Aid

Home Accidents

Accidental deaths in the home are gradually declining, but accidental injuries continue to be a major source of concern. As shown in Table 2, disabling injuries in the home exceed 3 million per year and 25 percent of injuries result in some form of permanent disability. Home accidents take a heavy toll on the elderly with both injuries and deaths. As a greater proportion of the U.S. population exceeds 75 years of age, this type of accident will threaten more individuals. The main categories of home accidents are as follows:

- *Falls*. The highest number of home accidents involve falls from one level to another (stairs, ladder, roof) or on the same level (ground, sidewalk, floor). By far, the age group experiencing the highest rate of serious injury and fatal falls is 75 years and older, accounting for more than two thirds. When considering home safety, it is easy to overlook hazards such as loose carpeting and objects on stairs that cause injury to elderly people. This segment of the population may have more difficulty dealing with wet floors, uneven walkways, ice on sidewalks, and other hazards that are not usually perceived as dangerous by younger people, whose flexibility, eyesight, and coordination may equip them to handle such hazards more easily.

- *Fires and burns*. Deaths from fires, burns, and asphyxiation primarily involve the very young and the elderly. More than half of all fire fatalities are people under the age of 4 or over age 65. The most common cause of fires in one- and two-family dwellings is faulty heating equipment followed by cooking mishaps, defective wiring, and malfunctioning appliances. The igniting of upholstery or bedding at night by smoking materials (primarily cigarettes) causes the greatest number of fire-related injury accidents.

- *Poisoning*. Accidental deaths from solid and liquid poisoning have been increasing since the early 1980s: more than 4,000 fatalities are recorded every year. Small children gaining access to harmful household chemicals are particularly at risk. Overdoses of prescription or illegal drugs and mixing drugs with alcohol are also common causes of death. The 25 to 44 age group accounts for more than 50 percent of accidental poisoning deaths. Elderly people are susceptible to poisoning resulting from overdoses of mistakenly ingested prescription drugs. Of course, many incidents of poisoning do not result in death. The American Association of Poison Control Centers estimates that more than 2 million people per year experience accidental poisoning from solids or liquids. Another type of home poisoning results from exposure to gases and vapors (usually carbon monoxide). Individuals exposed to faulty gas heaters or cooking stoves as well as to automobile exhaust vapors can be fatally injured.

- *Suffocation*. Fatal accidents from suffocation are most common in the very young and the very old. Children from infancy to the age of 4 years are at risk to be smothered by bed clothes or by plastic bags. Elderly people are susceptible to choking on food that obstructs the respiratory passages, but many younger people (about 4,000 annually) choke on food—often after drinking alcohol—by taking big bites of food while talking or laughing.

- *Drowning.* Home accidents occur in swimming pools and bathtubs. Between infancy and age 4 is the period of primary risk. When toddlers who cannot swim are left unattended, too often they fall or jump into home pools. Permanent brain damage or death can occur after only a few minutes of oxygen deprivation.

- *Firearms.* Fatal firearm accidents in the home and outdoors account for nearly 1,500 deaths per year. Cleaning and playing with weapons are the two most common causes of these accidents, which primarily strike the 5- to 24-year-old age group. One child under the age of 18 is accidentally killed by a firearm every day. Nearly 70 percent of the accidental shootings of young people take place when children are at home alone.

   Guns are very accessible in our nation today—U.S. citizens own 60 million handguns, 140 million rifles and shotguns, and one million assault rifles. Ownership of guns has become a major public issue, with con-

Fatal Attraction of Firearms

Gunshot wounds result in nearly 30,000 fatalities per year. Accidents are the cause of only about 5% of the fatalities; suicide, assault, law enforcement, and self-defense account for the remaining deaths. More Americans died from injuries inflicted by firearms in 1984 and 1985 (62,897 total) than during the entire Vietnam War.

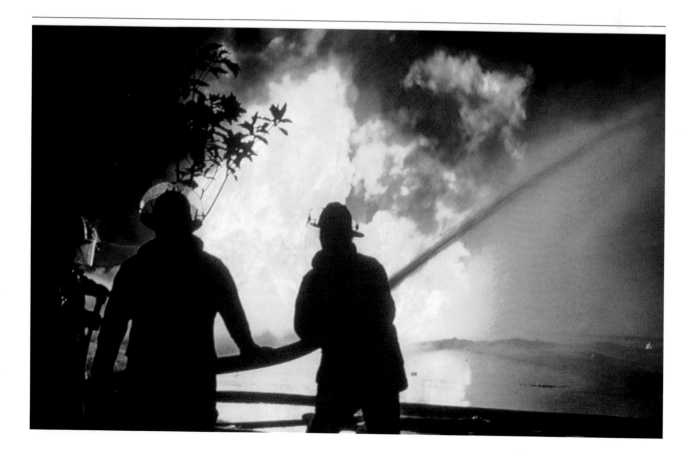

Earthquake!

The October 17, 1989, earthquake that struck the region from Santa Cruz to San Francisco, California, once again proved our vulnerability to the forces of nature. Unlike other natural phenomena, such as hurricanes and tornadoes, earthquakes strike with absolutely no warning and last only seconds. Geologists point out that wide areas outside of California experienced earthquakes of exceptional magnitude during the 1800s, and that millions of people are potentially exposed to future seismic action.

If you believe you are experiencing an earthquake, your most immediate danger is injury from falling debris or a collapsing ceiling. Get into a doorway or under a strong table or desk. Once the quake has subsided, the most serious threat is fire, usually caused by broken gas lines or downed electrical wires. If you smell gas, do not light a match. Vacate the premises and, if possible, turn off the gas main. Earthquake preparedness includes knowing where and how to shut off your utilities and stockpiling food and water to last for 72 hours. Battery-powered lights are essential, and a battery-powered radio will enable you to obtain information concerning the effects of the shock and possible disruption of your utilities and transportation network.

troversy raging between those who justify their gun ownership by the guarantees of the second amendment to the U.S. Constitution and their opponents, who strongly urge strict control over gun ownership and even suggest banning their sale. Safety experts agree that young people should receive gun safety education and that gun owners should keep their weapons unloaded, install trigger locks, and store firearms and ammunition in separate places, preferably in locked cabinets out of the reach of children. Guns should always be checked to make sure they are unloaded before cleaning; the user should never climb a fence or other obstacle while carrying a loaded gun; and above all other precautions, one should never point a gun at another person.

Preventing Home Accidents

Accident prevention at home requires constant awareness of the causes of accidents, and a willingness to take precautions to minimize risks. Whether you live in a family house, apartment, or residence hall, you are exposed to the hazards of falls, burns, fires, poisons, and electric shock. When handled improperly, firearms are extremely hazardous. Household appliances, tools, chemicals, and fuels are not inherently dangerous, but when used in a careless manner, they too can become agents for injury. The following is a partial list of suggested steps that you can take to eliminate unnecessary risks at home and reduce the chances of experiencing or causing an accident:

1. Inspect your living areas for potential electrical problems such as overloaded circuits, frayed electrical wiring, and electrical heaters close to flammable materials. Students often live in crowded quarters equipped with too few outlets for today's array of appliances. A multiple outlet box with built-in circuit breaker is both useful and safe.
2. Make certain that flammable or poisonous substances (e.g., solvents, cleaning supplies, charcoal lighter, and other petroleum-based chemicals) are properly labeled and safely stored.
3. Deal with the threat of fires by eliminating their causes as completely as possible. At parties, control the use of alcohol to reduce the risk of unwanted fires from fireplaces, barbecues, candles, oil burning lamps, and other open flames. Careless disposal of cigarettes and other smoking materials may result in a fire that, after smoldering for several hours, breaks out later when everyone is asleep.
4. Home smoke detectors have been very effective in reducing residential fire injuries and deaths, but the National Safety Council reports that up to one third of home smoke detectors are no longer operational. Whether you live at your family home or in a rented apartment, confirm that smoke detectors are properly installed and fully functional. Your residence hall or dormitory is required by law to have a fire warning system that works properly. In case a fire occurs, have a primary and an alternative escape route firmly fixed in your mind.

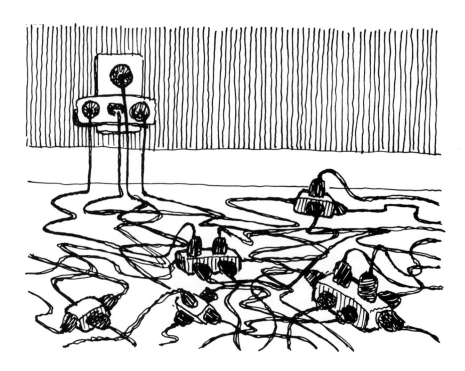

5. Reduce the possibility that you or someone else will fall as a result of loose carpeting, wet floor surfaces, or objects that obstruct hallways or stairwells. Other falls occur when chairs and boxes are unsuccessfully utilized as step ladders.

6. If you cook your meals or heat your living space with natural gas, check that the pilot lights are properly adjusted. If you detect the "rotten egg" odor of leaking gas, vacate the area and notify the utility company or fire department.

7. Accidental poisoning seems for most college students a very remote possibility. If small children have access to your hazardous chemicals (including such items as fingernail polish remover), then your carelessness may cause an accidental poisoning. The major risks for young adults involve mixing prescription medications with alcohol or other medications, swallowing overdoses of sleeping pills or other drugs, and taking someone else's medicine. More information on specific drugs and their effects is included in the chapter on **Alcohol and Other Drugs**.

Public Accidents

Public accidents account for nearly 20,000 deaths and over two million disabling injuries per year. These accidents include falls, drowning, firearms, and burns. The 15- to 24-year-old age group leads in fatal drowning, firearms, and boating accidents. The elderly are at greatest risk for falls and fires. Public accidents also include injuries sustained during travel by means other than motor vehicle.

Drowning   Drowning is the second most common cause of accidental death for the age 1 to 24 population, exceeded only by motor vehicle deaths. More than 2,500 young people drown each year, making up about half of the 5,300 U.S. total drownings. Many drowning victims do not know how to swim and, once in deep water, are unable to help themselves. Others drown when they become fatigued while swimming in a lake or are overpowered by river currents or ocean surf. The expression, "getting in over your head" certainly applies to swimming situations. Alcohol is frequently a contributing factor in swimming and boating tragedies.

Diving accidents, which result in 2,000 injuries per year, are a major cause of spinal cord injuries in the United States. Males from 15 to 29 years of age account for 90 percent of diving accidents. And 98 percent result in permanent paralysis. Diving accidents typically occur when people plunge head first into water that is too shallow or contains submerged obstacles. Checking the water depth and jumping feet first before diving reduces these risks.

Boating   In 1988, recreational boating accidents killed 946 people. Several types of boating activity often share the same limited water space—sailing, fishing, sport canoeing or kayaking, family outings, water skiing, informal racing, and so forth. The chance of collision is high; when alcohol is added to the situation, the risk of accidents is very great. "Drunken boaters are responsible for up to 50 percent of all the fatalities," says Captain Robert Melvin, the U.S. Coast Guard's Chief of Boating Safety in Portsmouth, Virginia. In response to the alarming boating accident rate, the Coast Guard will step up enforcement of alcohol regulations: legally drunk will be defined as a blood alcohol content of 0.10 percent or higher. Thirty-two states also have adopted BAC levels for boaters. Only three states had such rules in 1983.

In 1988 Florida ranked first in the nation in the number of recreational boating accidents with 1,203 and boating deaths with 94. Today, there are 700,000 registered boats (some of which can top 110 mph) in Florida, and authorities are concerned as the number of boats and boating accidents increases each year. Florida has implemented speed limits in many areas and will soon require boaters to have a license and to pass a boating safety course before receiving it.

States that have imposed tighter restrictions report a decrease in accidents. For example, after Michigan adopted training requirements and a speed limit, boating deaths decreased from 55 in 1987 to 30 in 1988. Other states are expected to follow suit and initiate boating restrictions to reduce the accident rate.

Water Scooters   Dubbed the "motorcycles of the waterways," water scooters have created "waves" throughout the accident prevention com-

---

A Deadly Mix

Alcohol and water don't mix. Even one or two beers can impair a person's ability to operate a boat safely. Alcohol also impairs your ability to swim, and it shortens cold-water survival time. A drinker may not be able to swim at all, or might swim downward in darkness. Ninety percent of boating deaths result from drowning.

Source: *USA Today*, August 15, 1989

In Florida a boat is not just a craft; it's an island kingdom, a floating assertion of independence.

Jeffrey Schmalz,

Special Correspondent to *The New York Times*,

August 30, 1989

---

munity. Also known as jet skis, water scooters travel at speeds up to 35 mph and weigh as much as 700 pounds, resembling snowmobiles. They are often ridden by youngsters more interested in speed and fun than safe operation. Already, 200,000 water scooters are buzzing the nation's waterways, and the accident rate is climbing. Water scooter accidents are 90 percent attributable to operator error. In the past five years, 640 accidents resulted in 20 fatalities. Florida is the leading accident state with 11 fatalities since 1987. Nearly 20 states now have safety requirements that include a minimum operator age of 14 years for privately owned scooters and 16 years for rentals, mandatory flotation vests for all drivers, an automatic cut-off switch, and operation restricted to daylight hours only.

All-Terrain Vehicles   All-terrain vehicles (ATVs) are three- or four-wheel motorized vehicles designed primarily for off-road use. With large, soft tires, ATVs have a relatively high center of gravity. Capable of speeds up to 50 miles per hour, ATVs have been involved in an alarming number of injuries and fatal accidents. During the past five years, more than 550 ATV-related deaths have occurred. Over 40 percent of those killed were children under the age of 16. ATV accidents have surpassed 85,000 per year, and children between the ages of 5 and 14 account for one third of those. Bruises, cuts, and broken limbs are common, but many serious head and spinal injuries have also been reported. As a result of these statistics, the Consumer Products Safety Commission has taken action to ban the sale of three-wheel ATVs. Four-wheel ATVs share similar

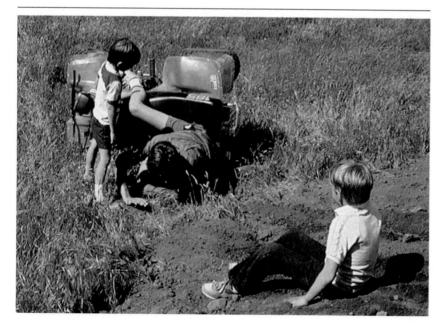

Accidents, Safety and First Aid

design features to the three-wheel variety. About 60 percent of the accidents involving four-wheel ATVs are a result of tipping and overturning. The use of alcohol and lack of safety equipment create additional risks. The American Academy of Orthopedic Surgeons recommends that the minimum age for ATV operation be set at 16 and that operators be required to wear safety equipment, most importantly, a helmet, since in 80 percent of ATV accidental deaths, the driver was not wearing one. Other safety recommendations would restrict ATV operation to daylight hours only, and limit their use to only one rider at a time.

The Consequences of Accidents

The consequences of any accident depend on such factors as the age and occupation of the individual and the extent and type of injury. Accident victims may be unable to attend school or work, they may lose some of their skills, or lose their source of income. If hospitalization and rehabilitation are required, they can be very costly in terms of both money and time. For the accident victim, an injury will probably result in physical pain, mental anguish, a visit to an emergency room or physician, and some type of treatment. There is often some loss of independence for the victim, who may have to decrease his or her activity level and may also require help with the simple necessities of daily living, such as eating, personal hygiene, and dressing.

Accidental death or injury has broad implications. The social impact is immense: for example, if one is handicapped or unable to function productively, the economic burdens may be enormous and affect many

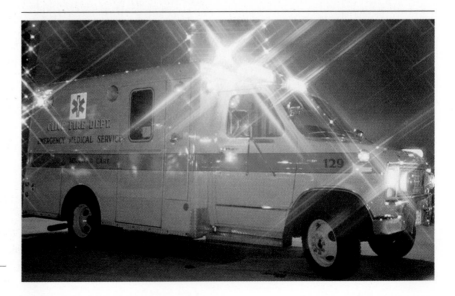

Accidents, Safety and First Aid

Seatbelts Really Save

The night of February 4, 1987, could have been my last. If I hadn't had my seatbelt on, it would have.

It was nearly midnight when I headed home to Santa Clara after visiting a friend in Berkeley. I was very tired from a heavy work schedule. The only thing I remember from that evening was being led to the freeway by my friend. My memory fades out from there. I drove 30 miles (approximately halfway home) when I dozed off. My car plunged off the road and tumbled down a 75 foot embankment through trees, shrubs, and finally a chain-link fence before landing upside down on the road below. According to numerous doctors, my survival was a miracle. During my hospital recovery, one of the paramedics who helped extract me from the car told me, "Grace, you do realize that if you hadn't had your seatbelt on, you wouldn't have survived the accident." I'll always wear my seatbelt and shoulder strap . . . please wear yours, too.

Grace E. Nino

Editor's Note: Grace Nino was still restrained by her lapbelt/shoulder harness when paramedics extracted her unconscious body from her demolished automobile. Her injuries included a fractured neck, concussion, smashed hand, internal injuries, and numerous cuts and bruises. During her recovery, Grace endured considerable pain and discomfort. She wore the halo traction device (pictured below) 24 hours per day for two periods of three months each. Today, she leads a busy life with few medical restrictions on her physical activities.

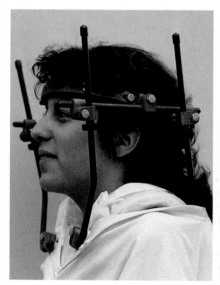

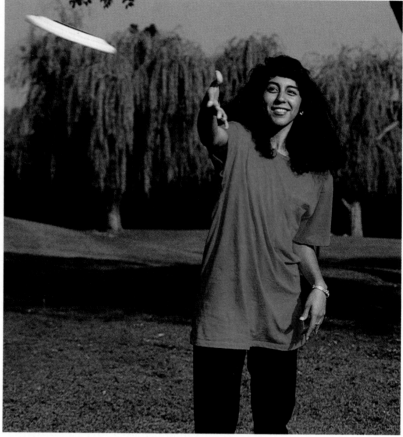

Costs of Accidents

The costs of accidents include loss of wages, medical expenses, insurance administration, and the costs to replace property damaged by fire and other causes (figures are for 1987).

Type of Accident	Cost in Billions
Motor vehicle	$ 64.7
Work	$ 42.4
Home	$ 16.7
Public	$ 11.5
Total	$133.3

Source: *Accident Facts*, 1988 edition, National Safety Council

people's lives. Most accidents are preventable, and if avoided could save millions of dollars and thousands of lives. (The economic costs of accidents are summarized in Table 3.) The complexity of living in today's world demands greater knowledge of the potential hazards that surround us and the development of more effective means of eliminating or compensating for these hazards without creating new ones. The fundamental goal of safety is the prevention of accidents.

Safety Is Everybody's Business

An accident, as defined by safety experts, is the occurrence of a sequence of events that usually result in unintended injury, death, or property damage. A realistic appraisal of accident data clearly shows that few events labeled as "accidents" really result purely from chance. Accidents result from unsafe acts or conditions. Each accident has a cause, although occasionally the cause is difficult to determine, especially when there are no witnesses to a fatal accident.

Safety is the prevention of accidents and the mitigation of personal injury or property damage which may result from accidents. Safety involves a judgment of the acceptability of risk, and risk is the relative probability and severity of harm to human health. Another consideration in avoiding accidents is danger, the relative exposure to a hazard or risk occurring from unsafe acts of people or conditions. For example, three college students—two swimmers and one nonswimmer—paddle a canoe across a deep lake. The hazard of deep water is a danger to all three, but the nonswimmer faces a potentially greater risk, should there be an accident. Due to the inherent instability of a canoe, behavior such as standing up increases the risk of capsizing. An approaching thunderstorm foretells danger and warns the students to take action to avoid the possible dangers of lightning, wind, and waves. To reduce the chance of a serious accident, all three students should wear a life jacket. Safety, therefore, is a highly relative condition that changes due to outside forces, human behavior, and specific actions that increase or decrease the danger factor.

The concept of safety, for most people, is the same as caution or precaution. Your attitude concerning safety is usually a reflection of your outlook on your overall health. Concern for your health means avoiding illness and injury by changing lifestyle actions when necessary. There are numerous ways in which you can incorporate safety into your life.

Risk

As previously defined, risk is the relative probability and severity of harm to human health. The relative probability of a head-on automobile crash is reduced by the design of a divided highway with one-way traffic in each lane. The severity of a head-on crash at high speed is normally much greater than a low speed rear-ender at a stop light. Two ways to reduce

Safety on Things That Roll

Riding cycles/boards/skates—things that roll, whether muscle-powered or motor-powered—can be fun. Riding for recreation and/or transportation requires learning and practicing safety. According to the Consumer Product Safety Commission, over one million people are injured annually in bicycle-related accidents, with over 400,000 requiring hospital emergency room treatment. *Accident Facts*, a publication by the National Safety Council, reports that more than 1,000 cycling fatalities occur annually. The National Electronic Surveillance System's data shows that roller skates cause more injury accidents than any other children's plaything, although tricycles, skateboards, toy cars, trucks, and boats cause their share, too.

In a review of the data regarding cycle accidents, it is readily evident that the major problem is not with the mechanical functioning of equipment, but usually with the unsafe behavior of the rider. Lack of visibility (riding without a pole, flag, rear and wheel spoke reflectors, or a functioning headlight, and not wearing reflectorized clothing) is the main contributing factor. In most crashes between motor vehicles and bicycles, the nearly universal comment by the vehicle operator is, "I didn't see the cyclist." In the United States, cars and trucks are almost always the only vehicles rolling on paved roads; cyclists are not expected. Therefore, the major responsibility for the prevention of motor vehicle and cycle collisions rests with the cyclist.

Although the Uniform Vehicle Code specifies that every person riding a bicycle shall have all rights applicable to the driver of any other vehicle, the responsibility to obey all traffic rules,

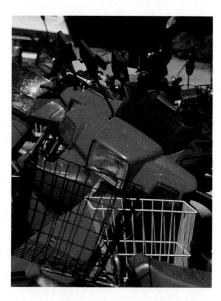

laws, and courtesies accompanies this right. According to "A Motorist's Guide to Bicycle Safety," published by the National Safety Council, four out of five accidents involving a bicycle and a motor vehicle are caused by cyclists who disregard traffic rules.

Obeying traffic laws includes signaling before turning or stopping, yielding to pedestrians and turning motorized vehicles, and stopping at all STOP signs/lights. Because any two-wheeled cycle is unstable, it offers little or no protection from environmental conditions such as rain, wind, or potholes. Wearing protective equipment (a helmet, gloves, and reflectorized material around the left arm, waist, and back of shoes) should be a part of the routine for any ride on the street.

Since an operator's license is not required in order to drive many cycles (bicycles, mopeds, ATV's), the primary responsibility for educating cycle drivers and passengers rests with

parents. The parents are usually responsible for buying the cycle, and the parents will be held liable for damages awarded in a court of law if the riders are under age.

The condition of the bicycle brakes, chainguard, and tires should be checked before every ride. Make sure your bike has the required reflectors and is equipped with functioning lights. To be even safer, riders may affix a five-foot pole with a flag at the top, so vehicles can recognize that a bicycle is just over the hill. Make yourself as visible as possible. When riding a bicycle with hand brakes, apply the rear wheel brake first. Never ride on sidewalks—they are reserved for pedestrians who cannot hear you approaching from the rear. Never assume you know when a pedestrian might stop, turn, or veer to the side. It is illegal and unsafe to hitch a ride by holding onto a rope or the rear of a motorized vehicle. Also, beware of parallel parked car doors opening into your path. When riding on the highway, stay on the right side of the road—go with the flow of traffic, never against—on pavement but near the right edge in single-file. It is recommended that you dismount and walk with pedestrians across busy city traffic intersections. It is dangerous and illegal for more than one person to ride on a single-seat bicycle. The luggage rack on the rear, the basket on the front, the bar between the seat and handle bars on a man's bike, and the handle bars are not meant to carry passengers.

Henry Baughman, HSD
Western Kentucky University

Safety Tips

Motor Vehicle Operators

- Obey posted speed limits.
- Observe traffic signs.
- Follow rules of the road.
- Use lap belt/shoulder harness.
- Do not drive under the influence of alcohol or other drugs.
- Drive defensively.
- Keep vehicle in good repair.

Motorcyclists

- Observe same rules as motor vehicle operators.
- Wear safety helmet and eye protection.
- Wear protective clothing.

Bicyclists

- Follow rules of the road.
- Make yourself visible day and night.
- Use rear view mirror.
- Wear safety helmet.
- Do not ride wearing headphones.

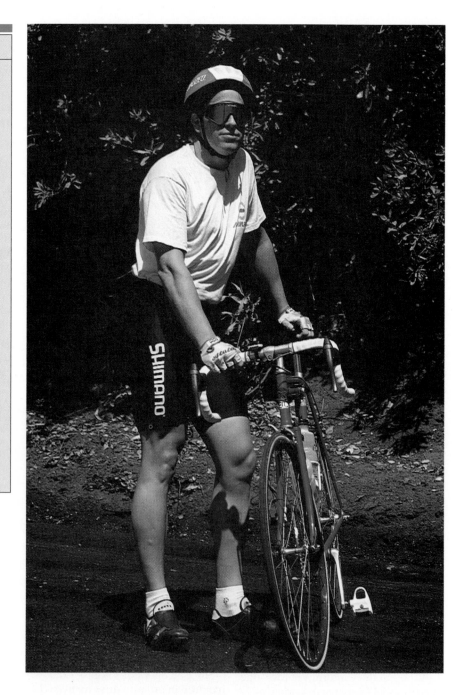

Accidents, Safety and First Aid

CHAPTER 20

the risk of, or prevent, an accident are to eliminate the potential cause or to compensate for the risk by modifying the environment or behavior of people. By using your automobile's lap/shoulder harness, you compensate for some of the risks inherent in motor vehicle operation. By reducing your driving speed to the posted limits, you are modifying your driving behavior. The federal government requires that manufacturers equip autos with certain safety equipment. The decision to use it responsibly rests with the individual driver or passenger.

Risks are an inherent part of life, but not all risks are equal. The risk of injury due to a fall is reduced when one uses a stepladder rather than climbing up the back of a rickety chair. Compensating for risks can be accomplished by one or a combination of three steps:

- Education: becoming aware of hazards, risks, and the potential for accidents, and informing others about accident risks.
- Engineering: modifying the environment (living, working, or leisure areas), utilizing safety equipment, or changing human behavior.
- Enforcement: making sure that people abide by rules and regulations established for accident prevention.

Safety education usually begins at an early age when children learn from their parents. However, much of this process is achieved through avoidance conditioning; that is, a child gets burned by touching a hot stove and avoids the stove thereafter. Learning by experience may be effective, but allowing injuries to occur as a teaching strategy is not ideal. An example of engineering to reduce accidents is the installation of smoke alarms and heat sensors to provide sufficient warning to enable you to escape the perils of fire. Workplace accidents have been substantially reduced by the introduction of safety regulations and their enforcement by such agencies as Occupational Safety and Health Administration (OSHA). In the final analysis, the process of preventing accidents is a daily challenge because physical danger threatens your health in so many ways. The ability to recognize danger, assess risks, and modify behavior are prerequisites to a safe lifestyle.

Safety precautions compete with many high risk lifestyle choices such as experiencing the thrill of adventure (diving off a cliff), yielding to group pressure (overconsumption of alcohol), or saving time (driving at excessive speeds). However, practicing safety need not diminish the fun of an event; this is sometimes given as an excuse for reckless behavior. Exercising caution, using safety equipment, and following other safety guidelines will enable you to enjoy activities with greatly reduced risks and much less chance of injury. Suffering an injury is no fun and may cause much pain and suffering for yourself and others. Preventing accidents is an important aspect of healthy living.

The Air Bag System

The air bag system works during the second collision—the "human" collision. In a frontal crash, the vehicle stops abruptly when it collides with another vehicle or a fixed object. But unrestrained occupants continue moving forward at the same speed that the vehicle was traveling just before the crash took place. The "human" collision occurs when the moving occupants slam into the hard interior surface of the abruptly stopped or nearly stopped vehicle—usually within $\frac{1}{8}$th of a second.

The air bag inflates in less than $\frac{1}{25}$th of a second and diffuses the potentially harmful forces of this collision by functioning as a pillow between the occupants and the vehicle's interior. Head, facial, and chest injuries are minimized.

First Aid

First Aid Defined

First aid is the immediate care given to an injured or ill person. It does not comprise total or even professional medical treatment; rather, it is temporary assistance given to a victim until competent medical care can be administered or the injured person recovers.

A knowledge of first aid may mean the difference between life and death, disability, or permanent injury. Knowledge of first aid skills is important for all members of this society. In an emergency situation, you may be the only person present who can administer first aid.

Legal Aspects of First Aid

In our "suit-happy" society, victims of accidents frequently file law suits as a result of experiencing even the most insignificant of injuries or mental distress. Certainly, negligence is a factor in many cases, but the basis of many claims seems to be a possible healthy out-of-court financial settlement.

When you observe an accident or arrive at the scene, your natural inclination is to help rescue victims and to provide emergency treatment. Fortunately, the legal aspects of first aid provide helpful guidelines and protection for both the victim and you, the provider of aid.

Emergency Response

A timely and appropriate response to an emergency situation can make the difference between life and death. Motor vehicle accidents, fires, and boating mishaps are examples of dramatic events but victims of heart attack, poisoning, electric shock, and accidental falls need assistance as well. The following suggestions are provided to help you be prepared to respond to emergencies.

- *Summon Help* Throughout most of the United States you can dial 911 to summon help in the event of a medical emergency, fire, or incident requiring law enforcement personnel or Coast Guard search and rescue. Make certain you know the emergency assistance telephone number used on your campus.
- *Know the Location of Emergency Resources* A very helpful and available resource is your telephone directory. Most directories provide a 10-to-12 page First Aid and Survival Guide containing helpful action steps in response to a wide range of common emergencies. Familiarize yourself with your telephone book's special emergency section.
  You should know the location of emergency fire fighting equipment and first aid supplies where you live, work, and study. A first aid kit in your home and automobile would be a valuable resource as would a fire extinguisher in your kitchen.

Legal Aspects of First Aid

- No one is duty bound to act by giving aid when no legal duty to do so exists.
- You do have a duty to administer first aid when there is a pre-existing contractual relationship (e.g., parent-child, teacher-student, driver-passenger, and so forth).
- If you do choose to administer first aid, obtain the victim's oral, informed consent prior to giving care, or risk possible charges of technical assault. Consent will be implied if the victim is unconscious.
- Once you begin to administer first aid, you cannot legally stop; you must not abandon the victim after administering first aid until competent or professional help arrives.
- When oral consent to receive first aid is refused by a conscious, rational adult victim, you may not give care. For your own protection, however, attempt to document the interaction and obtain the victim's signature.
- A few states offer protection to the first aid provider under a Good Samaritan law which protects those acting in good faith, without gross negligence, or willful misconduct. Some legal experts believe this law may create a false sense of security for the person administering first aid.

Airway and Rescue Breathing

Basic life support includes determining when a person is unconscious, establishing an open airway, assuring adequate breathing, and providing circulation if it is not present. These maneuvers are called cardiopulmonary resuscitation (CPR). To perform CPR adequately, you will need to take a certified course. This section will focus on establishing an airway, then, if the person does not breathe spontaneously, breathing for him.

Responding When Someone May Be Unconscious

1. Call out for help as you approach victim.
2. Check responsiveness by shaking shoulders and shouting "Are you OK?" This will help to determine whether victim is unconscious.
3. If no response, place victim on flat, firm surface and position self next to victim at about the same level.

Establish Airway

1. Tilt head by placing palm of hand on victim's forehead.
2. Press backward on forehead to open airway.
3. Lift chin by placing fingers of other hand under bony part of jaw on side nearest you until teeth are nearly closed.

Assess Victim's Breathing

1. Lean over victim's head, and look at chest to determine if chest rises and falls.
2. Place ear and cheek near victim's mouth and nose to listen and feel for air movement.
3. If you see or suspect an object blocking the airway, immediately perform the Heimlich maneuver discussed later in this chapter. If no object is suspected, begin mouth-to-mouth breathing.

Perform Rescue Breathing (Adult)

1. Pinch victim's nostrils closed.
2. Fully cover victim's mouth with your own to form mouth-to-mouth seal. Do not let air escape around the seal.
3. Take a deep breath and expel air into the victim's mouth. Take 1 to 1½ seconds to expel breath until you see chest rise.
4. If you do not see the chest rise, reposition airway and try again.
5. Release seal and turn your head to the side.
6. Take fresh breath and watch for victim's chest to fall.
7. Give second breath—repeat cycle every 5 seconds.
8. Check neck pulse for 5 to 10 seconds.
9. If pulse present, continue rescue breaths: one breath every 5 seconds.

Accidents, Safety and First Aid

For Choking—the Heimlich Maneuver

Like CPR, the Heimlich maneuver is an emergency procedure that can save a life. If food or another object lodges in the throat, it can block the airway, making breathing impossible. Such a victim will die in four minutes without help. Use of the Heimlich maneuver has saved more than 10,000 individuals from choking to death. After years of controversy, the American Heart Association and the American Red Cross finally agreed that the Heimlich maneuver is the single best treatment for choking. The new first-aid guidelines for this procedure show you how to save not only others, but also yourself—and what is more important than that?

Dr. Henry J. Heimlich first proposed this treatment back in 1974. He advocated that choking victims be saved by applying pressure with your fist below the rib cage and above the navel. This action forces the diaphragm upward, compresses the air in the lungs, and the food is expelled through force. After this procedure became popular, several experts suggested that back blows be included in the maneuver. New guidelines do not include back blows as part of the procedure.

Steps of the Heimlich Maneuver

Victim Is Standing or Sitting

1. The victim cannot speak or breathe and looks distressed.
2. Tell victim to hold hand to neck if he is choking.

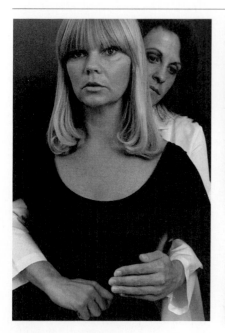 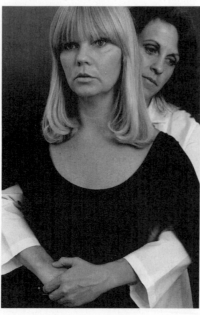 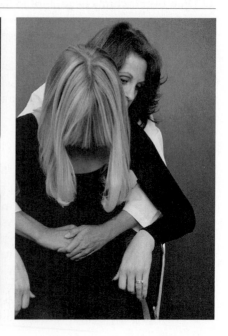

3. Stand behind victim and place hands around victim's waist.
4. Make a fist with one hand and place thumb side against victim's abdomen. It will be slightly above the navel and below rib cage.
5. Place other hand over your fist and press into victim's abdomen with a quick upward thrust
6. Repeat several times—you may have to use a rotating motion of the hands in an upward direction to assist in expelling foreign object.

Victim Is Lying on Back

1. Facing victim, kneel and place your legs astride victim's hips.
2. Place heel of one hand on victim's abdomen slightly above navel and below rib cage. Place other hand on top of first hand.
3. Press into victim's abdomen with a quick upward thrust.
4. Repeat this action several times if necessary.

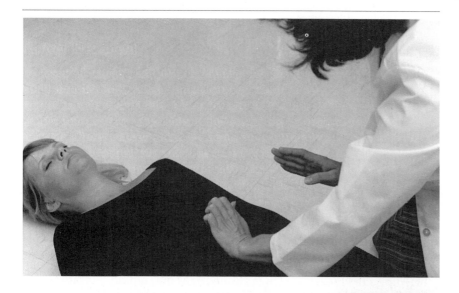

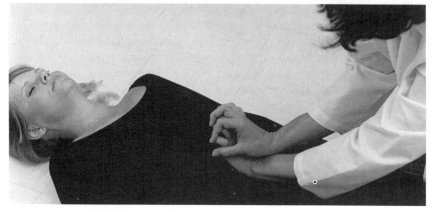

Heimlich Maneuver

Use if:

- Someone is choking, cannot cough or speak, and (perhaps) puts hand to throat.
- Victim has fallen or slumped over and you see or suspect object is blocking throat.
- You yourself are choking.

Your objective is:

- Apply pressure slightly above navel to force object out of throat.

Accidents, Safety and First Aid

If You Are Choking

Read the following material now so that you will be prepared if you are ever choking and you are by yourself. When you are actually choking, it will be too late to read directions.

1. Place your fist below your rib cage and above your navel (same position as if you were performing this on another person).
2. Use your dominant hand over the fist and press quickly upward and inward. Do this repeatedly.

   If this action does not work, try:

1. Placing your abdomen against a firm object—a sink, chair back, or table edge.
2. Use your full weight to press inward and upward—keep repeating until object is expelled.

   A final alternative:

1. Lie down on stairs or over a bed in the face down position so head is lower than feet.
2. Allow gravity to assist the food to fall out.

Bleeding Emergencies

When someone is bleeding profusely, you must take immediate action to preserve life. The rapid loss of more than 25 to 30 percent of the total blood volume may result in death. A person who has had an artery injured will bleed to death within minutes without an intervention.

External Bleeding

If you see external bleeding, do a quick assessment:

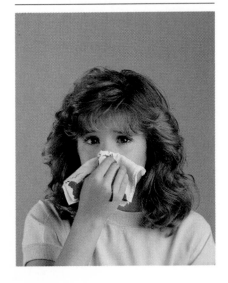

- Identify the exact source of the bleeding. Cut off victim's clothes to find bleeding site if necessary. Significant bright red, rapidly pulsating flow means an arterial injury, an urgent life-threatening condition.
- Assess the extent of the wound.
- Observe general condition of the person—color of skin, temperature and general condition.

   As soon as you complete this assessment, immediately and simultaneously take these emergency actions:

- Identify the artery nearest the top of the bleeding site (see accompanying diagram of arteries).
- Apply direct pressure to the artery using your fingers.
- If a limb is bleeding, raise it above the level of the heart about 30 degrees.

- Maintain direct pressure on the bleeding site or wound for at least five minutes. Do not remove pressure before five minutes, as clot formation has not had an opportunity to stabilize.
- If clean towels or cloths are available, apply these to the wound site, unless the wound contains glass particles.
- Wait for professional help to clean and dress wound.

If bleeding cannot be controlled by pressure and wound involves an arm or leg:

- Apply a tourniquet or tie to the limb. Use a piece of material, folded cloth or wide belt. Do not use a thin tie, rope or wire.
- Place tourniquet above bleeding site as close to the wound as possible and between wound and body.
- Loosen tourniquet every 15–30 minutes for a moment to protect circulation to the limb. Leaving blood supply cut off too long damages the arm or leg.
- If bleeding is severe, raise feet 20 degrees and keep head flat to prevent shock.

Massive Bleeding Is Life-Threatening
- Find bleeding site.
- Apply direct pressure to site.
- Get help.

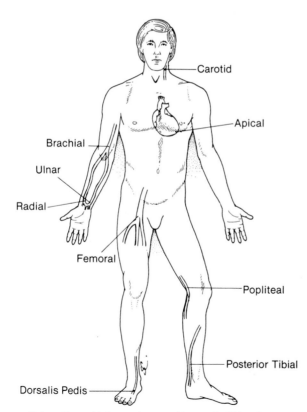

Pulse sites which may be used to control bleeding.

Accidents, Safety and First Aid

Internal Bleeding

Blood vessels, together with the heart, form a closed system. When damage results in leakage, the blood volume drops and the individual goes into shock. Medically, shock does not mean an emotional state, but a specific life-threatening condition in which circulation slows and blood flow is inadequate to provide vital organs with sufficient oxygen. If blood leakage is internal and there is no external sign of blood, you may not be able to identify the problem. Internal bleeding can occur as a result of a car crash, trauma, fall, or any type of accident. If you suspect this condition has occurred, immediately send for help and:

- Restrict the person's activity—the less exertion, the less blood will be lost.
- Elevate the involved body area above the heart, if possible.
- Minimize the person's stress, since any stimulation increases the heart rate.
- Keep the person warm, covered with blankets.

Puncture Wounds

It's a hot day and you and your friends are enjoying walking around campus barefoot. Suddenly one friend gouges her foot on a very long splinter. What should you do? Any sharp object can cause a puncture wound—a nail, tack, metal splinter, thin piece of wood, even a pen. Though most puncture wounds are minor, some are potentially dangerous and may lead to:

- Injury to an artery (loss of blood can be fatal).
- Injury to a tendon or nerve.
- Infection.
- Tetanus, resulting in lockjaw, paralysis and, potentially, death.

If victim has not had a tetanus immunization within five years, or if the wound is from a dirty or rusty object, see health service immediately.

If the wound is minor and the victim has had a tetanus immunization within five years, you may apply home treatment:

- Remove the object from the wound.
- Let wound bleed to clear away foreign material.
- When bleeding stops, wash the wound with water.
- Clean the wound with hydrogen peroxide (3%) or equivalent. Let it bubble and drain. Repeat this procedure.
- Soak wound in water several times a day for three or four days to keep wound clean. Follow with hydrogen peroxide application.
- If severe redness, swelling, pus, noxious smell, or fever occurs, notify your health center.

Broken Bones—Splinting a Fracture

You are backpacking with friends, when someone falls and breaks a leg. Can you splint the fracture until professional help comes? Read over these steps now and be prepared; you probably won't be carrying a first-aid manual with you.

Material Necessary for Splinting

- Splint: a flat piece of wood, strip of bark, pillow, magazine, or blanket.
- Padding: cloth, towels or blankets.
- Strapping materials: cloth, rope or tape.
- If splint material is not available, strap fractured limb to another unfractured body part for support:
- Splint legs together.
- Splint an arm to torso.
- Splint toes or fingers together.

How to Splint a Fracture

1. Control bleeding by applying direct pressure. (See Bleeding Emergencies in this chapter.)
2. Do not try to put a bone back into a wound—this could contaminate the wound.
3. Affix splint.

    - Splint arms in a flexed position
    - For broken wrist, support wrist from the hand to elbow.
    - Splint legs in an extended position. Use stiff object (piece of wood, tree limb, and so forth) along side of the leg.

4. Stabilize joint above and below fracture. Strap injured extremity to splint so that body part is immobile. Strap an arm to torso for support; strap legs together for support.
5. Check pulse and skin color or capillary refill below fracture to be sure blood flow is adequate.
6. Pad joints, bony prominences, and skin areas as much as possible to prevent skin damage. Be sure padding does not affect circulation. (For instance, avoid padding in the underarm.)
7. Elevate extremeties after splinting, and apply an ice pack to relieve pain and prevent swelling.
8. Check victim's circulation frequently by looking at color and temperature of extremity, feeling for pulse, and asking if extremity feels numb.

For Fractures

Your objectives are:

- Immobilize the extremity.
- Protect bone fragments, if present.
- Decrease pain.
- Reduce potential for shock (by minimizing blood loss and by keeping victim warm and calm).

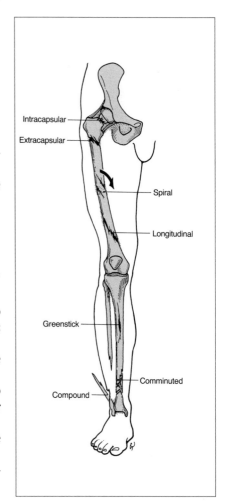

Intracapsular

Extracapsular

Spiral

Longitudinal

Greenstick

Comminuted

Compound

Too Hot or Too Cold— Dangerous Condition

Each person has a "set point," or critical body temperature. Regulatory mechanisms in the body attempt to maintain this temperature. Below the set point, heat-conserving and heat-producing operations are activated; above the level, heat-losing mechanisms are initiated. We have all experienced mild forms of the effects of these processes. If you're cold, you start to shiver, because your body is burning more oxygen and creating motion to warm itself up. If you're hot, you perspire, because your body is releasing fluid to the skin to produce evaporative cooling. The **Physical Fitness** chapter gives information on how to protect yourself from the extremes of temperature.

The body can cope with moderate temperature changes, but extreme heat or cold can result in a medical emergency, sometimes life-threatening. With too little heat (hypothermia), the core temperature of the body drops, causing the heart to beat more slowly. If this condition continues and becomes extreme, the vital organs receive insufficient oxygen, and death results. Too much heat (hyperthermia) is dangerous because the body's heat-regulating mechanism is overloaded. Extremely high body temperatures may cause seizures and other complications.

Hypothermia

Someone overexposed to severe cold is in extreme jeopardy. Vulnerability to cold injury increases if the person is drunk, exhausted, or already suffers from impaired cardiac function. Several key symptoms that can help you recognize hypothermia are:

- Shivering (increases oxygen consumption)
- Cold extremities—loss of control or movement in fingers
- Lethargy or extreme tiredness
- Slowed breathing and heartbeat
- Mental confusion
- Numbness and loss of feeling in extremities

If you identify that a person is suffering from overexposure to cold in any of these forms, immediate intervention is important:

- If possible, give a complete warm bath and oil the skin; massage skin frequently and dry skin thoroughly. (Old methods of slow warming or rubbing with snow are contraindicated.)
- Give victim hot drinks to warm internally. Do not give alcohol or caffeine, or allow the victim to smoke tobacco.
- Wrap victim in blankets or sleeping bag next to a warm body.
- Use a heating pad and/or hot water bottles to maintain warmth.
- Warning: Since the skin is partially anesthetized, the temperature of warming fluids or pads should not exceed 43° C or 110° F; otherwise, the skin may burn.

- Find professional help or a hospital as soon as possible to prevent complications.

Hyperthermia

Heat disorders are of several types: heat stroke or sunstroke, heat exhaustion, and heat cramps. Though these major conditions usually stem from prolonged exertion or exposure to high temperatures and humidity, they may have very different physical effects.

Heat Stroke or Sunstroke

Heat stroke or sunstroke is basically caused by failure to lose heat. This condition has an abrupt onset and is a serious emergency. It is important to notice the signs and symptoms immediately, so intervention can begin swiftly.

- Headache, dizziness and fatigue may occur first.
- Absence of sweating and a hot, dry, flushed skin are key signs.
- Rapid pulse and respirations usually increase.
- Disorientation may precede unconsciousness.

Once this condition is recognized, you must make vigorous efforts to decrease the temperature. Call for professional care as soon as possible. Until medical personnel take over, immediately institute the following procedure:

- Immerse victim in a cool bath or lake, or cool water from hose. If you are not near any body of water, use cool water on cloths and fan. The objective is to reduce the temperature, but not allow it to fall below 101° F. (Otherwise, the victim will go into hypothermia.)

Heat Exhaustion

Heat exhaustion results from excessive fluid loss. This condition does not have a rapid onset, so there is adequate warning, if you are aware of the signs and symptoms to look for:

- Gradual fatigue and weakness
- Anxiety and nausea
- Profuse sweating with cold, clammy, pale skin
- Slow, weak pulse
- Confusion, with some degree of disorientation

Because the primary cause of heat exhaustion is fluid loss, the treatment is to restore the normal blood volume as soon as possible.

- Have the person lie down flat or with feet slightly elevated.
- Offer small amounts of fluid (slightly salty if possible) every few minutes to gradually reverse dehydration.

Heat Cramps

Still another form of heat injury is heat cramps, which result from excessive sweating and the resultant loss of sodium chloride (salt). This condition is usually experienced by people doing strenuous activity in hot weather. The signs and symptoms are:

- Abrupt onset, with muscles in the legs and arms affected first
- Victim complains of cramping pain in the muscles
- Vital signs usually normal

If you experience heat cramps, drink fluids with a high salt content or eat salty foods. The problem will resolve after ingestion of enough salt.

Head Injuries

A head injury is caused by a trauma to the skull. It can result from an auto accident, fall, assault, or blow from a blunt object. Such an injury can result in a concussion, bruising of the brain, hemorrhage, or fracture of the skull. Of these, the most serious concern is bleeding inside the skull. As a non-medical person, you may not be able to tell whether a head injury is serious. If you even *suspect* that head injury is more than a minor bump on the head, obtain professional help as soon as possible. For a minor bump involving a bruise but no bleeding, apply ice to decrease swelling. In all other circumstances, here are some guidelines for applying emergency medical treatment while awaiting professional assistance:

- If there is bleeding from the scalp:

  Apply moderate, even pressure to wound; do not press too hard, because you cannot tell whether the scalp has been fractured.

  Observe for a change in consciousness (headache, pupil changes, nausea and vomiting) and report these changes to available medical personnel.

- If there is a severe head injury:

  Suspect a spinal cord injury; stabilize the victim against any movement.

  If there is bleeding from eyes, ears or mouth, or drainage from the nose or ear, do not clean but get help as soon as possible.

  Keep victim warm and calm. Tell victim not to blow nose.

If the victim is released after receiving medical assistance, check him or her every two hours. If there is a change in alertness, pupil size (they will be unequal after the injury), or severe vomiting, notify the physician again immediately.

Seizures

Seizures (also called convulsions) are a frightening sight if you have not been exposed to this condition. You may see the victim jerking uncontrollably, the eyes may roll up into the head, and breathing may become labored, with frothing at the mouth. In such circumstances, it is better to do almost nothing; just allow the seizure to run its course and protect the victim from injury.

- Never force an object between the victim's teeth; you may injure the person or yourself.
- Assist the victim to the floor if he or she is falling.
- Turn victim on his or her side to protect airway.
- Remove objects that may hurt the victim as he thrashes around (desk, chair, and so forth).
- Call for help.
- Observe the progression or pattern of the seizure so that you can report to a professional. (Knowledge of how the seizure progresses—from body part to body part—assists the physician in making an accurate diagnosis.)

Following the seizure:

- Check victim's breathing. If it has stopped or is very weak, give mouth-to-mouth breathing.
- If the victim is wearing a Medic Alert bracelet, check to see if there are instructions as to care.
- Remain with victim following a seizure; he may or may not be conscious. Keep warm and continue to check breathing.
- When victim is able to move and appears conscious, get medical follow-up care.

Poisoning

You may think of poisoning emergencies as accidents that happen to toddlers. Most such accidents do happen to small children, who are particularly vulnerable to poisons because they like to explore new things by putting them in their mouth. However, the college environment presents significant poison hazards. These include chemicals in science labs and art studios, ingestion of toxic wild plants, overdoses of medication, and alcohol and drug overdoses. Many people attempt suicide by taking excessive amounts of medications or other poisons. Any attempted suicide, whether or not it causes immediate significant physical damage, is an emergency condition—seek professional help immediately. For further information, see the **Depression and Suicide** chapter.

> ### For Poisoning
>
> Your objectives are:
>
> - Halt or blunt the action of the poison.
> - Get professional help.
> - Induce vomiting *only* on advice of medical professionals.

The American Association of Poison Control Centers estimates that more than 2 million people per year experience accidental poisoning from solids or liquids.

Initial Emergency Actions

Poisons may be inhaled, on the skin, in the eye, or swallowed. Whatever the type, your first action is to halt or blunt the action of the poison. The American College of Emergency Physicians and American Association of Poison Control Centers recommend these emergency steps:

Inhaled Poison Immediately get the person to fresh air. Avoid breathing fumes. Open doors and windows wide. If victim is not breathing, start artificial respiration.

Poison on the Skin Remove contaminated clothing and flood skin with water for 10 minutes. Then wash gently with soap and water and rinse. Brush or scrape dry chemicals from the skin; do not flood with water.

Poison in the Eye Flood the eye with lukewarm (not hot) water poured from a large glass 2 or 3 inches from the eye. Repeat for 15 minutes. Have victim blink as much as possible while flooding the eye. Do not force the eyelid open.

Swallowed Poison Maintain an open airway. If possible, identify the poison ingested, then call the local poison control center for advice on what action to take. Induce vomiting according to instructions. Vomiting should not be induced when corrosives or petroleum products have been ingested.

Getting Professional Help Fast

1. As soon as you have taken the emergency actions just recommended, call for professional help. (If possible, get someone else to make the call immediately.) If the victim is having an acute medical problem, such as unconsciousness, seizures, or acid burns, first call 911 or other appropriate number for paramedic assistance. Then call poison control center for further advice. Whether the situation is acute or moderate, accidental or deliberate, call the poison control center.
2. Try to identify what poison is involved. Look for clues if necessary. Save any vomit for emergency personnel to take for analysis.
3. Follow instructions of poison control center as to counteragents.
4. Induce vomiting only on advice of poison control center. Syrup of ipecac is effective to induce vomiting. Currently, activated charcoal is preferred because it absorbs the poison.

Drug and/or Alcohol Overdose

A drug or alcohol overdose is a type of poisoning, and one that can lead to death. It is important to recognize this condition as soon as possible, so you can facilitate an immediate intervention. Call for professional assistance immediately. Until help arrives:

- Check victim's breathing; if it has stopped or is very weak, give mouth-to-mouth breathing.
- Do not give anything by mouth; wait for professional help.
- Keep victim warm.
- Alcohol and PCP poisoning can result in violent behavior, so be watchful if victim is "coming to."

For more information, see overdose discussion in the **Alcohol and Other Drugs** chapter. If the overdose may have been attempted suicide, seek professional counseling immediately.

Burns

When a person is severely burned, the faster the intervention, the more the damage is controlled. Obtain help immediately. Taking these steps while waiting for professional help may limit the extent of injury:

- Immediately put limb or body part in cool water (sink, shower, tub, hose) to stop the burning process. Keep under cool water for 20 minutes (for 3rd degree burns do not do this—get help).
- Do not put butter or ointments on burned area. (They hold heat in, retarding cooling process, and increase possibility of infection.)
- Cover burned area with sterile dressing or clean cloth to transport.
- Check victim's breathing. If it has stopped or is very weak, give mouth-to-mouth breathing.
- Do not remove clothing from severely burned area unless burn is from caustic material.

For Burns

Your objectives are:
- Cut off oxygen to stop burning process.
- Minimize life-threatening consequences of extensive burns.
- Prevent infection.

If you are treating a skin burn on a small area and ice cubes are available, put about ten ice cubes in a bucket of water. Immerse burned area in bucket. Remove and reimmerse injured area in iced water as comfort indicates.

Seeking Professional Help

By their very nature, accidents sometimes involve life-threatening situations requiring immediate professional medical attention. Even less serious accidents may result in injuries that will heal more quickly if treated by health professionals.

When to Seek Help

Even if you have administered first aid and improved the patient's condition, sometimes only a trained medical professional can discern repercussions from trauma. Seek such help immediately if you have encountered:

- No pulse
- No breathing
- Choking
- Bleeding, arterial or extensive venous
- Broken bones
- Poisoning
- Shock
- Alcohol or drug overdose
- Overexposure to heat or cold
- Head injury that does not seem minor

Although you believe an accident or injury is not life threatening, call your student health center or an emergency clinic to find out if the problem should receive further attention.

Beyond the Text

1. Drunk driving laws in the U.S. are criticized as being rather ineffective when you consider the DWI accident statistics. What should be done to keep drinking drivers from killing and injuring themselves and others?

2. Respond to the statement: Nobody can make the world a completely safe place. In the end, you're on your own to protect yourself.

3. Your roommate blows a fuse whenever she turns on her electric popcorn popper. What are your risks and what should you do?

4. All states in the U.S. require automobile drivers to be licensed. What would be the advantages and disadvantages of extending similar requirements to operators of power boats, jet skis, and ATVs?

5. You are first on the scene of a two-vehicle crash in which several people appear to be injured. What are the first actions you would take?

6. Respond to the following statement: Accidents involving boats are most frequently caused by sailboats that can't get out of the way of power boats.

Supplemental Readings

First Aid Essentials by Alton Thygerson. Boston: Jones and Bartlett Publishers, Inc., 1989. Provides clear and concise instructions for responding to a wide variety of injuries. Includes helpful flow charts and diagrams. Endorsed by the National Safety Council.

Handbook of First-Aid and Emergency Care by the American Medical Association. New York: Random House, 1980. Provides information on how to prepare for medical emergencies (first-aid techniques you can practice), discusses life-threatening situations and how to cope with them, and provides a comprehensive alphabetical quick-reference list of injuries and illnesses.

Save a Life: The ABC's of CPR by Barbara W. Trefz. Park Ridge, IL: The American Academy of Orthopaedic Surgeons, 1988. Written by a certified American Heart Association Basic Life Support Instructor, this brief but very informative book provides general background information on how and why cardiopulmonary resuscitation (CPR) is vital to saving lives. The author cautions that the book is not a substitute for successful completion of an authorized CPR course.

Key Terms Defined

accident   that occurrence in a sequence of events that usually produces unintended injury, death, or property damage; two major categories of accidents are fatal (resulting in the death of the victim) and injury

CPR   acronym for cardiopulmonary resuscitation, an emergency treatment given to revive victims of heart attacks, drowning, and other life-threatening incidents

disabling injury   any degree of partial or total disability beyond the day of the accident, including permanent disability

DWI   acronym for driving while intoxicated; also called DUI, or driving under the influence; refers to operating a motor vehicle when one's blood-alcohol content exceeds the legally allowed level

first aid   emergency treatment administered to injured or sick persons before professional medical aid is available

injury   physical harm to the body, resulting from an exchange, usually acute, of mechanical, chemical, thermal, or other environmental energy that exceeds the body's tolerance

risk   the danger or probability of suffering harm or loss, such as from an accident

safety   the condition of being safe; freedom from risk of injury

suffocate   to impair or cut off the supply of oxygen for respiration

Environmental Health Issues

The decade of the 1990s will be a crucial period for progress on local, national, and global environmental issues. From getting rid of our daily trash to patching holes in the ozone layer, environmental problems are major topics of public and political attention.

This chapter covers a wide range of environmental health issues: air, water, and land pollution, radiation health hazards, and the global issues of the greenhouse effect and the ozone layer. As an individual you will be affected by legislation and regulation, and you will be required to help finance environmental programs through your tax payments.

This chapter will help you become informed concerning the issues and provide you with suggestions on how you can contribute to solving them.

Key Terms

Acid rain

Asbestos

Biodegradable

Carcinogen

Composting

Environmental Protection
   Agency

Greenhouse effect

Industrial Revolution

Ozone

Ozone layer

PCBs (polychlorinated
   byphenyls)

Pesticide

Pollutant

Radon gas

Smog

Toxics

Contents

Historical Perspective

The Rise of Environmental Pollution

For thousands of years, the earth's land masses, oceans, and surrounding atmosphere maintained a relatively stable ecological balance. The atmosphere readily absorbed smoke from natural fires, gases from volcanos, and dust from wind storms without lasting negative effects. Biodegradable wastes from animal and plant life were flushed by streams and rivers into lakes and oceans. But changes in human behavior upset this environmental balance. The Industrial Revolution of the 1800s changed the relationship between mankind and the environment. No longer could the environment readily assimilate and disperse the waste products generated by industry. The United States was blessed with seemingly endless resources, a hardworking population, and an appetite for economic gain. Settlers exploited our natural resources, especially timber and minerals, with little consideration given to conservation or restoration. The widespread use of fossil fuels—coal, coke, and later petroleum—to support economic growth and development resulted in new sources of atmospheric pollution. Waterways served as industrial pollution sinks, and the abundant land was used as a convenient, inexpensive place to dump industrial, commercial, and household wastes.

Following World War II, the United States experienced significant growth in population, industry, and prosperity. Environmental pollution

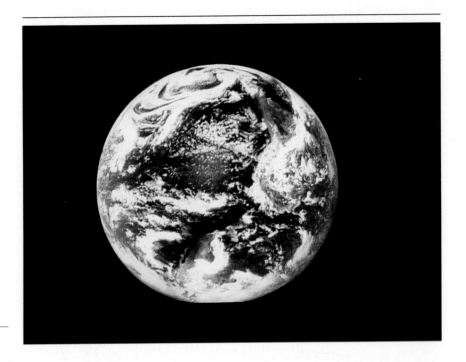

continued relatively unchecked; by the mid-1960s, it had reached staggering proportions and posed major health hazards to a large segment of the American population.

Responding to Environmental Problems

Response to air pollution in the United States began in the late 1800s when a few large cities passed laws to regulate smoke emissions. People could see that smoke-filled skies related to such problems as lack of visibility and abundance of soot. Society had very limited understanding of potential health hazards at that time. Not until after World War II did air pollution gain recognition as a serious problem. Killer fogs in Donora, Pennsylvania (1948), and in London (1952) focused public and government attention on the potential health hazards of air pollution. In 1963, Congress authorized studies of the effects of air pollution. The Clean Air Act of 1970 defined a comprehensive approach to regulating specific pollutants, particularly those resulting from automobile emissions. By this time, the contamination of lakes and streams had reached alarming levels. In 1972, Congress passed the Clean Water Act "to restore and maintain the chemical, physical, and biological integrity of the nation's waters." Subsequent legislation included the Safe Drinking Water Act of 1974 and the Water Quality Act of 1987. The potential health hazard of unsanitary land dumps was recognized and addressed by Congress with the enactment of the Resources Recovery Act of 1970.

The Clean Air Act of 1970

This legislation set maximum levels for specific pollutants: lead, sulfur dioxide, nitrogen dioxides, carbon monoxide, ozone, and particulate matter such as dirt, dust, and soot. Specific maximum levels were not established for 320 potentially toxic chemicals. The EPA was charged with assessing their risks and then drafting rules for controlling each one. By 1989, the agency had completed regulations on seven toxic chemicals. An EPA spokesman said in March 1989, "Little is known about the health effects of most of the chemicals surveyed." This aspect of pollution control—assessing health risks and balancing risks with benefits—is likely to be a major environmental issue of the 1990s.

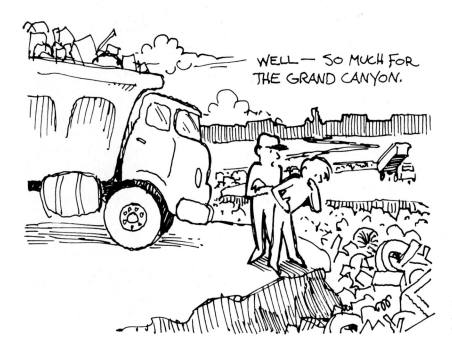

WELL — SO MUCH FOR THE GRAND CANYON.

Environmental Health Issues

> The United States is going to undergo significant changes in the years to come. Managing our environment will require major investments. It will require changes in behavior. It will require some reasonably significant changes in our lifestyles.
>
> William K. Reilly, Administrator,
> U.S. Environmental Protection
> Agency

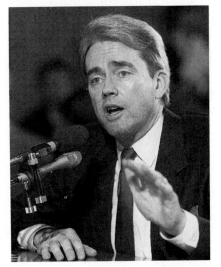

The Environmental Protection Agency (EPA), established by Congress in 1970, coordinates federal, state, and local enforcement of existing laws and addresses problems for which new programs or legislation may be needed on a national level. In response to newly defined problems such as acid rain, the global greenhouse effect, and depletion of the stratospheric ozone layer, the EPA coordinates the nation's international environmental protection programs.

Legislation provides the legal tools, and the EPA, with state and local governments, implements programs to control pollution and to assure that standards are met on a continuing basis. Major industrial polluters of the environment have spent billions of dollars to meet EPA standards. Purchasers of automobiles have paid additional costs for pollution control devices on new cars. Federal and state governments have budgeted billions of dollars for cleanup projects and new facilities to remove wastes before they become pollutants.

Some organizations argue that these existing regulations provide adequate protection; others lobby for more stringent measures. In spite of political and economic pressure from all sides, scientists cannot provide definitive evaluations of environment safety and risk for every chemical or process with which we deal. Certainly they have documented well the potential health hazards of any of these pollutants in their pure forms.

For example, asbestos is a known cancer agent, concentrated ammonia fumes can be fatal, a strong dose of chloroform will anesthetize you permanently, and sufficient lead in your system will damage your brain. The health threat varies greatly from substance to substance, and researchers must evaluate each chemical compound for its own characteristics and effects, as well as its effect in combination with other substances. Scientists are not yet able to accurately predict the long-term effects of human exposure to many potentially harmful substances. Some of the variables that analysts must consider include the following:

- Most toxicology studies are conducted on animals, and projecting their results on humans is very difficult.
- Certain substances, though relatively harmless in small doses, accumulate in the body's fatty tissue until sufficient concentrations are present to cause cancer or other illnesses.
- Prevailing winds may carry pollutants many miles from industrial facilities, rendering studies of local workers and neighboring residents meaningless.
- Some chemicals break down quickly in water, but others settle as sediment; the effects of the latter on waterlife may be difficult to analyze.
- Certain chemicals are relatively harmless alone, but when mixed with other chemicals, they react to create a toxic substance.

Evaluating Early Progress

The EPA points out that, although many urban areas do not yet meet EPA quality standards, the air in most of our cities today is far cleaner and healthier than it was in the 1960s. Thousands of miles of rivers and streams and thousands of acres of lakes have been restored and protected for swimming, boating, and fishing. However, many of our ocean beaches are still polluted. Steps have been taken to improve the management of toxic chemicals and other hazardous wastes. Some specific examples of early progress include the following:

- The levels of hazardous chemicals in urban air have been substantially reduced since 1977; lead levels are down 87 percent, sulfur dioxide has been lowered by 37 percent, and ozone and carbon monoxide levels are down by 13 percent and 32 percent, respectively.
- Municipal sewage treatment has improved so that pollution of rivers, streams, and bays has been dramatically reduced.
- Government agencies established disposal procedures for many hazardous wastes and initiated a major program to clean up existing toxic waste sites.
- The EPA terminated or restricted use of many dangerous pesticides, such as DDT, and hazardous materials, such as asbestos.

As summarized at the end of this chapter under the heading "Environmental Health Issues of the 1990s," the challenges ahead are formidable. More than 60 cities still do not meet federal air quality standards for ozone; hundreds of communities do not comply with requirements for more effective treatment of municipal sewage; disposal of urban garbage is a growing problem; several thousand hazardous chemical waste sites must be cleaned up; and issues of unhealthy indoor pollution must be addressed. In addition to the continuing domestic problems, the nation must deal with the potential health consequences of acid rain, global warming, and depletion of the ozone layer, each of which has international significance.

Air Pollution—A Continuing Problem

As the pace of industrialization, urbanization, and automobile use expanded, scientists and the public began to notice problems—smog, dirty air, and health complications. Beginning in the 1960s, research began to show that air pollution lead to several problems: decreased visibility and eye irritation, respiratory problems, and, in some cases, serious illness or death.

Industrial and commercial firms, utilities and transportation companies, and individuals cause a wide spectrum of substances to be released into the atmosphere. Some vapors, such as steam, are relatively harmless, but others, such as carbon monoxide, are potentially hazardous to one's health.

Air pollution results from the release of gases and particles into the atmosphere. Natural sources of air pollution include volcanos, forest and grass fires, and dust storms. However, the human race has added sub-

Cancer Risk Chemicals

Following is a list of the nine chemicals—and their common industrial usage—cited as cancer risks by the Environmental Protection Agency:

- *Arsenic*: a metal used in a wide variety of pesticides, medical products.
- *Butadiene*: an odorless gas used in production of synthetic rubber.
- *Chloroform*: a gas—odorless in small quantities—that is a common byproduct of pulp and paper production. It was a common anesthetic until linked to liver damage.
- *Carbon tetrachloride*: a widely used chemical ingredient and cleansing agent; odorless in small quantities.
- *Chromium*: a metal with a wide variety of industrial applications.
- *Ethylene dichloride*: a common solvent and a gasoline additive; used by the pharmaceutical industry.
- *Ethylene oxide*: a common industrial sterilizer.
- *Methylene chloride*: a volatile liquid solvent. Common uses: degreaser, paint remover.
- *Vinylidene chloride*: used to make latex for carpet backing, paints.

stantially to these natural phenomena by using the atmosphere as a giant dumping space for industrial and commercial waste products as well as the receptor for exhaust emissions from gasoline-powered engines.

Standards were set to protect human health, crops, livestock, vegetation, buildings, and visibility. Establishing the standards and continued monitoring of their levels is a complicated and expensive process.

Breathing Unhealthy Air

A serious effect of air pollution is its harmful impact on human health. Gases and particulates in the air can burn your eyes and irritate your nasal passages, lungs, and other parts of your respiratory system. Polluted air is potentially hazardous to the very young, the elderly, and to people who suffer from allergies or respiratory diseases, such as asthma, bronchitis, and emphysema. Health experts generally agree that polluted air may be a causal factor in lung cancer, birth defects, and certain heart problems. The EPA has estimated that toxic air pollution accounts for approximately 2,000 new cases of cancer each year. Carbon monoxide, a common pollutant in areas of heavy motor vehicle congestion, is potentially harmful to anyone, but it has particularly severe health consequences for people with heart and lung problems. Research studies indicate that high concentrations of ozone are potentially hazardous and that certain individuals, especially children, are much more vulnerable than others to its effects.

Air pollution is also harmful to plant life, and in certain regions of the nation, forests and vegetable gardens have experienced considerable damage from poison gases in the air. Unpleasant odors and reduced visibility are additional effects of air pollution. People living or working near an oil refinery, paper mill, or certain types of chemical plants may be subjected to odors of which the effect is more unpleasant than health-threatening. The inability to see surrounding hills or mountains deprives people of gaining enjoyment from their natural surroundings. The threat to health as well as odor and reduced visibility contribute to the stress of daily living for all people subjected to air pollution.

Sources of Air Pollution

Under provisions of the Clean Air Act of 1970, the EPA set national ambient air quality standards for "criteria" pollutants, substances commonly found throughout the country that posed the greatest overall threats to air quality: ozone, carbon monoxide, airborne particulates, sulfur dioxide, lead, and nitrogen oxides.

The Clean Air Act also required the EPA to analyze and determine the potential health hazards for another group of airborne toxics, termed "hazardous" pollutants because they are known to cause death or serious illness. Standards have been issued for asbestos, beryllium, mercury, vinyl chloride, and other chemicals. These air pollutants, and their potential health hazards, are listed in an accompanying table.

The EPA

The Environmental Protection Agency (EPA) was established in 1970 by Congress. Currently, the EPA employs 15,000 personnel and operates with a $5 billion budget. Appointed in late 1988 by President George Bush, William K. Reilly became EPA administrator on February 8, 1989.

Health Effects of the Regulated Air Pollutants

Criteria Pollutants	Health Concerns
Ozone	Respiratory tract problems such as difficult breathing and reduced lung function. Asthma, eye irritation, nasal congestion, reduced resistance to infection, and possibly premature aging of lung tissue.
Particulate Matter	Eye and throat irritation, bronchitis, lung damage, and impaired visibility.
Carbon Monoxide	Ability of blood to carry oxygen impaired. Cardiovascular, nervous, and pulmonary systems affected.
Sulfur Dioxide	Respiratory tract problems; permanent harm to lung tissue.
Lead	Retardation and brain damage, especially in children.
Nitrogen Dioxide	Respiratory illness and lung damage.
Hazardous Air Pollutants	
Asbestos	A variety of lung diseases, particularly lung cancer.
Beryllium	Primary lung disease, although also affects liver, spleen, kidneys, and lymph glands.
Mercury	Several areas of the brain as well as the kidneys and bowels affected.
Vinyl Chloride	Lung and liver cancer.
Arsenic	Causes cancer.
Radionuclides	Causes cancer.
Benzene	Lukemia
Coke Oven Emissions	Respiratory cancer.

Source: Environmental Protection Agency

Ozone and Carbon Monoxide Sunlight can trigger chemical reactions between naturally occurring atmospheric gases, volatile organic compounds (VOC's), and nitrogen oxides to produce ozone, the major component of smog. Visible as a yellowish-brown haze, smog is one of our more tenacious and potentially hazardous air quality problems. Petroleum refineries, gas stations, and motor vehicles are the main sources of VOC's and nitrogen oxides. Carbon monoxide, a colorless, odorless gas also primarily comes from motor vehicles; other sources are wood stoves, incinerators, and certain industrial processes.

Progress has been made in many geographic regions to reduce ozone and carbon dioxide levels. Because motor vehicles are a major source of

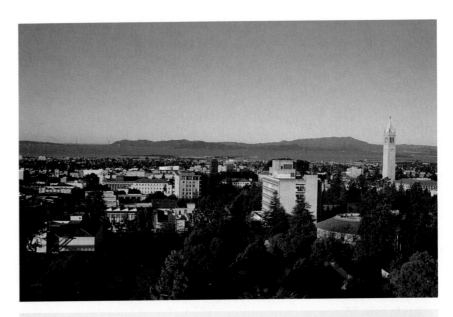

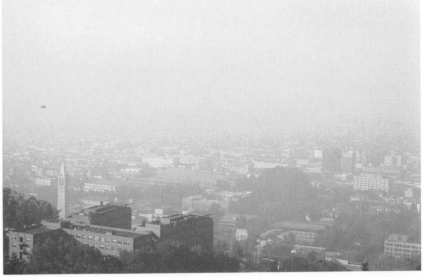

airborne wastes causing smog (nearly 40 percent), the government requires auto emission control devices. Under the Federal Motor Vehicle Control Program, the EPA sets national standards that automobile manufacturers must meet. State and local governments operate vehicle inspection programs to test auto tailpipe emission levels and to ensure that vehicle owners comply with emission control equipment requirements.

There are 55 percent more autos on the road today than there were in 1970 when the Clean Air Act was passed, and they are being driven more miles per year than ever before. The EPA estimates that 20 to 30 million

Air Quality—Best and Worst

Urban areas exceeding EPA standards for ozone and carbon monoxide by the most and least number of days in 1988.

| City | Number of Days Exceeding EPA Standards—1988 | |
	Ozone	Carbon Monoxide
Bakersfield, CA	54	—
Chicago, IL	16	—
Chico, CA	—	2
Colorado Springs, CO	—	2
Great Falls, MT	—	1
Greeley, CO	—	1
Jacksonville, FL	1	—
Las Vegas, NV	—	26
Los Angeles, CA	148	51
New York, NY	18	26
Philadelphia, PA	18	—
Spokane, WA	—	37
Steubenville, OH	24	31
Yakima, WA	—	1

ozone-sensitive people live in urban areas where ozone levels are 25 percent or more above the current health standard. Los Angeles is identified as having the worst air quality; contributing factors include the number of automobiles in the region, extremely congested freeways, high proportion of sunny days, lack of pollutant dissipating breezes, and a frequent inversion layer that keeps gases from escaping into the atmosphere. The four geographic regions most seriously affected by ozone are California, the Northeast, the Texas Gulf Coast, and the Chicago-Milwaukee area. The accompanying table lists cities that exceeded EPA standards for ozone and carbon monoxide by the greatest number of days in 1988. Several cities with the best air quality are listed as well.

Airborne Particulates   The most visible air pollution (other than smog) consists of smoke, dust, aerosols, and other particles. Major sources of particulates include steel mills, cement plants, electrical generating facilities, and diesel engines. In urban areas, demolition and construction create large quantities of dust. Wood stoves and fireplaces create particulate problems in populated regions where burning wood has become popular.

The EPA initially issued air quality standards in 1971 and later amended them in 1987. To comply, many industrial facilities installed pollution control devices such as filters. The ban on backyard burning by municipalities creates another waste disposal problem as increased amounts of leaves and yard trim threaten to overload many landfill dump sites. Forest and agriculture burning is now a political issue in states such as Oregon where economic dependence on the timber industry, which burns much of its wastes, clashes with the environmental objective of maintaining clean air. Many areas exceeding EPA standards are in the western states, where windblown dust is a natural, uncontrollable phenomenon.

Sulfur Dioxide   The burning of coal and fuel oil results in release of sulfur dioxide into the atmosphere. Today's primary sources of sulfur dioxide are electric power plants, accounting for two thirds of all emissions on a national basis. Coal-burning facilities account for 95 percent of all power plant emissions. Other sulfur dioxide pollution sources include pulp and paper mills, refineries, steel and chemical plants, and smelters. On a national level, efforts to control sulfur dioxide (by shifting to fuels with lower sulfur content and installing smokestack scrubbers) have resulted in a 37 percent decrease in ambient levels between 1977 and 1986.

However, recent recognition of and publicity surrounding the acid rain problem illustrates the complex nature of environmental pollution. Tall

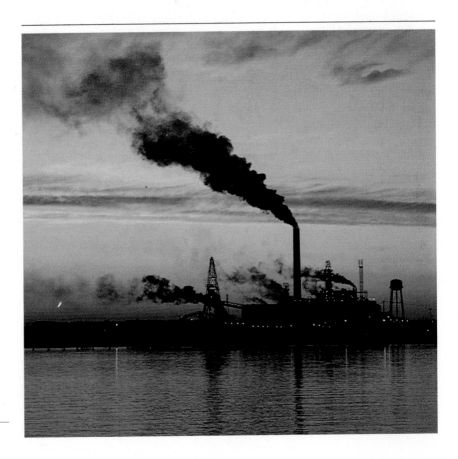

Industrial Pollution Survey

In December 1984, a toxic chemical leak from a United States-owned factory in Bhopal, India, killed 3,000 people and injured 50,000 others. Concerned about possible consequences of a similar episode in the United States, Congress ordered the EPA to conduct a survey of industrial toxic waste. Reports from 19,278 factories enabled analysts to pinpoint the source and amount of 328 toxic chemicals. The EPA concluded that 7 billion pounds of toxic chemicals were released into the air, water, and land during 1987. When considering this project, it is important to note that the above total did not include air pollution caused by motor vehicles nor did it account for several major sources of water pollution, such as farmland water runoff.

The EPA survey identified the leading producers of toxic chemical wastes as Texas, Louisiana, Indiana, Ohio, Florida, and Tennessee. States with the lowest amounts to report were Hawaii, North Dakota, South Dakota, and Vermont. Manufacturers of chemicals and paper were the nation's major producers of toxic chemical waste; both industries dispose of their toxic wastes into rivers and other waterways. Printing companies and furniture manufacturers dispose of 85 percent of their chemical wastes (mostly solvents) into the air while food processors and leather converters usually utilize the public sewage system.

Upon analyzing the EPA data, the National Resources Defense Council estimated that 361 million pounds of cancer-causing chemicals are pumped into the air yearly; these include asbestos (building materials), chloroform (fumigants, insecticides), and formaldehyde (fertilizers).

When the EPA survey was released in mid-1989, the results received widespread media coverage that substantially increased public awareness concerning the problems of toxic waste. President Bush announced plans to bolster the role of the federal government in establishing, monitoring, and enforcing stricter pollution standards. The longer-term benefits of this project will be determined during the early 1990s when follow-up actions as proposed by the 1989 amendments to the Clean Air Act will have taken effect.

---

smokestacks from power-generating plants in the upper Midwest carry sulfur dioxide emissions hundreds of miles eastward, where this chemical becomes a chief contributor to acid rain, snow, or fog. Its effects include killing of fish in lakes and streams and defoliation of forests. Lakes have shown high acid levels in the Upper Peninsula of Michigan and the Adirondacks of New York.

Because the U.S.-originated sulfur dioxide has damaged areas of southern Canada, the problem has taken on an international dimension. Producers of high-sulfur coal in West Virginia and Pennsylvania are fearful about the economic impact of new emission standards, because the most direct way to restrict emission would be to shift from high- to low-sulfur coal. Political, economic, and social factors, as well as the basic objective of reducing health hazards to humans, animal life, and vegetation, will play important roles in the process of solving this complicated problem.

Airborne Toxics   Waste products containing toxic chemicals pour into the atmosphere via smokestacks. Toxic pollutants are recognized as a serious problem that early environmental protection programs did not initially address because of the difficulty in accurately detecting their

Environmental Health Issues

presence in minute quantities and because scientists lacked hard data regarding their health hazards. Now the EPA and others recognize the potential seriousness of their effects. Many sources emit toxic substances into the atmosphere: manufacturing plants, municipal waste sites, metal refineries, sewage treatment plants, motor vehicles, and others. Plastics and chemical manufacturing plants are two major producers of airborne toxic wastes.

Environmentalists have voiced concern that several hundred potentially carcinogenic air pollutants are still dumped into the atmosphere without restriction. The EPA has targeted this area for concentrated analysis during the early 1990s.

Indoor Air Pollution   The problem of indoor air pollution is becoming a major health issue as the American public becomes more aware of daily exposure to pollutants in the home and at the workplace. The degree of risk associated with exposure to indoor pollutants depends on how poorly the buildings are ventilated and the type of pollutants to which individuals are exposed. Indoor pollutants of greatest health concern include the following:

- Radon, a naturally occurring gas resulting from the radioactive decay of radium, which is found in many types of soil and rocks. Additional information about radon appears later in this chapter.
- Environmental tobacco smoke has become a major health issue among nonsmokers who resent exposure to tobacco fumes from smokers. This topic is covered in more detail in Chapter 10, **Health Hazards of Tobacco**.
- Formaldehyde is used in the manufacture of furniture, foam insulation, and pressed wood products (particle board and some plywood). This chemical can present health hazards if its concentration level becomes too high in poorly ventilated indoor spaces.
- Asbestos has been a main ingredient in many building materials, especially insulation, ceiling and floor tiles, and wallboard. The EPA has banned the use of asbestos but continuing hazards will be associated with exposure to asbestos fibers during building remodeling or demolition.

Steps toward Cleaner Air

Cleaning up our atmosphere presents major challenges whose resolution will require political action, economic costs, and, for a significant portion of the population, lifestyle changes. Many regional and national problems defy the ability of local governments to implement effective antipollution measures. Federal and state governments must maintain the leaderership role in formulating new programs and enforcing stricter standards.

Urban Smog   In response to the increased number of days per year that many urban areas exceed EPA safe limits for carbon monoxide, ozone, and other pollutants, stricter standards and new strategies have been proposed, including the following:

- Improving the fuel economy of automobiles to 45 miles per gallon.
- Applying stricter controls to reduce automobile tailpipe emissions, using the current California requirements as the national standard.
- Requiring light trucks and vans to meet the same emission standards as autos.
- Shifting gradually to cleaner-burning fuels, such as methanol, ethanol, and compressed natural gas, for motor vehicles.
- Implementing stricter controls to reduce vapor releases from filling stations, dry cleaners, and other commercial establishments.
- Reducing emissions from millions of residential air pollution sources.

Toxic Air Pollution   As described earlier in this chapter, the unregulated release by industry of millions of pounds of toxic chemical wastes each year threatens the health of a significant number of people exposed to these chemicals. Proposals for reducing this problem include the following:

- Continuing to research and document health hazards associated with toxic air pollution.
- Requiring industrial firms to recover greater portions of their wastes by using currently available technology.
- Developing more efficient smokestack scrubbers and vapor recovery devices and requiring industrial plants to meet stricter emission standards.

Acid Rain   In response to pressures from environmentalists in the United States and Canada, the U.S. government has proposed the following steps to reduce the 20 million tons of sulfur dioxide emitted per year.

- Require power-generating plants to reduce their emissions of sulfur dioxide by shifting from high-sulfur to low-sulfur coal and/or to install effective smokestack scrubbers.
- Longer-term solutions include reevaluation of alternative fuel sources for generating electricity; these include nuclear power and renewable energy. Potential sources of renewable energy are solar, wind, biomass, and geothermal.

Protecting Our Water Quality

Since 1970, significant progress has been made to restore the quality of our water. The badly polluted lakes and streams of the 1960s have largely given way to waterways now safe for swimming, fishing, and other recreational activities. The EPA, in partnership with state and local governments, is responsible for improving and protecting our water quality. The three problems receiving the most attention during the 1970s and 1980s

Methanol: Panacea or Problem

The candidate to become America's favorite alternative to automobile gasoline is methanol. This clean burning liquid has the potential to cut our smog-forming emissions in half. There are several concerns about methanol though: it burns without a flame, dissolves in water, and is highly poisonous. In the event of a leak from a storage tank, something which is already a serious problem with gasoline, methanol could be very harmful to nearby underground water supplies.

were the quality of drinking water, the pollution of surface waters (lakes and streams), and the destruction of wetlands, the productive wildlife habitats that link the land and the waterways.

Water Quality and Health

Polluted water puts you at risk for various diseases, including gastrointestinal disorders (from drinking water contaminated by untreated sewage) and cancer (from ingesting carcinogenic residue from agricultural, industrial, or commercial wastes). Untreated sewage, agricultural drainage, heated water expelled from processing plants, and industrial waste are all potential poisons to animal and plant life and upset the natural cycles that balance the aquatic environment.

People living near toxic waste dumps are gravely concerned about the safety of their drinking water, especially if ground water is their household source. Residue from heavy metals waste can cause neurological, heart, and kidney damage. The health effects related to the ingestion of lead include increased blood pressure, brain damage, premature birth, low birth weight, and nervous system disorders.

If wetlands and rivers become contaminated, then animals consume those pollutants. Those toxins move through the food chain, finally contaminating the fish, birds, and plants we eat. For instance, in the 1970s dumping by Japanese industry in one rural area caused a rise in mercury levels in fish, leading to blindness and deformity in many local residents.

Sources of Water Pollution

U.S. consumers obtain their water from two main sources: surface water and ground water. Surface water (rivers, lakes, and reservoirs) supplies about half the population, and ground water (slow-moving, underground rivers that feed wells and springs) supplies the remainder.

Waste products enter our waterways by means of direct dumping, from accidental spills, through seepage from landfill, or by being carried by rain or irrigation into streams and rivers. A major unsolved problem is runoff from farmers' fields, lawns, streets, and other paved areas. Pesticides used by agriculture are carried into nearby streams; oil, grease, and rubber residue is swept into storm drains and deposited into rivers. This is referred to as "nonpoint" pollution because a single source, or point, cannot be identified. The impact of water pollution on the natural food chain can be devastating when poisoned microorganisms are eaten by fish that either die or pass the poison on to the next "consumer."

The EPA has established maximum levels for 26 drinking water pollutants, and the agency receives testing data from 58,000 public water systems. In 1986, 87 percent of the public water systems that provide more than 80 percent of the nation's drinking water were meeting federal standards. The EPA plans to establish standards for 83 additional contaminants by the early 1990s. Tracing a contaminant from the water system

---

Reducing Your Exposure to Lead in Your Drinking Water

To have your drinking water tested for lead or other possible contaminants, contact your local water utility or your local health department for assistance.

To minimize your exposure to lead in your drinking water, you should take the following steps:

- Before using water for drinking or cooking, "flush" the cold water faucet by allowing the water to run until you can feel that the water has become as cold as it will get. This allows water that has been standing in contact with lead pipes or solder to be replaced by fresh water. Use the flushed water—usually one or two gallons—for nonconsumptive purposes such as washing dishes or clothes.

- Never cook with or consume water from the hot water tap. Hot water dissolves lead more quickly than cold water. So, do not use water taken from the hot water tap for drinking or cooking and especially not for making baby formula. For instant coffee, tea, cocoa, and other hot beverages, heat cold water to desired temperature on the stove or in a microwave oven.

Source: Environmental Protection Agency

back to its source is often a difficult process. And, drinking water samples may contain several contaminants from multiple sources. The most common pollution sources are as follows:

- Animal waste and runoff from pesticides and fertilizers: Between 50 and 75 percent of all surface water pollution problems stem from runoff from farms and urban and suburban lawns and streets. Hydrocarbons (including oil and grease) and metallic and rubber particles are washed from streets into streams and lakes. Farmers spread millions of tons of fertilizers and pesticides on the land each year. Natural rainfall and irrigation water wash residue from the fields into our water supplies.
- Surface water absorbs pollutants from industrial discharges, mining waste, agricultural chemical runoff, and accidental petroleum spills.
- Leaking underground tanks: The EPA estimates that hundreds of thousands of the nation's 5 to 6 million underground storage tanks are leaking gasoline or other hazardous chemicals. This source may account for 40 percent of all ground water contamination.
- Toxic chemicals buried in the earth or dumped down dry wells threaten ground water and have become a major concern to many people who live in rural areas or in small towns using wells.
- Toxic waste sites: Approximately 85 percent of the 29,000 toxic waste sites in the United States are present or future polluters of ground and surface water. Waste products from metal refineries are particularly hazardous when their residue seeps into ground water supplies.
- Lead: Corrosion of such plumbing materials as lead pipes and solders is the primary source of lead in drinking water. Although lead pipes have

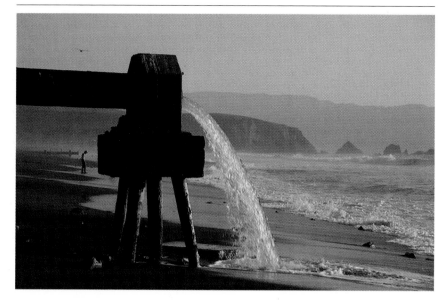

Environmental Health Issues

been replaced by copper in recent years, solder continues to contain some lead, and most faucets are made of materials that can contribute small amounts of lead to our drinking water.

Steps toward Cleaner Water

To continue the process of cleaning up the nation's waterways and keeping them habitable for wildlife and safe for recreation, federal and state government agencies will share the burden of setting standards and enforcing them. The EPA's 1988 toxic chemical survey identified many sources of water pollution; political and economic pressure will require increased responsiveness from industry to reduce pouring toxic wastes into waterways. Proposals include the following:

- Enforcing stricter regulations covering underground storage tanks containing gasoline or other hazardous chemicals to reduce the frequency of underground leaks.
- Accelerating the cleanup of toxic waste dumps that qualify for treatment under the Superfund program.
- Continued monitoring of drinking water systems for unhealthy contaminants.
- Enforcing regulations prohibiting municipalities from dumping untreated sewage and hazardous chemicals into waterways.
- Prohibiting industrial firms and commercial establishments from pouring even small quantities of toxic substances into their local sewer systems.

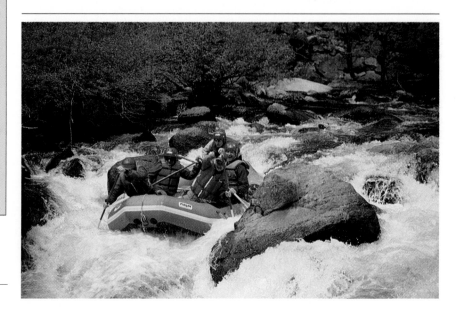

Because industry in the past was not required to dispose of its own toxic wastes, the technology to accomplish this task is just now being developed. Various thermal, solidification, vacuum, and biological methods are presently under development. One device is a plasma torch that effectively destroys both organic compounds (e.g., PCP's) and industrial solvents (e.g., carbon tetrachloride). Another treatment method uses steel rods and high voltage electrical charges to convert a buried toxic dump into a solid glassy substance resembling obsidian, a black igneous stone.

Polluting the Soil with Solid Waste

Until recently, the United States seemed to be a nation of unlimited space and resources. Until the twentieth century, neither conservation of natural resources nor environmental pollution were major concerns. In the same tradition of plentiful resources and space, industrial firms dumped their wastes in the most convenient and least expensive manner: through smokestacks into the air, via pipes into waterways, and by dumping it on the land. Often a nearby gully or dry riverbed served as a disposal site. When manufacturers had toxic wastes, they put the chemicals in barrels and buried them in the ground. Meanwhile, a growing population dumped its solid waste products into landfill sites that expanded to accommodate the continual inflow. Now the nation faces major problems of finding alternative methods of disposing of solid waste and of cleaning up existing toxic waste dumps.

In 1986, Americans generated solid waste (garbage) at a rate of 3.58 pounds per person per day.

Sources of Solid Waste

Solid waste creates problems by its very mass. Although quantity is a big issue, the form, chemical composition, and disposal method of solid wastes all play roles in determining the environmental risk such waste poses.

Municipal Solid Waste   What government calls municipal solid waste, almost everyone else calls garbage. In 1988, Americans produced 160 million tons of municipal solid waste; this could fill a convoy of 10-ton trucks 145,000 miles long—enough to circle the equator nearly six times. At its present rate, garbage production is projected to reach 190 million tons by the year 2000.

More than 40 percent of our solid waste consists of paper and paper products we discard in our homes, offices, and schools. Yard wastes—lawn clippings and leaves—make up another 18 percent of the total. The other major ingredients of the garbage deluge are metals, glass, food waste, broken furniture and appliances, old tires, and many other items of human refuse that characterize our modern industrial society. Symptomatic of our "throwaway society" are the many disposable prod-

What's in Our Trash

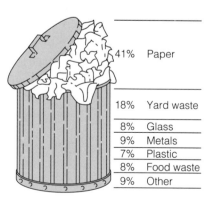

41%	Paper
18%	Yard waste
8%	Glass
9%	Metals
7%	Plastic
8%	Food waste
9%	Other

What Did You Say? Noise Pollution?

Noise pollution is often over-looked, but many people experience this form of "interference" on an almost daily basis. Noise pollution is both a stressor and a physiological hazard. When your study or sleep time is disrupted by excessive noise, whether loud music or neighboring conversation, your reaction will be similar to what it is in response to many other stressors. Noise can cause fatigue, irritability, anger, tension, and anxiety. From a physiological standpoint, noise levels exceeding 85 decibels (the unit of measurement of sound intensity) present a threat to your hearing mechanisms.

The nearby chart shows the relative decibel strength of several commonly experienced noise producers. Workers are required by OSHA to wear protective devices when performing many job functions where the noise level is dangerous. However, you do not have to operate a jack hammer or work on the flight line of a jet airport to need protection.

One of the most common hazards is amplified sound, namely music whose decibel level may reach as high as 130 decibels. The incidence of hearing loss among rock musicians is alarmingly high. As a frequent listener to live or amplified music, you are at risk when the volume exceeds the 85 decibel safe limit.

Noise Sources	Decibels
Jet take-off	140
Rock music	130
Auto horn	110
Motorcycle	100
Garbage truck	100
Jackhammer	90
Heavy traffic	80
Vacuum cleaner	75
Normal conversation	60
Library	40
Whisper	30

ucts that are manufactured or imported, sold, used, and thrown away; for example, we discard 1.6 billion pens, 2 billion razors and razor blades, and 16 billion diapers every year.

Eighty percent of garbage becomes landfill; that is, the refuse is compressed and then covered with dirt by huge tractors. About 10 percent of the refuse is burned in special incinerators, and the remaining 10 percent is recycled. Ineffective or irresponsible disposal of our solid waste has the potential to degrade the environment and cause risk to public health. For example, landfill sites may give off substantial quantities of methane gas. Household solvents and pesticides, lead from discarded batteries, and other heavy metal residues may leech into nearby water tables or streams. The gases given off by large incinerators may create air pollution and contain highly toxic substances. More than one third of the nation's existing

Environmental Health Issues

CHAPTER 21

552

landfills will be full within the next three years as a result of this space problem. Many cities are experiencing difficulty locating sites for new landfills and incinerators. The common citizen reaction to proposed new sites has been "not in my backyard" (NIMBY). Some American cities are shipping their trash to other counties, states, and even foreign countries.

Toxic Waste   The 1987 EPA survey indicates that 3.9 billion pounds of toxic wastes were buried on-site in landfills, stored in ponds, or injected into deep wells. A nearly equal amount was shipped off for treatment or disposal at public sewage plants or private chemical waste sites. Some of these waste products are highly hazardous chemicals that leech into local water supplies or into nearby waterways. Other wastes contain toxic metals that will remain in the soil for many years and are potential causes of cancer if humans come in contact with the residue. Residents of homes constructed on former toxic chemical waste sites (for example, the Love Canal area in Niagara Falls, New York, where 21,800 tons of chemical wastes were buried in the 1940s and 1950s), have experienced extremely high incidences of cancer, birth defects, and other illnesses.

In spite of common perception, big industry is not the only source of toxic waste. Many households and small businesses also have toxic wastes. Old paint, weed killer, rat poisons, insecticides, household cleaners, and dozens of other common products have harmful effects when they leach into groundwater or are incinerated. Some sanitary services now prohibit the dumping of household toxic wastes with ordinary trash. They offer special times and places for dropping off such waste, so they can handle it properly.

Dealing with Solid Waste Pollution

Solving the problems of solid waste pollution will require individual commitments on the part of citizens and the combined interventions from federal, state, and local governments. Consumers must participate in recycling programs, municipalities need more space for trash disposal, industrial firms must develop safer methods of toxic waste disposal, and toxic waste sites must be cleaned up.

Recycling   The most promising solutions to the solid waste dilemma are recycling and composting. In 1986, only 11 percent of our nonhazardous solid wastes were recycled. The EPA estimates that recycling and composting together could reduce solid waste by 25 percent.

Recycling is economically viable for newspapers, corrugated boxes, and other paper products as well as glass, aluminum, and some plastic products. Steps to reduce the quantity of waste plastics and incentives to recycle them are high on the environmental agenda for the 1990s. Composting biodegradable yard waste converts it to an enriching product for gardens and parks.

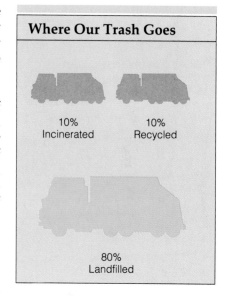

Where Our Trash Goes

10% Incinerated

10% Recycled

80% Landfilled

Environmental Health Issues

Hazardous Waste Disposal on College Campuses

Colleges and universities throughout the United States face rising costs, increased regulation, and greater public scrutiny regarding the problems of collecting, storing, and disposing of chemical wastes produced by laboratories and maintenance operations. Compared with industry, colleges do not generate large quantities of specific hazardous waste, rather they have relatively small amounts of a great number of substances. Iowa State University reported disposing of 3,000 different items in one year. Common wastes include solvents used in research laboratories, pesticides used by grounds maintenance, and heavy metals in glazes from art departments. On-campus problems include limited knowledge about handling materials, lack of commitment to safe handling, and inadequate funds budgeted for waste disposal.

Larger universities are allocating up to $300,000 per year for hazardous waste disposal which, in many cases, represents ten times what was spent only a few years ago. A common practice at many institutions is to pour waste chemicals down the drain and let them "disappear" through the sewer system. This issue is one of both safety and health. Institutions expose themselves to law suits from government agencies, employees, students and others whose health may have been affected by the wastes. As a student, you need to be aware of the hazards of handling various health-threatening substances and the guidelines for their safe storage or disposal.

Landfill Dump Sites Every American contributes an average of 1,300 pounds of garbage per year. In many highly populated areas, landfill sites are nearing capacity, and available space for expansion is limited. Because many landfill dumps are located in or near wetlands or other ecologically sensitive areas, environmentalists are opposing expansion of present landfills. Neighboring residents tend to oppose construction of giant incinerators designed to burn solid wastes, and foreign countries are no longer willing to accept barges loaded with waste products.

The Superfund Program Created by Congress in 1970 and funded with $8.5 billion, the EPA-administered Superfund program was initiated to supervise the cleanup of nearly 1200 of the most dangerous toxic waste dumps in the United States. By mid-1989, several hundred cleanups were under way. At a typical site, the cleanup process will require 10 to 20 years depending upon the nature of the soil and ground water contamination. After the EPA cleans up a dump area, the agency seeks to recover the costs from the responsible polluters.

Radiation Health Hazards

Radiation poses a potentially hazardous, yet invisible, environmental threat. Sources of potential ionizing radiation include nuclear power plants, nuclear weapons facilities, and radon gas. Another type of radiation is electromagnetic. Sources of this potentially hazardous radiation are high-voltage electrical transmission lines and certain electrical appliances.

Sources of Radiation Hazards

Nuclear Power Plants   Radioactive discharges in March 1979 from the nuclear power plant at Three Mile Island in Pennsylvania and from the nuclear power plant in Chernobyl, USSR, in April 1986 increased public concern about nuclear safety, and raised the specter of radioactive fallout and its health consequences. Long-term effects of nuclear radiation include increased rates of cancer and birth defects.

In the United States, the debate rages over the operation of nuclear power plants and facilities where nuclear weapons are manufactured. Environmentalists are especially concerned about the threat of radioactive particles in the atmosphere resulting from malfunction of a nuclear power plant located near a highly populated area. Nuclear power plants have been plagued by problems that caused regulatory agencies to restrict their operations and antinuclear activist organizations to call for their shutdown. In June 1989, residents of Sacramento, California, voted to shut down Rancho Seco, their utility's only nuclear power plant. This was the first time voters had decided to close down a working nuclear reactor. The decision was based more upon economics than safety. Operating costs of the plant were substantially higher than alternative coal-burning facilities. People concerned with the potential problems of acid rain and global warming are in a dilemma—do long-term clean air objectives outweigh the costs and possible hazards of nuclear power?

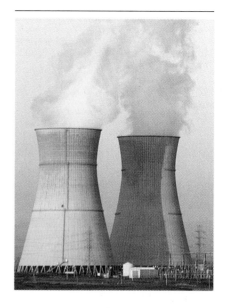

The Nuclear Regulatory Commission has issued operating licenses for 112 nuclear reactors throughout the United States, but the task of storing and disposing of highly radioactive waste from nuclear power plants has not yet been solved. The Department of Energy is analyzing potential sites such as Yucca Mountain in Nevada, but no repository will be ready to receive waste products until after the year 2000. Meantime, environmentalists continue to voice concern about the safe storage of nuclear waste.

Nuclear Weapons Facilities   Management of the nation's nuclear weapons plants, traditionally shrouded in secrecy, has come under the scrutiny of governmental officials and concerned citizen groups. The potential health hazards to workers exposed to on-the-job radiation, as well as hazards to neighboring residents and the environment, are not fully

Radon Survey

Average Levels

Highest	Lowest
Indiana	Alaska
New Mexico	California
Pennsylvania	Delaware
Washington	Louisiana
Wyoming	Vermont

documented. Waste disposal from nuclear weapons facilities poses serious safety problems for workers and, potentially, for population centers through which such waste must be safely transported en route to its final storage site. Economic and political pressures clash with environmental concerns. For example, the pay and benefits for the 6,000 workers employed at the Rocky Flats, Colorado, nuclear weapons facility total $300 million per year. Closing the facility would have a significant economic impact on the surrounding area.

Since World War II, chemical and radioactive wastes have been accumulating at our nation's 16 nuclear weapons sites which are scattered through 12 states. A serious environmental threat from nuclear weapons facilities is seepage of chemical and radioactive wastes into streams and underground water. The cleanup task will take several decades, and cost estimates run from $100 to $200 billion.

Radon   Outdoors, radon gas dissipates harmlessly into the atmosphere. However, radon can accumulate to unhealthy levels indoors, especially in basements. Radon seeps into basements through cracks in foundations and through openings around pipes.

In late 1988, the EPA set off a furor when it released a warning that occupants of more than eight million homes may be at risk due to the presence of radon. A subsequent report revealed that radon levels in many school classrooms exceed EPA-recommended safe levels. The evidence linking radon with lung cancer is based on studies of uranium miners who were exposed to excessive quantities of radon over an extended number of years. When inhaled, radon particles release ionizing radiation that can damage sensitive lung tissue and lead to lung cancer. The EPA estimates that radon may be responsible for 5,000 to 20,000 lung cancer deaths each year.

Household radon levels usually are very low; nevertheless, the EPA recommends all home owners test the radon level in their basements. Professional testing costs from $10 to $50, and hardware stores sell do-it-yourself test kits for about $25. Consumer protection groups warn against some of the less expensive kits because they may be unreliable and inaccurate. Radon problems can usually be solved by sealing cracks and installing basement ventilators.

Electromagnetic Radiation   Experts agree that of all the types of radiation, the least understood is electromagnetic. Recent studies have increased the public's awareness regarding potentially hazardous effects of electromagnetic radiation: the emissions from television sets, high-power electric lines, and various household or workplace electronic devices.

Possible health hazards associated with exposure to extra-low-frequency (ELF) radiation have been clouded in controversy. For more than 15 years, independent researchers have cautioned that electromagnetic radiation of 450 mHz modulated at 16 hertz (cycles per second) may be associated with higher than normal incidences of cancer. The main sources of ELF waves are high-voltage overhead transmission lines, certain defense department antenna systems, and home appliances, such as electrically heated water beds and electric blankets. Scientists do not know the exact reaction of the human body to ELF radiation but several independent studies point to some forms of cancer, particularly leukemia, lymphoma, and brain tumors.

Officials representing public utilities and the U.S. Air Force have responded to this concern with skepticism, saying that the research findings are not convincing. Consumer health advocates maintain that building high-voltage transmission lines through densely populated areas should cease until further studies are completed.

Global Atmospheric Issues

The Greenhouse Effect

The 1980s have experienced the four hottest years on record. Recent world-wide droughts and heat waves have focused public awareness on a much publicized concept described as the greenhouse effect. Certain gases in the atmosphere trap heat and keep the earth warm, just as the glass of a greenhouse keeps the air inside warm. Without an atmospheric blanket, the earth would be much colder and uninhabitable. Recent global warming is considered to be caused by release of increased amounts of heat-trapping gases into the atmosphere.

Causes of the Greenhouse Effect

Several factors account for most of the greenhouse effect: fossil fuel combustion, increase in other heat-trapping gases, and deforestation.

Fossil Fuel Combustion The great increase in burning of fossil fuels (coal and petroleum products) to support the Industrial Revolution disturbed the natural carbon dioxide equilibrium. Today's atmospheric carbon dioxide levels are 25 percent higher than they were just 100 years ago. Carbon dioxide released from fossil fuel combustion accounts for nearly 60 percent of the greenhouse effect. The United States contributes one fifth of the carbon dioxide added to the atmosphere on a worldwide basis.

Other Heat-trapping Gases The levels of other heat-trapping gases have increased as well: methane from bacterial decomposition of organic matter in open-air garbage dumps, chlorofluorocarbons from refrigerants and cleaning solvents, nitrous oxide from fertilizers, and ground-level ozone from power generating plants that burn coal or petroleum. All these gases absorb infrared energy reflected by the earth.

Destruction of Rain Forests and Savannas Facing problems caused by population growth and inadequate food supplies, the governments of

---

Atmospheric CO_2 Increases

By analyzing air bubbles trapped in glacial ice, climatologists have determined that levels of atmospheric CO_2 rose 26 percent between 1860 and 1986. At current rates of increase, CO_2 concentration could cause global temperature to rise by about 7° F by the year 2050.

Environmental Health Issues

Rain Forest Destruction

The edge of a smoke cloud that obscured almost a third of South America in late September, 1988, is shown here as it trails off in the valleys of foothills of the Andes Mountains.

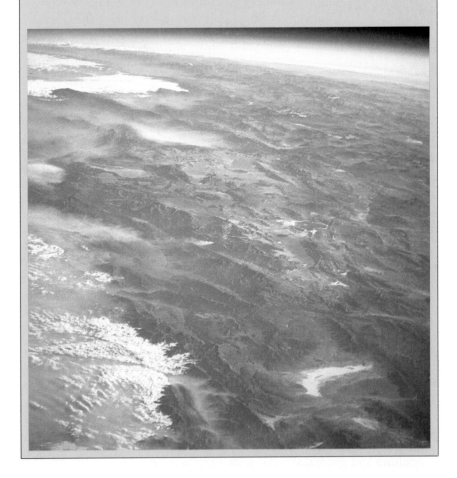

many underdeveloped nations have allowed the systematic destruction of vast areas of virgin rain forest and grassy savannas. In Brazil, nearly 30,000 square miles—an area the size of Maine—were burned in one year. Using data collected by infrared sensors in satellites, scientists counted 5,000 fires burning on the same day. In Central Africa, farmers and herdsmen have ignited the grassy savannas to clear shrubs and stimulate the growth of grass. Such fires cause massive quantities of gases and smoke to pour into the atmosphere. This intensifies the greenhouse effect already created by the industrial nations' burning of fossil fuels.

Consequences of the Greenhouse Effect

The overall temperature of the earth has stayed within a relatively narrow range for at least 3.5 billion years because of the continuous self-adjusting ebb and flow of cloud cover and polar ice packs. Both clouds and ice reflect sunlight back into space, and carbon dioxide in the atmosphere helps "insulate" the earth. Living organisms play an important role in keeping the carbon dioxide in proper balance. Scientists estimate that for the last 100,000 years, atmospheric carbon dioxide has remained quite stable because of its natural generation and consumption by animal and plant life. However, fossil fuel combustion and other industrial, consumer, and agricultural practices have increased the concentration of heat-trapping gases in the atmosphere.

As the sun continues to warm the earth and the greenhouse effect retains the reflected heat, the overall temperature of the planet increases. Some scientists predict that if this trend continues for the next 50 to 75 years, the average global temperature could increase by three to nine degrees Fahrenheit. Exactly how fast or how much the temperature will rise is uncertain, as are the precise consequences of the rise. Two most probable consequences are a rise in the ocean level and changing weather patterns.

- *Rising Oceans*: As the ocean temperature increases, the water will expand and the polar and alpine ice packs will partially melt. Some scientists predict that the sea level will rise one to three feet by the year 2050, causing severe coastal erosion, destroying irreplaceable wetlands, and contaminating fresh water supplies with sea water. Several cities built on low-lying islands—Miami, Galveston, Atlantic City—will be especially vulnerable to a rise in sea level.
- *Changing Climate*: A severe warming trend will enable deserts of the American Southwest to extend northward into the midwestern states. Decreased rainfall would have a devastating effect on U.S. grain production. Because of warmer water temperatures, tropic storms are predicted to be more intense and would pose a greater threat to low-lying coastal cities. A warmer, drier climate will reduce the snowfall in certain mountainous regions where reservoirs and runoff provide water for agriculture and general consumption by cities and towns.

Reducing the Greenhouse Effect

Strategies to clean up the atmosphere will also help reduce the greenhouse effect. The overwhelming dependence on fossil fuels to generate our electricity, power our automobiles, and support our industrial production will result in a continued worsening of the greenhouse effect unless steps are taken to develop and use alternative fuel sources. Additional information is included earlier in this chapter under the heading "Steps toward Cleaner Air."

Environmental Health Issues

A continuing problem is the vast burning of forests and grasslands in many underdeveloped nations. These countries are more concerned with present problems posed by explosive population growth and severe food shortages than with the long-term threat of global warming. Proposed actions on the part of industrial nations to reduce the damaging effects of smoke and gases from intentionally set fires include forgiving international debt repayments in return for reductions in burning and commencement of major reforestation projects.

The Ozone Layer—Our Planet's Sunscreen

Ozone is a form of oxygen with a split personality. When it is close to the ground, ozone is a potentially harmful ingredient in smog. But in the stratosphere, this gas serves as a lifesaving sunscreen. The chemical symbol O_3 signifies that an ozone molecule consists of three oxygen atoms compared to the two atoms comprising an oxygen molecule (O_2).

In the lower regions of the earth's atmosphere, ozone increases when sunlight acts on nitrogen oxides most commonly found in automobile exhaust fumes. Ground-level ozone, potentially dangerous to our health, is totally separate from the more concentrated layer that surrounds the earth 15 to 20 miles above the surface. Stratospheric ozone shields the earth from much of the sun's ultraviolet (UV) light. Because UV rays harm living tissues, plants and animals probably could not survive on earth without a protective ozone shield. UV radiation causes sunburn, eye damage, snow blindness, and skin cancer.

The Ozone Culprits   The two most effective destroyers of ozone are chlorofluorocarbons (CFC's) and halons. CFC's contain chlorine, and halons contain bromide. Under normal conditions, chemical reactions triggered by sunlight continuously balance the ozone content. The human community upset this natural balance by introducing products containing chlorine and bromine. These chemicals can survive intact in the atmosphere for 100 years. When they finally break down, each chlorine and bromine atom initiates a chain reaction that can destroy tens of thousands of ozone molecules.

- *Chlorofluorocarbons*: The versatility and low cost of CFC's resulted in their extensive use in aerosol spray cans, air conditioning units, and foam insulation. In Western Europe, aerosol cans are the largest source of CFC emissions. In the United States, where the chemical has been banned for use in aerosols, 45 percent of the production is used for refrigerants and 15 percent as cleaning agents for computer chips, metals, and fabrics. The remaining U.S. production is used for styrofoam and other products.
- *Halons*: Many fire extinguishers contain halons, a very effective chemical for fighting fires. Halons are also utilized in fire suppressant systems installed to protect sensitive equipment spaces such as computer rooms

Population Growth Threatens Environmental Stability

There is a very close relationship among population growth, the depletion of resources, and pollution of the environment. As more people inhabit the earth and as their life expectancy increases, the demands upon the planet's resources grow as well.

The world's population is increasing at the rate of 255,000 people per day or 90 million per year. Nonrenewable resources, such as mineral ores and petroleum, are being depleted while renewable resources, such as timber and seafood, are being consumed at a rate faster than they can regenerate. Protection of the environment is generally recognized as necessary in the industrialized nations, although the political strength to enforce pollution control may be lacking. The priority to feed, clothe and shelter the populations of the underdeveloped countries, where 90 percent of new population occurs, supercedes longer-term goals of environmental protection.

As a result, burning of rain forests to gain agriculture space in South America and burning of savannas in Africa are likely to continue. The resulting impact on the atmosphere will be experienced not only as local smoke but also as a global problem of ozone depletion and the greenhouse effect.

The controversy over population control raises social, political, moral, and religious issues. Some experts recommend that the industrialized nations make foreign aid to underdeveloped countries contingent upon local population control measures. The problem is not simple and its implications are far-reaching. It has taken from the beginning of time until the present to reach today's world population of 5.2 billion. At the current rate we will add another billion in only ten years, and another 2 billion by 2020.

Source: *National Geographic*, December 1988

and telephone exchanges. Testing fire suppressant systems releases more halons than does fighting fires. Until more efficient and cost-effective chemicals are developed, halons will probably continue to be used.

Protecting the Ozone Layer

While the complicated nature of the ozone layer continues to be researched and analyzed, steps have commenced to protect our upper atmosphere sunscreen.

- The United States and the 12 nations of the European Community agreed in mid-1989 to ban the production and use of CFC's by the year 2000. This is a major step because these 13 nations account for 75 percent of the world's CFC production. Environmentalists are concerned

Environmental Health Issues

that nations such as India and China, which have refused to sign the agreement, may contribute substantial CFC's into the atmosphere as their economies develop greater industrial complexity.

- Federal, state, and local programs designed to reduce our dependence on fossil fuels will also result in less air pollution and contribute to protecting the ozone layer.
- Two ozone destroyers not covered in the 1989 international agreement are methyl chloroform and carbon tetrachloride. Together, they contribute nearly 15 percent of total annual ozone depleting emissions, and experts have targeted them for stricter controls.

You Can Make A Difference

Environmental pollution is a major global problem. Solutions seem to require so much time, effort, and money you may wonder what you can do, as an individual, that makes any difference. You can (1) become an informed citizen, (2) minimize your personal pollution, and (3) become involved on a national or international scale.

Making Informed Choices

Newspapers, television, radio, magazines, and other media cover environmental issues. They describe problems of environmental pollution, identify health hazards, and propose action plans. By reading and listening you can become aware of national and global problems. You can learn about situations unique to your local area, such as health-threatening water or atmospheric contamination. Certainly any person who suffers from respiratory or cardiovascular disease should remain acutely aware of local air quality.

It's important to be able to sort out objective information from scare tactics and scientifically based data from rumor. Similar to other public action groups, environmental organizations usually state their positions in very strong terms. Politicians often use strongly worded arguments and gross oversimplifications to catch the attention of the voting public. Government officials responsible for implementing pollution regulations are often handicapped by lack of funds. Manufacturers are now incorporating environmental themes into their product advertisements. Be receptive to new information, but take note of both its content and source. Then you will be able to interpret the basic positions of various special interest groups and the editorial slant of specific publications on important issues.

Your Contributions Are Important

Your lifestyle choices can help reduce environmental pollution, and your example will influence others. Specific daily actions that contribute to a healthier environment include the following:

- Reduce your personal contribution to air pollution by using an automobile less frequently and cutting down on the total number of miles you drive. Use a bicycle or public transportation; walk instead of drive; carpool when possible.
- Participate in your community's recycling program. Recycle paper, glass, aluminum, and plastics. This reduces demands on landfill dump sites and helps prolong our supply of trees, minerals, petroleum, and other resources for future needs.
- Do not pour solvents, cleaners or other toxic chemicals down the drain because they may contaminate the water supply. Take them to a hazardous waste collection center or call your sanitation department for disposal instructions.
- Purchase products in biodegradable containers when they are available. For example, at least one major corporation is now packaging liquid soap in a biodegradable plastic container.
- Put grass clippings, leaves, and vegetable waste into a compost heap. If you do not have a lawn or trees, give your vegetable waste to someone who has a compost heap. This action also reduces the demands on landfill sites, and compost is an effective substitute for chemical fertilizers.
- Use low-phosphate dish and laundry detergent to keep difficult-to-dispense phosphates out of our water supply.
- Minimize your purchases of food packed in plastic or foil when paper, cardboard, or other biodegradable alternatives are available.
- Purchase products made from recycled material.
- When having your automobile's air conditioning system serviced, ask the mechanic to drain the coolant into containers rather than allowing it to evaporate.
- Limit the use of pesticides and, when possible, use organic fertilizers and insecticides.
- Insulate your home with fiberglass or cellulose (wood fiber) insulation instead of rigid urethane foams containing CFC's.
- Minimize your use of gasoline-powered lawn mowers (use an electric or manual one), charcoal lighter fluid (use newspaper or other starter), and chemical paint thinners (use water-soluble latex paint).

Get Involved

You can participate in solving environmental problems by getting involved on a local level and by supporting organizations dedicated to specific environmental issues.

- Participate in or start a voluntary recycling program at your college or in your neighborhood.
- Urge other people to recycle their waste, reduce their automobile miles, and conserve energy.
- Write letters to local, state, and federal legislators urging them to support legislation aimed at solving environmental issues. Elected officials

What Is Recyclable?

At present, approximately 11 percent of all U.S. solid waste is recycled, but experts estimate that its full potential may be as high as 50 percent.

Recyclables

Materials:

- Paper (newspapers, corrugated boxes, office papers, mixed papers)
- Plastics (milk, soft drink, and other containers)
- Glass (bottles and jars)
- Aluminum (cans and other aluminum products)
- Steel (appliances and other steel products)
- Wood (pallets, lumber, etc.)

Compost:

- Leaves, grass, and brush
- Food wastes
- Some other organic materials, such as paper contaminated with food

Nonrecyclables

- Wastes heavily contaminated by food residues, household chemicals, or dirt
- Composite materials, e.g., aseptic boxes made of paper, foil, and adhesives, plastic-coated paper, furniture and appliances (other than their metal content)
- Miscellaneous inorganics, such as street sweepings

Source: Environmental Protection Agency

Environmental Protection Groups

	Members	Purpose
Clean Water Action 317 Pennsylvania Ave. S.E. Washington, D.C. 20003	500,000	Protection of waterways, coasts and drinking water; works to reduce toxic wastes and emissions.
Environmental Defense Fund 257 Park Ave. South New York, N.Y. 10010	100,000	Combining efforts of scientists, economists and attorneys to devise practical solutions to environmental problems.
Greenpeace 1436 U Street N.W. Washington, D.C. 20009	3 million	Environmental protection through direct action, education and lobbying. Emphasis: endangered species; ocean ecology; toxic waste; nuclear disarmament.
National Audubon Society 950 Third Avenue New York, N.Y. 10022	560,000	Conservation of plants, animals and habitats. Emphasis: saving the Platte River; protecting the Arctic National Wildlife Refuge; conserving wetlands; saving old-growth forests; clean air.
National Wildlife Federation 1400 18th Street, N.W. Washington, D.C. 20036	5.8 million	To promote the wise use of natural resources through conservation education, lobbying and litigation.
Sierra Club 730 Polk Street San Francisco, CA 94109	505,000	Promote conservation by influencing public policy decisions. Emphasis on Clean Air Act; Arctic refuge protection; parkland protection; toxic waste regulations; global warming.

keep track of their incoming mail and telephone calls, and they usually are responsive to their constituents' demands.

- Join one or more of the nonprofit organizations dedicated to protecting our environment. The accompanying list identifies several of the most active national organizations. More information is contained in the Resources appendix at the back of this text. Many local or regional groups focus on local conservation and/or environmental problems, and they need your support as well. Nonprofit organizations rely heavily on membership dues and voluntary contributions. In return for paying nominal annual dues, you will usually receive a periodic newsletter or magazine that keeps you informed about current issues.

In Search of Solutions

The tasks of formulating and implementing solutions to the problems of environmental pollution are complex and costly. Government intervention is required to reverse practices of dumping wastes into the atmosphere, waterways, and earth that have prevailed for many decades. Some pollution control measures have been very effective. For example, mandatory auto emission controls have reduced air pollution per automobile but the gains in attaining cleaner air have been largely nullified by the great increase in the number of automobiles on the nation's streets and highways. Population growth and industrial development continue to burden the environment with greater amounts of waste products. As described earlier in this chapter, specific laws were enacted in the early 1970s to control environmental pollution. Health experts agree that too many people continue to be subjected to unhealthy air or water. There appears to be a renewed commitment in the 1990s to solve pollution problems, including many still unresolved from the 1970s (smog) and others more recently defined (depletion of the ozone layer).

Environmentalists were critical of President Reagan's administration for lax enforcement of existing environmental protection laws and failure to adequately respond to new problems. However, proposals made in 1989 by the administration of President George Bush addressed critical environmental issues and indicated a renewed commitment on the part of the administration to seek solutions to these problems.

Environmental Issues for the 1990s

The environmental health issues that confronted the American population during the 1980s will continue into the 1990s and beyond. The problems are complex and will require comprehensive solutions. In addition to continuing to make our air cleaner and our water more pure, the specific issues demanding attention in the 1990s will include the following:

- *Unhealthy air*: More than 75 million Americans live in metropolitan areas with unhealthy levels of ozone and/or carbon monoxide. Population growth and the public's dependence on the automobile limit the ability of mechanical devices to keep pace with the increased emissions. Lifestyle changes such as reduction in miles driven, greater use of public transportation, and utilization of alternative fuels will be issues for the coming decades.
- *Municipal waste disposal*: The garbage deluge continues and cities are running out of space. Mandatory recycling, composting of yard waste, and the banning of certain hazardous substances, such as asbestos and benzene, from the home, will become common.
- *Hazardous waste disposal*: Industrial and commercial firms will be required to dispose of their hazardous waste products using methods that do not pollute our air or water, or endanger our health. Greater em-

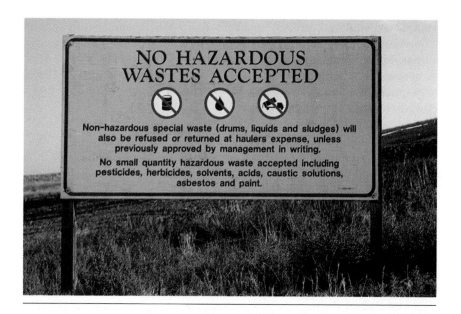

phasis will be placed on balancing the benefits we derive from many chemicals (and chemical products) against the risk to our health from exposure to them. Reducing the risk may require giving up the convenience of certain products made from plastics or other materials.

- *Global environmental threats*: International cooperation is a prerequisite to solving such problems as global warming, ocean pollution, acid rain, and the stratospheric ozone layer. These issues will be the topic of international conferences, and cooperative agreements may be reached.

The key factors to environmental protection in the 1990s will be commitment, cooperation, and costs. These are interrelated because unless all three are considered, progress will be limited.

- *Commitment*: Federal, state, and local governments must reaffirm their commitments to regulate, legislate, and enforce policies aimed at protecting the nation's environment. The commitment of the American public is essential because political action reflects public opinion and voter preferences. Progress during the 1970s and 1980s on solving environmental issues was quite substantial given the magnitude of the problems, the continued population and industrial growth of the two decades following the first major commitment to reversing the problems, and the limited technological resources available to apply to pollution control.
- *Cooperation*: On several levels cooperation is essential for problem solving. Federal, state, and local governments have been coordinating their efforts quite effectively, and the regulated industrial firms have complied with environmental standards for the most part. To continue to advance, the EPA needs to develop standards for hazardous substances

not yet regulated, and the multitude of small businesses and home owners must follow new, restrictive guidelines in a cooperative manner. Programs such as recycling and conservation of resources are essential, but their success rests largely upon voluntary cooperation of the population at large. Lifestyle changes may be required, but the inconvenience of minor cutbacks in energy consumption and waste production has great potential to reduce our environmental problems.

■ *Costs*: Administration officials estimate that for industry to accomplish a major environmental cleanup, costs would total $14 to $18 billion per year for the next decade. Heavy investments for new pollution-reducing equipment by electric utilities, oil and chemical companies, and other industries will be reflected in our monthly electric bills and the price we pay for many of our consumer products. At the same time, an effective clean air program could reduce a major portion of direct and indirect health care costs associated with air pollution, estimated by the American Lung Association to be $16 to $40 billion annually.

To clean up our environment and keep it in a healthy state will cost billions of dollars during the next several decades. The buildup of waste products in our atmosphere, waterways, and on our land cannot be accomplished without substantial payments on the part of industry, commercial enterprises, and the general public. Use of alternative fuels may increase our heating or automotive bills; responsible waste management may result in our paying higher fees for garbage collection. We may need to sacrifice some elements of convenience by giving up certain forms of packaging or by using public transportation in place of driving our cars. However, the costs to our economy and our lifestyle may be substantial in the long term if we fail to pay the price of progress in the immediate future.

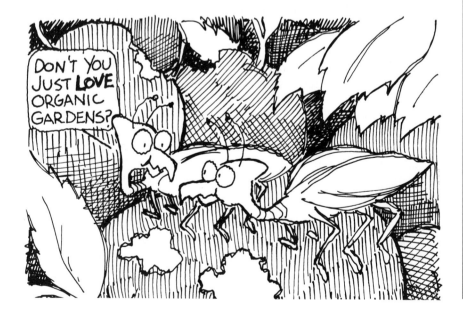

Seeking Professional Help

Environmental health encompasses a wide range of local, regional, and global issues. Your most likely need for professional help will apply to your immediate environment and threats to your health.

Seek Help If:

■ You suspect that you or someone else has been exposed to a toxic chemical due to an industrial spill, transportation accident, or workplace incident
■ Your workplace or living quarters is located in a "sick building" suffering from poor ventilation, excessive noise, or chemical pollution
■ You suffer from respiratory or cardiovascular disease and live in an area characterized by high levels of air pollution
■ Your residence is located in an area where radon testing is recommended
■ You wish to dispose of waste products containing potentially hazardous chemicals, such as solvents, pesticides, or discarded automobile batteries

Types of Help Available

Most help in the environmental area is government: federal, state, county, and local. In case of an emergency stemming from accidental exposure to a toxic substance, call 911. Your local telephone directory contains numbers for the EPA and local hazardous waste disposal and environmental protection agencies.

Beyond the Text

1. Mary says, "Don't cut down the trees for food packaging when plastic is cheaper." John argues, "Plastics involve petroleum and their manufacture results in air pollution." Whose side would you take and what other arguments would you use?

2. As a society, we're creating holes in the ozone layer, polluting the air, ruining our food with pesticides, and creating garbage we can't get rid of. As one individual, what can you do about it?

3. Respond to the statement: We should rely on nuclear energy production because it is environmentally less harmful than generating plants using oil or coal.

4. Respond to the following question: Why should I care how my fast-food is packaged, when industrial polluters are the real offenders?

5. If various industries are required to invest funds in antipollution devices, who ultimately will pay for this expense?

Supplemental Readings

Fifty Simple Things You Can Do To Save The Earth by The Earthworks Group. Berkeley, CA: The Earthworks Press, 1989. Practical tips for resource conservation, energy saving, and recycling for the everyday, average person.

Global Warming: Are We Entering the Greenhouse Century by Stephen H. Schneider. San Francisco: Sierra Club books, 1989. The clearest, most complete scientific assessment of climate change yet written for a general audience. A specialist in atmospheric science, the author suggests several options for forestalling global warming.

Health Risks of Radon by The National Research Council. Washington, DC: National Academy Press, 1987. Comprehensive report summarizing extensive research on genetic, carcinogenic, and other biological effects of radon and other internally deposited alpha-emitters.

Life in the Balance by David R. Wallace. New York: Harcourt Brace Jovanovich Pub-

lishers, 1987. A thorough explanation of the state of the earth's ecosystems, the threats to them (acid rain, overpopulation, and industrial waste), and measures designed to solve these problems.

Secrets of the Soil by Peter Tompkins and Christopher Bird. New York: Harper & Row, 1989. A strong indictment against the use of synthetic chemical fertilizers to restore soil fertility. Instead, the authors recommend the alternative of using humus (compost) prepared from animal and vegetable wastes.

The Hole in the Sky by John Gribbin. New York: Bantam, 1988. Describes the ozone layer and the consequences of its potential destruction by mankind.

The State of the World by Lester Brown. Washington, DC: Worldwatch Institute, 1989. Describes the major environmental problems faced by the world today and provides recommendations for resolving them.

Key Terms Defined

acid rain   rain with a high concentration of acids produced by air pollutants emitted during combustion of fossil fuels

asbestos   fibrous nonburning compound used in roofing and insulating materials; causal factor for lung cancer

biodegradable   capable of being decomposed by natural biological processes

carcinogen   substance that produces cancerous cells or enhances their development

composting   mixing organic material together and allowing it to decay to be used for fertilizer

Environmental Protection Agency   federal government agency responsible for protecting natural resources and the quality of the environment

greenhouse effect   gradual warming of the earth's surface; produced when solar heat becomes trapped by layers of carbon dioxide and other gases

Industrial Revolution   social and economic changes that marked the transition from agricultural and commercial society to industrial society

ozone   form of oxygen naturally present in the upper atmosphere; sometimes present in lower atmosphere as a component of air pollution

ozone layer   upper layer of the earth's atmosphere that protects the earth from harmful ultraviolet radiation

PCBs (polychlorinated byphenyls)   cancer-causing industrial chemicals used in

electrical transformers, lubricants, and plastic

pesticide   any toxic substance used to kill pests or vermin

pollutant   substance or agent in the environment that is the byproduct of human industry or activity and that is injurious to plant, animal, or human life

radon gas   naturally occurring radioactive gas produced by the decay of uranium

smog   grayish or brownish fog caused by the presence of smoke and/or chemical pollutants in the air

toxics   poisonous chemicals associated with air, water, or soil pollution

Consumer Health Choices

As a health care consumer, you have many choices; how you make these choices can greatly influence your overall health and well-being. The first major decision is whether you will play an active or passive role in managing your health care. The active individual concentrates upon education and prevention to maintain his or her health and to avoid the inconvenience, discomfort, and expense of illness. The last factor, expense, has become a major national issue due to the tremendous increase in the costs of both health care and health insurance.

This chapter summarizes many of the choices you have in terms of health care providers, facilities, and services. The challenges of obtaining quality health care and adequate health insurance are also addressed. Tips on controlling your health care costs are included as well.

Key Terms

Catastrophic health insurance

Consent

Diagnostic Related Group (DRG)

Extended care facility

Health care provider

Health Maintenance Organization (HMO)

Holistic health

Medical or Medicaid

Medicare

Patient's Bill of Rights

Preferred Provider Organization (PPO)

Preventive medicine

Public hospitals

Wellness

Contents

The Health Care Industry

Health care has become a major industry in the United States during the past two decades. Total health care expenditures increased from less than $100 billion in 1970 to over $500 billion in 1988. This represents a phenomenal growth rate. As 12 percent of our nation's annual gross national product (GNP), health costs surpass our current expenditures for national defense.

Funds to finance this thriving industry have largely come from two federal programs, Medicare and Medicaid. Medicare (for the elderly) and Medicaid (for the poor) were created in 1965. Since then, government has become the leading purchaser of health services. When state and local funds are combined with federal, more than 40 percent of medical costs are government supported. Private insurance and individuals pay about 30 percent each. Although initially resisted by physicians as "socialized medicine," Medicare had become the leading source of physicians' income by 1985, with current annual payments to doctors approaching $30 billion. The government paid the bills, but no one effectively controlled the costs. During the 1970s, hospital construction and expansion proliferated, and the health care industry began a rampage of growth. The costs for private health insurance soared as well, regardless of whether it was employer-paid or purchased by individuals. To put some limits on runaway health care expenses, in 1983 the federal government initiated a new funding mechanism for Medicare: the diagnosis-related groups (DRG's). The immediate result was to slow down the increases in Medicare payments to hospitals; however, this widened the gap in the ability of many individuals to pay the difference between their medical bills and their insurance reimbursements. Meanwhile, hospitals, clinics, and laboratories became accustomed to obtaining state-of-the art, high-technology equipment with expensive purchase prices and operating costs. Physicians became accustomed to top-dollar fees as well. In response, health insurance premiums doubled from 1980 to 1986, when their total reached nearly $145 billion.

Your Role as a Health Care Consumer

Enrollment in college for many students means a great number of changes in daily life, such as moving to a new location, giving up a full-time job, or assuming new responsibilities. Students must often manage their own time, money, academic commitments, social life, and health care. This chapter deals with your role as an informed health care consumer, a critical aspect of managing your overall health care. Ideally, you would maintain your health at such a high level that you would not require medical treatment. However, most people find this is an unrealistic expectation.

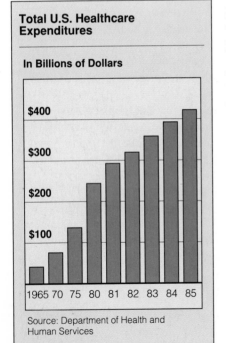

Total U.S. Healthcare Expenditures

In Billions of Dollars

$400

$300

$200

$100

1965 70 75 80 81 82 83 84 85

Source: Department of Health and Human Services

You cannot predict when you will need health care—you may develop viral pneumonia, suffer an ankle sprain while jogging, need to talk to some one about dealing with stress, or develop a strange rash on a part of your body not usually displayed in public. A family member or roommate may be injured in a bicycle accident or take a bad fall on an icy walkway. When illness or injury strikes, you should be prepared to react effectively to care for yourself or to help others. It is impossible to be prepared for every potential situation, but you can become familiar with your health care options and how to make best use of them.

As a college student, you may have access to your college health services. But, if you live off campus, you may elect to use community services for the sake of time and convenience in urgent situations. College health services cannot deal with all medical illnesses or conditions, so they provide students with referrals. You should know how to evaluate referrals and medical advice. And who will have responsibility to pay your medical bills? Today's health care is expensive, so it is important to be aware of your insurance status at all times. If your parents' health insurance does not cover you at college, if you travel overseas, drop out of school temporarily or have dependents, you may no longer have appropriate health insurance coverage for your specific needs.

The role of the health care consumer has changed significantly in the past decade. The consumer was traditionally called a "patient," which implied a passive accepting role; now the consumer is a "client," a term that connotes partnership, participation, and mutual respect. Medical care has become very specialized and, in many areas, "high-tech." Government impacts health care through regulations and insurance programs. Understanding the health care system will enable you to care for your own health effectively while minimizing the costs. Learn to be an informed health care consumer. You play a crucial role in obtaining the benefits.

Health Care Alternatives—Many Choices

Doctors, clinics, and hospitals may seem intimidating, especially if you have had little experience dealing with health care providers. You can minimize your discomfort by familiarizing yourself ahead of time about how professional health care operates. This section describes the system's facilities, services, and personnel. Suggestions for selecting your health care provider follow.

Health Care Professionals and Their Services

Health care professionals—medical doctors, nurses, medical technicians, and others—provide a wide range of services in health promotion, illness prevention, diagnosis and treatment of illness and injury, and rehabilita-

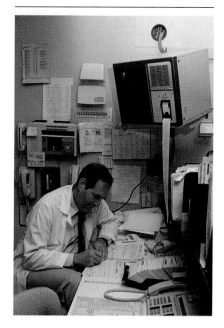

Health Care Practitioners

Doctors have training and skills that make them uniquely qualified to provide health care. However, other health care practitioners have specialized knowledge in areas of concern to specific populations, such as college students. Each type of provider plays a valuable role in the delivery of health care.

Physicians

General Practitioner A GP, or primary care physician, uses a wide range of medical knowledge to monitor the overall health of clients, often with particular emphasis on health promotion.

Family Practitioner Similar to a GP with, perhaps, more emphasis on child health.

Gynecologist Specializes in women's reproductive health. Most often seen for pelvic exams, contraceptive advice, and maternity care. Though actually a specialist, serves as primary care physician for many women.

Internist A specialist in internal organs, who also often functions as a primary care physician.

Specialist Physician When situations warrant detailed knowledge in a particular area, a primary care physician makes a referral to a specialist physician. Medicine has five basic types of specialities: Internal medicine, surgery, pediatrics, obstetrics/gynecology and psychiatry. In turn, each of these has further subspecialities. For instance, a surgeon may be a general surgeon, orthopedic surgeon (bones and joints), cardiac surgeon (heart), plastic surgeon (skin and other outer body areas), or neurosugeon (brain and nervous system) among other choices.

Mental Health Professionals

Several types of practitioners specialize in mental health care. When you request professional counseling, you may receive an appointment with a psychologist, psychiatrist, or social worker. One of the most important considera-

tions in choosing this caregiver is whether you can communicate well with him or her. Another factor to be aware of is that some insurance policies cover mental health care only by licensed psychiatrists, not psychologists.

Psychiatrists Licensed medical doctors, authorized not only to counsel clients but also to diagnose physical causes of mental problems (such as brain tumors and chemical imbalances) and to prescribe medication.

Psychologists Qualified with Ph.D.'s and state licensing. Often have specialities, such as marriage, family, and child counseling (MFCC), hypnosis, or psychological testing. Because they cannot prescribe medications, psychologists often work with people who are less severely affected or do not require drugs to recover or improve.

Social Workers Receive graduate degrees and licensing. May have

tion. In all aspects of health care services, information is a primary component.

The goal of health promotion is to help clients lead healthy lifestyles and maintain their own health with minimal professional intervention. Health promotion includes lifestyle changes, nutrition and weight counseling, and physical fitness programs. Another objective is community education through public information campaigns that focus on specific illnesses, such as AIDS, lung cancer or heart disease. Health promotion and illness prevention overlap. Other illness prevention measures offered by health services include immunizations and periodic physical examinations.

special skills in such areas as family, alcohol and other drugs, nutrition, stress, sexual relations and contraception, and AIDS.

Peer Counselors Individuals with special training in providing information and informal counseling on a particular health issue. Many students feel more comfortable talking about sexual issues or alcohol and other drugs with fellow students. Peer counselors do not provide medical services but can usually give information, answer questions, and help explore options.

Dental Practitioners

Dentists Receive a DDS degree and are eligible for a licensing exam. Within the general area of tooth, mouth, and jaw care, some dentists receive additional training and specialize in such areas as orthodontics (straightening teeth) or oral surgery (tooth extraction, root canals, and so forth).

Dental Hygienists Provide teeth cleaning, usually in a dentist's office, though sometimes at their own practice. Other members of the dental health team include dental assistants and dental lab technicians.

Medical Professionals

Nurses Provide health treatment and carry out physicians' orders. They also provide health-care information, counseling, support, and care in doctors' offices, clinics, hospitals, and sometimes their own facilities. Different nursing titles reflect different education and licensing levels. A registered nurse (RN) is a professional who completes a four year (BSN), three year (Diploma), or two year nursing program (ADN) prior to passing a licensing examination. A nurse practitioner is an RN with advanced training, through either a master's degree or a specialized nurse practitioner program. A licensed vocational nurse (LVN) usually has a high-school degree, completes a nine to eighteen month program

and passes a licensing examination. Only nursing aides and orderlies do not need licensing. LVN's, aides, and orderlies are all support staff to the RN.

Emergency Medical Technicians Provide emergency medical services in critical situations, such as motor vehicle accidents, fires, rescues and medical emergencies. Trained in cardiopulmonary resuscitation and other lifesaving procedures, EMT's administer IV's and certain medications under supervision of a physician. Highest level of preparation is EMT-P (Paramedic).

Physical Therapists Work with a client's body to help increase mobility and strength, and decrease pain. Clients are usually referred to a PT by a physician for treatment of a congenital problem, an injury, or other pain problem.

Occupational Therapists Supervise creative and fine-motor activities to mentally and physically promote recovery.

In spite of vigorous prevention measures, some people do sustain injuries and contract illnesses. Self-care suffices sometimes, but to provide care you need to identify the problem. Is your persistent sore throat caused by a virus or a strain of bacteria? Are your headaches a response to academic stress, or do they signal a need for new prescription contacts or eye glasses? Perhaps you need a brief visit to a health care facility where you can consult with a physician and perhaps other health care professionals. To diagnose your problem, a physician will assess your health history, signs and symptoms, and appropriate tests such as throat culture or eye exam. The doctor will then recommend a treatment program to manage the symptoms, protect your body from further complications,

Consumer Health Choices

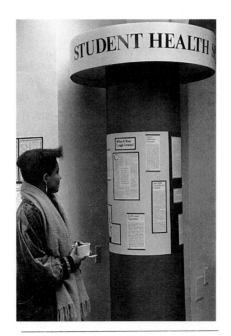

and increase the rate of recovery. Your treatment may include prescription or nonprescription medication, use of special equipment, or in rare cases, surgery. If appropriate, your complete recovery may include a period of physical therapy.

Health Care Facilities

U.S. health consumers spend billions of dollars per year on health care. This money is divided among many types of providers. These range from the traditional doctor's office to a massive regional medical center. Health care alternatives have diversified considerably in the last few years, with the proliferation of walk-in emergency clinics and home health care. Knowing the right place to obtain help can make obtaining health care quicker, more cost-effective, and less traumatic.

Physician's Offices   Some physicians operate their practices independently, with a nurse or medical assistant and receptionist as support staff. The physician may share space with other independent practitioners who provide off-hours backup and referrals for one another. Overhead costs and increasing rates of malpractice insurance make this type of practice more expensive and, therefore, less attractive than group practice for many physicians.

Group-Practice Clinics   A clinic is an association of physicians and other health care providers working together in a single facility to share overhead costs and information. Among the 60 percent of America's doctors who are office-based, the number of group practitioners doubled between 1969 and 1980. A clinic may have a few physicians, all with the same specialty (such as family practice, pediatrics, or ophthalmology), or it may have a full range of both primary physicians and specialists. Sometimes a clinic is associated with a local hospital.

College Health Centers   Approximately 80 percent of colleges and universities offer health services for students and staff. College health centers tend to operate as group-practice clinics, with physicians and staff as employees. College health centers provide services, information and counseling in response to the needs of their student clients. Some colleges offer all services in one clinic; others have several facilities or use off-campus providers. If you need a specialist not available at your health center, the staff will refer you to a practitioner in the community. Learn what kinds of treatment and information services your student health center offers by reading materials that come in the college's registration packet or by contacting the health service directly.

Community Clinics   A community clinic usually operates as a nonprofit organization, employing physicians and other health care professionals to provide a wide range of basic services to the community. Some community clinics specialize in low-income clients who cannot otherwise afford adequate health care services.

Public health clinics, usually sponsored by the city or county, provide services such as family planning, prenatal care, pediatrics, and general health care to low-income residents. Some offer specialized functions such as immunizations or testing for sexual transmitted diseases (STD's). Public health clinics may be free-standing, usually in a low-income area, or share a facility with the public hospital. Some public health departments operate mobile units that come to neighborhoods, work sites, and child care facilities.

Emergency Clinics   In the past decade, emergency clinics have opened throughout the country. Many of these clinics operate without hospital affiliation. To meet the needs of cost-conscious two-worker families, the clinics are often located in or near shopping malls and other commercial areas. They offer extended working hours, including weekends, holidays, and evenings. Clients walk in without appointments and receive a wide range of on-site services including X-ray and laboratory, and a pharmacy. Clients see whichever staff member is on duty. Many hospitals have an emergency department where the client can receive walk-in care. Hospital emergency care may take longer and cost more than a walk-in clinic; however, all of the hospital support services are available.

Outpatient Clinics   Also called surgi-centers or ambulatory care centers, simple surgeries and procedures formerly done in hospitals are now available at these clinics on a one-day basis. Hospitals that operate outpatient centers may perform as many as 40 percent of their surgeries on an outpatient basis. Though the public initially resisted this change, most people now welcome it as a safe, less stressful, and less costly alternative. Clients do not have to go through a lengthy admission process, overnight stay or extensive evaluation or tests.

Hospitals   The major health care centers in this country are hospitals. The mandate of hospitals is to provide treatment services and comprehensive care to the acutely ill. To accomplish this, hospitals offer diagnostic tests and treatment services in surgery, maternity, pediatrics, psychiatry, and other subspecialties. Hospitals offer various levels of care. For example, they have surgery recovery rooms, intensive care units, cardiac care facilities, step-down care for recovery, rehabilitation, and coordination of home health services. They also provide in-house services such as X-ray, laboratory analysis, blood bank, and pharmacy.

There are three hospital types—public, nonprofit, and private. Cities and counties operate nonprofit public hospitals for both community members with private insurance and clients who cannot afford medical services. Private hospitals, run independently or as part of a nationwide

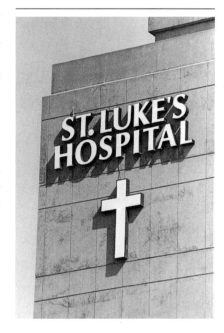

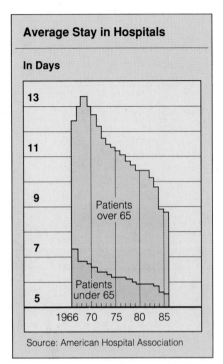

Average Stay in Hospitals

In Days

13

11

9

Patients over 65

7

Patients under 65

5

1966 70 75 80 85

Source: American Hospital Association

chain of health-care facilities, are for-profit organizations and accept only clients with insurance coverage. Every hospital must obtain a state license. Only about 75 percent have received accreditation from the Joint Commission on Accreditation of Hospitals (JCAH) which assures certain standards of sanitation, medical supervision, and diagnostic and laboratory services.

Larger hospitals have board-certified specialists in a wide range of areas. Teaching hospitals, affiliated with medical schools, usually offer the most sophisticated medical services, which are useful in cases of serious illness or injury. On the other hand, many community hospitals also offer excellent care. Some hospitals limit their care to specific clinical specialties such as psychiatry, child birth or cancer.

Counseling Centers   Many facilities offer supportive services and programs designed for specific problems. These include drug and alcohol rehabilitation, crisis intervention, hospice, and AIDS centers. Some counseling centers have live-in facilities; others offer specialist physicians, referral, and assistance with their clients' daily living.

Home Health Care Agencies   For individuals well enough to live at home but not well enough to care for themselves, a home health care agency or visiting nurse association can provide assistance. Personnel range from licensed nurses to homemaker services who assist clients with medication, physical therapy, and help with day-to-day activities on a short-term or long-term basis. Rates for these services are usually much lower than hospital fees. Most insurance companies have strict criteria that limit payments for home health care services.

Working with Health Care Providers

As a "client," your responsibilities include selecting and interacting with your health care provider. By planning who you will see, why and what you want your visits to accomplish, you can increase the provider's success in helping you regain and maximize your health.

Choosing a Provider

If you have always been healthy, you may not have your own doctor. If you get injured or suddenly become ill, you may take whatever health care is convenient. Ideally, you may want to interview several potential health care providers when you are feeling well to select the right one. If you have an ongoing health problem or concern (such as diabetes or severe acne), make sure you have appropriate care for your specific needs. Check the services available at your college health clinic. The three most important factors in selecting a health care provider are (1) particular knowledge of the specialty area that includes your medical condition, (2) good credentials, and (3) a manner compatible with yours.

Consumer Health Choices

Alternative Treatment Methods

Acupuncture An ancient Chinese method of relieving pain and treating disease. Based on the belief that energy flows along certain lines or meridians in the body creating a balance between two principles of nature called Yin and Yang. It is believed that lack of energy flow or blocked energy along the meridians leads to illness. Acupuncture treatment involves inserting sharp needles under the skin along the meridian lines, thereby unblocking energy, stimulating flow and restoring balance and health of internal organs. Since the 1960s Chinese doctors, as well as some U.S. physicians, have performed major surgery with acupuncture as the only anesthetic.

Applied Kinesiology A form of treatment based on the theory that the condition of a person's muscles reflect certain internal disorders or problems. Body imbalances or disorders are identified when certain muscle groups are tested and appear weak.

Certain foods, medications, or herbs, are held in a person's hand or placed next to their skin. If the substance is not appropriate for the body, the muscles will respond to testing by appearing weak. When the substance is removed, the muscles will regain their strength.

Chiropractic Originating from ancient Greece, literally meaning "done by the hands." This method of treating illness suggests the cause of disease and dysfunction in the body is misalignment of the spinal column which interferes with proper nerve function. These conditions cause or contribute to some diseases and lower the body's resistance to others. Spinal adjustments and manipulation will restore structural integrity, thus enabling the body to heal itself. Studies have shown that chiropractic can relieve pain and structural disorders in the joints and muscles.

Reflexology This method of treatment, also called "zone therapy," proposes that diseases and organ dysfunction can be both diagnosed and treated by pressing on certain areas of the hands or feet. Each area of the body is represented by a corresponding area on the feet or hands; pressing on specific points increases blood, nutrients, and energy flow to the diseased area of the body.

Energy Medicine A contemporary view of medicine that views the human body as made up of electronic vibrations. A new healing paradigm suggests that twenty-first century care will be based on principles of energy where interventions involving the mind and body will interface with environmental, spiritual, and vibrational aspects of healing.

Homeopathy Based on the early 1800s work of a German physician, Dr. Samuel Hahnemann, this system of treatment rests on the theory that small doses of certain substances, usually herbal or chemical, can cause a response in a person that mimics a particular disease. These substances or homeopathic remedies are then administered to a person with a disease exhibiting a similar symptom pattern, stimulating the body's natural healing response. This is called "treatment by similars or like cures like." The practice of homeopathy is becoming more popular; there is even a software package designed to assist physicians in the homeopathic diagnosis and treatment of disease.

Iridology A diagnostic method based on the premise that each particular area in the eye represents a specific area or organ in the body. Examination of the color, texture, and pigment in the iris of the eye can reveal conditions of related body area.

Naturopathy According to this school of thought, diseases are the body's attempt to heal itself through release of impurities. Treatment is oriented toward increasing the client's "vital force" by eliminating the toxins, allowing the body to heal. Methods utilized include anything drugless such as nutrition, herbs, massage, and exercise.

577

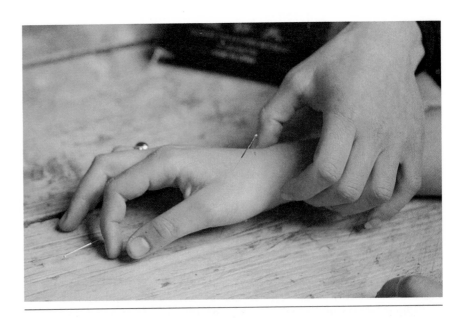

Choose the Right Provider   Many health care professionals recommend that you have a primary-care physician who provides or coordinates all your medial care. A primary-care physician is usually a general practitioner, family practitioner, gynecologist, or internist. For many conditions, you will want to start with this physician, to get an overall view of your health status. What you think of as stress may turn out to be a nutritional deficiency. A backache may signal a kidney infection, and so forth.

Student health services and other clinics often have clients first see a primary-care physician who then provides referrals to specialists as necessary. Gynecologists, dermatologists, and some other specialists usually receive clients without a referral from a primary physician. To find a good specialist, talk not only with your primary care physician but also with people who have experienced a similar health condition.

Certain specialty services are offered in college centers. For instance, because sexual health is a frequent concern to many students, college health centers often include a sexual health or women's clinic. For contraceptives, STD's, AIDS, or other sexual health issues, students often choose to start with these resources.

Consider Credentials   Most health care professionals are required to obtain specialized training and certification. Ask about such qualifications if you are not sure. Specialist physicians should be board-certified, which means they have received further clinical training and passed advanced exams in their specialty area. Find out at which hospital the physician has admitting privileges and be sure your insurance will cover that hospital's charges. Find out how the physician or clinic handles off-hour emergencies. Ask about fees, especially if your insurance will not pay for all charges.

Consumer Health Choices

C H A P T E R   22

Choose a Provider You Can Work With   Talk with other people about their experiences with various physicians and other providers at on-campus and community health services. If you have an ethnic background, lifestyle or other situation you feel some health care providers might not understand, talk with others who share your perspective to identify health professionals most likely to meet your needs.

It is your right to be informed concerning your medical condition, so choose a physician and/or nurse who will communicate clearly with you. If you are more comfortable being examined by someone of the same gender, make that request when you set up appointments. In the final analysis, the quality of your health care is more important than the verbal style or outward appearance of the provider.

When to Seek Help

No one wants the doctor's opening line to be, "Why didn't you come to me sooner?" On the other hand, you have wasted your time and might feel like a fool if the doctor offers home treatment advice that you could have learned in five minutes from a book or free phone call. Each chapter in this book describes circumstances under which you should seek professional help. The accompanying list summarizes guidelines for when to seek help.

In case of an immediately life-threatening injury or symptom, dial your area's emergency telephone number for fast medical aid. The most common emergency number in the United States is 911. The 911 operator will dispatch emergency medical services to your location.

If the situation is serious but not acute, you may be able to talk with your physician or an advice nurse. If possible, contact your physician or clinic for advice about when to come in for prompt, appropriate care. You may be directed to go to walk-in services, either at the doctor's office or through your college health clinic, a freestanding clinic, or a hospital emergency room. However, remember that hospital emergency rooms are designed to respond to emergency conditions; clients with nonacute problems must often wait a long time in uncomfortable surroundings and pay higher fees than at their regular doctor's office. So avoid the emergency room when a same-day appointment would also address the problem.

Clinics and doctors often have certain times of the day reserved for clients with sudden medical problems. In less severe cases, you may have to wait days or even weeks for an appointment; ask to be called if the doctor has a cancellation. If your symptoms worsen, call to ask if you should come in sooner.

Consent

When an individual enters a hospital, some of the person's basic legal rights are affected. In order to ensure that these rights are not violated, the client must give permission (consent) for all treatment. Routine care is accepted when the client signs the hospital's "Conditions of Admission." Certain procedures, such as injections, are treatments ordered by the physician and agreed to by the client. There are many rules and regulations governing consents. The age of consent varies according to state and also according to specific situations, such as being away from the family and supporting yourself. If you are under 18, a health care provider must usually have authorization from your parent or guardian to perform medical services. In some cases, children and adolescents brought to emergency rooms after automobile accidents have not received assistance because no one has been available who could consent to treatment. If you (or your dependents) are under 18, make sure that a signed consent form is on file with the regular physician and authorized school staff.

Talking with Your Health Care Provider

The average physician lets the client talk for less than a minute without interrupting. To make your visit with the health care provider as productive as possible, take the following steps:

- Prepare notes beforehand (or while you are waiting, if you come in without an appointment) regarding:

    Symptoms: Be as specific as possible about the frequency, duration, severity, and location of your problem. Consult the Wellness and Illness chart in this book for types of observations to consider. Are you dizzy all the time or only when you stand up from a sitting position? Where do you hurt? When you feel feverish, take your temperature. Did some major stress take place just before or at the same time as your symptoms, such as finals week, an airplane trip, or a change in medication? Were you in close contact with others who have recently had similar symptoms or a diagnosed infectious disease?

    Current medical status: What steps have you taken to treat these symptoms? Note over-the-counter medications you have taken. List the medications you have been taking for other medical conditions.

    Relevant family history: Your doctor will probably ask you about this, depending on your medical record and what is already on the forms you filled out after admission to college. Be sure to indicate any allergic reactions to medications you have experienced.

    Questions: A busy physician may not give you a full explanation of the causes, treatment, and control of your condition unless you ask. Think about what you want and need to know to take responsibility for following through with prescribed treatment. Do you need bed rest? Is your condition contagious? Will you be quarantined so that you will miss classes? Should you be on a special diet? What level of physical exercise is appropriate? Will reducing stress improve your condition? What are the chances that this condition will recur, and what can you do to prevent its recurrence?

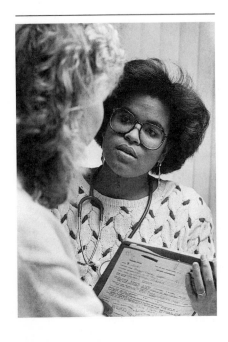

- Make sure you get a chance to explain your symptoms and concerns to your health care provider. In 70 percent of cases, a correct diagnosis depends solely on what you tell your doctor, according to an analysis by the American Society of Internal Medicine.
- If you do not understand something your health care provider says, ask for clarification. Make sure you understand what he or she says about diagnosis, treatment (especially medications), and prognosis. Do not be too embarrassed to ask questions. You have a health consultant; take full advantage of his or her knowledge.
- Discuss diagnostic and treatment alternatives. If you are fearful, shy or hesitant about the risks of any procedure, communicate your point of view and ask about other options. Get adequate information about prescribed medication, especially concerning possible side effects, such as drowsiness or nausea.
- Bring a friend if you would feel more comfortable. In most cases, a friend or family member can help you relax, remind you about topics to discuss, and support you later in following recommended treatments. If possible, let your doctor know ahead of time, in case there is a legitimate reason not to bring someone along.
- If you are concerned about confidentiality, say so. The clinician can assure you about procedures for confidentiality. Normally, only persons directly involved in your health care will have access to your records. However, there are legal requirements regarding reporting of certain communicable diseases, such as STD's, to the public health department.
- Have realistic expectations. Physicians are knowledgeable, but sometimes diagnosis is difficult. The doctor may not have an immediate answer. Some situations will require more than one test to find the underlying cause, or more than one treatment to find the best solution. Sometimes only time can heal a specific condition. Expect to participate in recovering your health.
- If new symptoms appear or your condition worsens, do not hesitate to call your physician, clinic or health service to talk with the provider on duty. You can also leave a message for the person who saw you earlier.

Hospitalization

Very few people look forward to spending time in a hospital. Some clients need hospitalization because they have had surgery or given birth. Others experience hospital admission in an emergency situation, such as an injury. Under normal conditions, your assigned hospital will be the one at which your physician has admission privileges. Your health insurer may be a Health Maintenance Organization (HMO) or a Prepaid Health Plan (PHP) that has preselected hospitals for its members. Many people select a hospital after receiving a recommendation from a friend or family member. If you live in a rural area, there may be only one hospital within a reasonable distance. Under emergency conditions, the ambu-

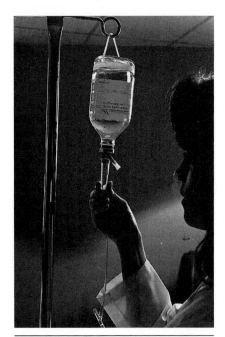

lance company will take you to the emergency room of the closest hospital.

Participating in Your Return to Good Health

After an office visit or a hospital stay, you will probably receive follow-up directions. Take careful note of these instructions. To make your visit worthwhile, you must now take the major responsibility. Your "prescription for health" may include:

- Lifestyle changes (cutting down on alcohol or caffeine, practicing stress-reduction techniques)
- Physical activities (physical therapy, regular exercise)
- Medication (prescription or OTC) and instructions
- Specific healing behaviors (bedrest, using crutches)
- Nutritional actions or limitations (increased fiber, reduction of fat intake)
- Actions to avoid transmission of the illness (quarantine, frequent hand-washing, abstinence from sex)
- Follow-up appointments

If the provider does not find anything wrong but your symptoms persist, you may want to try another provider. If your condition is serious or you are not satisfied with the diagnosis or recommendations you receive, arrange for a second opinion from another physician. Be certain to get a second (or third) opinion if recommendations include a major decision such as surgery. Find out your insurance carrier's policy on covering these consultations before obtaining them.

Keeping Track of Your Health

As long as you continue with the same provider, his or her office maintains your records. The quality of future care you receive may depend on your next health care provider's knowing your previous conditions and treatments. When you change doctors (such as when moving away from home to college), ask your previous care provider to send your records to your new physician or clinic. Past medical history is important for accurate assessment and subsequent treatment. Keep your own set of medical records. Important data includes the following:

- Baseline information (weight, blood pressure, ECG readings, urine and blood analyses)
- Immunizations
- Major illnesses and injuries (date, treatment, and location of treatment)
- Allergies to medicine, foods, or other substances
- Current medications and prescriptions (including corrective lenses)
- Significant family health history

Diagnostic Tests and Exams

Even apparently healthy persons should have certain medical tests on a periodic basis. Such tests serve important purposes in identifying potential problems early, facilitating more effective, simpler treatment. Common diagnostic tests and their recommended frequency are as follows.

Physical exam

Birth to 2 years:	Frequently, starting with every two weeks, progressing to every six months, according to physician's recommendation.
2 years to 17 years:	Every 1 to 2 years.
18 years to 35 years:	Every 4 years.
36 to 45 years:	Every 3 years.
46 to 55 years:	Every 2 years.
After 55:	Every year, or as physician advises.

Blood tests For glucose (for diabetes) and for anemia. At every physical.

Breast exam Self-exam every month and with periodic physical exam.

Cholesterol test Every year.

Colorectal exam For cancer detection. After age 50, every 3 years for women, every 5 years for men.

Dental exam Exam and cleaning. Every 6 months.

Glaucoma test Eye test. Every 2 years after age 35.

Mammogram Breast X-ray to detect cancer. One baseline mammogram for women between ages 35 to 40; then every 1 to 2 years.

Pap smear Cervical cancer screening for women. Once between 18 to 24 years, then every five years (unless sexually active, then every year).

Prostate exam For men, after age 40 years, annually.

Stool blood test For cancer detection. After age 50 years, annually.

TB test Every 3 to 5 years; more often if exposed.

Testicular exam Self-exam every month and with periodic physical exam.

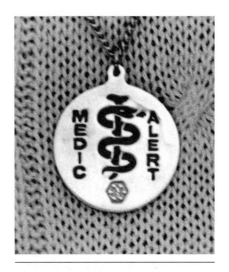

If you have a special medical condition such as diabetes, consider wearing a MedicAlert® tag. MedicAlert is a system designed primarily (though not exclusively) for individuals with potentially life-threatening conditions, such as diabetes, epilepsy, heart conditions, or allergies to medications. A metal emblem on a necklace or bracelet is embossed with your specific condition, a unique registration number, and a collect phone number. Medic Alert Foundation keeps a file with more detailed medical information and emergency contact numbers. Most emergency services personnel are trained to look for MedicAlert tags.

Even if you are perfectly healthy, you may want to consider carrying an Emergicard®. The Emergicard is a plastic wallet-sized card containing a microfilm copy of your important medical records and a built-in magnifying lens, so the microfilm can be read without special equipment. The microfilm contains not only medical data but emergency contact information and authorization for emergency medical treatment. For instance, if you were seriously injured or rendered unconscious in a car accident, the Emergicard would allow emergency room personnel to reach your relatives quickly and to provide immediate medical treatment without waiting for further authorization.

The Challenge of Quality Health Care

The rate of change in U.S. health care has been outpacing our ability to keep up. The complexity of health-care technology, the magnitude of medical malpractice suits and resulting cost of physicians' malpractice insurance, and the increased incidence of long-term medical conditions have led to increasingly expensive health care. Health insurance premiums have increased and policies are becoming more restrictive.

More enterprises are competing for consumers' health care dollars—from pharmaceutical companies and health product manufacturers to freestanding emergency clinics, and nontraditional care options. These changes underscore your responsibility for making sure you are receiving cost-effective medical care. But in today's environment, even doctors are challenged to keep up with the pace of medical knowledge. The media coverage is extensive regarding studies, research, and recommendations. So it is no wonder consumers are sometimes confused.

Elements of Good Health Care

Though opinions may differ about doctors, medications, and treatments, some factors are common to providers who give high quality care. Whether you go to the college health center, a private physician, a public health clinic, or a leading medical research center, you have the right to evaluate the care you receive. The American Hospital Association has developed a "Patient's Bill of Rights." Its guidelines apply to professional health care in all health care settings, not just hospitals. It is summarized in the accompanying box.

Here are some additional points to consider in evaluating your relationship with a specific physician or other health care professional. A good provider should be aware of your previous medical history, reviewing your chart before starting to talk with you. He or she should listen to you and answer your questions in understandable terms. The provider should also take the necessary time to perform exams and keep good records on a routine basis.

When issuing a prescription, the physician should give you complete directions and precautions. Medication is not the answer to all problems; usually it is useful, but sometimes it just masks symptoms or the devastating side effects outweigh its benefits. When a physician recommends surgery, a responsible client (you) understands the role of a second or even a third opinion. As appropriate, your provider should explain the options and encourage you to participate in decision-making. Many health insurance policies will pay for such consultation.

Avoiding the Quacks

The snake-oil salesman doesn't come around anymore. Now we encounter mass media promotions for allergy relief, weight loss miracles, and cancer cures. Every year, people spend millions of dollars on pills, procedures, and potions whose only real achievement is to make money for their promoters. A well-educated consumer can usually spot the difference between a genuine treatment and a baseless approach. Beware of medical "cures" that are delivered via direct mail, door-to-door solicitation, or television/magazine advertising. Do not be persuaded by scare tactics that suggest this is the only cure, your only opportunity to purchase, or your only weapon against the powerful medical establishment, which wants to suppress this cure.

Research a new health product or procedure before buying or trying it. Ask for written, scientifically based evidence of claims, including published reports of studies. Talk with your health care provider before substituting new products or treatments for his or her recommendations. Helpful resources include health-oriented magazines and newsletters, professional journals, and consumer reports. Your local library should be able to provide you with current references.

Consumer Advocates for Health

When you receive a diagnosis and have questions about what to expect, you probably will want to talk with someone supportive and knowledgeable. You can obtain advice and assistance from many private, state, and federal organizations. Several are listed in the resource section for this chapter.

Patient's Bill of Rights

Developed by the American Hospital Association, the Patient's Bill of Rights provides useful guidelines for quality health care. In summary, it states that each patient has the right to:

- Considerate and respectful care.
- Complete diagnostic, treatment, and prognosis information.
- Information to allow for informed consent.
- Refuse treatment to the extent permitted by law.
- Privacy concerning medical care program.
- Confidential medical communication.
- Reasonable response to request for services.
- Information about relationships among health care institutions and individuals.
- Information about experimentation affecting care; right to refuse participation in research projects.
- Reasonable continuity of care.
- Examine and receive explanation of bill.
- Know rules and regulations applying to patient conduct.

If you have a problem or question about student health services, find out if your campus clinic has a health educator or ombudsperson. This person has specific responsibility to help clients understand the system and to resolve problems and disputes. Community clinics, hospitals, and large group practices also often have a clients' ombudsperson. If your problem involves your health insurance policy, you may want to contact your state's department of insurance. This agency licenses insurance companies and mediates disputes between consumers and insurance companies. States usually have a department of consumer affairs to handle complaints about all types of products, businesses, and advertisements.

Paying For Health Care

Types of Health Insurance

The first step in determining your health insurance needs is to check what kinds of coverage you already have through your college, your employer, your parents, or your spouse. Then you should consider what type of coverages you really need—accident, illness, disability, and so forth. Although many colleges include basic health care coverage in their student fees, these plans typically include only care at the health center, not off-campus or during the summer. You may conclude that you need supplementary insurance. Consumers usually get lower insurance rates by purchasing group coverage through a school, employer, union or other organization. You may be eligible to participate in a group that already includes your parents or spouse.

Health insurance is available on the basis of fee-for-service or prepaid. Fee-for-service insurance requires you to choose which physician, hospital, or other care provider to use. With basic health insurance, the consumer pays a certain amount of each health-care bill; the insurance company pays the remainder. Basic coverage pays hospital and medical expenses only up to a certain dollar amount. Buying additional insurance, called major medical insurance, gives consumers more protection from the extremely high expenses that occur in cases of serious injury or prolonged illness.

Prepaid insurance covers a greater share, or perhaps even all, of the expenses associated with health-care bills. The two most common forms of prepaid insurance are the preferred provider organization (PPO) and the health maintenance organization (HMO). An individual who subscribes to a PPO avoids virtually all charges by using doctors and hospitals who have contracted with the PPO to accept fixed fees.

In an HMO plan, individuals receive care from a preselected group or groups of providers. These providers agree to accept a set monthly fee for each client or to charge for services at a lower fee schedule. You pay only a token amount for each actual visit, procedure or prescription. Though

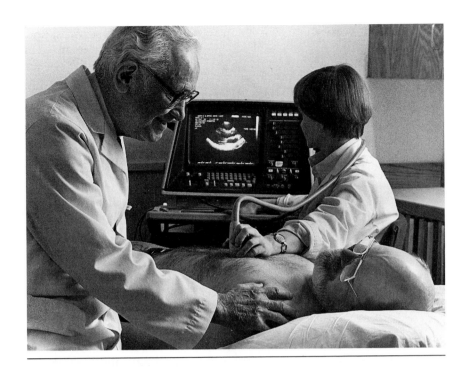

HMO coverage may have a higher monthly cost than other plans, it may have lower overall costs for services. HMO's also emphasize preventive care. They range in size from Kaiser-Permanente Medical Program's more than 5.6 million members to local HMO's that have just 50 members.

The Federal government sponsors two health care insurance programs—Medicare and Medicaid. Medicare covers individuals 65 years old or older, or disabled. Part A of this program provides hospitalization insurance funded through social security. Participants may also voluntarily pay for Part B coverage, which covers nonhospital medical costs, such as physicians, outpatient care, and ambulance services. Medicaid assists low-income people who otherwise could not pay for medical care. Though the federal government pays for Medicaid, each individual state administers its own program.

For government claims, the physician must place the medical condition or treatment into one of 467 diagnosis-related groups (DRG's). This DRG categorization determines the amount of reimbursement the doctor or hospital will receive from Medicare or Medicaid. If a client stays more days than the DRG covers, the hospital must cover the additional expense or expect the client to pay the additional charges. Similarly, if the client leaves the hospital before the DRG reimbursement expires, the hospital makes money. Faced with this incentive to minimize length of stay, many hospitals are sending clients home on schedule, often with a requirement for subsequent home health care.

Choosing Your Plan

Upon enrollment in college or acceptance of full-time employment, you may be provided with health insurance. Almost all colleges (96 percent) make health-insurance benefits available to their students. Group health insurance plans vary greatly in terms of items covered and required deductibles. For example, some policies include dental care and eye examinations or psychological counseling while others do not. You may have the option of supplementing the basic group plan or even selecting among two or more group plans. Many employer health plans require deductions from your pay when you select special additional coverage above the basic group plan.

If you have no coverage or your college does not offer you an adequate plan, you may wish to purchase your own plan. Over 1700 commercial firms sell health insurance. In selecting a plan you should consider the following factors: recommendations of your health care provider, coverage, exclusions, deductibles, payments, dependent coverage, and coverage continuity. Nearly all new policies involve a waiting period between the date you sign the policy and the time when it goes into effect.

Choice of Health Care Provider   Determine which physicians, clinics, and hospitals will accept your plan, especially if you select a PPO or HMO. Suggestions from your physician, friends, and family members may be helpful.

Coverage and Exclusions   When comparing plans, pay close attention to what items each plan includes and excludes. Review the restrictions (waiting time) concerning previously diagnosed health problems, for example, anything relating to chronic back conditions for which you have received prior medical attention. As your life situation changes, your health care needs will change as well. For example, maternity coverage may not be a factor now, but when you plan to become a parent, you may wish to make sure your insurance includes maternity benefits.

Deductibles   Look carefully at how much you will have to pay annually before insurance starts to cover any costs, and for what proportion of each visit you will have to pay. A policy might have a $250 deductible per year, meaning that the insured person will have to cover the first $250 of approved medical expenses before the carrier starts to pay. If you have dependents, ask about family deductibles. Once the policy starts providing coverage, the carrier may pay only a portion of covered expenses, such as 80 percent. This percentage often varies for different types of treatment, such as 80 percent for doctor's visits, and 50 percent for outpatient psychiatric care.

Limits   Some plans cover costs only up to a certain dollar limit. These limits apply to overall costs, or to costs per illness or injury, per individual, per day, or per year. College plans typically have a limit of $20,000 to $25,000, though some colleges supplement with a voluntary extra-cost plan that covers an additional $50,000.

Payments   Find out if you will have to pay insurance premiums, or whether your coverage is included in college fees or employment benefits. Employers and schools usually charge the individual for dependent coverage; if relevant, find out what these costs will be.

Dependent Coverage   It may be appropriate to ask about dependent coverage. Some companies extend such coverage to a spouse and to unmarried children under 19 years old; others include children up to a specified age if they are full-time students. They may exclude children who are full-time college students or on active military duty. The term "dependent" also includes stepchildren, foster children, and legally adopted children who depend on the insured person for support and maintenance.

Coverage Continuity   If you are considering insurance offered specifically to students, check the enrollment conditions you must meet to continue coverage. Some college policies cover students on campus, but not during summer break, travel (even out of town), residence at an overseas campus, holidays or vacations. Find out if you can change from full-time to part-time, or if you can take a semester or two off and keep your coverage. If your status changes from full-time to less than half-time employment, employer-provided insurance probably will not continue to cover you. Students returning to college frequently overlook this situation or do not realize that coverage included in their student fees may be considerably less than the amount provided by former employers.

Controlling Your Health Care Costs

Even with insurance, health care can drain your bank account. You can help to keep these costs down. Though the advice may sound simplistic, the most effective tactic is to stay healthy in the first place. This book contains many suggestions designed to help you make informed choices and stay healthy. By focusing on wellness, you will strengthen your body's reserves enough to minimize the seriousness and duration of most health problems that arise. The following suggestions can help you minimize the cost of your health care.

Use Phone-in Advice.   Find out if your college health service or other health care provider has phone-in advice. If it does, keep the number handy; by using it you will save yourself discomfort and unnecessary trips to the doctor. Other telephone sources of health information are listed in specific chapters and in the accompanying box.

What Your Insurance Policy Covers

When considering a health insurance policy, find out which of the following services the policy includes (or includes for an extra fee).

- Physician's fees
- Prescriptions
- Preventive care
- Alternative health care (chiropractic, acupuncture, and so forth)
- Hospital room and board
- Preadmission tests
- Second surgical opinions
- Fees for assistant surgeon, anesthetist
- X-ray, laboratory expenses
- Outpatient services
- Ambulance services
- Emergency-room treatment
- Psychiatric care
- Other forms of mental-health counseling
- Treatment for substance abuse
- Home health care
- Maternity
- Dental care (including orthodontics, crowns)
- Vision care (including eye glasses and contacts)

Buy Generic Prescriptions. If your physician prescribes medication, discuss whether a brand name or a generic one would be preferable. When a pharmaceutical company's patent expires, other companies may manufacture that same drug under a generic name or their own brand. Both generic and the brand name versions must meet federal standards for safety, purity, and effectiveness. Because generic usually costs less than original brand name, consumers often prefer generic prescriptions. However, many doctors believe that different brands of medications have varied levels of effectiveness and side effects. Ask for your physician's recommendation.

Use Community Health Resources. If your policy covers health care at a specified facility (such as the college health center or another HMO), use those services whenever appropriate. However, not all health care costs money. As discussed in other chapters, self-help groups assist millions to cope more effectively with problems such as alcohol and drug dependence, diabetes, stroke, heart disease, cancer, and sexual abuse. Such aid is usually free and confidential. Support from others who have gone through similar circumstances provides healing in ways professionals cannot. Other free services include community blood pressure and cholesterol screenings, community family planning clinics, and immunization programs. Your physician or the county public health department should know about such services.

Understand Your Insurance Coverage. Knowing your plan thoroughly and selecting and scheduling medical treatment in accordance with your coverage can save you hundreds or thousands of dollars. Know how to ensure that your plan will cover services in case of emergency. The back of most health plan cards gives such information, as well as a phone number for more information. Refer to your policy if you have the choice of inpatient or outpatient care, or a choice of when to schedule a procedure.

After you obtain insurance, you will probably receive an identification card. Carry this with you at all times. If you are injured or suddenly become seriously ill, an emergency clinic or hospital will want assurance that you are financially covered.

Choose Outpatient Procedures Instead of Hospitalization. In some ways, a hospital bed looks inviting—plenty of rest, meal delivery, a television in the ceiling, and a call button if you need anything. But hospital stays are expensive: nonprofit hospital charges can average $700 to $800 per day (without physician's fees). For the average client under 65 years old whose average length of stay is five and one-half days, that total is over $4,000. You will often rest better, recuperate more quickly, and have less risk of infection at home. So, to minimize disruption and costs, use outpatient clinics whenever possible. If you must be hospitalized, arrange to have diagnostic tests and other preparatory work done on an outpatient basis before admission.

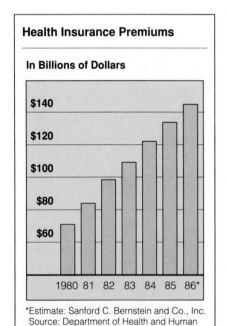

Health Insurance Premiums

In Billions of Dollars

$140	
$120	
$100	
$80	
$60	
	1980 81 82 83 84 85 86*

*Estimate: Sanford C. Bernstein and Co., Inc.
Source: Department of Health and Human Services

File Claim Forms Properly. One of the requirements of some types of insurance coverage is filing claims. If you use the college health service, belong to an HMO, or use PPO-approved services, you may not need to fill out claim forms. However, if your policy requires that you make some payment, then you will probably have to file a claim form for every doctor's visit, test, or other procedure.

You may either pay the care provider's bill yourself and have the insurance company reimburse you, or you can assign the carrier's payment to the care provider when you file the claim. If you must pay a certain deductible amount before insurance begins to cover expenses, send proof of payment for those charges you cover, so the insurance company will have records of how much you have paid. Keep copies of all claim forms you submit. It takes a few weeks to a few months for insurance carriers to pay claims.

Keep Track of Health Care Charges. Maintain complete and well-organized records of health-related transactions. Keep a file of all health care expenses and payments, particularly if you must pay deductibles. Under certain conditions, you may qualify for a medical deduction on your year-end federal income tax return. Taking notes on conversations with providers and insurance representatives can minimize confusion and help you document your points clearly and persuasively if you encounter a health complication.

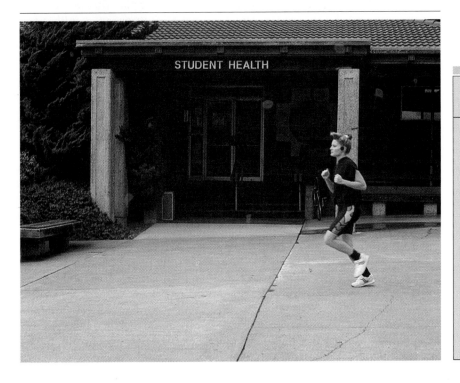

Mandatory Health Insurance for Students

A new Massachusetts law will require all full-time and part-time students enrolled in public or private institutions of higher education to participate in a qualifying student health insurance plan. Each student will pay an average of $250 a year for health insurance, although at the University of Massachusetts at Amherst, the annual premium will be $392 for the year.

Source: *Chronicle of Higher Education,* August 2, 1989

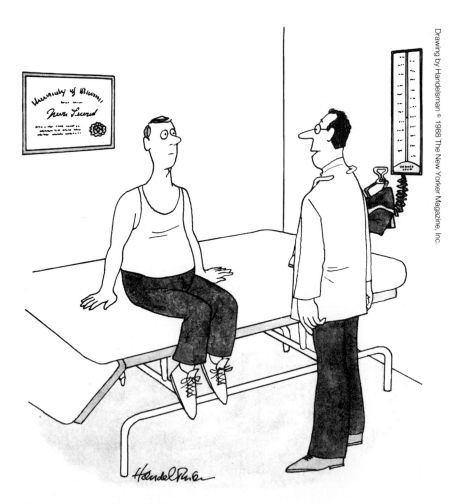

"We medical practitioners do our very best, Mr. Nyman. Nothing is more sacred to us than the doctor-plaintiff relationship."

Review Bills. If you take issue with any charge, review the back of the health care bill, which usually details payment requirements and late charges. If the provider's billing office admits an error, ask to receive a corrected bill promptly. If needed, write a letter supporting your position, enclosing copies of supporting evidence.

The Crisis in Student Health Insurance

Faced without coverage on their parents' policies, many college students are choosing to go without insurance rather than pay for it out of their own pockets. Nearly 3 million students (24 percent) have no health insurance at all, and an equal number have inadequate coverage. Student health administrators point out that the average premium of $250 to $350 for a year's health insurance is nominal compared to automobile insurance premiums, or to other items commonly purchased by students, such as stereo equipment and microwave ovens. In response, more colleges and universities are requiring students to sign up for the school's sponsored health plan or to prove comparable coverage from a private policy. About 40 percent of four-year institutions now have health insurance requirements. The trend is toward a stricter policy for mandatory insurance.

Proposals to Control National Health Care Costs

Consumer advocate organizations, including the American Association of Retired Persons, are very concerned that elderly clients will be spending a major share of their fixed incomes on medical expenses unless costs are controlled. The problems associated with providing health care to people without any insurance have become a major public concern, as well. Proposals include universal health insurance and limiting doctors' fees.

Controlling Doctors' Fees   In mid-1989, the U.S. Congress opened hearings on various proposals aimed at controlling the rapid rise in Medicare fees paid to doctors. These payments tripled from $9 billion to $28 billion between 1980 and 1988. They are expected to surpass $30 billion by 1990. Many of the nation's 553,000 licensed physicians are less than enthusiastic about such regulatory measures.

Universal Health Insurance   The elderly are only one of several important segments of the health consumer population. The 37 million Americans under the age of 65 with no public or private health insurance include 12 million children under the age of 18 and an estimated 3 million college students. Minorities are strongly represented in those lacking coverage: 22 percent of African Americans and 32 percent of Hispanics have no health insurance. Many workers in part-time or low-paying jobs (a high proportion are minority workers) are not included in company health care plans. Current proposals under debate range from mandatory insurance coverage financed by employers for all workers to a federally sponsored program. In a recent Louis Harris and Associates survey, 81 percent of Americans said they would prefer a health-care system similar to Canada's, where government-funded insurance sets fees charged by doctors and hospitals. Canadians select their own physicians and hospitals and are guaranteed care at no charge. The main financing comes from taxes paid by individuals, plus a small portion from employers. The American Medical Association has voiced its opposition to this kind of plan.

Seeking Professional Help

Seek Help If:

You have questions or disputes in your dealings with your physician, college health center, hospital, insurance carrier, or other health care provider that you do not feel is working out satisfactorily. Your concerns might include:

- Finding the most appropriate provider for your needs
- Getting a second opinion about diagnosis or treatment
- Believing that you are getting too little information from your health care provider about diagnosis, treatment, or prevention
- Unprofessional behavior or possible malpractice
- Disagreement about charges for procedures or services
- Adequacy or affordability of health insurance

Types of Assistance

Many college health centers, medical centers, and hospitals now have an ombudsperson on staff specifically skilled in answering health care questions and resolving conflicts. This person acts as a consumer advocate, but knows how the larger organization functions.

In cases involving unprofessional behavior or potential malpractice, you may also want to file a complaint with your state board of medical examiners (look in your phone book, ask your health center, or contact your state legislative representative's office).

Beyond the Text

1. Who pays or who should pay for the health care costs incurred by the 37 million people in the United States with no health insurance?

2. Ben Franklin once observed that "an ounce of prevention is worth a pound of cure." How would you apply this to your own health care situation?

3. You have been suffering from "tennis elbow." Your doctor recommends a cortisone injection, but a friend suggests acupuncture. Which treatment would you take and why?

4. Your physician recommends surgery to correct an old knee injury that continues to trouble you. What questions would you ask in order to decide what to do?

5. What steps can you take to protect yourself from fraudulent claims of promoters of health products?

Supplemental Readings

An Introduction to the U.S. Health Care System by M. I. Roemer. New York: Springer Publishing, 1986. Describes the history, structure, and operation of the U.S. health care system and suggests changes for the future.

Extended Health Care at Home by Evelyn M. Baulch. Berkeley, CA: Celestial Arts, 1988. An excellent resource for families facing long-term illnesses or injuries.

HMO's: The Revolution in Health Care by Jill Bloom. Tucson, AZ: The Body Press, 1987. Analyzes strengths and weaknesses of five types of health maintenance organizations, and provides a helpful checklist for use in selecting an HMO.

Take Care of Yourself by Donald M. Vickery, MD, and James F. Fries, MD. Reading, MS: Addison-Wesley, 1986. A consumer's guide to medical care, this book is one of the most popular and easy-to-follow medical guides. Useful, sensible advice for over 100 medical problems.

The Alternative Health Guide by B. Inglis and R. West. New York: Springer Publishing, 1986. A comprehensive description of over fifty alternative therapies.

The AMA Family Medical Guide edited by Jeffrey Kunz, MD. New York: Random House, 1982. Answers questions about all the most common diseases and their symptoms. Extensive use of self-analysis charts. Very comprehensive.

The People's Book of Medical Tests by Tom Ferguson, MD, and David Sobel, MD. New York: Summit Books, 1985. The first comprehensive guide to which tests are reliable and which are not.

Key Terms Defined

catastrophic health insurance covers illnesses whose costs exceed coverage provided by any other insurance policy

consent in law, voluntary agreement with an action proposed by another; written informed consent is generally required before nonemergency medical procedures

Diagnostic Related Group (DRG) classification of patients according to medical diagnosis for purposes of paying medical costs

extended care facility provides long term medical care for patients who are not acutely ill

health care provider any organization or individual who provides health care or instruction

Health Maintenance Organization (HMO) broad term encompassing a variety of health care delivery systems based on offering comprehensive care to a prepaid, identifiable population

holistic health concept of medical care in which the emotional and social needs of the client are dealt with as well as the physical needs

Medical or Medicaid state-operated program providing medical care to qualifying low-income persons, subsidized by the federal government

Medicare program of the Social Security Administration that provides funding for medical care for the elderly and certain others

Patient's Bill of Rights published by the American Hospital Association in 1973, a document that outlines and specifies the rights attributed to a person seeking health care

Preferred Provider Organization (PPO) group of physicians who arrange their fees with insurance companies prior to treatment

preventive medicine prophylactic medical care aimed at preventing disease

public hospitals hospitals operated by government agencies and supported by taxes

wellness sum total of behaviors, activities, and attitudes that improve health and the quality of life

Appendix 1: Communicable Diseases

Disease	Symptoms and Incubation Period	Transmission and Communicability	Treatment and Home Care
Chickenpox (varicella)	Acute viral disease; onset is sudden with high fever; maculopapular rash and vesicular scabs in multiple stages of healing. Incubation is 10 to 21 days.	Spread by droplet or airborne secretions; scabs not infectious. Communicable: 1 day before rash to 5–6 days after eruption.	Isolate. Treat symptomatically: fluids for fever, Tylenol. Prevent scratching. Observe for signs of complications—notify physician.
Mumps	Acute viral disease, characterized by fever, swelling, and tenderness of one or more salivary glands. Potential complications, including meningoencephalitis.	Spread by droplet and direct and indirect contact with saliva of infected person. Communicable: 5 days before to 9 days after swelling appears. Most infectious 48 hours prior to swelling.	Prevent by vaccination. Isolate. Treat symptomatically: ice pack and encourage fluids, Tylenol. Watch for symptoms of neurological involvement: fever, headache, vomiting, stiff neck.
Measles (rubeola)	Acute viral disease, characterized by conjunctivitis, bronchitis, Koplik's spots on buccal mucosa. Dusky red and splotchy rash 3 to 4 days. Usually photophobia. Complications can be severe in respiratory tract, eye, ear, and nervous system. Incubation is 10 to 12 days.	Spread by droplet or direct contact. Communicable: 5th day of incubation to first few days of rash (5–7 days).	Treat symptomatically: bedrest until cough and fever subside; force fluids, dim lights in room; tepid baths and lotion to relieve itching. Observe for signs of neurological complications.
German Measles (rubella)	Viral infection. Slight fever, mild coryza and headache. Discrete pink-red maculopapules that last about 3 days. Incubation is 14 to 21 days.	Spread by direct and indirect contact with droplets. Fetus may contract measles in utero if mother has the disease. Check rubella titer in women who may become pregnant. Communicable: 7 days before rash to 5 days after rash appears.	Basically a benign disease. Treat symptomatically: bedrest until fever subsides. Encourage fluids and give Tylenol.
Diphtheria	Local and systemic manifestations. Malaise, fever, cough with stridor. Toxin has affinity for renal, nervous and cardiac tissue. Incubation 2 to 6 days or longer.	Spread by droplets from respiratory tract or carrier. Communicable: 2–4 weeks if untreated; 1–2 days with antibiotic treatment.	Antitoxin must be given early; give antibiotic therapy to kill toxin. Strict bedrest; prevent exertion. Liquid or soft diet. Observe for respiratory complications. Hospitalization may be required for suctioning and oxygen; emergency tracheotomy may be necessary.
Whooping Cough (pertussis)	Dry cough occurring in paroxysms. Dyspnea and fever may be present. Lymphocytosis. Incubation is 5 to 21 days.	Direct contact or droplet from infected person. Communicable: 7 days after exposure to 3 weeks after onset.	Treat symptomatically: rest, warm, humid air. Maintain nutritional status. Protect from secondary infections.

Appendix 2: Wellness and Illness Reference Guide

Condition and Symptoms	Traditional Medical Care
Athlete's Foot Athlete's foot is caused by a fungus that thrives in a warm, moist environment. It is most common in hot, humid areas. Common symptoms are redness, cracks in the skin between toes, burning, itching, and peeling skin.	Usually treated at home, the MD will suggest OTC (over-the-counter or nonprescription) medications such as Desenex powder between the toes to keep them dry. A stronger antifungal medication may be required to actually control the fungus. Tinactin in either cream or lotion works effectively. A prescription called Nystatin taken by mouth will help correct the problem.
Bleeding Gums—Gingivitis Bleeding gums or periodontal disease affects 20 million Americans. It is the result of bacteria lodging in your mouth between your teeth and along the margins of teeth and gums. Bacteria live in plaque that hardens into tartar. Bacterial buildup causes gum irritation, swelling and bleeding. Long-term problems result in bone involvement and loss of your teeth.	Frequent dental care to remove plaque. Brushing teeth two times a day with tartar-control toothpaste. Daily flossing until teeth are squeaky clean.
Blisters Blisters on the skin may result from allergic reactions to internal causes (food or medication) or to external causes (plant oils or insect bites). Blisters also result from injuries such as friction, heat or pinched skin. Viral infections may also cause blisters. Blisters form a raised area of skin filled with fluid.	Blisters from burns: current medical treatment suggests that they not be punctured—even under sterile conditions—due to danger of infection. Do nothing (unless caused from an infection) and allow skin to heal naturally. If blister breaks, cover with bandage. If infection present, antibiotics or antiviral medication will be prescribed.
Body Odor Sweat glands, imbedded in your skin, produce a liquid as your body gets hot. Evaporation of the liquid cools the body, keeping your body's temperature regulated. This perspiration usually has a distinctive odor, but it is not terribly offensive. If yours is, read the Holistic column. Offensive odor is often caused by bacteria on the skin and clothing.	This is a normal process, and there is no medical care suggested.
Canker Sores Acute, painful ulcers that occur singly or in groups. They appear as painful, raw, open sores on the lips, tongue or lining of the mouth.	Rinse orally with topical anesthetic, such as lidocaine, every few hours. A dental protective paste will decrease irritation. For severe ulcers, oral tetracycline is given by prescription. Occasionally, this treatment results in oral candidiasis, a yeast infection.

Holistic or Nontraditional Care	Prevention
Ask your pharmacist to make up a solution of 30% aluminum chloride and apply twice daily to dry up the fungus.	Wash feet twice a day and keep them dry, especially between the toes. Use your hair dryer to be sure skin is dry.
Dust with cornstarch between toes to keep them dry. Sprinkle cayenne pepper in your shoes.	Wear absorbent cotton socks. Change them *every day*.
Open a clove of fresh garlic and rub on the affected areas; it may sting but it will help.	If possible, keep feet bare in open sandals. Don't wear sneakers, because they make your feet perspire.
Try raw honey smeared between your toes on all affected areas; put on a light cotton sock and leave on all night.	Don't go barefoot in locker room showers.
	Put vinegar on a cotton ball and dab between your toes morning and night.
Rinse mouth four times a day with one tablespoon aloe vera juice. Swish it around and spit it out.	Frequent and good dental care as well as daily hygiene practices (cleaning and flossing) are critical.
Another rinse is hydrogen peroxide. Rinse, allow to bubble and spit out. *Do not swallow.*	Diet is important for prevention: eat fibrous foods such as celery, carrots and apples; limit sugar; eat fruits for Vitamin C; and maintain a well-balanced diet.
Nutrient supplements that have positive effects: Organic germanium (150–200 mg per day), CoQ_{10} (50–100 mg per day), calcium gluconate or calcium carbonate (500 mg two times per day). Available at your health food store.	Vitamins and minerals, especially Vitamin A to strengthen gum tissue.
	CoQ_{10}, 60 mg per day, is great for maintenance.
Do not break blister with a needle. Allow it to remain intact to avoid infection.	Wear moleskin on areas that tend to blister.
Vitamin E on area, three times a day, lessens soreness and protects the skin.	Wear shoes with correct fit.
	If your hands are tender, wear gloves when you do manual labor.
If you already have good personal hygiene habits (you shower and use deodorant) and body odor persists, zinc tablets (30 mg a day) may alleviate the problem.	Wash your underarms and your feet with antibacterial soap daily because the offensive odor is usually caused by the action of bacteria, not the perspiration itself. If you are a woman, shave your underarms frequently and use deodorant and powder.
Zinc also helps foot odor; dusting cornstarch on feet keeps them dry; or try soaking them daily in warm water with white vinegar added.	If sensitive to one product, switch to another.
To relieve pain for several hours, dissolve two aspirin in four ounces of warm water and rinse mouth, or hold aspirin tablet directly on lesion.	Because deficiencies of iron, Vitamin B_{12} and folic acid increase susceptibility, prevention involves eating a well-balanced diet or taking these supplements.
Eat fresh pineapple and apply pineapple juice to canker sores (improvement in one day).	Limit intake of sugar and fatty foods.
	Increase intake of Vitamin C and A.

Condition and Symptoms	Traditional Medical Care

Colds

A viral infection of the respiratory tract—may include both nose and throat.

Colds usually appear gradually—your nose runs, you feel a little stuffed up, and you may have a headache. (On the other hand, flu appears quickly and hits you like a Mac truck. Suddenly you have a fever, cough, and can hardly make it out of bed. Nausea and vomiting may be part of the flu.)

Stuffy nose: Viruses (any of 200 varieties, according to scientists) have invaded cells in your nose, and the tissue becomes inflamed.

Runny nose: Mucous membranes increase secretions to try to fight the viral infection.

Symptom Alert: Call MD if:

- Pain in your ear—may indicate ear infection.
- Sinus pain—may indicate sinus cavity infection.
- High fever—secondary infection.
- *Heavy* yellow or green mucus—may indicate bacterial infection.
- Difficulty breathing.
- Symptoms persist beyond two weeks.

See also Cough, Fever and Chills, Flu, Sore Throat.

There is no cure for the common cold (which usually lasts seven days), so treatment is supportive.

A cold is caused by a virus; antibiotics are not necessary, and are even contraindicated.

Runny nose: decongestants decrease secretions and open nasal passages. Use only if necessary.

Stuffy nose: antihistamines reduce swelling.

Self-care suggestions:

- Rest and keep warm.
- Drink lots of fluids.
- Some studies suggest Vitamin C lessens severity of cold symptoms.
- Vaporizer or humidifier.

Now available are intranasal Interferon sprays. When begun within 48 hours of cold onset, 40 to 50 percent of cases improve significantly.

Constipation

Constipation is characterized by irregular, infrequent or very difficult bowel movements. There is no one normal pattern. If your schedule of bowel movements changes from one a day to one every three days, you may be constipated. Correction of constipation may just require a change of diet, taking more time to be regular, or correction of hemorrhoids that inhibit bowel activity through pain or fear.

Symptom Alert: Call MD if:

- Weight loss and thin, pencil-like stools (may suggest a tumor).
- Bloating and abdominal pain (may be a bowel obstruction).
- Blood in the stool.
- Constipation lasts more than two weeks.

The first approach is usually to encourage a healthy diet—one that includes fresh fruits and vegetables for laxative action and fiber to add bulk to the stool.

Laxatives may be prescribed, such as Metamucil or Milk of Magnesia; enemas for acute problems.

Cough

Coughing is usually your body's best defense mechanism—it is the body's way of clearing secretions and foreign material from the throat and lungs.

Cough may be a symptom of many illnesses, so it is important to distinguish an irritating cough from a serious one.

See also Colds, Fever and Chills, Sore Throat.

Usually this involves self-care and the doctor will advise bedrest, hot fluids (to thin mucus), a humidifier to increase moisture in the air, and avoiding dairy products (especially milk) that thicken secretions.

For a productive cough, doctors advise not trying to suppress the cough—the sputum or mucus needs to be cleared from the lungs.

Since the cold virus often finds a home in your nasal passages and prefers a cooler environment (85 to 95 degrees), warm air will inhibit growth. Use a viralizer or your hair dryer on low—breathe warm air for three minutes.

One study showed duration of cold reduced by two-thirds when subjects took 20 to 30 mg zinc gluconate per day.

When cold symptoms appear, try an enhanced immune system formula to help your body fight the invading organisms: CoQ_{10} is a miracle immune system booster. Take this natural element (50–100 mg/day), along with Vitamin C (3000–5000 mg/day), beta-carotene (50,000 units/day), and zinc gluconate (minimum of of 30 mg/day).

Drink black tea; the tannin in tea binds iron, which the cold virus needs for reproduction. (Remember to increase your iron intake after you've recovered from the cold.)

Nose drops: dissolve one-quarter teaspoon salt in eight ounces warm water; sniff solution to relieve congestion. Dissolve 20 mg tablet zinc gluconate in eight ounces warm water and sniff. Zinc is believed to kill the cold virus.

Try garlic, three capsules three times per day. Eat fresh parsley to eliminate garlic odor from breath.

Diminish airborne spread of virus as much as possible by covering mouth and nose with disposable tissue when sneezing or coughing. This followed by frequent handwashing with hot water and soap is the best preventive measure—since many colds are spread through touching hands or objects that carry the infecting virus.

Keep your immune system healthy.

Vitamin A is as important as Vitamin C for prevention; it keeps the mucous membranes in the nose and mouth strong to resist invasion by germs or viruses.

Humidify the air if you spend time in air-conditioned or dry, heated rooms.

Yearly, U.S. expenditure on laxatives is 200 million dollars. Most people are not truly constipated—they just think they are. If you fall into this group, read the Prevention column. If you really need help, continue reading.

Daily supplements of bran (see also Prevention).

A supplement of Vitamin B complex or brewer's yeast in your daily diet helps treat constipation. (Deprivation of thiamin and niacin results in constipation.)

Morning blend for regularity: prune juice and bran, two teaspoons each in unsweetened applesauce.

Chronic constipation allows certain toxins to recirculate in the system. An excellent remedy is natural or organic apple cider vinegar (from an old Vermonter, Dr. Jarvis). Drink one tablespoon in pure warm water every morning.

Bran is not a laxative, but it is a bowel normalizer. Every day, take unprocessed bran—either tablets or flakes—to provide bulk and fiber to the diet. Begin with one or two teaspoons a day. Take it with lots of fluid. Try oat bran as opposed to wheat, as studies show this type of bran to be more effective. It is delicious as hot cereal every morning.

Other foods that assist in preventing constipation are high fiber foods, whole fruit, dried fruit, raw vegetables and blackstrap molasses.

Regular exercise helps—especially the kind that conditions the stomach and back muscles.

Do not resist the call of nature—it may stop calling regularly. Go to the bathroom at the same time every day and relax. Try not to make this a stressful experience.

Holistic care involves all the steps of traditional care, with these additions:

Hot fluids: drink chicken soup—helps to loosen secretions.

Drink at least eight glasses of hot fluids every twenty-four hours. (Avoid cold drinks.)

If you don't have a vaporizer, use a hot shower.

The best prevention is a strong immune system, enhanced daily with:

- Vitamin C: 5,000 mg
- Beta-carotene: 25,000 units
- Zinc: 20–30 mg
- CoQ_{10}: 30–50 mg

Condition and Symptoms	Traditional Medical Care

Cough (continued)

Productive cough: Following a virus infection, this cough clears mucus from the respiratory tract. May be a good sign your lungs are clearing.

A physical exam, perhaps a chest x-ray, will determine if you have a viral cough or another illness.

Antibiotics will not be prescribed for a viral infection. For bronchitis (a bacterial infection), you may take both antibiotics and corticosteroids (to reduce inflammation).

For a nonproductive cough, doctor's advice is similar, except that you try to minimize a dry cough, which may prolong irritation of throat passage. You *may* try OTC cough suppressants (dextromethorphan) to relieve irritated passageways and encourage sleep.

Cough drops or hard candy will help keep throat moist.

Symptom Alert: Call MD if:

- Cough produces green, yellow or thick mucus or blood in the mucus.
- Cough causes difficulty in breathing, wheezing or pains in the chest.
- Cough is accompanied by elevated temperature, over 102°, or if fever of 100° persists more than four days.
- Persists for more than two to three weeks without improving.

Diarrhea

Diarrhea is frequent elimination of stools that are abnormally watery.

Causes are:
- Viral or bacterial infections.
- Parasites.
- Drinking to excess (fraternity parties).
- Side effect of medication.
- Stress or anxiety disorders.

Symptoms include cramps, bloating and general discomfort, nausea and vomiting, and fever.

Over-the-counter medications include Kaopectate and Pepto-Bismol (suggested as the best prevention for "turista").

Prescriptive drugs such as Lomotil, anticholinergics such as belladonna or atropine.

Bulking agents such as psyllium seed to decrease fluid content in stools are often advised.

Traveler's diarrhea cure: sulfonamide trimethoprim cures diarrhea so fast there is no need to take preventive doses of antibiotics. Since all antibiotics have side effects, try Pepto-Bismol first.

Stool culture may be necessary to determine cause.

Symptom Alert: Call MD if:

- Black or bloody stools.
- Consistent pain in your abdomen accompanied by fever.
- Severe diarrhea lasting longer than two days.
- Persistent, chronic bouts of diarrhea.

Fever and Chills

Fever is a symptom—not a disease. The most common cause is an infection—viral or bacterial.

Fever is the way the body has of defending itself against infection—the higher the body temperature, the more inhospitable the environment for the invading organism. Chills and shivering generate even more heat.

Recent research indicates aspirin or acetaminophen should *not* be automatically given to reduce fever.

The fever is a healthy sign the body is fighting the infection. Allow a fever to run its course if it remains under 104°. If fever goes above 104°, medical advice is necessary.

Supportive care suggestions include lots of fluids and juice, bedrest and sponging with luke warm water if fever rises above 102°F.

Symptom Alert: Call MD if:

- Fever goes above 104° and home measures do not bring it down.
- Fever is associated with a stiff neck or other symptoms such as rash, sore throat, earache, breathing difficulties or severe headache.
- Fever lasts for more than 4–5 days.

Holistic or Nontraditional Care	Prevention

Avoid irritants: smoke, very dry air, very cold air.

Sucking on hard candies will relieve your throat irritation. Avoid medicated throat lozenges. (Studies have shown that overuse of such lozenges can result in fungus infection.)

Ginger root capsules for chronic cough.

Golden seal tea also seems to help.

Fenugreek tea, one cup per hour for the first day, then four cups per day.

Wash your hands frequently when you are around others who are coughing or have a cold.

Take as much fluid as possible to compensate for fluids lost and to prevent dehydration.

After a bout of diarrhea, add lactobacillus acidophilus—either tablet or yogurt—to your diet every day to replace the "good" bacteria.

What helps?
- Apples, bananas and carob for pectin content
- Carrots, either raw or in soup
- Bran to add fiber
- Blueberries—several bowls a day

A diet rich in protein, carbohydrates, vitamins and minerals to compensate for the nutrients that are lost.

Activated charcoal tablets help to control diarrhea (and gas).

Raw garlic after each meal (this might not be your first choice if you are dating someone special). Peel and swallow a garlic clove with hot tea with lemon (don't add sugar).

Diet: eliminate highly spiced foods, food preservatives, sugar, too many starches, fried foods, and milk. Include more fruits and fiber.

Stress is a major cause of diarrhea—methods of stress reduction will be beneficial.

Don't over-do sugarless gum—it has been known to cause diarrhea.

The primary prevention for traveler's diarrhea is to not drink water unless you are certain it is clean and chlorinated. Also, do not brush your teeth in it or use ice cubes. Boil the water, add two percent tincture of iodine to water, or use a water filter. Peel all fruit. Avoid lettuce. Avoid street food unless fresh-cooked and still hot.

Fluids (not food) are the nutritional key to coping with a fever. Drink eight ounces of water, broth, juice, or herbal tea every two hours.

Exercise is contraindicated—it will result in overheating and sweating and may lead to more dehydration.

If you can stand to chew fresh garlic cloves (like the old Italians did), garlic will immediately decrease symptoms.

Fever is only a symptom; you can prevent its cause—invasion by a viral or bacterial agent—by keeping your immune system strong.

Condition and Symptoms	Traditional Medical Care

Flu

Influenza, like the common cold, is a viral infection. There are types A, B and C.

Type A acts like a cold at first but is much more virulent. With the appearance of symptoms you feel *very* ill. (This is the flu type that has caused thousands of deaths in this century.) You will note a sudden onset of symptoms: headache, high fever, cough, congestion, muscle aches, and fatigue. You will feel terrible and probably won't make it out of bed. This flu may take ten or more days to resolve.

Type B acts like a cold and it is difficult to distinguish between the two. Type C rarely manifests major symptoms.

Do not take aspirin when you have the flu. One study found that aspirin doubled time required for recovery.

Usual treatment is supportive: rest, drink fluids, keep warm, and follow other cold-type remedies.

The only medication found to work for Type A is Symmetrel, prescribed by your doctor.

Headaches

There are many types of headaches, each with its own symptoms, treatments and preventive measures. If you develop a headache, try to determine what kind you have. *Sinus or vasomotor rhinitis headache:* Nose feels full, dull pain and tenderness above eyes (occurs with change in the weather, pollution or allergies).

OTC decongestants and/or anti-inflammatory medications. Caution: Prolonged use can lead to dependency.

Aspirin, acetaminophen or medications to dry up your sinuses (Sinutab, and so forth).

Antibiotics necessary if sinus is infected.

Symptom Alert: Call MD if:
- Pain, fever and discharge through nose (indicate acute infection).

Hypoglycemia

This disorder is often misdiagnosed. It is, in fact, low blood sugar, and from a clinical standpoint, very few people actually have this condition. If you suspect you are suffering from hypoglycemia, have a five-hour glucose tolerance test.

Symptoms that may be present are weakness, faintness and feeling shaky. There may also be confusion, headache, and muscle weakness, rapid heartbeat, and dizziness.

Involves correct diagnosis—establishing the fact that true hypoglycemia does exist.

Correction of diet and eating habits. Including more protein and less sugars and carbohydrates.

Avoid eating candy, drinking coffee or other caffeine drinks or alcohol.

If you are prone to attacks, the doctor may advise you to carry glucose tablets or sugar lumps.

Menstrual Cramps

Menstrual cramps are not always present with menstruation. Painful cramps, called dysmenorrhea, are considered to be caused by normal hormonal changes during menstruation.
Weight gain, breast tenderness, irritability, headache, bloating, depression, edema, and, of course, painful cramps are associated symptoms that women may experience before or during menstruation.

Providing heat to the abdominal area or lower back with a heating pad or warm bath often relieves intense cramps.

Drugs that counter prostaglandin action have been found to be effective. Some drugs now available are Motrin, Anaprox and Ponstel.

Aspirin, a mild antiprostaglandin, also works.

If your menstrual flow is unusually heavy, the health center clinician will check the amount of iron in your blood; heavy loss of blood can lead to an anemic condition.

If pain and bleeding are much more severe than normal, or menstruation is absent, physician will perform examination to rule out any underlying disorder.

Symptom Alert: Call MD if:
- Pain is more severe than usual.
- Bleeding is unusually heavy.
- Menstruation is absent when it would regularly occur.

Holistic or Nontraditional Care	Prevention
It is better not to overmedicate your body when it is fighting the influenza virus. Holistic care is the same as traditional treatment (rest, fluids, and so forth) plus added nutrients: ■ Vitamin C: 5,000 to 10,000 mg/day ■ Beta-carotene: 50,000 units/day ■ CoQ_{10}: 50–100 mg/day ■ Zinc: 30–50 mg/day unless you are dissolving them in your mouth for a sore throat. Another alternative is an herbal tea formulated by a famous herbalist, Maria Trebin from Germany. It is called "Swedish Bitters" and is available at health food stores.	Vaccination with Type A vaccine is available and has few side effects. However, unless you have a chronic illness or are over 65, it is usually not given. The best general prevention is to maintain a healthy immune system.
Inhale steam either in a shower or by creating a tent by placing a towel over your head as you lean over a container of simmering water. Put one-quarter teaspoon salt in a cup of warm water and inhale through nostrils. Apply fingerpoint pressure on tender areas around your eye—relieves clogged sinuses.	Because air pollution is a cause, use an ionizer or air purifier. If allergies seem to be responsible, consider allergy shots. A mucus-free diet dramatically improves sinus problems. Eliminate white flour, sugar, milk products, eggs, fats, potato chips, corn chips, and so forth.
The best self-care approach is to modify your diet. Begin the day with protein—not sugar, simple carbohydrates, or fats. Avoid foods listed under traditional medical care. Take vitamin and mineral supplements to promote a well-balanced diet.	Prevention is also dietary. See Holistic column for dietary approach.
Some movement and mild exercise can ease cramps; vigorous exercise will be too uncomfortable; use simple yoga-type movements. Cramping may be relieved by taking extra calcium, iron, and niacin. Add to this a Vitamin B complex (which includes B_6 and folic acid). Current research indicates that taking an amino acid, DLPA, several days before the period begins works very well. Ask in your local health food store for details. Flaxseed (linseed) oil on a regular basis.	Limit salt and fluid intake a few days before your period. Take extra Vitamin A or beta-carotene to relieve general symptoms. Exercising consistently helps to rid the body of toxins and excess water. Stress-reducing activities. The higher your stress level, the more you experience problems with cramps. If you retain water, try cranberry juice, watercress, parsley, or kelp a few days before your period.

Condition and Symptoms	Traditional Medical Care

Muscle Cramps—Legs

Cramps in the leg muscles may be just painful or they may be caused from inflammation (the latter is less frequent).

Pain or cramps in the muscle can be due to tension, vigorous exertion, or there may be no obvious cause.

Suggested treatment for leg cramps at night is usually rest, exercise and warm baths, in addition to two aspirin tablets.

If the condition is long-lasting and debilitating, the doctor may do a physical examination and prescribe pain medications or muscle relaxants.

If there is a particular area of pain, a cortisone injection will relieve it.

Sore Throat

Sore throat is often caused by virus infection. Resolves in five to seven days.

Soreness begins slowly and gradually worsens. Accompanied by low-grade fever, headache, runny nose, and lethargy.

Sore throat may be caused by a bacteria (the most common is streptococcal). A "strep" throat requires antibiotics; know when to call the doctor.

Supportive care at home: fluids, gargle with salt water (¼ teaspoon in eight ounces water), aspirin, and a humidifier or vaporizer. Limited medicated lozenges also help.

There is no specific treatment for viral sore throat, just the same supportive care as for bacterial.

To determine if sore throat is caused by strep, a throat culture may be done. If result is positive, antibiotics will be prescribed.

Symptom Alert: Call MD if:

- Difficulty breathing or severe problem with swallowing.
- Sore throat lasts longer than one week and is not improved.
- A fever over 101°, hoarseness, cough, swollen glands, and earache.
- You have had rheumatic fever.

Vomiting

Vomiting occurs when the gastrointestinal tract sends partially digested stomach contents back up through the esophagus into the mouth, which are then expelled. Causes vary. Common causes include alcohol intoxication, flu and other intestinal infections, poisoning.

Vomiting is the body's way of ridding itself of toxins. Dangers include dehydration and fluid imbalance, or damage to the intestinal tract if vomiting is prolonged.

Self-care suggestions:

- No food.
- Start liquid intake with sucking ice cubes; gradually increase fluids—herbal tea, carbonated sugar drink, 7-Up, Ginger Ale (no caffeine).
- If vomiting does not recur within two hours of adding fluid, then start on simple foods such as the BRAT Diet: bananas, rice, applesauce, toast. Later add soft-boiled eggs.

Symptom Alert: Call MD if:

- Severe abdominal pain is present for more than one hour and is not relieved by vomiting.
- Head injury has occurred in the past 24 hours.
- Vomiting is accompanied by eye pain, blurry vision, pain when bending head forward, or light intensifies discomfort.
- Vomit contains blood or dark coffee grounds-like material.
- Poison ingestion, food poisoning or flu suspected.
- Vomiting is recurring and self-induced.

For serious or prolonged vomiting the doctor will assess for dehydration and, if necessary, replace fluids intravenously.

To determine cause of condition, a patient history, physical examination, blood and urine tests, and possibly x-ray will be completed. (May be related to allergy, stomach disease, hypovitaminosis, especially B vitamins, endocrine disorders, heart disease.)

Treatment will be based on underlying cause.

Holistic or Nontraditional Care	Prevention

Vitamin E capsule (200–400 mg) before bedtime.

Calcium lactate or calcium gluconate with magnesium and Vitamin C and Vitamin D before bedtime significantly help abolish night cramping.

If you wake up in pain with a leg cramp, curl your toes up and stretch the muscle: try walking around in bare feet or massage the knotted muscle. (Do not point your toes; this only increases the cramping.) If all this fails, place a warm, wet cloth over the muscle to help it relax.

Eat more fruits and vegetables and grains to increase mineral intake.

An exercise to prevent leg cramps: walk on your tip toes (barefeet) with your arms straight up. Do this several times across the room—it will stretch the leg muscles.

Beware of the chair you use while studying; if it cuts into your lower thigh, it may impede circulation and cause cramps.

Strep throat requires antibiotics—no holistic care can replace this treatment.

An important adjunct is to take lactobacillus acidophilus to replace the "good" bacteria killed by antibiotics. Continue immune boosters of Vitamin C, beta-carotene, zinc, and CoQ_{10}.

Dissolving a zinc gluconate tablet in your mouth every two to three hours helps harsh throat symptoms. (Study showed that zinc decreased severity and duration of symptoms by two-thirds.) Zinc tastes bad; the most palatable form is zinc lozenges, available at your local health food store.

To soothe symptoms and provide needed fluids, try apple cider vinegar with honey dissolved in a cup of hot water or fenugreek tea.

Gargle every four hours with aloe gel mixed in warm water or with warm salt water.

If a close friend or family member has strep throat, be aware that you are vulnerable. If symptoms appear, have a throat culture.

The most effective way to prevent a viral sore throat is to have a strong immune system.

Follow traditional self-care diet suggestions.

One of the best anti-vomit aids is an over-the-counter medication called Emetrol. With nothing in your stomach, take 1 to 2 teaspoons every 15 minutes ×4. If vomiting persists, seek professional help.

If connected to bulimia, seek professional care.

Avoid alcohol intoxication.

Avoid wild mushrooms; follow rules for avoiding food poisoning.

Keep immune system strong.

If you suspect pregnancy, take a home test.

Appendix 3: Your College Medicine Chest

Antacids

Tums, Rolaids, Alka-Seltzer or equivalent
Stomach upset, indigestion or heartburn

Antibacterial creams

Polysporin, Neosporin or equivalent
Minor wounds, cuts, skin irritations

Antihistamines and decongestants

Benadryl, Actifed, Sudafed, Contac or equivalent
Allergies, colds

Antifungal creams

Desenex, Tinactin or equivalent
Athlete's foot or jock itch

Antimotion medication

Dramamine, Bonine or equivalent
(May cause drowsiness.)

Anti-inflammatory medications

Cortaid, Lanacort or equivalent
(0.5% hydrocortisone cream)
Skin rashes and irritations

Constipation aids

Mitrolan, Metamucil, Milk of Magnesia or equivalent
Constipation

Cough suppressants/expectorants

Robitussin-DM, Benylin DM or equivalent
Coughs

Diarrhea medication

Pepto-Bismol, Kaopectate or equivalent
"Turista," stomach flu

Disinfectants

Hydrogen peroxide, Betadine or equivalent
Wound cleansers

Eye drops

Murine, Visine or equivalent
(Use with caution as these products may cause damage and retard healing. Recommended alternative: artificial tears.)
Eye irritation, bloodshot eyes

Fever, headache, and muscle ache medication

Aspirin, Excedrin or equivalent
Take aspirin for inflammation; otherwise use acetaminophen or ibuprofin. Many aspirin products contain caffeine.

Tylenol or equivalent
(Do not combine with heavy alcohol intake; both substances processed by your liver.)

Advil, Nuprin or equivalent, ibuprofin
Fever, cold, flu, stress headache, minor aches and pain

Nasal decongestants, spray or drops

Afrin or equivalent
Stuffy nose due to allergies or cold

Nausea and vomiting

Emetrol, for vomiting; Pepto-Bismol or equivalent
Upset stomach, vomiting

General Supplies

Adhesive tape (minor injuries)

Bandaids, Curaids or equivalent (minor wound protection)

Corn pads (minor corn removal)

Elastic bandages (sprains and muscle strain)

Eye cup (foreign object removal)

Heating pad (minor pain, chills)

Humidifier or mist machine (flu, stuffy nose and dry skin in winter)

Ice pack (minor injuries, sprains)

Moleskin (blisters or abrasions)

Needles, matches to sterilize, and tweezers (splinter removal)

Thermometer (evaluate fever)

Bibliography

Accident Facts, 1988 Edition. Chicago: National Safety Council, 1988.

AIDS Health Project, San Francisco General Hospital. "AIDS and Substance Abuse Program," 1986.

American Academy of Orthopaedic Surgeons. *Emergency Care and Transportation of the Sick and Injured.* Chicago: American Academy of Orthopaedic Surgeons, 4th ed., 1987.

American Medical Association. *Family Medical Guide.* New York: Random House, 1982.

American Medical Association. *Handbook of First-Aid and Emergency Care.* New York: Random House, 1980.

American Medical Association. *The AMA Handbook of First Aid and Emergency Care.* New York: American Medical Association, 1984.

Anderson, Bob. *Stretching.* Bolinas CA: Shelter, 1980.

Bailey, Covert. *The Fit-or-Fat Target Diet.* Boston: Houghton Mifflin, 1984.

Basini, Richard. *How to Cut Down on Your Social Drinking.* New York: Putnam, 1985.

Beck, Aaron T., et al. *Anxiety Disorders and Phobias: A Cognitive Perspective.* New York: Basic Books, 1985.

Beck, Aaron T., et al. *Cognitive Therapy of Depression: A Treatment Manual.* New York: Guilford, 1979.

Bennett, William, MD, and Joel Gurin. *The Dieter's Dilemma: Eating Less and Weighing More.* New York: Basic Books, 1982.

Benson, Herbert, MD. *The Relaxation Response.* New York: Avon, 1975.

Berger, Gilda. *Addiction: Its Causes, Problems, and Treatments.* New York: Franklin Watts, 1982.

Berkow, Robert, ed. *The Merck Manual of Diagnosis and Therapy.* Rathway NJ: Merck, 1987.

Berkowitz, Alan D., and H. Wesley Perkins. "Problem Drinking Among College Students: A Review of Recent Research," Journal of American College Health, Vol 35, Jul 1986.

Beverly, Peter, and Quentin Sattentau. "ABC of AIDS," British Medical Journal, Vol 294, Jun 1987.

Bloomfield, Harold, MD, and Robert B. Kory. *The Holistic Way to Health and Happiness.* New York: Simon and Schuster, 1978.

Bonner, Joseph, PhD, and William Harris. *Healthy Aging: New Directions in Health, Biology, and Medicine.* Claremont CA: Hunter House, 1988.

Borysenko, Joan, PhD. *Minding the Body, Mending the Mind.* Reading MA: Addison-Wesley, 1987.

Boston Women's Health Book Collective, Inc. *The New Our Bodies, Ourselves.* New York: Simon and Schuster, 1985.

Brallier, Lynn. *Successfully Managing Stress.* Los Altos CA: National Nursing Review, 1982.

Branden, Nathaniel. *Honoring the Self.* New York: Bantam, 1985.

Brody, Jane. *Jane Brody's Nutrition Book.* New York: Bantam, 1987.

Brody, Jane. *Jane Brody's The New York Times Guide to Personal Health.* New York: Avon, 1982.

Brown, Lester. *The State of the World.* Washington: Worldwatch Institute, 1989.

Brownell, K. D., and J. P. Foreyt, eds. *Handbook of Eating Disorders.* New York: Basic Books, 1986.

Brownmiller, Susan. *Against Our Will: Men, Women and Rape.* New York: Simon and Schuster, 1975.

Burns, David, MD. *Feeling Good: The New Mood Therapy.* New York: William Morrow, 1980.

Burns, David, MD. *The Feeling Good Handbook.* New York: William Morrow, 1989.

Carlinsky, Dan. *Stop Snoring Now!* New York: St. Martin's, 1987.

Carson, Robert C., et al. *Abnormal Psychology and Modern Life.* 8th ed. Glenview IL: Scott, Foresman, 1988.

Cauwells, Janice M. *Bulimia: The Binge-Purge Compulsion.* New York: Doubleday, 1983.

Centers for Disease Control. *Recommendations for Prevention of HIV Transmission in Health Care Settings.* Vol 36. No. 2S, Aug 1987.

Chatlos, Calvin, MD. *Crack: What You Should Know About the Cocaine Epidemic.* Perigee, 1987.

Chew, Robyn T. et al. *The Fitness and Health Handbook.* University of California at Berkeley, 1985.

Claydon, Peter. *Setting the Right Course: Alcohol and Drug Education on the College Campus.* University of California at Santa Barbara, 1984.

Cooke, Cynthia W., and Susan Dworkin. *The Ms. Guide to a Woman's Health.* New York: Anchor/Doubleday, 1979.

Cooper, Kenneth H., MD. *The Aerobics Program for Total Well-Being.* New York: Bantam, 1982.

Cooper, Kenneth H., MD. *The Aerobics Way.* New York: Bantam, 1977.

Cooper, Robert K., PhD. *Health and Fitness Excellence. The Scientific Action Plan.* Boston: Houghton Mifflin, 1989.

Corry, James, and Peter Cimbolic. *Drugs: Facts, Alternatives, Decisions.* Belmont CA: Wadsworth, 1985.

Cousins, Norman. *Anatomy of an Illness as Perceived by the Patient.* New York: Bantam, 1981.

Cousins, Norman. *The Healing Heart. Antidotes to Panic and Helplessness.* New York: W. W. Norton, 1983.

Dass, Ram, and Paul Gorman. *How Can I Help?* New York: Alfred A. Knopf, 1985.

Davis, Martha, et al. *The Relaxation and Stress Reduction Workbook.* Richmond CA: New Harbinger Publications, 1981.

Douglass, Merrill E., and Donna N. Douglass. *Manage Your Time, Manage Your Work, Manage Yourself.* New York: AMACOM, 1985.

Edelstein, Scott. *College: A User's Manual.* New York: Bantam, 1985.

Erasmus, Udo. *Fats and Oils: The Complete Guide to Fats and Oils in Health and Nutrition.* Vancouver, Canada: Alive, 1986.

Ericson, Eric, et al. *Vital Involvement in Old Age: The Experience of Old Age in Our Time.* New York: W. W. Norton, 1988.

Farquhar, John W. *The American Way of Life Need Not Be Hazardous to Your Health.* Stanford CA: Stanford Alumni Association, 1978.

Farrell, Barbara. "AIDS Patients: Values in Conflict," *Critical Care Nursing*, Vol 10, No. 2, Sep 1987.

Ferguson, Tom, MD, and David Sobel, MD. *The People's Book of Medical Tests.* New York: Summit Books, 1985.

Fix, James, and David Daughton. *The Odds Almanac.* Chicago: Follett Publishing, 1980.

Francis, Donald P., and James Chin. "The Prevention of Acquired Immunodeficiency Syndrome in the United States. An Objective Strategy for Medicine, Public Health, Business and the Community," *Journal of the American Medical Association*, Vol 257, No. 10, Mar 1987.

Garrick, James, MD, and Peter Radetsky. *Peak Condition.* New York: Crown, 1986.

Goodwin, Donald, MD. *Anxiety.* New York: Ballantine, 1986.

Gordon, Sol. *Why Love Is Not Enough.* Boston: Bob Adams, Inc., 1988.

Gray, John. *What You Feel, You Can Heal.* Mill Valley CA: Heart Publishing, 1984.

Grieco, Alan. "Cutting the Risks for STDs," *Medical Aspects of Human Sexuality*, Mar 1987.

Hastings, Arthur C., James Fadiman, and James S. Gordon. *Health for the Whole Person.* Boulder CO: Westview, 1980.

Hatcher, Robert A. et al. *Contraceptive Techniques 1986–1987.* New York: Irvington, 1986.

Haynes, Marion E. *Personal Time Management.* Los Altos CA: Crisp, 1987.

Herzfeld, John. "Their Smoke in Your Lungs." *American Health*, Nov 1987.

Hoffman, David. *Successful Stress Control.* Rochester VT: Thorsons, 1986.

Holl, Lindsay, and Leigh Cohn. *Bulimia: A Guide to Recovery.* Santa Barbara CA: Gürze Books, 1989.

"Is There Really a Cancer Epidemic?" *The Johns Hopkins Medical Letter, Health After 50.* Fernandina Beach FL: Medletter Assoc., Apr 1989.

Jaffey, Dennis T. *Healing From Within: Psychological Techniques to Help the Mind Heal the Body.* New York: Fireside, 1980.

Kart, Cary, Eileen Metress, and Seamus Metress. *Aging, Health & Society.* Boston: Jones and Bartlett, 1988.

Keegan, Lynn, and Barbara Dossey. *Self Care: A Program to Improve Your Life.* Temple TX: BodyMind Systems, 1987.

Kenton, Leslie. *The Joy of Beauty.* London: Century Publishing, 1983.

Kirsch, M. M. *Designer Drugs.* Minneapolis: CompCare Publications, 1986.

Kirsta, Alix. *Stress Survival.* New York: Simon and Schuster, 1986.

Klagsbrun, Francine. *Too Young to Die. Youth and Suicide.* New York: Pocket Books, 1981.

Kline, Nathan S., MD. *From Sad to Glad.* New York: Ballantine, 1981.

Koestenbaum, Peter. *Is There an Answer to Death?* Englewood Cliffs NJ: Prentice-Hall, 1976.

Krause, Barbara. *Calorie Guide to Brand Names and Basic Foods.* New York: Signet, 1987.

Kübler-Ross, Elizabeth. *Death, The Final Stage of Growth.* Englewood Cliffs NJ: Prentice-Hall, 1975.

Kübler-Ross, Elisabeth. *Questions and Answers on Death and Dying.* New York: Macmillan Publishing, 1974.

Kunz, Jeffrey, MD, ed. *The AMA Family Medical Guide.* New York: Random House, 1982.

Lamberg, Lynne. *Straight Talk No-Nonsense Guide to Better Sleep.* New York: Random House, 1984.

Lappé, Francis M. *Diet for a Small Planet.* New York: Ballantine, 1982.

Lark, Susan, MD. *Dr. Susan Lark's Premenstrual Syndrome Self-Help Book.* Los Angeles: Forman Publishing, 1984.

Lawson, John. *Friends You Can Drop: Alcohol and Drugs.* Boston: Quinlan Press, 1986.

Lesko, Wendy, and Matthew Lesko. *The Maternity Sourcebook.* New York: Warner Books, 1984.

Levy, Stephen J. *Managing the Drugs in Your Life: A Personal and Family Guide to the Responsible Use of Drugs, Alcohol, and Medicine.* New York: McGraw-Hill, 1983.

Liebman-Smith, Joan. "New-Style First Aid," *American Health*, May 1986.

Litt, Jerome Z., MD. *Your Skin, From Acne to Zits.* New York: Dembner Books, 1989.

Locke, Steven, MD, and Douglas Colligan. *The Healer Within: The New Medicine of Mind and Body.* New York: E. P. Dutton, 1986.

Mason, L. John. *Guide to Stress Reduction.* Culver City CA: Peace Press, 1980.

Miller, Emmett, MD. *Software for the Mind.* Berkeley: Celestial Arts, 1987.

Moody, Raymond A., MD. *Life After Life.* New York: Bantam Books, 1975.

Morra, Marion, and Eve Potts. *Choices: Realistic Alternatives in Cancer Treatment.* New York: Avon Books, 1987.

National Research Council. *Diet and Health: Implications for Reducing Chronic Disease Risk.* Washington: National Academy Press, 1989.

Nutrition Almanac. New York: McGraw-Hill, 1979.

Orbach, Susie. *Fat Is a Feminist Issue: The Anti-Diet Guide to Permanent Weight Loss*. New York: Berkley Books, 1987.

Osborn, June E. "The AIDS Epidemic: Multidisciplinary Trouble," *The New England Journal of Medicine*, Vol 314, No. 12, Mar 1986.

Ouseley, S. G. J. *Color Meditations*. Essex England: L. N. Fowler and Co., 1949.

Oyle, Irving. *The New American Medicine Show*. Santa Cruz: Unity Press, 1979.

Parachini, A. "The California Humane and Dignified Death Initiative." *Hastings Center Report*, 1989. 19:1 10–12.

Peck, M. Scott. *The Road Less Traveled*. New York: Simon and Schuster, 1978.

Pelletier, Kenneth. *Holistic Medicine*. New York: Delacorte, 1976.

Pelletier, Kenneth. *Mind as Slayer—Mind as Healer: A Holistic Approach to Preventing Stress Disorders*. Magnolia MA: Peter Smith, 1984.

Pomidor, William J. "Pap Tests, What Every Woman Must Know Now." *Medical SelfCare*, Mar 1989.

Ratto, Trish. "The 'Four Food Groups' Revisited," *Medical SelfCare*, Jul–Aug 1987.

Ratto, Trish. "The New Science of Weight Control," *Medical SelfCare*, Mar–Apr 1987.

Ratto, Trish. "The Truth About Protein," *Medical SelfCare*, Nov–Dec 1986.

Refkin, Arthur, MD. "Panic Disorder—and its Many Complications," *Medical Update*, Vol XI, No. 6, Dec 1987.

Rippe, James M., and William Southmayd. *The Sports Performance Factors*. New York: Putnam, 1986.

Robbins, John. *Diet for a New America*. Walpole NH: Stillpoint Publishing, 1987.

Roemer, M. I. *An Introduction to the U.S. Health Care System*. New York: Springer Publishing, 1986.

Rogers, Carl. *Becoming Partners*. New York: Delacorte Press, 1972.

Saltman, Paul, Joel Gurin, and Ira Mothner. *The California Nutrition Book: A Food Guide for the '90s From Faculty at the University of California and the Editors of American Health*. Boston: Little, Brown, 1987.

Sarrel, Lorna J., and Philip M. Sarrel. *Sexual Turning Points: The Seven Stages of Adult Sexuality*. New York: Macmillan, 1984.

Scarf, Maggie. *Intimate Partners*. New York: Random House, 1987.

Scharf, Diana, and Pam Hait. *Studying Smart*. New York: Barnes and Noble, 1985.

Selye, Hans, MD. *Stress Without Distress*. New York: Signet, 1974.

"Sex on Campus: A Special Issue." *Journal of American College Health*, May 1989.

Shanghold, Mona, and Gabe Mirkin. *The Complete Sports Medicine Book for Women*, New York: Simon and Schuster, 1985.

Shealy, C. Norman, MD, PhD, and Caroline M. Myss, MA. *The Creation of Health*. Walpole NH: Stillpoint Publishing, 1988.

Shell, Ellen Ruppel. "How to Talk to Your Doctor . . . in 18 Seconds," *American Health*, Jan–Feb 1987.

Shelley, Florence D. *When Your Parents Grow Old*. New York: Harper & Row, 1988.

Shephard, Bruce D. and Carroll A. Shephard. *The Complete Guide to Women's Health*. New York: Plume, 1985.

Shilts, Randy. *And the Band Played On: Politics, People, and the AIDS Epidemic*. New York: St. Martin's, 1987.

Siegel, Bernard, MD. *Love, Medicine and Miracles*. New York: Harper & Row, 1986.

Sloane, Beverlie Conant. *Partners in Health: Sexuality: Contraceptive and Reproductive Health Issues*. Columbus OH: Charles E. Merrill, 1986.

Smith, Lendon. *Dr. Lendon Smith's Diet Plan for Teenagers*. New York: McGraw-Hill, 1986.

Smith, Sandra F., and Donna Duell. *Clinical Nursing Skills*. 2nd ed. Los Altos CA: National Nursing Review, 1988.

Smith, Sandra F., et al. *Review of Psychiatric and Psychosocial Nursing*. Los Altos CA: National Nursing Review, 1984.

Spielberger, Charles. *Understanding Stress and Anxiety*. New York: Harper & Row, 1979.

Squire, Susan. *The Slender Balance*. New York: Putnam, 1983.

Stavish, Philip C. "Psychoimmunology: Something to Think About," *Let's Live*, Nov 1987.

Student Health Strategies. Claremont CA: The Claremont Colleges, 1985.

"Students, Alcohol, and College Health: A Special Issue," *Journal of American College Health*, Vol 36, No. 2, Sep 1987.

Suitor, C. W., and M. F. Crawley. *Nutrition: Principles and Application in Health Promotion*. Philadelphia: J. B. Lippincott, 1984.

Taintor, Jerry F., DDS. *The Consumer's Common Sense Guide to Better Dental Care*. New York: Ballantine Books, 1989.

Tenney, Louise. *Today's Herbal Health*. Provo UT: Woodland, 1983.

Tenney, Louise. *Health Handbook*. Provo UT: Woodland, 1987.

The Earthworks Group. *Fifty Simple Things You Can Do To Save The Earth*. Berkeley: The Earthworks Press, 1989.

The Stanford Health and Exercise Handbook. Stanford CA: Stanford Alumni Association, 1987.

Thygerson, Alton. *Fitness and Health*. Boston: Jones and Bartlett, 1989.

Timm, Paul R. *Successful Self-Management*. Los Altos CA: Crisp, 1987.

Tompkins, Peter, and Christopher Bird. *Secrets of the Soil*. New York: Harper & Row, 1989.

U.S. Bureau of the Census. *Statistical Abstract of the United States: 1989*. Washington: U.S. Government Printing Office, 1989.

U.S. Department of Health and Human Services. *III International Conference on AIDS*, Jun 1987.

U.S. Environmental Protection Agency. *A Management Review of the Superfund Program*. Washington: U.S. Government Printing Office, 1989.

U.S. Environmental Protection Agency. *Environmental Progress and Challenges: EPA Update*. Washington: U.S. Government Printing Office, 1988.

U.S. Public Health Service. *A Report of the Surgeon General on the Health Consequences of Using Smokeless Tobacco*. Washington: U.S. Government Printing Office, 1986.

U.S. Public Health Service. *The Surgeon General's Report on the Health Consequences of Involuntary Smoking*. Washington: U.S. Government Printing Office, 1986.

U.S. Public Health Service. *The Surgeon General's Report on the Health Consequences of Using Tobacco*. Washington: U.S. Government Printing Office, 1964.

Vickery, Donald M., MD, and James F. Fries, MD. *Take Care of Yourself: The Consumer's Guide to Medical Care*. Reading MA: Addison-Wesley, 1986.

Viorst, Judith. *Necessary Losses*. New York: Ballantine, 1986.

"Weight Kit," Stanford Heart Disease Prevention Program, 1984.

Weil, Andrew, and Winifred Rosen. *From Chocolate to Morphine: Understanding Mind-Active Drugs*. Boston: Houghton Mifflin, 1983.

Werner, David. *Where There is No Doctor: A Village Health Handbook*. Palo Alto CA: Hesperian Foundation, 1977.

Witters, Weldon, and Peter Venturelli. *Drugs and Society*. Boston: Jones and Bartlett, 1988.

Woititz, Janet G. *Adult Children of Alcoholics*. Deerfield Beach FL: Health Communications, Inc., 1983.

"Women and AIDS: Questions and Answers," *Health Letter*, Public Citizen Health Research Group, Feb 1988.

Zilbergeld, Bernie, PhD, and Arnold A. Lazarus, PhD. *Mind Power: Getting What You Want Through Mental Training*. Boston: Little, Brown, 1987.

Zimbardo, Philip V. *Shyness*. New York: Jove, 1986.

Index

and diet, 135, 146, 449–450
early detection of, 453, 456
hotlines, 461
incidence of, 457
liver, 453, 454
lung, 456, 459, 556
melanoma, 242–244, 453, 462
Pap smear test for, 304–305
prevention of, 453
prostate, 292, 475
and radiation, 452–453
risk factors for, 9, 447–450, 452–454
seven warning signs of, 456
skin, 240–242, 453
and smoking, 393, 431, 448
statistics, 457, 459, 460
treatment for, 456, 459–461
Candida albicans, 150
Cannabis. See Marijuana
Cannon, Dr. Walter B., 19
Carbohydrates, 128–131
defined, 128, 176
and starches, 161
types of, 128
Carbon dioxide, 557
Carbon monoxide, 430–431, 442, 448, 540, 541, 543
poisoning, 508
Carbonated soft drinks, 143
Carcinogens, 430, 434, 442, 448, 453, 462, 546, 568
Cardiac catheterization, 459
Cardiopulmonary resuscitation (CPR), 521, 534
Cardiovascular disease, 443, 444
and smoking, 431
decline in, 454
early detection of, 454–455
and fat intake, 135
hotlines, 461
prevention of, 453
treatment of, 456–458
Cardiovascular system, 444–445, 462
Career choice, and stress, 27–28
Carrier, 352
Cataracts, 472, 477
Catastrophic health insurance, 594
Cellular death, 486
Cellulite, 238
Cerebral vascular accident (CVA). See Stroke
Cerebrovascular disease, and smoking, 431
Cervical cancer, 304–305
Cervical cap, 308, 311
Cervical os, 285
Cervix, 284, 285, 286
infection of, 288
Chamomile tea, 237

Chemicals, and cancer, 453
Chemotherapy, 459
Chernobyl, 555
Chest pain, and the detection of heart disease, 455
Chewing tobacco. See Smokeless tobacco
Childbirth, 373–377
theories of, 373–374
Children
and accidents, 507, 508, 509, 512
of alcoholics, 418, 421–422
effect of divorce on, 278–279
reaction to death, 490
See also Adolescence, Infants
China white, 400
Chiropractic, 577
Chlamydia, 288, 291, 295–297
Chlorofluorocarbons (CFCs), 557, 560
Chloroform, 538, 539
Choice, process of, 13–15
Choking, 508–509
Cholesterol, 133–136, 161, 176, 205
and cancer and heart disease, 443, 449, 455
kinds of, 455
measurement of, 454–455, 583
sources of, 134, 135
Chromosomes, 355, 356, 357, 384
Chronic bronchitis, and smoking, 431
Cigar smoking, 432
Cigarettes. See Smoking, Tobacco
Circadian rhythm, 97–98, 126, 108
disorders of, 103–104
Circumcision, 290
Clean Air Act of 1970, 537, 540
Clean Water Act, 537
Clean Water Action, 564
Climate changes, 559
Clinical death, 486, 502
Clinics, health, 574–576
Clitoris, 284
Clocks, biological, 97, 103, 105, 112
Clove cigarettes, 432
COA's (Children of Alcoholics), 418
Coal-tar formula, 248
Cocaine, 341, 393–395, 397, 424
Cocaine Anonymous, 423
Codeine, 397, 425
Codependency, 420, 426
Coffee drinking, 154–155
Cognitive-behavioral therapy, 64, 93
Cohabitation, 275–276, 280
Cohen, Dr. Sidney, 395
Cold, overexposure to. See Hypothermia
Cold sore, 299
Colon cancer, 456, 459
Color, 42
effect on mood, 34

Colorectal exam, 583
Commitment, 271–272, 280
Community clinics, 574–575
Complementary proteins, 176
Complete proteins, 176
Complex carbohydrates, 128–131, 161
Composting, 563, 568
Comprenhsive Drug Abuse Control Act, 392
Compulsion, 61, 66
Compulsive eating, 88–89, 93, 94
Compulsive exercise, 92
Conception, 384
Condoms, 337, 338–340
advantages and disadvantages of, 308
choosing, 339
effective use of, 311–312, 340
Confidentiality, defined, 343
Conflict, interpersonal, 57, 270–271, 280
Congenital heart disease, 445
Congestive heart failure, 447, 462
Conroy, Claire, 494
Consent (for health care), 579, 594
Consumer health care. See Health care
Consumer information, nutritional, 164
Contraception, 306–312, 328
responsibility for, 306
types of, 308–312
Contraceptive sponge, 308, 311
Contractions, during labor, 374
Conditioning, during exercise, 222
Contact lenses, 251
Cooking, 159
Cooper, Dr. Kenneth, *The Aerobic Program for Total Well-Being, Aerobics*, 200, 204, 226
Coping
with divorce, 277–279
with dying, 487
with loss, 498–501
Coronary angiography, 455
Coronary arteries, 445, 459, 462
and cholesterol, 134, 135
Coronary heart disease, 200, 445–446, 448, 459
and diet, 134, 135, 449
prevention of, 455
Cortex, 245
Cosmetics, 238–240, 258
and contact lenses, 251
natural vs. synthetic, 238
Counseling, genetic, 355–357, 366
Counseling centers, 576
Cousins, Norman, *Anatomy of an Illness*, 9–10
CPR, 521, 534
Crabs, 303–304
Crack, 393–395, 426

effect of aging on, 465
importance of relationships to, 260
in treatment of cancer, 459
Immunotherapy, 459
Impotence, 293, 328, 475
Indoor air pollution, 546
Industrial pollution, 545. *See also* Environmental pollution
Infants, 260, 377, 380, 381
Infertility, 358–359, 384
Inhalants, 425
Injuries
disabling, 504, 506, 507
head, 530
prevention of, 5, 219–222
from sports, 207–208, 217–225
See also Accidents
Inpatient treatment, 418–419
Insomnia, 99–100, 108
Insulin, 176, 198
Insurance, health, 586–593
Intellectual ability
and aging, 473–474
effect of exercise on, 206
Intercourse. *See* Sexual relations
International drug problems, 407
Internist, 572
Interpersonal conflicts, 57, 270–271, 280
Intimacy, 261, 263, 266–269, 280
Intoxication, 386–387, 388, 390–391, 426
Intraamniotic injection, 315
Intrauterine device, 308, 310
In-vitro fertilization, 359, 384
Involuntary smoking, 433–434
Iodine, 172–173
Ionizing radiation, 452–453
Ions, negative, 33, 35, 240
Iridology, 577
Iron, 74, 77, 144, 172–173
supplements, during pregnancy, 369
Irrational ideas, 64
Isolation. *See* Loneliness
IV drug users, 332, 335, 337, 340–341
Izumi, Shigechiyo, 470, 481

Jet lag, 97, 98
Jet skis accidents, 513
Job-training program for the aged, 467
Jogging, 204, 206, 214, 215
Jojoba oil, 247, 248

Kaposi's sarcoma, 333, 341, 352, 454
Kastenbaum, Robert, *Is There an Answer to Death?*, 488, 489
Kennedy, John F., 226
Keratin, 245
Kreteks, 432

Kübler-Ross, Dr. Elisabeth, *On Death and Dying*, 486–487, 498

Labia majora and minora, 284
Labor and delivery, 373–377
Lamaze, 373
Landfill dump sites, 552, 554
Laryngeal cancer, 448
Laxative, 88, 90, 108
Lazarus, Richard, 22
LDL. *See* Low-density lipoproteins
Lead, 538, 541, 548, 549
Leboyer, Frederick, 376
Left-overs, storing, 159, 164
Leukemia, 454, 456, 459
Librium, 396
Lice, pubic, 303–304
Life expectancy, 464, 469–470, 484
Lifestyle
and health, 443
and nutrition, 153, 188–192
and pollution, 562–564
and stress, 30
and weight control, 188–194
Life-sustaining devices, withdrawal of, 494–495
Life-threatening events. *See* Accidents, First aid, Suicide
Light, effect of, on mood, 35, 70
Lindemann, Erich, 499
Lip sores. *See* Herpes simplex
Lipoproteins, 134–135
Lips, protection of, from sun, 243, 244
Liquid lady, 393
Lithium, 70, 81
Liver cancer, 453, 454
Living Will, 495–496
Loneliness, 49, 260, 262, 263
of the aged, 478, 482
Longevity, 469–470, 479–483
Loss, 498–499
coping with, 499, 500–501
Love, 265–266, 267, 280
and conflict, 270–271
Low-calorie fat substitutes, 133
Low-calorie versus reduced-calorie, 131
Low-cholesterol fat substitutes, 133
Low-density lipoproteins (LDL), 134–135, 176
Low-fiber foods, 147
Low-salt substitutes, 148
Low-tar cigarettes, 433
LSD, 399–400, 425
Lung cancer, 456, 459, 556
and smoking, 431, 448
Luteinizing hormone, 285
Lymphoma, 459

Lysergic acid diethylamide (LSD), 399–400, 425

Macular degeneration, 477
MADD, 506
Magic mushrooms, 400
Magnesium, 172–173, 231, 449–450
Male
menopause, 475
obesity pattern, 451–452
problems with sexual functioning, 293–294
reproductive health problems, 291–292
sexual anatomy, 290–291
testicular examination, 292–293
Malignant tumors, 447, 462
Mammogram, 328, 583
Mammography, 453, 456
Manic behavior, 70, 81
Marathons, 226–227
Marijuana, 341, 397, 398–399. 425. 426
Marriage, 272–274, 280
alternative, 274–277
Mascara, 240
contact lenses and, 251, 252
Maslow, Abraham, 7, 11, 260, 261
Massage, scalp, 248
Masturbation, 294, 323
McDonald's job-training program for the aged, 467
McGuire, Ted, 410–411
McMasters, 467
MDMA (3,4 methylenedioxymethamphetamine), 393, 397, 400–401
Meal preparation, 159
Meat, buying and preparing, 163
Medical care. *See* First aid, Health care
Medical or Medicaid, 587, 594
Medical professionals, 573
Medical tests, 583
Medicare, 587, 594
Medication therapy, 4, 65
for cancer, 459
for depression, 74
for high-blood pressure, 447, 454
for strep throat, 446
See also Holistic health
Medications. *See* Drugs
Meditation, 41–42, 44, 123
Medulla, 244
Mehl, Dr. Lewis, 492
Melanoma, 242–244, 453, 462
Melatonin, 240–241
Men
and aging, 475–476. *See also* Male
and coronary heart disease, 445
and loneliness, 275

617

RICE, 222–223, 228
Richart classification system, 305
Right to die, 494–496
Right to life. *See* Prolife.
Risk-taking, 6, 47, 516–519, 534
Rite of passage, 497
Roe vs. Wade, 319–320
Rogers, Carl, 271–272
Roller skates, accidents involving, 517
Romance, 264–265, 272, 277, 280
Roommates, 35
Rowing, 204
RU 486 (abortion pill), 315
Running, 204, 205, 206, 219, 226–227
Rush, dry, 413

SAD. *See* Seasonal affective depression
Sadness, 70
Safe Drinking Water Act, 537
Safety helmets, 505, 517
Safety precautions, 503–519, 534
    all-terrain vehicle, 514
    boating, 512
    on campus, 33–35
    while driving, 506
    during exercise, 220
    with guns, 510
    when handling food, 162–164
    in the home, 510–511
    motor-scooter, 513
    during sex, 337, 338, 352
    at work, 507
Sai Baba, Sathya, 486
Salmonella, 162, 163, 164
Salt, 148, 161, 447, 450, 454
Sandwich generation, 464, 479, 484
Saturated fats, 131–133
    and cancer and heart disease, 449
    sources of, 135
Scabies, 303–304
Scarf, Maggie, *Intimate Partners*, 270
Schedule, study, 115–120
Schizophrenia, 78–80, 81
Schutz, Will, *Profound Simplicity*, 14, 269
Scrotum, 290
Seasonal affective depression, 70, 240–241, 258, 346
Seat belts, 481, 507, 515
Sebaceous glands, 230, 231, 234, 258
Sebum, 235, 258
Second-hand smoke, 434
Second-trimester, 363, 364, 366
    abortion during, 314, 315–316
Segal, Erich, 226
Seizures, 531
Selenium, 174–175, , 231, 248, 449
Self-acceptance, 46–48
Self-actualization, 7, 16

Self-confidence, 38
Self-esteem, 46–49, 57, 66, 178–179, 202, 262, 280
Self-image, 183–184, 258
Self-responsibility, for health, 3, 7–8
Selye, Dr. Hans, 18–20, 27
Semen, 285, 291
Senescence, 465
Senility, 477
Sensitivity, 47
Setpoint, 184, 198, 528
Sexual assault, 322–327
    hotlines, 323
Sexual relations
    effect of alcohol and drugs on, 391, 402
    importance of communication in, 305, 348–350
    precautions during, 332, 336–341, 348–350
    during pregnancy, 371
    short of intercourse, 307
    See also Contraception
Sexuality, 265, 267, 275
    and the aged, 474–475
    and drugs, 391
    learning stages of, 282–283
    orientation, 321–322
Sexually transmitted diseases (SIDs), 288, 291, 294–304, 328, 334
    chlamydia, 288, 291, 295–297
    genital warts, 301–302
    gonorrhea, 297–298
    hepatitis B, 302–303, 454
    herpes simplex type I and II, 299–301
    during pregnancy, 371
    prevention of, 295, 303
    pubic lice, 303–304
    syphilis, 298–299
    See also AIDS
Shaman, 2, 16
Shampoo, 247, 248
Sheehy, Gail, *Pathfinders*, 467
Shock and disbelief stage of grief, 499
Shyness, 48
Sickle cell anemia, 356
Sidestream smoke, 434
Sigmoidoscopy, 456, 462
Silicon, 231
Simon, Sidney, 47
Simonton, Carl O. and Stephanie, 3
Simplesse, 133
Single people, 275
Skateboarding, 220
Skiing, 204, 207, 215, 220
    protection of eyes during, 243
Skin
    aging, 33, 448
    anatomy, 230–231

cancer, 240–242, 453
care, 230–234, 235, 240–244
pH balance, 231
rash, 255
See also Acne, Cosmetics
Sleep
    and biological rhythms, 95–98
    importance of, 119
    improving quality of, 104–107
    and mental fitness, 54
    stages of, 96
Sleep apnea, 101–102, 108
Sleep disorders, 83, 99–107
    circadian rhythm, 103–104
    excessive sleep, 99–100
    insomnia, 99–100
    parasomnia, 102–103
    professional help for, 107
Sleeping pills, 100, 106–107
Sleepwalking, 103
Smog, 542, 546–547568
Smoke detectors, 510
Smokeless tobacco, 430, 432–433, 442, 448
Smoking, 481
    decline in, 429
    hazardous effects of, 370, 428–434, 448–449
    history of, 428
    increased costs of, 437–438
    involuntary, 433–434
    quitting, 439–440, 448
    restrictions on, 437
    versus nonsmoking, 429, 434, 438
    voluntary, 434–436
Smuts, Jan, 3
Snacking, 157–159
Snoring, 101–102
Snow blindness, 244
Soccer, 204, 220
Social drinking, 386, 389
Social phobia, 60–61
Social relationships. *See* Relationships
Social security benefits for the aged, 475, 478
Social workers, 572–573
Sodium, 148–149
Soft drinks, 143
Softball, 215, 220
Soil pollution, 551–554
Solid waste, pollution with, 551–554
Sonography, 365, 384
Space management, 125
"Spanish fly," 387
Speed (drug), 341, 392
Speed and motor-vehicle accidents, 506
Speedball, 393
Sperm, 285, 290, 291
Spermatocele, 293
SPF. *See* Sun protection factor

Photo/Illustration Credits

Acknowledgments

Page 96 From Hauri, Peter. *The Sleep Disorders*. Copyright © 1977 by the Upjohn Company.

Page 132 From Liebman, Bonnie. "Ferreting Fat From Your Diet," *Nutrition Action Healthletter*, Sep 1982, page 24. Copyright © 1988, Center for Science in the Public Interest.

Page 138 From "Protein Content of Selected Foods," *University of California, Berkeley Wellness Letter*, Vol 2, No. 9, June 1986, page 5. Copyright © 1986 by Health Letter Associates.

Page 158 From "Newsweek on Campus Poll: Food, Tolerable Food," *Newsweek on Campus*, Mar 1987, page 19. Copyright © 1987, Newsweek, Inc. All rights reserved. Reprinted by permission.

Page 180 Metropolitan Height and Weight Tables. Courtesy, Statistical Bulletin, Metropolitan Life Insurance Company.

Page 181 Frame Size Table. Courtesy, Statistical Bulletin, Metropolitan Life Insurance Company.

Page 214 From "Burning Calories: How Walking Stacks Up," *The Walking Magazine*, Feb–Mar 1986. Reprinted with the permission of The Walking Magazine, copyright © 1986, Raben Publishing Company.

Page 215 From Delhagen, Kate, "Total Fitness," *Runner's World*, Feb 1988, page 26. Copyright © 1988 by Runner's World. Reprinted with permission.

Page 251 From "Contact Lenses and Cosmetics," *Healthwise*, Feb 1988. Copyright © 1988 by Healthwise.

Page 305 From "Breaking the STD Chain", Cowell Student Health Center and Office of Residential Education. Copyright © 1986 by The Trustees of Stanford University.

Page 310 From "Oral Contraceptive Failures," *Healthwise*, Sep 1984, page 4. Copyright © 1984 by Healthwise.

Page 336 Brochures courtesy of American College Health Association.

Page 394 Excerpted from Willis, Dr. L. R. "A Hard Look at Cocaine," *San Francisco Chronicle*, Aug 1987, page A-10. Copyright © 1987 by L. R. Willis. Reprinted with permission of the author.

Page 404 Poster courtesy of Clement Communications Substance Abuse Program, Concordville, PA.

Page 405 From Ewing, J.A. "Detecting Alcoholism: The CAGE Questionnaire," *Journal of the American Medical Association*, (14) 1984, pages 1905–1907. Copyright © 1984, American Medical Association.

Page 408 *Yale Alumni Magazine*, Mar 1987. Copyright © 1987 by Yale Alumni Magazine.

Page 417 From *Dealing With Alcohol at Dartmouth*, Dartmouth College.

Pages 428–441 Data courtesy of U.S. Department of Health and Human Services.

Pages 504–512 Data courtesy of National Safety Council.

Pages 538–561 Data courtesy of U.S. Environmental Protection Agency.